Models for Assessing Drug Absorption and Metabolism

Pharmaceutical Biotechnology

Series Editor: Ronald T. Borchardt
The University of Kansas
Lawrence, Kansas

Models for Assessing Drug Absorption and Metabolism

Edited by

Ronald T. Borchardt
The University of Kansas
Lawrence, Kansas

Philip L. Smith
SmithKline Beecham Pharmaceuticals
King of Prussia, Pennsylvania

and

Glynn Wilson
Tacora Corporation
Seattle, Washington

Plenum Press • New York and London

Library of Congress Cataloging-in-Publication Data

Models for assessing drug absorption and metabolism / edited by Ronald
T. Borchardt, Philip L. Smith, and Glynn Wilson.
    p.   cm. -- (Pharmaceutical biotechnology ; v. 8)
  Includes bibliographical references and index.
  ISBN 0-306-45243-X
    1. Pharmacokinetics--Research--Methodology. 2. Drugs--Metabolism-
-Research--Methodology.   I. Borchardt, Ronald T. II. Smith, Philip
L., 1949-   . III. Wilson, Glynn. IV. Series.
    [DNLM: 1. Pharmacokinetics. 2. Drugs--metabolism. 3. Models,
Biological.   W1 PH151N v.8 1996]
  RM301.5.M63   1996
  615'.7--dc20
  DNLM/DLC
  for Library of Congress   96-28902
                                                                CIP

ISBN 0-306-45243-X

Contributors

Kenneth L. Audus • Department of Pharmaceutical Chemistry, The University of Kansas, Lawrence, Kansas 66045

Ronald T. Borchardt • Department of Pharmaceutical Chemistry, The University of Kansas, Lawrence, Kansas 66045

Claire M. Brett • Department of Anesthesia, University of California, San Francisco, California 94143

Robert L. Bronaugh • Office of Cosmetics and Colors, Food and Drug Administration, Laurel, Maryland 20708

Kim L. R. Brouwer • Division of Pharmaceutics, School of Pharmacy, University of North Carolina, Chapel Hill, North Carolina 27599

Peter L. Bullock • Department of Pharmacology, Toxicology, and Therapeutics, University of Kansas Medical School, Kansas City, Kansas 66160

James P. Cassidy • Ciba-Geigy Corporation, Summit, New Jersey 07901

William N. Charman • Department of Pharmaceutics, Victorian College of Pharmacy, Monash University, Parkville, Victoria 3052, Australia

Edward D. Crandall • Department of Medicine and Pathology, School of Medicine, University of Southern California, Los Angeles, California 90033

Mohammed Eljamal • Inhale Therapeutic Systems, Palo Alto, California 94303

Joseph A. Fix • Alza Corporation, Palo Alto, California 94304

T. C. Ganguly • Graduate Center for Toxicology, University of Kentucky, Lexington, Kentucky 40503

Kathleen M. Giacomini • Department of Biopharmaceutical Sciences, University of California, San Francisco, California 94143

Robin Griffiths • SmithKline Beecham Pharmaceuticals, DMPK, The Frythe, Welwyn, Herts AL6 9AR, United Kingdom

Marcelo M. Gutierrez • Forest Laboratories Inc., New York, New York 11696

Ismael J. Hidalgo • Drug Metabolism and Pharmokinetics (NW12), Rhone-Poulenc Rorer, Collegeville, Pennsylvania 19427

Jerome H. Hochman • INTERx Research/Merck Research Laboratories, Lawrence, Kansas 66047

Phillip Jeffrey • SmithKline Beecham Pharmaceuticals, DMPK, The Frythe, Welwyn, Herts AL6 9AR, United Kingdom

Kwang-Jin Kim • Departments of Medicine, Physiology and Biophysics, and Biomedical Engineering, Schools of Medicine and Engineering, University of Southern California, Los Angeles, California 90033

Edward L. LeCluyse • INTERx Research/Merck Research Laboratories, Lawrence, Kansas 66047, and the Department of Pharmacology, Toxicology, and Therapeutics, University of Kansas Medical School, Kansas City, Kansas 66160

Vincent H. L. Lee • Department of Pharmaceutical Sciences, School of Pharmacy, University of Southern California, Los Angeles, California 90033

Harry Leipold • Emisphere Technologies, Inc., Hawthorne, New York 10532

Ann Lewis • SmithKline Beecham Pharmaceuticals, DMPK, The Frythe, Welwyn, Herts AL6 9AR, United Kingdom

Y. Liu • Graduate Center for Toxicology, University of Kentucky, Lexington, Kentucky 40503

Sudha Nagarajan • Inhale Therapeutic Systems, Palo Alto, California 94303

Lawrence Ng • Department of Pharmaceutical Chemistry, The University of Kansas, Lawrence, Kansas 66045

Noriko Okudaira • Pharmaceutical Research Center, Meiji Seika Kaisha, Ltd., 760 Morooka-cho, Kohoku-ku, Yokohama 222, Japan

Andrew Parkinson • Department of Pharmacology, Toxicology, and Therapeutics, University of Kansas Medical School, Kansas City, Kansas 66160

John S. Patton • Inhale Therapeutic Systems, Palo Alto, California 94303

Doreen Pierdomenico • Pharmaceutical Technologies, SmithKline Beecham Pharmaceuticals, King of Prussia, Pennsylvania 19406

Christopher J. H. Porter • Department of Pharmaceutics, Victorian College of Pharmacy, Monash University, Parkville, Victoria 3052, Australia

Elizabeth Quadros • Ciba-Geigy Corporation, Summit, New Jersey 07901

Patricia M. Reardon • Amgen, Inc., Thousand Oaks, California 91320

Jim E. Riviere • Cutaneous Pharmacology and Toxicology Center, North Carolina State University, Raleigh, North Carolina 27606

Joseph R. Robinson • School of Pharmacy, University of Wisconsin, Madison, Wisconsin 53706

Philip L. Smith • Department of Drug Delivery, SmithKline Beecham Pharmaceuticals, King of Prussia, Pennsylvania 19406

Quentin R. Smith • Neurochemistry and Brain Transport Section, National Institute on Aging, National Institutes of Health, Bethesda, Maryland 20892

Yuichi Sugiyama • Faculty of Pharmaceutical Sciences, University of Tokyo, Tokyo 113, Japan

Ronald G. Thurman • Laboratory of Hepatobiology and Toxicology, Department of Pharmacology, University of North Carolina, Chapel Hill, North Carolina 27599

M. Vore • Graduate Center for Toxicology, University of Kentucky, Lexington, Kentucky 40503

Doris Wall • Pharmaceutical Technologies, SmithKline Beecham Pharmaceuticals, King of Prussia, Pennsylvania 19406

Wen Wang • Department of Pharmaceutical Chemistry, The University of Kansas, Lawrence, Kansas 66045

Carla B. Washington • Department of Pharmacy, University of California, San Francisco, California 94143

Glynn Wilson • Tacora Corporation, Seattle, Washington 98105

Sy-Juen Wu • School of Pharmacy, University of Wisconsin, Madison, Wisconsin 53706

Preface

A major challenge confronting pharmaceutical chemists is the rational design of drug molecules to optimize pharmacological interactions with their therapeutic targets and to enable them to circumvent biological barriers (e.g., intestinal mucosa, liver, blood–brain barrier) that separate the site of drug action from the site of drug administration. The inability to circumvent such barriers often prevents leading drug candidates from being clinically developed (see Volume 4 in this series, *Biological Barriers to Protein Delivery*, edited by K. L. Audis and T. J. Raub).

Therefore, in the 1980s, scientists in the pharmaceutical industry began to employ *in situ* (e.g., perfused organ) and *in vitro* (e.g., tissue and cell culture) systems in the drug discovery process in order to optimize the pharmaceutical properties of drug candidates. These systems also started to play an important role in the evaluation of individual components of novel drug delivery formulations that had the potential to facilitate drug transport.

While the applications of these *in situ* and *in vitro* models are now being widely described in the scientific literature, the experimental details necessary to set up these systems in a research laboratory are not always provided in the primary publications. Furthermore, as these methodologies stem from a number of biological disciplines, the primary scientific literature will not be the normal purview of many pharmaceutical scientists.

Therefore, the editors of this book decided to provide pharmaceutical scientists ready access to these experimental methodologies. The first chapter, which is written by Ronald T. Borchardt, Philip L. Smith, and Glynn Wilson, provides an overview of the general principles for characterizing and using *in situ* and *in vitro* model systems for biopharmaceutical studies. Chapters 2 through 6 describe methodologies for studying drug absorption and metabolism after oral administration. These chapters describe the use of intestinal mucosal tissue (Chapter 2, Philip L. Smith), cultured intestinal epithelial cells (Chapter 3, Ismael J. Hidalgo), intestinal rings and isolated intestinal mucosal cells (Chapter 4, Joseph A. Fix), and *in situ* and conscious animals (Chapter 5, Robin Griffiths, Ann Lewis, and Phillip Jeffrey) for evaluating a drug candidate's ability to permeate the intestinal epithelium. In addition, Chapter 6 (Christopher J. H. Porter and William N. Charman) describes models for studying the intestinal lymphatic transport of drugs.

Methodologies are also described for studying other epithelial barriers, including the buccal epithelium (Chapter 7, Elizabeth Quadros, James P. Cassidy, and Harry Leipold), nasal epithelium (Chapter 16, Patricia M. Reardon), respiratory epithelium (Chapter 17, Kwang-Jin Kim and Edward D. Crandall), alveolar epithelium (Chapter 18, Doris Wall and Doreen Pierdomenico), pulmonary epithelium (Chapter 19, Mohammed Eljamal, Sudha Nagarajan, and John S. Patton), skin epithelium (Chapter 20, Robert L. Bronaugh; Chapter 21, Jim E. Riviere), vaginal epithelium (Chapter 22, Sy-Juen Wu and Joseph R. Robinson), and the ocular epithelium (Chapter 23, Vincent H. L. Lee).

This volume also describes methodologies for studying elimination barriers, such as the liver, by using isolated hepatocytes (Chapter 8, M. Vore, Y. Liu, and T. C. Ganguly), cultured hepatocytes (Chapter 9, Edward L. LeCluyse, Peter L. Bullock, Andrew Parkinson, and Jerome H. Hochman), and isolated perfused liver (Chapter 10, Kim L. R. Brouwer and Ronald G. Thurman). Methodologies are also provided for studying drug elimination in the kidney using isolated renal brush border and basolateral membrane vesicles and cultured renal cells (Chapter 11, Marcelo M. Gutierrez, Claire M. Brett, and Kathleen M. Giacomini) and isolated perfused kidney (Chapter 12, Noriko Okudaira and Yuichi Sugiyama).

Finally, included in this book are chapters describing the methodologies used to study drug transport and metabolism at the level of the blood–brain barrier (Chapter 13, Kenneth L. Audus, Lawrence Ng, Wen Wang, and Ronald T. Borchardt; Chapter 15, Quentin R. Smith) and the blood–cerebrospinal fluid barrier (Chapter 14, Carla B. Washington, Kathleen M. Giacomini, and Claire M. Brett).

Lastly, we thank all the authors, who are experienced practitioners in the development and use of the various model systems, for their valuable and timely contributions. We hope that the methodologies described in this book will facilitate the *in situ* and *in vitro* evaluation of drug candidates by scientists in the pharmaceutical/biotechnology industry and ultimately will lead to the expedited discovery of novel drugs together with formulations for improving their delivery.

Contents

Chapter 3

Cultured Intestinal Epithelial Cell Models

Ismael J. Hidalgo

Chapter 4

Intestinal Rings and Isolated Intestinal Mucosal Cells

Joseph A. Fix

Chapter 5

Models of Drug Absorption *in Situ* and in Conscious Animals

Robin Griffiths, Ann Lewis, and Phillip Jeffrey

Chapter 6

Model Systems for Intestinal Lymphatic Transport Studies

Christopher J. H. Porter and William N. Charman

Chapter 7

Buccal Tissues and Cell Culture

Elizabeth Quadros, James P. Cassidy, and Harry Leipold

Chapter 8

Isolated Hepatocytes

M. Vore, Y. Liu, and T. C. Ganguly

Chapter 9

Cultured Rat Hepatocytes

Edward L. LeCluyse, Peter L. Bullock, Andrew Parkinson, and Jerome H. Hochman

Chapter 10

Isolated Perfused Liver

Kim L. R. Brouwer and Ronald G. Thurman

Chapter 11

**Isolated Renal Brush Border and Basolateral Membrane Vesicles and
Cultured Renal Cells**

Marcelo M. Gutierrez, Claire M. Brett, and Kathleen M. Giacomini

Chapter 12

Use of An Isolated Perfused Kidney to Assess Renal Clearance of Drugs: Information Obtained in Steady-State and Non-Steady-State Experimental Systems

Noriko Okudaira and Yuichi Sugiyama

Chapter 13

Brain Microvessel Endothelial Cell Culture Systems

Kenneth L. Audus, Lawrence Ng, Wen Wang, and Ronald T. Borchardt

Chapter 14

Methods to Study Drug Transport in Isolated Choroid Plexus Tissue and Cultured Cells

Carla B. Washington, Kathleen M. Giacomini, and Claire M. Brett

Chapter 15

Brain Perfusion Systems for Studies of Drug Uptake and Metabolism in the Central Nervous System

Quentin R. Smith

Chapter 16

In Vitro Nasal Models

Patricia M. Reardon

Chapter 17

Models for Investigation of Peptide and Protein Transport across Cultured Mammalian Respiratory Epithelial Barriers

Kwang-Jin Kim and Edward D. Crandall

Chapter 18

Drug Transport across *Xenopus* Alveolar Epithelium *in Vitro*

Doris Wall and Doreen Pierdomenico

Chapter 19

In Situ and *in Vivo* **Methods for Pulmonary Delivery**

Mohammed Eljamal, Sudha Nagarajan, and John S. Patton

Chapter 20

In Vitro **Viable Skin Model**

Robert L. Bronaugh

Chapter 21

Isolated Perfused Porcine Skin Flap Systems

Jim E. Riviere

Chapter 22

Vaginal Epithelial Models

Sy-Juen Wu and Joseph R. Robinson

Chapter 23

Ocular Epithelial Models

Vincent H. L. Lee

Chapter 1

General Principles in the Characterization and Use of Model Systems for Biopharmaceutical Studies

Ronald T. Borchardt, Philip L. Smith, and Glynn Wilson

1. INTRODUCTION

A major challenge confronting pharmaceutical chemists in the future will be the design of drug candidates having structural characteristics adequate to circumvent the biological barriers [e.g., intestinal mucosa, liver, blood–brain barrier (BBB)] that often prevent the clinical development of potentially useful drug candidates (Audus and Raub, 1993). Through rational drug design, medicinal chemists are capable of synthesizing very potent and very specific drug candidates (Morgan and Gainer, 1989; Greenlee, 1990; Huff, 1991; Doherty, 1992; Bondinell *et al.*, 1994). These drug candidates are developed with molecular characteristics that permit optimal interaction with the specific macromolecules (e.g., receptors, enzymes) that mediate their pharmacological effects. However, rational drug design, as currently practiced in many pharmaceutical companies, does not necessarily ensure optimal delivery of the drug to its site of action. Optimal delivery can be achieved by incorporating the drug candidate into a delivery system (e.g., formulation strategies) and/or by designing the

Ronald T. Borchardt • Department of Pharmaceutical Chemistry, The University of Kansas, Lawrence, Kansas 66045. *Philip L. Smith* • Department of Drug Delivery, SmithKline Beecham Pharmaceuticals, King of Prussia, Pennsylvania 19406. *Glynn Wilson* • Tacora Corporation, Seattle, Washington 98134.

Models for Assessing Drug Absorption and Metabolism, Ronald T. Borchardt *et al.*, eds., Plenum Press, New York, 1996.

1

drug candidate to have the structural characteristics (rational drug design strategies) that will provide optimal transfer between the point of administration and the pharmacological target in the body (Lee, 1991).

During the 1970s and 1980s, pharmaceutical scientists dedicated a significant amount of time and effort to the development of delivery systems that could potentially facilitate this transfer process (Borchardt *et al.*, 1985; Anderson and Kim, 1986). However, it became very apparent in the mid to late 1980s that delivery systems alone could not always ensure optimal transfer of the drug candidate to its pharmacological target in the body (Humphrey and Ringrove, 1986; Lee and Yamamoto, 1990; Taylor and Amidon, 1995). Many potentially useful drug candidates were never developed clinically because these molecules lacked the structural features needed to circumvent the epithelial (e.g., intestinal mucosa), endothelial (e.g., BBB), and elimination (e.g., liver) barriers that limit the access of the drug to its site of action.

Therefore, in the late 1980s, pharmaceutical scientists began to place increased emphasis on designing drug candidates to have the structural features necessary for interaction with the pharmacological target as well as those structural features necessary to circumvent the epithelial, endothelial, and elimination barriers (Taylor and Amidon, 1995). This increased focus on designing the drug candidate to ensure optimal discovery required several significant changes in the drug delivery and development process within pharmaceutical companies.

One major change was a need for increased communication and expanded interactions between discovery scientists (e.g., medicinal chemists) and development scientists (e.g., drug metabolism and formulation scientists). Excellent examples of the success of this approach were the design and development of an orally bioavailable renin inhibitor by a multidisciplinary team of scientists at Abbott Laboratories (Kleinert *et al.*, 1992) and the design and development of an orally bioavailable platelet fibrinogen receptor (GPIIb/IIIa) antagonist (Bondinell *et al.*, 1994).

The second major change was the need to adapt existing methodologies or to develop new methodologies in order to facilitate the rapid characterization of the pharmaceutical properties (e.g., transport, metabolism) of a drug candidate (Audus *et al.*, 1990; Wilson *et al.*, 1991; Miller *et al.*, 1995; Hillgren *et al.*, 1995). While some scientists in the pharmaceutical industry recognized the need to characterize both the pharmaceutical and the pharmacological properties of a drug candidate, the assays which existed in the late 1980s for characterizing the pharmaceutical properties of a drug candidate were more suitable for development than for research. These tended to be animal-based assays, which were time-consuming, required large amounts of a drug candidate, and were not suitable for high-throughput screening. In contrast, assays based on tissues, cells, or macromolecules were needed. These types of assays tend to be more rapid, require smaller amounts of a drug candidate, and are more suitable for automation. Using data generated from organ-, tissue-, cellular-, and molecular-based assays and an iterative process, medicinal chemists, working in collaboration with molecular pharmacologists, cell biologists, immunologists, and biochemists, have been very successful in optimizing the pharmacological properties of drug candidates. The availability of similar *in situ* and *in vitro* assay systems for biopharmaceutical assessment would allow the medicinal chemists to use this same iterative process to define the pharmaceutical properties of a drug candidate.

Therefore, in the late 1980s, scientists in the pharmaceutical industry began to employ *in situ* (e.g., perfused organ) and *in vitro* (e.g., tissue and cell culture) systems in drug discovery to characterize the pharmaceutical properties of drug candidates (e.g., transport, metabolism). With the recent advances in combinatorial approaches by medicinal chemists, the need for more rapid throughput screens to assess the pharmaceutical properties of drug candidates will become even more acute. Fortunately, many of these systems could be adapted from preparations used for decades by physiologists and cell biologists to study these epithelial, endothelial, and elimination barriers from a physiological and/or a developmental biology perspective.

While the applications of these *in situ* and *in vitro* models are described widely in the scientific literature, the experimental details necessary to set up these systems in one's laboratory are not always provided. In addition, since these methodologies cross discipline lines (physiology–cell biology–pharmaceutical sciences), the primary literature is not always readily available to an investigator. Therefore, the editors of this book decided to provide a one-stop location for the experimental methodologies needed to establish, validate, and implement these commonly used *in situ* and *in vitro* model systems for biopharmaceutical studies.

2. BIOLOGICAL BARRIERS TO DRUG DELIVERY

The biological barriers to drug delivery can basically be divided into epithelial, endothelial, elimination, and target cell barriers (Audus and Raub, 1993). This volume will not describe methods used to assess target cell penetration; thus, the barrier properties of the target cell will not be discussed in this section. Instead, attention will be focused on the properties of epithelial, endothelial, and elimination barriers.

The barriers that restrict access of drugs to the systemic circulation include the intestinal epithelium (Neutra and Kraehenbuhl, 1993), rectal epithelium (Muranishi *et al.*, 1993), oral epithelium (Merkle and Wolany, 1993), nasal and respiratory epithelium (Johnson and Boucher, 1993), vaginal epithelium (Muranishi *et al.*, 1993), ocular epithelium (Lee and Robinson, 1986), and dermal epithelium (Banga and Chien, 1993). While these epithelia differ morphologically, they all serve to restrict the permeability of drugs into the systemic circulation by serving as both physical and biochemical barriers. They serve as physical barriers because the epithelial cells form tight cellular junctions, which thus restrict paracellular flux of solutes. Therefore, solutes that can penetrate these epithelial barriers must possess either the optimal physicochemical characteristics (size, charge, lipophilicity, hydrogen-bonding potential, conformation) that allow them to passively diffuse via the transcellular route (Burton et al., 1991) or the structural features necessary to serve as a substrate for one of the endogenous transporter systems (e.g., peptide transporter) (Smith et al., 1993). Another common feature of these epithelia is that they possess a low level of transcytotic activity, which restricts the permeability of macromolecules (e.g., proteins). These epithelia also serve as biochemical barriers because of their ability to metabolize drugs. However, in addition, it has recently been shown that some of these epithelia (e.g., intestinal mucosa) contain apically polarized efflux systems that can restrict the passive diffusion of drugs (Burton et al., 1993; Hunter et al., 1993).

If a drug successfully penetrates one of the epithelia mentioned above and enters the systemic circulation, or if the drug is administered directly into the systemic circulation, endothelial barriers may restrict its distribution to its site of action. One of the most significant endothelial barriers from a drug delivery perspective is the BBB (Audus et al., 1992; Broadwell, 1993; Malik and Birmboim, 1993). Like the epithelial barriers described above, the BBB serves as both a physical and a biological barrier to drug delivery. As a physical barrier, its tight cellular junctions restrict the paracellular flux of solutes. Again, drugs must have optimal physicochemical characteristics for passive diffusion via the transcellular route or the structural features necessary to serve as a substrate for one of the endogenous transporters. Vascular trafficking of macromolecules (e.g., proteins) is also highly restricted. The BBB is also a biochemical barrier having not only a high metabolic capacity but also apically polarized efflux systems that restrict blood-to-brain flux of certain solutes (Tsuji et al., 1992; Chikhale et al., 1995).

Finally, the efficacy of drugs can be substantially reduced by the elimination barriers, which include the liver (Meijer and Ziegler, 1993) and the kidney (Rabkin and Dahl, 1993). While morphologically and functionally very different, the liver and the kidney both possess mechanisms for removal of drug substances from the systemic circulation and the secretion of these drugs (or their metabolites) into bile and urine, respectively. The net result is a reduced blood level of the drug and thus reduced efficacy.

3. DESIRABLE CHARACTERISTICS OF A MODEL SYSTEM

The ideal model system for biopharmaceutical assessment of drug transport and metabolism should have certain characteristics. The model should be physiologically reflective of the specific biological barrier of interest in humans. For example, if the barrier of interest is a specific segment of the human intestinal tract (e.g., ileum), the model system should consist of a monolayer of highly polarized human intestinal mucosal cells that exhibit the physiological characteristics (e.g., thickness of the mucus layer) of the region of interest (Madara and Trier, 1987). The model should also exhibit all of the biochemical characteristics of the specific biological barrier of interest in humans. For example, if the barrier is again a specific segment of the human intestinal tract (e.g., ileum), it should express transporters (e.g., peptide transporters), efflux systems (e.g., P-glycoprotein), and metabolic enzymes (e.g., aminopeptidases) at the same level as the region of interest (Alpers, 1987; Hopfer, 1987; Shiau, 1987). In addition, the model system should require a low to moderate level of technical expertise to set up and maintain, and, if possible, the system should be amenable to automation, so that a large number of studies can be done rapidly and inexpensively (screening mode). However, it should also be sufficiently sophisticated that it can function as a valuable research tool. For example, if the barrier is the intestinal mucosa, the model should be sufficiently flexible to permit determination of uptake, efflux, and transcellular transport of a drug candidate so that mechanisms of transport can be elucidated. As an example, Burton *et al.* (1993) and Hunter *et al.* (1993) recently used a cell culture model (Caco-2 cells) of the intestinal mucosa to identify apically polarized efflux systems that restrict the transcellular permeability of some molecules.

Finally, an ideal model for biopharmaceutical assessment would be one in which the viability could be maintained using "simple" media (e.g., Hanks' balanced salt solution). This would allow the investigator to use standard methodology (e.g., HPLC) to determine the disposition of the drug. Ideally, when using these models in a screening mode, one would like to avoid the use of radiolabeled material or the need to spend significant time and resources to develop analytical methodologies for each compound of interest. However, it should be noted that advancement in optimizing the use of LC-MS-MS analysis of biological fluids will dramatically reduce our dependence on radiolabeled compounds and simple buffers.

Unfortunately, there are very few, if any, *in situ* and *in vitro* model systems that satisfy all of the characteristics described above. However, this does not mean that the available models are not useful for biopharmaceutical studies. It simply means that the investigator using the model system needs to be fully aware of the limitations of the model in order not to overinterpret the data being generated.

4. CHARACTERIZATION OF MODEL SYSTEMS

Once a model system has been established in a laboratory, the investigators should conduct some characterization experiments even if they are duplicating literature data. These characterization experiments will vary, depending upon the nature of the model (perfused organ and isolated tissue vs. cell culture). For example, if the model system consists of a perfused organ or an isolated tissue, the major issue is the viability of the preparation. There are two aspects to the viability issue with perfused organs or isolated tissues. One of these deals with whether the preparation, upon isolation from the animal, retains both its physical and its biochemical barrier properties. The second issue deals with the viability of the preparation during a typical transport or metabolism experiment. Both of these viability issues can be addressed experimentally by using light microscopy and transmission and scanning electron microscopy to detect physical damage to the preparation and by conducting transport experiments using radiolabeled markers that can detect whether the barrier properties of the preparation have been compromised during isolation or experimentation. For example, [^{3}H]inulin or [^{3}H]mannitol is often used as an impermeable hydrophilic marker in perfused organs and isolated tissues and cell culture systems to check for the integrity of the barrier (Marks *et al.*, 1991; Raeissi and Borchardt, 1993; Tang *et al.*, 1993; Chikhale *et al.*, 1994). Alternatively, transepithelial electrical resistance (TEER) values are often used in tissue preparations to measure the integrity of the barrier (Pierdomenico *et al.*, 1992). However, in epithelia, TEER values are sufficiently variable that inclusion of a permeability marker provides the most accurate method for evaluating tissue integrity. In addition, the integrity of the barrier is often characterized by measuring the activity of transporters or enzymes known to be present in the biological barrier. For example, radiolabeled amino acids (e.g. [^{3}H]leucine) are often used in perfused organ and isolated tissue preparations to measure the activity of the large neutral amino acid transporter observed in some biological barriers (e.g., BBB) (Smith *et al.*, 1984).

If the model being employed by the investigator is a cell culture system, then two major issues need to be addressed. First, one must determine if the cell culture system has fully differentiated and thus has expressed all of the physical and biochemical characteristics of the biological barrier *in vivo*. This requires that the investigator use light microscopy and transmission and scanning electron microscopy to ensure that the cell culture system has all the morphological characteristics of the biological barrier *in vivo*. For example, cell culture models of the intestinal mucosa should be columnar in shape, have occluding functional complexes, and have a well-defined brush border with microvilli (Hidalgo *et al.*, 1989). Histochemical localization studies are also required to demonstrate the cell polarity. For example, cell culture models of the intestinal mucosa should exhibit an asymmetric distribution of alkaline phosphatase on their luminal side (Hidalgo *et al.*, 1989). The barrier properties of a cell culture model can be determined by using impermeable hydrophilic markers (e.g. [^{3}H]inulin) and by measuring TEER values (Hidalgo *et al.*, 1989) in a manner similar to the experiments described above for perfused organs and isolated tissue preparations. The functional integrity of the barrier can be determined by measuring the transport of specific substrates for endogenous transporters (Hidalgo and Borchardt, 1990a,b) or efflux systems (Burton *et al.*, 1993; Hunter *et al.*, 1993) and by measuring the activity of metabolic enzymes (Chikhale and Borchardt, 1994).

The second major issue that needs to be addressed with cell culture systems concerns ensuring the viability of the cells and the integrity of the barrier during experimentation. This can be accomplished, for example, with intestinal tissues through measurement of the transport rates for actively transported solutes such as glucose or amino acids (e.g., villus cell integrity) or through measurement of the secretory rate for chloride (e.g., crypt cell function). Both these techniques provide a measure of functional viability since they are dependent on cellular generation of ATP (Swaan *et al.*, 1994; Yeh *et al.*, 1994).

5. APPLICATIONS TO PHARMACEUTICAL PROBLEMS

In each of the chapters that follow, specific examples are provided to show how the *in situ* or *in vitro* model system considered has been employed to address pharmaceutical problems. However, we provide here a listing of various potential applications of these models in the pharmaceutical sciences. These applications include: (a) estimation of the permeability characteristics of drug candidates through a particular biological barrier, thus conserving compounds that are available only in limited quantities; (b) elucidation of pathways of drug transport (e.g., paracellular vs. transcellular, passive vs. carrier-mediated diffusion); (c) determination of the structure–transport relationship for carrier-mediated pathways (e.g., peptide transporters, bile acid transporters) of drug transport; (d) determination of how components of the media can influence the transport of drug candidates (e.g., protein binding); (e) determination of the optimal physicochemical characteristics (e.g., size, charge, lipophilicity, hydrogen bonding potential, conformation) of a drug for passive diffusion; (f) determination of the structure–transport relationships for the apically polarized efflux mechanisms that limit the transcellular flux of drugs across some biological barriers (e.g., intestinal, BBB); (g) rapid assessment of chemical strategies (e.g., prodrugs) designed to enhance the membrane permeability of a drug or to minimize its metabolism; (h) rapid assessment of formulation strategies (e.g., adjuvants) designed to enhance membrane permeability; (i) rapid assessment of potential toxic effects of drug candidates or formulation components on the biological barrier; and (j) elucidation of potential pathways of drug metabolism and/or elimination. In addition, these *in situ* and *in vitro* model systems are being used to elucidate the physical and biological characteristics of epithelial and endothelial barriers and to evaluate the relative roles of physical or biochemical/metabolic factors in the transport of drug molecules across these barriers. For example, several research groups (Tsuji *et al.*, 1992; Burton *et al.*, 1993; Hunter *et al.*, 1993) have recently used cell culture systems of the intestinal mucosa and the BBB to identify and partially characterize the properties of apically polarized efflux systems in these biological barriers which appear to play important roles in limiting the permeability of certain drug candidates. These model systems have also been used as a resource from which proteins involved in drug transport and metabolism can be identified and characterized. To illustrate, Dantzig *et al.* (1994) have recently deduced the amino acid sequence for a putative peptide transporter in Caco-2 cells, an *in vitro* model of the intestinal mucosa. Some of the systems (e.g., cell culture models) also afford the exciting possibility of screening combinatorial libraries for lead compounds that possess both pharmacological and pharmaceutical properties that are desirable.

In addition to the convenience of these *in situ* and *in vitro* model systems in rapidly carrying out both basic and applied research, some of these systems (e.g., cell culture models) also afford the opportunity to minimize time-consuming, expensive, and sometimes controversial animal studies. In addition, some of these systems (e.g., cell culture models) are of a human origin, which could ultimately permit better predictability of the behavior of a drug in humans, particularly from the standpoint of metabolism, and some of these systems (e.g., tissues) can provide information concerning regional differences in intestinal permeability, which is valuable for designing controlled-release formulations.

6. FUTURE DIRECTIONS

In spite of the advances that have been made in recent years, a substantial amount of research is needed before many of the model systems described in this volume become a routine part of the drug discovery process. For example, more effort must be dedicated to (a) establishment of *in situ–in vivo* and *in vitro–in vivo* correlations of drug permeability data; (b) establishment of *in situ–in vivo* and *in vitro–in vivo* correlations of drug elimination data; (c) further characterization of the metabolic potential of these model systems, particularly the cell culture models; (d) establishment of *in situ–in vivo* and *in vitro–in vivo* correlations of the metabolic potential of these model systems; (e) establishment of standardized methods for quantitation of permeability data; (f) genetic, hormonal, and/or biochemical manipulation of the cell culture models to achieve the permeability and metabolism characteristics that most accurately reflect the biological barrier *in vivo*; (g) configuration of more complex cell culture models (e.g., co-culture of intestinal mucosa cells and goblet cells) that would most accurately reflect the biological barrier *in vivo*; (h) automation of the cell culture systems that would allow their greater involvement in the early phases of a drug discovery project; and (i) adaptation of these systems to handle insoluble compounds and/or complex formulations.

Finally, efforts should be made to more actively publish data generated by industrial scientists using these model systems. Since some of these models have become an integral part of the drug discovery process in pharmaceutical companies, publication of important new data in the open literature is dictated by proprietary issues. Of particular concern is the lack of data in the open literature on *in situ–in vivo* and *in vitro–in vivo* correlations of permeability and metabolism. Many companies that have embraced the idea of using cell culture systems to characterize the pharmaceutical properties of drug candidates have conducted or are currently conducting internal validation studies. Unfortunately, this process is being repeated over and over again throughout the pharmaceutical industry. Hopefully, in the near future, some of these studies will be published in the open literature so that this duplication of effort can be minimized.

7. CONCLUSIONS

In conclusion, the introduction of these model systems into drug discovery represents an exciting new advance in the pharmaceutical sciences. The use of these model systems could not only lead to an improved understanding of the biological barriers that often limit the efficacy of a drug candidate but could also have the potential to expedite the process of drug discovery and development, thus improving the efficiency of the pharmaceutical industry. Hopefully, by optimizing both the pharmacological and the pharmaceutical properties of a drug candidate by structural manipulation, the pharmaceutical industry will ultimately see an improvement in the number of drug candidates that succeed in clinical trials, thus reducing costs and the time necessary to introduce a new therapeutic agent into clinical practice. If properly established, validated, and implemented in a pharmaceutical company, the models described in this volume have the potential to expedite the discovery and development process and make it more cost-effective.

REFERENCES

Alpers, D. H., 1987, Digestion and absorption of carbohydrates and proteins, in: *Physiology of the Gastrointestinal Tract*, Vol. 2 (L. R. Johnson, ed.), Raven Press, New York, pp. 1469–1487.

Anderson, J. M., and Kim, S. W., 1986, *Advances in Drug Delivery Systems*, Elsevier, Amsterdam.

Audus, K. L., and Raub, T. J. (eds.), 1993, *Biological Barriers to Protein Delivery*, Plenum Press, New York.

Audus, K. L., Bartel, R., Hidalgo, I., and Borchardt, R. T., 1990, The use of cultured epithelial and endothelial cells for drug transport and metabolism studies, *Pharm. Res.* **7:**435–451.

Audus, K. L., Chikhale, P., Miller, D., Thompson, S. E., and Borchardt, R. T., 1992, Brain uptake: Influence of chemical and biological factors, in: *Advances in Drug Research* (B. Testa, ed.), Academic Press, London, pp. 1–64.

Banga, A. K., and Chien, Y. W., 1993, Dermal absorption of peptides and proteins, in: *Biological Barriers to Protein Delivery* (K. L. Audus and T. J. Raub, eds.), Plenum Press, New York, pp. 179–197.

Bondinell, W. E., Keenen, R. M., Miller, W. H., Ali, F. E., Allen, A. C., DeBrosse, C. W., Eggleston, D. S., Erkard, K. F., Haltwanger, R. C., Huffman, W. F., Hwang, S. M., Jakas, D. R., Koster, P. F., Ku, T. W., Lee, C. P., Nichols, A. J., Ross, S. T., Samanen, J. M., Valocik, R. E., Vaska-Moser, J. A., Venslavsky, J. M., Wang, A. S., and Yuan, C.-K., 1994, Design of a potent and orally active nonpeptide platelet fibrinogen receptor (GPIIb/IIIa) antagonist, *Bioorg. Med. Chem.* **2:**897–908.

Borchardt, R. T., Repta, A. J., and Stella, V. J. (eds.), 1985, *Directed Drug Delivery: A Multidisciplinary Approach*, Humana Press, Clifton, New Jersey.

Broadwell, R. D., 1993, Transcytosis of macromolecules through the blood–brain fluid barrier *in vivo*, in: *Biological Barriers to Protein Delivery* (K. L. Audus and T. J. Raub, eds.), Plenum Press, New York, pp. 269–296.

Burton, P. S., Conradi, R. A., and Hilgers, R. A., 1991, Mechanism of peptide and protein absorption. 2. Transcellular mechanism of peptide and protein absorption: Passive aspects, *Adv. Drug Deliv. Res.* **7:**365–386.

Burton, P. S., Conradi, R. A., Hilgers, R. A., and Ho, N. F. H., 1993, Evidence for a polarized efflux system for peptides in the apical membrane of Caco-2 cells, *Biochem. Biophys. Res. Commun.* **190:**760–766.

Chikhale, P. J., and Borchardt, R. T., 1994, Metabolism of α-methyl-DOPA in cultured intestinal epithelial (Caco-2) cells: Correlation with metabolism *in vivo, Drug Metab. Dispos.* **22:**592–560.

Chikhale, E. G., Ng, K. Y., Burton, P. S., and Borchardt, R. T., 1994, Hydrogen bonding potential as a determinant of the *in vitro* and *in vivo* blood–brain barrier permeability of peptides, *Pharm. Res.* **11:**412–419.

Chikhale, E. G., Burton, P. S., and Borchardt, R. T., 1995, The effects of P-glycoprotein on the transport of peptides across the blood–brain barrier in rats, *J. Pharmacol. Exp. Ther.* **273:**298–303.

Dantzig, A. H., Hoskins, J. A., Tabas, L. B., Bright, S., Shepard, R. L., Jenkins, I. L., Duckworth, D. C., Sportsman, J. R., Mackensen, D., Rosteck, P. R., and Skatrud, P. L., 1994, Association of intestinal peptide transport with a protein related to the cadherin superfamily, *Science* **264:**430–433.

Doherty, A. M., 1992, Endothelin: A new challenge, *J. Med. Chem.* **35:**1493–1508.

Greenlee, W. J., 1990, Renin inhibitors, *Med. Res. Rev.* **10:**173–236.

Hidalgo, I. J., and Borchardt, R. T., 1990a, Transport of a large neutral amino acid (phenylalanine) in a human intestinal epithelial cell line: Caco-2, *Biochim. Biophys. Acta* **1028:**25–30.

Hidalgo, I. J., and Borchardt, R. T., 1990b, Transport of bile acids in a human intestinal epithelial cell line: Caco-2, *Biochim. Biophys. Acta* **1035:**97–103.

Hidalgo, I. J., Raub, T. J., and Borchardt, R. T., 1989, Characterization of a human colon carcinoma cell line (Caco-2) as a model system for intestinal epithelial permeability, *Gastroenterology* **96:**736–749.

Hillgren, K. M., Kato, A., and Borchardt, R. T., 1995, *In vitro* systems for studying intestinal drug absorption, *Med. Res. Rev.* **15:**83–109.

Hopfer, U., 1987, Membrane transport mechanisms for hexoses and amino acids in the small intestine, in: *Physiology of the Gastrointestinal Tract*, Vol. 2 (L. R. Johnson, ed.), Raven Press, New York, pp. 1499–1526.

Huff, J. R., 1991, HIV protease: A novel chemotherapeutic target for AIDS, *J. Med. Chem.* **34:**2305–2314.

Humphrey, M. J., and Ringrove, P. S., 1986, Peptides and related drugs: A review of their absorption, metabolism and excretion, *Drug Metab. Rev.* **17:**383–410.

Hunter, J., Jepson, M. A., Tsuruo, T., Simmons, M. L., and Hirst, B. H., 1993, Functional expression of a P-glycoprotein in apical membranes of human intestinal Caco-2 cells: Kinetics of vinblastine secretion and interaction with modulators, *J. Biol. Chem.* **268:**14991–14997.

Johnson, L. G., and Boucher, R. C., 1993, Macromolecular transport across nasal and respiratory epithelia, in: *Biological Barriers to Protein Delivery* (K. L. Audus and T. J. Raub, eds.), Plenum Press, New York, pp. 161–178.

Kleinert, H. D., Rosenberg, S. H., Baker, W. R., Stein, H. H., Klinghofer, V., Barlow, J., Spina, K., Polakowski, J., Kovar, P., Cohen, J., and Denissen, J., 1992, Discovery of a peptide-based renin inhibitor with oral bioavailability and efficacy, *Science* **257:**1940–1943.

Lee, V. H. (ed.), 1991, *Peptide and Protein Delivery*, Marcel Dekker, New York.

Lee, V. H. L., and Robinson, J. R., 1986, Topical ocular drug delivery: Recent developments and future challenges, *J. Ocul. Pharmacol.* **2:**67–108.

Lee, V. H. L., and Yamamoto, A., 1990, Penetration and enzymatic barriers to peptide and protein absorption, *Adv. Drug Deliv. Res.* **4:**171–207.

Madara, J. L., and Trier, J. S., 1987, Functional morphology of the mucosa of the small intestine, in: *Physiology of the Gastrointestinal Tract*, Vol. 2 (L. R. Johnson, ed.), Raven Press, New York, pp. 1209–1249.

Malik, A. B., and Birmboim, A. S., 1993, Vascular endothelial barrier and its regulation, in: *Biological Barriers to Protein Delivery* (K. L. Audus and T. J. Raub, eds.), Plenum Press, New York, pp. 231–267.

Marks, G. J., Ryan, F. M., Hidalgo, I. J., and Smith, P. L., 1991, Mannitol as a marker for intestinal integrity in *in vitro* adsorption studies, *Gastroenterology* **100:**A697.

Meijer, D. K. F., and Ziegler, K., 1993, Mechanisms for the hepatic clearance of oligopeptides and proteins: Implications for rate of elimination, bioavailability and cell-specific drug delivery in the liver, in: *Biological Barriers to Protein Delivery* (K. L. Audus and T. J. Raub, eds.), Plenum Press, New York, pp. 339–408.

Merkle, H. P., and Wolany, G. J. M., 1993, Intraoral peptide absorption, in: *Biological Barriers to Protein Delivery* (K. L. Audus and T. J. Raub, eds.), Plenum Press, New York, pp. 131–160.

Miller, D. W., Ng, L., Kato, A., Chikhale, E., and Borchardt, R. T., 1995, Cell culture models for examining peptide absorption, in: *Peptide-Based Drug Design: Controlling Transport and Metabolism* (M. Taylor and G. Amidon, eds.), American Chemical Society Books, Washington D.C., pp. 475–500.

Morgan, B. A., and Gainer, J. A., 1989, Approaches to the discovery of non-peptide ligands of peptide receptors and peptidases, *Annu. Rep. Med. Chem.* **24:**243–252.

Muranishi, S., Yamamoto, A., and Okada, H., 1993, Rectal and vaginal absorption of peptides and proteins, in: *Biological Barriers to Protein Delivery* (K. L. Audus and T. J. Raub, eds.), Plenum Press, New York, pp. 199–227.

Neutra, M., and Kraehenbuhl, J. P., 1993, Transepithelial transport of proteins by intestinal epithelial cells, in: *Biological Barriers to Protein Delivery* (K. L. Audus and T. J. Raub, eds.), Plenum Press, New York, pp. 107–129.

Pierdomenico, D., Madonna-Langen, M., Smith, P. L., and Wall, D. A., 1992, An *in vitro* model for pulmonary epithelial permeability, *Proc. Intl. Symp. Controlled Release Bioact. Mater.* **19:**228–229.

Rabkin, R., and Dahl, D. C., 1993, Renal uptake and disposal of proteins and peptides, in: *Biological Barriers to Protein Delivery* (K. L. Audus and T. J. Raub, eds.), Plenum Press, New York, pp. 299–338.

Raeissi, S., and Borchardt, R. T., 1993, Cultured human adenocarcinoma cells (Caco-2) as a model to study the mechanism by which adjuvants enhance intestinal permeability of drugs, *S. T. P. Pharm. Sci.* **3:**56–62.

Shiau, Y. F., 1987, Lipid digestion and absorption, in: *Physiology of the Gastrointestinal Tract*, Vol. 2 (L. R. Johnson, ed.), Raven Press, New York, pp. 1527–1556.

Smith, G. R., Takasato, Y., and Rapoport, S. I., 1984, Kinetic analyses of L-leucine transport across the blood-brain barrier, *Brain Res.* **31:**167–170.

Smith, P. L., Eddy, E. P., Lee, C.-P., and Wilson, G., 1993, Exploitation of the intestinal oligopeptide transporter to enhance drug absorption, *Drug Deliv.* **1:**103–111.

Swaan, P. W., Marks, G. J., Ryan, F. M., and Smith, P. L., 1994, Determination of transport rates for arginine and acetaminophen in rabbit intestinal tissues *in vitro*, *Pharm. Res.* **11:**283–287.

Tang, A. S., Chikhale, P. J., Shah, P. K., and Borchardt, R. T., 1993, Utilization of a human intestinal epithelial cell culture system (Caco-2) for evaluating cytoprotective agents, *Pharm. Res.* **10:**1620–1626.

Taylor, M., and Amidon, G. (eds.), 1995, *Peptide-Based Drug Design: Controlling Transport and Metabolism*, American Chemical Society Books, Washington D.C.

Tsuji, A., Terasaki, T., Takabatake, Y., Tenda, Y., Tamaj, I., Yamashita, J., Moritani, S., Tsuruo, T., and Yamashita, T. 1992, P-glycoprotein as the drug efflux pump in primary cultured bovine brain capillary endothelial cells, *Life Sci.* **51:**1427–1437.

Wilson, G., Davis, S. S., Illum, L., and Zweibaum, A. (eds.), 1991, *Pharmaceutical Applications of Cell and Tissue Culture to Drug Transport*, Plenum Press, New York.

Yeh, P.-Y., Smith, P. L., and Ellens, H., 1994, Effect of medium-chain glycerides on physiological properties of rabbit intestinal epithelium *in vitro*, *Pharm. Res.* **11:**1148–1154.

Chapter 2

Methods for Evaluating Intestinal Permeability and Metabolism *in Vitro*

Philip L. Smith

1. INTRODUCTION

Oral administration of therapeutic agents is often desired for convenience to the patient and therefore enhanced compliance. Successful design of orally bioavailable molecules requires that the molecules (1) be stable to chemical and enzymatic degradation (e.g., within the intestinal lumen, intestinal wall, liver, and circulation); (2) are able to traverse the intestinal epithelial barrier to the portal circulation; and (3) can pass through the liver and enter the systemic circulation intact at a concentration sufficient to elicit the appropriate pharmacologic response. *In vitro* methods can be employed to determine whether molecules have the required permeability and stability characteristics to traverse the gastrointestinal wall and enter the portal circulation. Compared to *in vivo* absorption studies, evaluation of intestinal permeability *in vitro* (1) requires less compound; (2) is relatively easier and, in the case of segmental absorption studies, avoids complicated surgery and maintenance of surgically prepared animals; (3) is more rapid and has the potential to reduce animal usage since a number of variables can be examined in each experiment; (4) provides insights into the mechanisms (e.g., carrier-mediated vs. passive), routes (e.g., transcellular vs. paracellular), and segmental differences (e.g., small vs. large intestine) involved in transepithelial transport; and (5) is analytically more simple because compounds are

Philip L. Smith • Department of Drug Delivery, SmithKline Beecham Pharmaceuticals, King of Prussia, Pennsylvania 19406.

Models for Assessing Drug Absorption and Metabolism, Ronald T. Borchardt *et al.*, eds., Plenum Press, New York, 1996.

being analyzed in an aqueous buffer solution as opposed to whole blood or plasma. In addition to their utility in defining intestinal permeability of compounds, *in vitro* methods can also be employed to study metabolism of molecules during transport across the intestinal epithelium and to aid in formulation design and provide information to medicinal chemists about molecular features which impede or enhance the absorption of compounds, thereby allowing rational approaches to the design of orally active molecules (Bondinell *et al.*, 1994; Samanen *et al.*, 1996).

The *in vitro* techniques to be described in this chapter resulted from the pioneering work of Ussing and co-workers, who in the late 1940s and early 1950s published a series of papers describing the measurement of ion fluxes employing radioisotopes in "short-circuited" frog skin (Ussing, 1949; Koefoed-Johnson *et al.*, 1952; Ussing, 1950; Ussing and Zerahn, 1951; Koefoed-Johnson *et al.*, 1953; Koefoed-Johnson and Ussing, 1953). These techniques have subsequently been applied not only to frog skin but to a variety of epithelia including intestine (Field *et al.*, 1971; Schultz and Zalusky, 1964), trachea (Smith *et al.*, 1982), lung (see Chapters 18 and 19), nasal mucosa (see Chapter 16), buccal mucosa (see Chapter 7), and cultured epithelial cells (see Chapters 3, 7, 11, 16, and 18).

2. METHODS

2.1. Materials

2.1.1. BUFFERS

Experimental procedures will be presented for studying rabbit intestinal tissues. Males have been employed in these studies to avoid complications that may arise from hormonal fluctuations in females. However, as discussed in Section 2.2, intestinal transport/metabolism studies have been conducted in epithelia from a variety of animals. For studies with tissues from animals other than the rabbit, the references cited in Table I may be consulted. A description of the Ussing chamber procedure which depicts the conventional Ussing chamber setup together with the associated electrical setup for monitoring the voltage and current of the epithelial preparation has recently been presented by Hegel *et al.* (1993).

Buffers employed for studying intestinal tissues from the rabbit contain (in mM): Na^+, 141; K^+, 5; Ca^{2+}, 1.2; Mg^{2+}, 1.2; Cl^-, 122; HCO_3^-, 25; $H_2PO_4^-$, 0.4; and HPO_4^{2-}, 1.6. A procedure for preparation of stock solutions and for preparation of the working buffer is presented in Table II. This buffer solution has a pH of ~7.4 when gassed with 5% CO_2 in O_2. Alternate buffers have been employed for experiments in which the effect of pH or ion dependence on permeability or stability of molecules is to be examined (Hidalgo *et al.*, 1993; Roden *et al.*, 1991).

Table I
Tissue Preparations Employed for Studying Intestinal Permeability

Tissue preparation	Reference
Amphiuma small intestine (stripped vs. unstripped)	White, 1977
Amphiuma duodenum and jejunum (stripped)	White *et al.*, 1984
Bovine colon (stripped)	McKie *et al.*, 1991
Bullfrog (*Rana catesbieana*) small intestine (unstripped)	Quay and Armstrong, 1969
Bullfrog (*Rana catesbieana*) small intestine (stripped)	Armstrong *et al.*, 1979
Canine duodenum, jejunum, ileum, and colon (unstripped)	Jezyk *et al.*, 1992
Chicken (*Gallus domesticus*) duodenum, jejunum, ileum, colon (unstripped)	Grubb *et al.*, 1987
Flounder (*Pseudopleuronectes americanus*) intestine (stripped)	Field *et al.*, 1979
Frog colon (unstripped)	Cooperstein and Hogben, 1959
Guinea pig ileum (unstripped)	Cooke *et al.*, 1983
Guinea pig colon (stripped)	Clauss *et al.*, 1985
Human cecum/proximal colon (stripped)	Hubel *et al.*, 1987
Human transverse colon (stripped)	Sellin and DeSoignie, 1987
Human sigmoid colon (stripped)	Sandle, 1989
Human colon (unstripped)	Rask-Madsen and Hjelt, 1977
Human ileum (stripped)	Hubel and Shirazi, 1982
Human jejunum (stripped)	Smith and Field, 1980
Monkey duodenum, jejunum, ileum, and colon (unstripped)	Jezyk *et al.*, 1992
Ovine colon (stripped)	McKie *et al.*, 1991
Porcine jejunum (stripped)	Hildebrand and Brown, 1990
Porcine colon (stripped)	Traynor *et al.*, 1991
Rabbit duodenum, jejunum (stripped)	Guandalini *et al.*, 1980
Rabbit ileum (stripped)	Field *et al.*, 1971
Rabbit ileum (unstripped)	Schultz and Zalusky, 1964
Rabbit cecum (stripped)	Guandalini *et al.*, 1980
Rabbit proximal colon (stripped)	Sellin and DeSoignie, 1984
Rabbit distal colon (stripped)	Frizzell *et al.*, 1976
Rat jejunum (unstripped)	Munck and Rasmussen, 1977
Rat ileum (unstripped)	Curran, 1960
Rat colon (stripped and unstripped)	Binder and Rawlins, 1973
Turtle colon (stripped)	Sarracino and Dawson, 1979

2.1.2. EQUIPMENT

The basic components of the Ussing chamber setup include (1) thermostatically controlled reservoirs which maintain the temperature of the bathing solutions and which have ports for oxygenation and circulation of the buffer solutions (Precision Instrument Design, Tahoe City, CA; WPI, New Haven, CT; Costar, Cambridge, MA); (2) half-chambers for exposing the tissue to the bathing solutions (Precision Instrument Design, Tahoe City, CA; WPI, New Haven, CT; Costar, Cambridge, MA); and (3) voltage clamps (JWT, Kansas City, KS; Precision Instrument Design, Tahoe City,

Table II

Composition of Stock Solutions Employed for Preparing Intestinal
Bicarbonate Buffer Solution for *in vitro* Transport Studies[a]

Components of stock solutions	Molecular weight	Grams added to one liter
Stock A		
Sodium chloride (NaCl)	58.4	130.82
Potassium chloride (KCl)	74.6	7.46
Stock B		
Calcium chloride (CaCl$_2$ · 2H$_2$O)	147.02	3.52
Magnesium chloride (MgCl$_2$ · 6H$_2$O)	203.3	4.88
Stock C		
Sodium phosphate (NaH$_2$PO$_4$ · H$_2$O)	137.99	1.104
Sodium phosphate (Na$_2$HPO$_4$)	142.0	4.54
Stock D		
Sodium bicarbonate (NaHCO$_3$)	84.0	42.0

[a]For preparation of the working buffer, add approximately 750 ml of distilled water to a 1-l volumetric
flask. Add 50 ml of each of the stock solutions, and adjust the volume to 1 l with distilled water. If the
solution is cloudy, bubble 5% CO$_2$ in O$_2$ through the solution until it clears. The pH of the final buffer
will be ~7.4.

CA; WPI, New Haven, CT) for monitoring the spontaneous transepithelial potential
difference (PD) and short-circuit current (I_{sc}) or for clamping the PD or current to any
desired level for examining the effect of electrical driving force on the transport/
permeability of molecules (Tomita *et al.*, 1992). The gas for oxygenation is first
passed through water to reduce evaporation from the bicarbonate buffer bathing the
tissue. The gassing ports are arranged to provide a lift system for circulation of
bicarbonate buffer across the tissue surfaces. This circulation system provides a
mechanism for rapid mixing of materials added to the bathing solutions and also acts
to reduce the thickness of the unstirred water layer at the surface of the epithelial
preparation (Anderson *et al.*, 1988; Barry and Diamond, 1984; Hidalgo *et al.*, 1991).
The unstirred water layer can be significant, and transport across this layer may
become the rate-limiting step when the permeability of hydrophobic molecules is
being determined (Dietschy and Westergaard, 1975; Westergaard and Dietschy, 1974).
The composition of the buffer and the gas can be altered to accommodate the
experimental design (e.g., effects of pH or ion replacement studies) or alternate tissue
preparations (e.g., amphibian or avian intestine). Over the years, the design of the
Ussing setup has been modified to incorporate the water-jacketed reservoirs and tissue
chamber into one piece (Grass and Sweetana, 1988; Sutton *et al.*, 1992), to accommodate different tissue surface areas (White, 1982), and to allow for alternative experimental procedures such as determination of the cell membrane potential or intracellu-

lar ion activities or for uptake studies (Rose and Schultz, 1971; Nellans *et al.*, 1974; Frizzell *et al.*, 1979). However, the majority of transport/metabolism studies described in the literature have been conducted with a setup essentially identical to that described by Ussing and Zerahn (1951).

2.2. Tissue Preparation

Techniques for preparation of intestinal tissues for use in Ussing chambers vary with the animal and segment being studied. Table I lists references which describe the preparation and use of intestinal tissues from a variety of animals. Studies have been conducted with both "unstripped" and "stripped" tissues. Unstripped tissues are prepared by opening the intestine along the mesenteric border and placing pieces of the intact mucosa in the Ussing chamber (see Section 2.2.1). From unstripped tissues it is possible to evaluate the effects of mediators released from the enteric nervous system on intestinal ion transport (Hubel and Shirazi, 1982; Hubel *et al.*, 1987; Hubel, 1978; Cooke *et al.*, 1983). For stripped tissues, the intestine is prepared by opening along the mesenteric border, removing the circular and longitudinal muscle layers, and then placing these muscle-deficient tissues in the Ussing chamber (see Section 2.2.1). For studies designed to determine the mechanisms and rates of drug transport and metabolism, stripped tissues are preferable because they more closely resemble the *in vivo* situation (e.g., drug absorption into the intestinal vasculature does not involve permeation through the intestinal smooth muscle).

Rabbit intestinal tissues are viable for several hours as judged by their electrical properties and constant passive and active transport properties (Hidalgo *et al.*, 1993; Swaan *et al.*, 1994; Yeh *et al.*, 1994; Ryan *et al.*, 1988; Marks *et al.*, 1991), are easily stripped, and have been reported from a number of studies to have permeabilities which predict absorption in humans (Fig. 1; Lee *et al.*, 1993; Smith *et al.*, 1988; Swaan *et al.*, 1994).

2.2.1. SMALL INTESTINAL TISSUES

New Zealand white male rabbits, weighing between 2 and 3 kg and maintained on standard rabbit chow and water *ad libitum*, are killed by cervical dislocation. The duodenum (a 10-cm segment from 2 to 12 cm distal to the pylorus), jejunum (a 20-cm segment beginning 30 cm distal to the pylorus), and ileum (a 15-cm segment beginning 10 cm proximal to the *sacculus rotundus*) are quickly removed, cut along the mesenteric border, and rinsed clean with ice-cold bicarbonate buffer (Table II). The two major muscle layers are then removed by employing a modification of the technique described by Field and co-workers (Field *et al.*, 1971; Guandalini *et al.*, 1980). The segment of tissue for study is placed serosal surface facing up on a Plexiglas plate and kept moist with bicarbonate buffer. With a scalpel blade, a

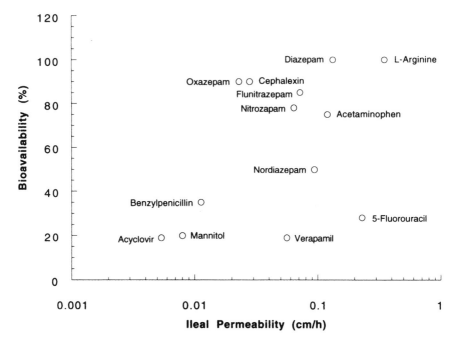

Figure 1. Bioavailability in humans vs. *in vitro* rabbit ileal permeability. Human bioavailabilities are taken from the literature. Permeability data are from studies conducted at SmithKline Beecham employing the techniques described in Section 2 (Swaan *et al.*, 1994; Smith *et al.*, 1988; Lee *et al.*, 1993; Hidalgo *et al.*, 1993).

transverse incision is made through the circular and longitudinal muscle layers, and then these muscle layers are removed with fine curved forceps. As shown previously, this stripped preparation consists of the epithelium, the underlying lamina propria, and the muscularis mucosae (Field *et al.*, 1971).

2.2.2. COLONIC TISSUES

Rabbit proximal and distal colonic segments are opened along the mesenteric border and rinsed of luminal contents with ice-cold bicarbonate buffer (Table II) as described above for small intestinal tissues. The proximal colon is stripped of the serosa and outer muscle layers as described previously (Sellin and DeSoignie, 1984). Briefly, the tissue is placed serosal surface up on a Plexiglas plate, which is kept moist with bicarbonate buffer. An incision is made through the muscle layers with a scalpel blade. The muscle layers are then removed with fine curved forceps. Distal colonic segments are stripped of the outer muscle layers as described previously (Frizzell *et al.*, 1976). The tissue is placed mucosal surface up on a Plexiglas plate, which is kept moist with bicarbonate buffer. The tissue is placed on pins at one end of the Plexiglas plate, stretched lengthwise, and held with a glass microscope slide. A second glass microscope slide is used to gently scrape the muscle layers from the mucosa.

2.3.   Transport Studies

2.3.1.   ELECTRICAL MEASUREMENTS

Tissues (or cells grown as confluent monolayers; see Chapters 3, 7, 11, 16, and 18) are placed between half-chambers and perfused separately on either side with 5–12 ml of bicarbonate buffer. Ideally, the chambers are equipped with ports located adjacent to the tissue which allow for measurement of the spontaneous transepithelial potential difference (PD). If the chamber is connected to calomel half-cells through salt/agar bridges, the agar bridges should be filled with the buffer that is being employed for transport studies to avoid generation of diffusion potentials. For agar bridges, polyethylene tubing is filled with a combination of agar (4.5 g) in buffer (90 ml) which has been brought to a slow boil with stirring. Upon cooling, the polyethylene tubing is cut to approximately 6-in. lengths. At the distal ends of the chamber, ports are provided for placement of current-passing bridges. These bridges are constructed as described for potential-sensing bridges and are connected to electrodes (e.g., Ag/AgCl or carbon bar) for passing current from the current/voltage clamp. Current is injected into the solution at the distal end of the chamber to allow for equal current spread at the tissue surface. With a current/voltage clamp, the PD can be clamped to zero (e.g., the short-circuit condition) or any desired value. The current required to nullify the PD is the short-circuit current (I_{sc}) and is equivalent to the sum of all active ion transport processes. Thus, the PD or I_{sc} is a measure of tissue viability since active ion transport requires energy production, generally in the form of ATP. Tissue viability in small and large intestinal tissues can be evaluated from the basal I_{sc} or from the change in I_{sc} resulting from addition of an absorptive or secretory stimulus [e.g., glucose or prostaglandin in small intestinal preparations (Swaan *et al.*, 1994) or amiloride or prostaglandins in distal colonic preparations (Frizzell and Turnheim, 1978; Frizzell and Heintze, 1979)]. From these values or from any measured change in PD resulting from passage of current (I), the transepithelial resistance (R_t) or transepithelial conductance (G_t) of the epithelial preparation can be determined employing Ohm's law (Eq. 1 or 2):

$$PD = I \cdot R_t \tag{1}$$

$$PD = I/G_t \tag{2}$$

The value of R_t, in ohms $\cdot$ cm^2, is obtained by dividing PD (in millivolts) by I (in microamps per square centimeter) and multiplying by 1000. For G_t in millimohs per square centimeter (or millisiemens per square centimeter), no correction is required. For comparison of data from different laboratories employing different chamber sizes, I, R, and G are normally corrected for surface area. Transepithelial conductance or resistance is a measure of tissue integrity. However, in "leaky" epithelia such as small intestine, significant increases in permeability can occur with no measurable changes in R_t. Thus, it is standard practice in many laboratories to include a permeability marker such as mannitol (or lucifer yellow) to evaluate tissue integrity (Marks et al., 1991; Swaan et al., 1994; Reardon et al., 1993; LeCluyse et al., 1993). Prior to initiating experiments with tissues, the offset potential is eliminated with the reservoirs containing only the buffer to be used in the experiment, and the fluid resistance between the bridge tips is determined so that a correction can be made when the tissue is in place during the experiment. Voltage clamps are set prior to placing tissues in the chambers to automatically correct for the offset potential and fluid resistance.

2.3.2. EXPERIMENTAL PROTOCOLS

After the tissue chambers are connected to the perfusion reservoirs, tissues are allowed to equilibrate for 30–60 min to allow reestablishment of ion-transport processes. During this equilibration period, PD (arbitrarily referenced to either the serosal or mucosal bathing solution) rapidly changes and in some cases reverses sign before stabilizing. With rabbit small and large intestinal tissues, the PD will usually be positive with respect to the mucosal bathing solution because these tissues are actively absorbing sodium. Throughout the equilibration and experimental periods, the tissues are bathed with bicarbonate buffer to which has been added 10 mM mannitol in the mucosal bathing solution and 8 mM glucose and 2 mM mannitol in the serosal bathing solution.

Transmural fluxes of molecules are determined on paired tissues taken from the same segment of intestine. Tissues can be paired on the basis of their electrical resistance and, as originally described by Field et al. (1971), should have electrical resistances which differ by less than 25%. In addition to electrical measurements or when electrical measurements are not being conducted, it is imperative to monitor the permeability of a small molecule such as mannitol. Mannitol permeability values can then be used as the selection criterion for acceptable tissues (Marks et al., 1991).

Following the equilibration period, the molecule to be studied is added to the mucosal (m) or serosal (s) bathing solution, and, at defined time intervals (normally >15 min), samples (0.5–1 ml) are removed from the bathing solution that did not initially receive the test molecule. Following removal of this sample, a volume of buffer identical to that removed (except for the transported molecule) is added back to the appropriate bathing solution to maintain a constant volume, ionic composition, and hydrostatic pressure. Additionally, a sample (0.05–0.1 ml) is removed from the bathing solution to which the test molecule was initially added. Samples are generally taken from the "donor" bathing solution at the beginning and end of the flux period to verify that the concentration in the donor solution does not change by more than 10% during the course of the experiment. This condition is required for the calculation of unidirectional fluxes (Schultz and Zalusky, 1964). These samples are not replaced.

When radiolabeled fluxes are being determined, unlabeled material is added to both bathing solutions. The presence of unlabeled material in both bathing solutions will not alter the permeability properties being determined because it is the radiolabel that will be monitored. The presence of unlabeled material avoids problems which may result from nonspecific binding of the radiolabel. When radiolabeled material is being studied, it is important to verify that the material being monitored is not being degraded or metabolized during the course of the transport experiments (Matuszewska *et al.*, 1988; Smith *et al.*, 1988).

2.3.3. CALCULATIONS

The apparent permeability coefficient (P_{app}, cm/hr) is calculated from the following equation (Grass and Sweetana, 1989):

$$P_{app} = (V_r \cdot dC_r)/(A \cdot C_o \cdot dt) \tag{3}$$

where V_r is the volume of the receiver chamber, A is the exposed tissue surface area, C_o is the concentration of the donor chamber, and dC_r/dt is the change in concentration of the receiver bathing solution with time.

Fluxes of solutes are often presented in units of mol/(hr $\cdot$ cm^2) or %/(hr $\cdot$ cm^2) and can be calculated according to previously described methods (Field *et al.*, 1971; Schultz and Zalusky, 1964).

2.4. Metabolism Studies

For studies to determine rates of intestinal metabolism, there are three compartments that can be monitored (i.e., the mucosal and serosal bathing solutions and the tissue). Metabolism studies are conducted as described for transport studies (see Section 2.3.2) with the exception that samples may be taken at different time intervals in order to monitor the time course of appearance of metabolites in the mucosal or serosal bathing solutions or in the tissue compartment. Prior to removal of tissues, the chambers are quickly drained of bathing solutions and rinsed with ice-cold buffer that does not contain the molecule of interest, and the tissues are then quickly excised from the chambers. Removal of tissues from the chambers can be accomplished by opening the half-chambers, quick-freezing the tissue, and cutting the exposed tissue surface with a scalpel blade. The tissues are then digested and analyzed with appropriate methods. The major advantage of evaluating intestinal metabolism employing the Ussing technique is that transport and metabolism can be monitored simultaneously

(Smith *et al.*, 1988; Back *et al.*, 1989; Matuszewska *et al.*, 1988; Rogers and Back, 1989). This approach can also be employed in the evaluation of prodrug approaches to enhance intestinal absorption. Ideally, the prodrug will increase apical membrane permeability; it will then undergo hydrolysis within the epithelial cells of the intestinal wall and subsequently be released into the portal circulation as the parent drug.

3. APPLICATIONS FOR ABSORPTION AND METABOLISM

3.1. Mechanistic/Segmental Transport Studies

Transport of solutes may occur by a variety of routes (Smith *et al.*, 1992), and the mechanisms involved in solute transport can vary depending on the location of the solute within the intestine (e.g., jejunum vs. ileum or small vs. large intestine).

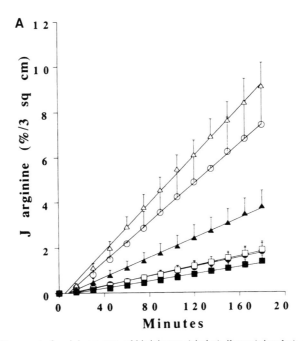

Figure 2. (A) Transport of arginine across rabbit jejunum (circles), ileum (triangles), and distal colon (squares) in the mucosal-to-serosal (open symbols) and the serosal-to-mucosal (filled symbols) direction. (B) Concentration dependence of arginine fluxes in the mucosal-to-serosal (squares) and the serosal-to mucosal (circles) direction across rabbit jejunum in the absence (open symbols) or presence (filled symbols) of serosal ouabain. (C) Concentration dependence of arginine fluxes in the mucosal-to-serosal (squares) and the serosal-to-mucosal (circles) direction across rabbit distal colon in the absence (open symbols) or presence (filled symbols) of serosal ouabain. Data are from Swaan *et al.* (1994), with permission.

However, for systemic delivery of organic molecules from the gastrointestinal tract, the pathways involved are passive paracellular or transcellular transport, which occurs in both the small and large intestine, and carrier-mediated energy-dependent or energy-independent transcellular transport, which occurs predominantly, if not exclusively, in the small intestine. With *in vitro* tissues, it is possible to determine which pathways are involved in the transport of a molecule and to establish structure–transport relationships. A comparison of arginine transport in the small versus the large intestine illustrates an active carrier-mediated process that exists only in the small intestine (Swaan *et al.*, 1994). As seen in Fig. 2A, transport of arginine in the

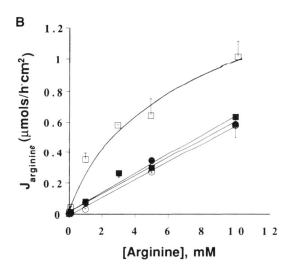

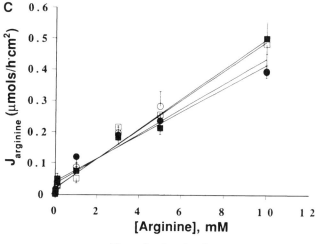

Figure 2. (*continued*)

mucosal (m)-to-serosal (s) direction is much greater than transport in the s-to-m direction. This is a characteristic of a carrier-mediated, actively transported molecule. Thus, the observation that the m-to-s flux is greater than the s-to-m flux suggests a carrier-mediated transport pathway for arginine in the small intestine. Further support for a carrier-mediated mechanism in the small intestine is provided by the finding that the m-to-s flux of arginine is a saturable function of concentration whereas the s-to-m flux is a linear function of concentration (Fig. 2B). The active nature of the m-to-s flux of arginine is demonstrated by the finding that arginine transport becomes a linear function of concentration when the tissues are pretreated with the Na^+/K^+-ATPase inhibitor ouabain (Fig. 2B). Taken together, these results indicate that arginine is transported in the m-to-s (absorptive) direction in the small intestine by an energy-dependent, carrier-mediated process. Results from ion replacement studies with amino acids have demonstrated that the uptake of amino acids across the apical membrane of intestinal cells is a Na^+-dependent process (Munck, 1980). From Fig. 2C, it can be seen that in the distal colon, transport of arginine is a linear function of concentration and is not altered by the presence of ouabain in the bathing solution. These data clearly demonstrate the regional differences in absorption of arginine. From these studies, it can be concluded that the most efficient absorption of arginine will occur in the small intestine. Similar types of studies have been conducted with peptidomimetics such as the β-lactam antibiotics, cephalosporins, and angiotensin converting enzyme inhibitors (Smith *et al.*, 1993). From studies with cephalexin, it has been demonstrated that, like arginine, cephalexin is transported by an active, carrier-mediated mechanism (Hidalgo *et al.*, 1993). Like arginine transport, the transport mechanism for cephalexin exists in the small but not the large intestine (Fig. 3) although, as shown in Fig. 3, the uptake mechanism for cephalexin is a proton-dependent process and not a sodium-dependent process as is the case for arginine.

Examples of passively transported transcellular and paracellular molecules are presented in Figs. 4 and 5, respectively. Acetaminophen and mannitol transport across tissues from small and large intestine are similar in both the m-to-s and s-to-m directions (Figs. 4 and 5). However, comparison of the transport rates for these two molecules reveals that the fluxes of acetaminophen are much greater than those of mannitol. These results are consistent with a much greater surface area for transport of acetaminophen via the transcellular route and a limited number of permeability pathways for mannitol via the paracellular route.

3.2. Evaluation of Formulation Approaches

One strategy proposed to overcome the limited oral bioavailability of potential therapeutic agents has been to increase the permeability of the gastrointestinal mucosa through the use of enhancers (Muranishi, 1990; Swenson and Curatolo, 1992). Effects of enhancers on morphology, nutrient and ion transport, and solute per-

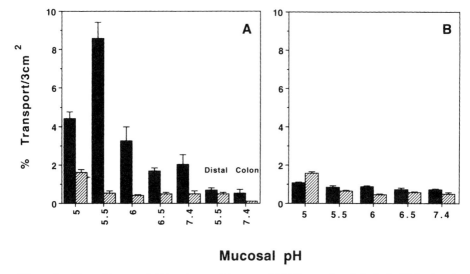

Mucosal pH

Figure 3. Mucosal-to-serosal (A) and serosal-to-mucosal (B) fluxes of cephalexin (solid bars) and mannitol (hatched bars) across rabbit ileum and distal colon with varying mucosal bathing solution pH. Serosal pH remains constant at 7.4. Data are from Hidalgo *et al.* (1993), with permission.

meability of the intestinal mucosa have been evaluated by a number of laboratories employing the Ussing chamber technique (LeCluyse *et al.*, 1993; Yeh *et al.*, 1994; Moore *et al.*, 1989; Tomita *et al.*, 1992; Yamashita *et al.*, 1985). From these studies, it has been demonstrated that enhancer molecules transiently denude the villus regions of the intestinal mucosa, thereby increasing intestinal permeability and reducing

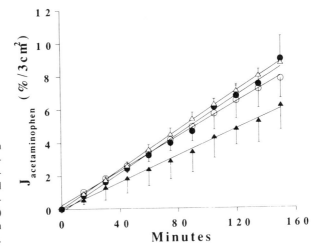

Figure 4. Acetaminophen fluxes across rabbit ileum (triangles) and distal colon (circles) in the mucosal-to-serosal (open symbols) and the serosal-to-mucosal (filled symbols) direction. Data are from Swaan *et al.* (1994), with permission.

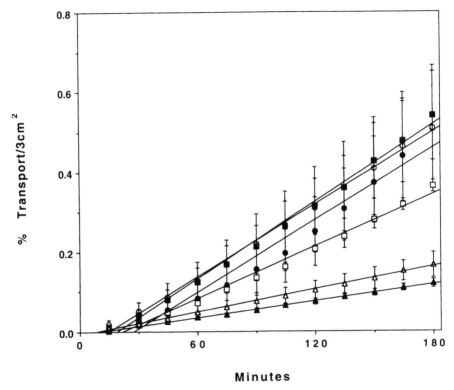

Minutes

Figure 5. Mannitol fluxes across rabbit jejunum (squares), ileum (circles), and distal colon (triangles) in the mucosal-to-serosal (open symbols) and the serosal-to-mucosal (filled symbols) direction. Data are from Hidalgo *et al.* (1993), with permission.

normal absorptive processes of the villus cells of the small intestine or surface cells of the colon (Moore *et al.*, 1989; LeCluyse *et al.*, 1993; Yeh *et al.*, 1994). Following removal of the enhancer, the intestinal mucosa has the capacity to rapidly reverse the epithelial damage and regain its original barrier function (Moore *et al.*, 1989; Yeh *et al.*, 1994). An example of changes in R_t produced by CapMul MCM and the reversibility of these effects is presented in Fig. 6. From Fig. 6 it can be seen that Cap-Mul MCM produces concentration-dependent changes in R_t of rabbit distal colon, which, at low concentrations, can be reversed following removal of CapMul MCM. In addition to identifying the effects of enhancers on gastrointestinal morphology and physiology, the *in vitro* Ussing chamber technique has also been shown to have the potential to predict which molecules will have enhanced bioavailability *in vivo* (Ryan *et al.*, 1993).

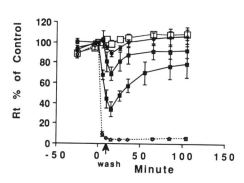

Figure 6. Changes in transepithelial resistance (R_t) in rabbit distal colon in the absence (□) or presence of mucosal addition of CapMul MCM [0.05% (◆); 0.1% (▣); 0.3% (■); 1% (◇)] and the time course of reversibility of these changes. Data are from Yeh *et al.* (1994), with permission.

3.3. Metabolism Studies

In addition to its utility for evaluating intestinal transport mechanisms, the Ussing technique or modifications of this technique have also been employed to study intestinal metabolism (Rogers and Back, 1989; Back *et al.*, 1989; Sund and Lauterbach, 1986, 1987; Smith *et al.*, 1988; Matuszewska *et al.*, 1988; Back *et al.*, 1981; Ryan *et al.*, 1988). In the study of Rogers and Back (1989), human intestinal tissues were employed to determine whether intestinal metabolism of paracetamol could be detected. Results from these studies demonstrated formation of the glucuronide and sulfate conjugates of paracetamol in both the small and large intestine although metabolism was greater in the small intestine (Rogers and Back, 1989). From these results, it is apparent that the Ussing technique has the potential to provide information regarding the metabolism of molecules during transport across the gastrointestinal mucosa. Thus, as our understanding of the role of intestinal metabolism in limiting bioavailability advances, this technique may find increasing use.

An approach to enhancing intestinal permeability has been the synthesis of prodrugs or conjugates in an attempt to increase intestinal permeability either through an increase in hydrophobicity, an increase in stability, or targeting to a specific membrane transporter (Moss *et al.*, 1990; Swaan *et al.*, 1993; Lundin *et al.*, 1991). The effectiveness of these approaches has been monitored with *in vitro* transport studies employing either tissues or cells (Moss *et al.*, 1990; Swaan *et al.*, 1993; Lundin *et al.*, 1991; Kahns *et al.*, 1993). One potential problem with this approach is that there are not sufficient data with animal tissues or cultured cells to ensure that metabolism by these systems will be qualitatively or quantitatively similar to that seen in humans. Although human tissue has been used in the Ussing system, safety concerns have limited the amount of data that has been generated.

3.4. Discovery Screening

We have employed the Ussing technique to screen molecules from the medicinal chemists in early stages of discovery to determine (1) structures having a permeability which is appropriate for evaluation in animals and (2) features in a molecule which are responsible for low (or high) intestinal permeability (Samanen *et al.*, 1996). This *in vitro* permeability screen provides a rapid feedback to the medicinal chemists, thereby allowing them to monitor both activity (through binding assays or pharmacodynamic studies) and the potential for oral bioavailability. In addition, we have also been able to evaluate molecules with low oral bioavailability to determine whether intestinal permeability and/or metabolism is the rate-determining step. This approach has allowed us to determine changes in intestinal permeability produced by prodrug approaches, to identify molecules that are recycled at the apical cell membrane, and to evaluate strategies to avoid this recycling mechanism.

3.5. Evaluation of Drug-Related Pathophysiology

In addition to the applications described above, the Ussing technique has also been important for the identification of mechanisms involved in drug-related patho-physiology. An example of this is provided by the studies done to investigate the mechanisms involved in auranofin-associated gastrointestinal intolerance (e.g., diar-rhea). Hardcastle *et al.* (1989) conducted a series of studies to examine the effects of auranofin on the electrical properties and sodium and chloride fluxes across stripped rat small intestine. From these studies, it was demonstrated that addition of auranofin to either the mucosal or serosal bathing solution stimulated a change in the short-circuit current which was consistent with stimulation of electrogenic chloride secre-tion (Hardcastle *et al.*, 1989). Support for the hypothesis that auranofin stimulated electrogenic chloride secretion was provided by the findings that removal of chloride from bathing solution or preincubation of the tissues with the cotransport inhibitor furosemide reduced the auranofin-induced increase in short-circuit current and that direct measurement of chloride fluxes demonstrated an increase in the s-to-m flux of chloride following addition of auranofin to the serosal bathing solution (Hardcastle *et al.*, 1989). Furthermore, it was demonstrated that the effects of auranofin on the small intestine were calcium dependent and appeared to be elicited by the gold in the auranofin molecule since the electrical effects of auranofin could be reproduced by chlorauric acid (Hardcastle *et al.*, 1989). From these results, it was concluded that the intestinal secretion elicited by auranofin could be partly responsible for the diarrhea associated with auranofin administration.

Madara and co-workers have employed the Ussing technique with both tissues and cells to investigate regulation of the barrier function of the intestine, with particular emphasis on the permeability of the tight junctional complexes (Madara,

1990; Parkos *et al.*, 1994; Moore *et al.*, 1992; Madara and Carlson, 1991). From these studies, they have suggested that tight junctional permeability may be regulated by cellular events such as nutrient-stimulated sodium absorption and have presented data to suggest that an increase in oligopeptide permeability can be induced by coadministration with glucose (Atisook and Madara, 1991). Further studies are required to determine the significance of these *in vitro* observations. Perhaps these observations provide an explanation for the enhanced absorption seen with some molecules when they are dosed with a meal.

From the above discussion, it is obvious that the Ussing technique is a versatile tool for studying intestinal permeability.

4.   ADVANTAGES AND DISADVANTAGES OF TISSUE TECHNIQUES

The utility of a technique for evaluating intestinal absorption/transport is related to its ease of use, the range of information that can be generated (e.g., transport and metabolism), and, of greatest significance, the reliability of the results generated to predict bioavailability in humans.

Identification of a drug candidate with high oral bioavailability in humans results from synthesis of a chemically, metabolically, and enzymatically stable molecule that can traverse the intestinal epithelial cell barrier to enter the portal circulation, pass through the liver, and enter the systemic circulation. Thus, lack of oral bioavailability may result from instability of the molecule, low epithelial permeability, or hepatic first-pass effects. The *in vitro* Ussing technique does not provide information on the potential for hepatic first-pass effects or instability in any compartment other than the intestinal epithelial cells. However, the *in vitro* Ussing technique does provide a method for comparing intestinal epithelial permeability of molecules as well as monitoring intestinal viability and integrity. Molecules with sufficient membrane permeability may not have adequate oral bioavailability owing to any of the other complicating factors listed above. However, molecules that do *not* have adequate intestinal permeability will *not* be orally bioavailable. Thus, evaluation of intestinal permeability by this rapid screening procedure provides a method for selecting molecules to evaluate in animals and thus will dramatically reduce the time and resources required to identify an oral development candidate. Advantages of this technique include the ability to (1) monitor viability and integrity; (2) determine mechanisms involved in transepithelial transport; (3) compare segmental differences in transport; (4) evaluate sites and types of metabolism and/or degradation; (5) identify interaction of molecules with apical recycling mechanisms; (6) determine effects of potential enhancers on the barrier properties and viability of the epithelium; and (7) identify structural features of molecules that allow them to interact with a transporter or are responsible for reducing their intestinal permeability.

The major disadvantage of the Ussing technique in particular and the use of *in vitro* techniques in general for predicting human bioavailability is the limited database that is currently available. With the molecules that have been evaluated and reported, there is in general a good agreement between the *in vitro* permeability of molecules and their bioavailability in humans. Exceptions to the predictive value of the technique appear to be related predominantly to first-pass clearance mechanisms. As the potential utility of this technique has become more widely known, its use has increased. We should therefore anticipate that more data will be appearing in the literature to allow a better understanding of the predictability of the system with various classes of molecules.

ACKNOWLEDGMENTS

I would like to thank my family for their support during the preparation of this chapter and acknowledge the constructive suggestions regarding the content of this manuscript provided by Harma Ellens and Chao-Pin Lee.

REFERENCES

Anderson, B. W., Levine, A. S., Levitt, D. G., Kneip, J. M., and Levitt, M. D., 1988, Physiological measurement of luminal stirring in perfused rat jejunum, *Am. J. Physiol.* **254:**G843–G848.

Armstrong, W. McD., Bixenman, W. R., Frey, K. F., Garcia-Diaz, J. F., O'Regan, M. G., and Owens, J. L., 1979, Energetics of coupled Na^+ and Cl^- entry into epithelial cells of bullfrog small intestine, *Biochim. Biophys. Acta* **551:**207–219.

Atisook, K., and Madara, J. L., 1991, An oligopeptide permeates intestinal tight junctions at glucose-elicited dilatations, *Gastroenterology* **100:**719–724.

Back, D. J., Bates, M., Breckenridge, A. M., Ellis, A., Hall, J. M., MacIver, M., Orme, M. L'.E., and Rowe, P. H., 1981, The *in vitro* metabolism of ethinyloestradiol, mestranol and levonorgestrel by human jejunal mucosa, *Br. J. Clin. Pharmacol.* **11:**275–278.

Back, D. J., Orme, M. L.'E., and Rogers, S. M., 1989, Intestinal metabolism of contraceptive steroids in man, in: *Progress in Pharmacology and Clinical Pharmacology: Intestinal Metabolism of Xenobiotics,* Vol. 7 (A. S. Koster, E. Richter, F. Lauterbach, and F. Hartmann, eds.), Gustav Fischer Verlag, New York, pp. 289–297.

Barry, P. H., and Diamond, J. M., 1984, Effects of unstirred layers on membrane phenomena, *Physiol. Rev.* **64:**763–872.

Binder, H. J., and Rawlins, C. L., 1973, Electrolyte transport across isolated large intestinal mucosa, *Am. J. Physiol.* **255:**1232–1239.

Bondinell, W. E., Keenan, R. M., Miller, W. H., Ali, F. E., Allen, A. C., DeBrosse, C. W., Eggleston, D. S., Erhard, K. F., Haltiwanger, R. C., Huffman, W. F., Hwang, S.-M., Jakas, D. R., Koster, P. F., Ku, T. W., Lee, C. P., Nichols, A. J., Ross, S. T., Samanen, J. M., Valocik, R. E., Vasko-Moser, J. A., Venslaky, J. W., Wong, A. S., and Yuan, C.-K., 1994, Design of a potent and orally active nonpeptide platelet fibrinogen receptor (GPIIB/IIIA) antagonist, *Bioorg. Med. Chem.* **2:**897–908.

Clauss, W., Durr, J., and Rechkemmer, G., 1985, Characterization of conductive pathways in guinea pig distal colon *in vitro, Am. J. Physiol.* **248:**G176–G183.

Cooke, H. J., Shonnard, K., and Wood, J. D., 1983, Effects of neuronal stimulation on mucosal transport in guinea pig ileum, *Am. J. Physiol.* **245:**G290–G296.

Cooperstein, I. L., and Hogben, C. A. M., 1959, Ionic transfer across the isolated frog large intestine, *J. Gen. Physiol.* **42**:461–473.

Curran, P. F., 1960, Na, Cl and water transport by rat ileum *in vitro*, *J. Gen. Physiol.* **43**:1137–1148.

Dietschy, J. M., and Westergaard, H., 1975, The effect of unstirred water layers on various transport processes in the intestine, in: *Intestinal Absorption and Malabsorption* (T. Z. Csaky, ed.), Raven Press, New York, pp. 197–206.

Field, M., Fromm, D., and McColl, I., 1971, Ion transport in rabbit ileal mucosa. I. Na and Cl fluxes and short-circuit current, *Am. J. Physiol.* **220**:1388–1396.

Field, M., Karnaky, K. J., Smith, P. L., Bolton, J. E., and Kinter, W. B., 1979, Ion transport across the isolated intestinal mucosa of the winter flounder, *Pseudopleuronectes americanus*, *J. Membr. Biol.* **46**:265–293.

Frizzell, R. A., and Heintze, K., 1979, Electrogenic chloride secretion by mammalian colon, in: *Mechanisms of Intestinal Secretion* (H. J. Binder, ed.), Alan R. Liss, New York, pp. 101–116.

Frizzell, R. A., and Turneim, K., 1978, Ion transport by rabbit colon: II. Unidirectional sodium influx and the effects of amphotericin B and amiloride, *J. Membr. Biol.* **40**:193–211.

Frizzell, R. A., Koch, M. J., and Schultz, S. G., 1976, Ion transport by rabbit colon. I. Active and passive components, *J. Membr. Biol.* **27**:297–316.

Frizzell, R. A., Smith, P. L., Vosburgh, E., and Field, M., 1979, Coupled sodium-chloride influx across brush border of flounder intestine, *J. Membr. Biol.* **46**:27–39.

Grass, G. M., and Sweetana, S. A., 1988, *In vitro* measurement of gastrointestinal tissue permeability using a new diffusion cell, *Pharm. Res.* **5**:372–376.

Grass, G. M., and Sweetana, S. A., 1989, A correlation of permeabilities for passively transported compounds in monkey and rabbit jejunum, *Pharm. Res.* **6**:857–862.

Grubb, B. R., Driscoll, S. M., and Bentley, P. J., 1987, Electrical PD, short-circuit current and fluxes of Na and Cl across avian intestine, *J. Comp. Physiol. B* **157**:181–186.

Guandalini, S., Kachur, J. F., Smith, P. L., Miller, R. J., and Field, M., 1980, *In vitro* effects of somatostatin on ion transport in rabbit intestine, *Am. J. Physiol.* **238**:G67–G74.

Hardcastle, J., Hardcastle, P. T., and Kelleher, D. K., 1989, Effect of auranofin on ion transport by rat small intestine, *J. Pham. Pharmacol.* **41**:817–823.

Hegel, U., Fromm, M., Kreusel, K.-M., and Wiederholt, M., 1993, Bovine and porcine large intestine as model epithelia in a student lab course, *Adv. Phys. Ed.* **10**:S10–S19.

Hidalgo, I. J., Hillgren, K. M., Grass, G. M., and Borchardt, R. T., 1991, Characterization of the unstirred water layer in Caco-2 cell monolayers using a novel diffusion apparatus, *Pharm. Res.* **8**:222–227.

Hidalgo, I. J., Ryan, F. M., Marks, G. J., and Smith, P. L., 1993, pH-dependent transcellular transport of cephalexin in rabbit intestinal mucosa, *Int. J. Pharm.* **98**:83–92.

Hildebrand, K. R., and Brown, D. R., 1990, Intrinsic neuroregulation of ion transport in porcine distal jejunum, *J. Pharmacol. Exp. Ther.* **255**:285–292.

Hubel, K. A., 1978, The effects of electrical field stimulation and tetrodotoxin on ion transport by the isolated rabbit ileum, *J. Clin. Invest.* **62**:1039–1047.

Hubel, K. A., and Shirazi, S., 1982, Human ileal ion transport *in vitro*: Changes with electrical field stimulation and tetrodotoxin, *Gastroenterology* **83**:63–68.

Hubel, K. A., Renquist, K., and Shirazi, S., 1987, Ion transport in human cecum, transverse colon, and sigmoid colon *in vitro*: Baseline and response to electrical stimulation on intrinsic nerves, *Gastroenterology* **92**:501–507.

Jezyk, N., Rubas, W., and Grass, G. M., 1992, Permeability characteristics of various intestinal regions of rabbit, dog, and monkey, *Pharm. Res.* **9**:1580–1586.

Kahns, A. H., Buur, A., and Bundgaard, H., 1993, Prodrugs of peptides. 18. Synthesis and evaluation of various esters of desmopressin (dDAVP), *Pharm. Res.* **10**:68–74.

Koefoed-Johnson, V., and Ussing, H. H., 1953, The contributions of the passage of D2O through living membranes: Effect of neurohypophyseal hormone on isolated anuran skin, *Acta Physiol. Scand.* **28**:60–76.

Koefoed-Johnson, V., Levi, H., and Ussing, H. H., 1952, The modes of passage of chloride ions through the isolated frog skin, *Acta Physiol. Scand.* **25**:150–263.

Koefoed-Johnson, V., Ussing, H. H., and Zerahn, K., 1953, The origin of the short-circuit current in the adrenaline stimulated frog skin, *Acta Physiol. Scand.* **27**:38–48.

LeCluyse, E., Sutton, S. C., and Fix, J. A., 1993, *In vitro* effects of long-chain acylcarnitines on the permeability, transepithelial electrical resistance and morphology of rat colonic mucosa, *J. Pharmacol. Exp. Ther.* **265**:955–962.

Lee, C.-P., Chiossone, D. D., Hidalgo, I. J., and Smith, P. L., 1993, Comparison of *in vitro* permeabilities of a series of benzodiazepines and correlation with *in vivo* absorption, *Pharm. Res.* **10**:S-177.

Lundin, S., Pantzar, N., Broeders, A., Ohlin, M., and Westrom, B. R., 1991, Differences in transport rate of oxytocin and vasopressin analogues across proximal and distal isolated segments of the small intestine of the rat, *Pharm. Res.* **8**:1274–1280.

Madara, J. L., 1990, Pathobiology of the intestinal epithelial barrier, *Am. J. Pathol.* **137**:1273–1281.

Madara, J. L., and Carlson, S., 1991, Supraphysiologic L-tryptophan elicits cytoskeletal and macromolecular permeability alterations in hamster small intestinal epithelium *in vitro*, *J. Clin. Invest.* **87**:454–462.

Marks, G. J., Ryan, F. M., Hidalgo, I. J., and Smith, P. L., 1991, Mannitol as a marker for intestinal integrity in *in vitro* absorption studies, *Gastroenterology* **100**:A697.

Matuszewska, B., Liversidge, G. G., Ryan, F., Dent, J., and Smith, P. L., 1988, *In vitro* study of intestinal absorption and metabolism of 8-L-arginine vasopressin and its analogues, *Int. J. Pharm.* **46**:111–120.

McKie, A. T., Goecke, I. A., and Naftalin, R. J., 1991, Comparison of fluid absorption by bovine and ovine descending colon *in vitro*, *Am. J. Physiol.* **261**:G433–G442.

Moore, R., Carlson, S., and Madara, J. L., 1989, Rapid barrier restitution in an *in vitro* model of intestinal epithelial injury, *Lab. Invest.* **60**:237–244.

Moore, R., Madri, J., Carlson, S., and Madara, J. L., 1992, Collagens are required for epithelial migration in restitution of native guinea pig intestinal epithelium, *Gastroenterology* **101**:119–130.

Moss, J., Burr, A., and Bundgaard, H., 1990, Prodrugs of peptides. 8. *In vitro* study of intestinal metabolism and penetration of thyrotropin-releasing hormone (TRH) and its prodrugs, *Int. J. Pharm.* **66**:183–191.

Munck, B. G., 1980, Transport of sugars and amino acids across guinea pig small intestine, *Biochim. Biophys. Acta* **597**:411–417.

Munck, B. G., and Rasmussen, S. N., 1977, Paracellular permeability of extracellular space markers across rat jejunum *in vitro*. Indication of a transepithelial fluid circuit, *J. Physiol.* **271**:473–488.

Muranishi, S., 1990, Absorption enhancers, *Crit. Rev. Ther. Drug Carrier Syst.* **7**:1–33.

Nellans, H. N., Frizzell, R. A., and Schultz, S. G., 1974, Brush-border processes and transepithelial Na and Cl transport by rabbit ileum, *Am. J. Physiol.* **226**:1131–1141.

Parkos, C. A., Colgan, S. P., and Madara, J. L., 1994, Interactions of neutrophils with epithelial cells: Lessons from the intestine, *J. Am. Soc. Nephrol.* **5**:138–152.

Quay, J. F., and Armstrong, W. McD., 1969, Sodium and chloride transport by isolated bullfrog small intestine, *Am. J. Physiol.* **217**:694–702.

Rask-Madsen, J., and Hjelt, K., 1977, Effect of amiloride on electrical activity and electrolyte transport in human colon, *Scand. J. Gastroenterol.* **12**:1–6.

Reardon, P. M., Gochoco, C. H., Audus, K. L., and Smith, P. L., 1993, *In vitro* transport across ovine mucosa: Effects of ammonium glycyrrhizinate on electrical properties and permeability of growth hormone releasing peptide, mannitol and lucifer yellow, *Pharm. Res.* **10**:553–561.

Roden, M., Paterson, A. R. P., and Turnheim, K., 1991, Sodium-dependent nucleoside transport in rabbit intestinal epithelium, *Gastroenterology* **100**:1553–1562.

Rogers, S. M., and Back, D. J., 1989, The use of Ussing chambers for the study of intestinal metabolism *in vitro*, in: *Progress in Pharmacology and Clinical Pharmacology: Intestinal Metabolism of Xenobiotics*, Vol. 7 (A. S. Koster, E. Richter, F. Lauterbach, and F. Hartmann, eds.), Gustav Fischer Verlag, New York, pp. 43–53.

Rose, R. C., and Schultz, S. G., 1971, Studies on the electrical potential profile across rabbit ileum: Effects of sugars and amino acids on transmural and transmucosal electrical potential differences, *J. Gen. Physiol.* **57**:639–663.

Ryan, F. M., Newton, J. F., Eckardt, R. D., and Smith, P. L., 1988, Transport and metabolism of SK&F 104353 in rabbit intestine *in vitro*: Preferential absorption by ileum, *Pharm. Res.* **5**:S-104.

Ryan, F. M., Welzel, G., Smith, P. L., Yeulet, S. E., Citerone, D. R., and Ellens, H. E., 1993, Correlation between *in vivo* bioavailability enhancement and *in vitro* transport enhancement by medium chain glycerides, *Pharm. Res.* **10**:S-182.

Samanen, J., Wilson, G., Smith, P. L., Lee, C.-P., Bondinell, W., Rhodes, G., Peishoff, C., Bean, J., and Nichols, A., 1996, Chemical approaches to improve the oral bioavailability of peptidergic molecules, *Pharm. Sci. Commun.*, *J. Pharm Pharmacol.* **48**:115.

Sandle, G. I., 1989, Segmental heterogeneity of basal and aldosterone-induced electrogenic Na transport in human colon, *Pflügers Arch.* **414**:706–712.

Sarracino, S. M., and Dawson, D. C., 1979, Cation selectivity in active transport: Properties of the turtle colon in the presence of mucosal lithium, *J. Membr. Biol.* **46**:295–313.

Schultz, S. G., and Zalusky, R., 1964, Ion transport in isolated rabbit ileum. I. Short-circuit current and Na fluxes, *J. Gen. Physiol.* **47**:567–584.

Sellin, J. H., and DeSoignie, R., 1984, Rabbit proximal colon: A distinct transport epithelium, *Am. J. Physiol.* **246**:G603–G610.

Sellin, J. H., and DeSoignie, R., 1987, Ion transport in human colon *in vitro*, *Gastroenterology* **93**:441–448.

Smith, P., Mirabelli, C., Fondacaro, J., Ryan, F., and Dent, J., 1988, Intestinal 5-fluorouracil absorption: Use of Ussing chambers to assess transport and metabolism, *Pharm. Res.* **5**:598–603.

Smith, P. L., and Field, M., 1980, *In vitro* antisecretory effects of trifluoperazine and other neuroleptics in rabbit and human small intestine, *Gastroenterology* **78**:1545–1553.

Smith, P. L., Welsh, M. J., Stoff, J. S., and Frizzell, R. A., 1982, Chloride secretion by canine tracheal epithelium: I. Role of intracellular cAMP levels, *J. Membr. Biol.* **70**:217–226.

Smith, P. L., Wall, D. A., Gochoco, C. H., and Wilson, G., 1992, Routes of delivery: Case studies (5) Oral absorption of peptides and proteins, *Adv. Drug Deliv. Rev.* **8**:253–290.

Smith, P. L., Eddy, E. P., Lee, C.-P., and Wilson, G., 1993, Exploitation of the intestinal oligopeptide transporter to enhance drug absorption, *Drug Deliv.* **1**:103–111.

Sund, R. B., and Lauterbach, F., 1986, Drug metabolism and metabolite transport in the small and large intestine: Experiments with l-naphthol and phenolphthalein by luminal and contraluminal administration in the isolated guinea pig mucosa, *Acta Pharmacol. Toxicol.* **58**:74–83.

Sund, R. B., and Lauterbach, F., 1987, 1-Naphthol metabolism and metabolite transport in the small and large intestine. II. Effects of sulphate and phosphate ion omission, and of 2,6-dichloro-4-nitrophenol in the isolated guinea pig mucosa, *Pharmacol. Toxicol.* **60**:262–268.

Sutton, S. C., Forbes, A. E., Cargill, R., Hochman, J. H., and LeCluyse, E. L., 1992, Simultaneous *in vitro* measurement of intestinal tissue permeability and transepithelial electrical resistance (TEER) using Sweetana-Grass diffusion cells, *Pharm. Res.* **9**:316–319.

Swaan, P. W., Stehouwer, M. C., Blok, R. I. C., and Tukker, J. J., 1993, Prodrug approach using the intestinal peptide carrier, *Pharm. Res.* **10**:S-295.

Swaan, P. W., Marks, G. J., Ryan, F. M., and Smith, P. L., 1994, Determination of transport rates for arginine and acetaminophen in rabbit intestinal tissues *in vitro*, *Pharm. Res.* **11**:283–287.

Swenson, E. S., and Curatolo, W. J. 1992, Means to enhance penetration. (2) Intestinal permeability enhancement for proteins, peptides and other polar drugs: Mechanisms and potential toxicity, *Adv. Drug Deliv. Rev.* **8**:39–92.

Tomita, M., Sawada, T., Ogawa, T., Ouchi, H., Hayashi, M., and Awazu, S., 1992, Differences in the enhancing effects of sodium caprate on colonic and jejunal drug absorption, *Pharm. Res.* **9**:648–653.

Traynor, T. R., Brown, D. R., and O'Grady, S. M., 1991, Regulation of ion transport in porcine distal colon: Effects of putative neurotransmitters, *Gastroenterology* **100**:703–710.

Ussing, H. H., 1949, Transport of ions across cellular membranes, *Physiol. Rev.* **29**:127–155.

Ussing, H. H., 1950, The distinction by means of tracers between active transport and diffusion: The transfer of iodide across the isolated frog skin, *Acta Physiol. Scand.* **19:**43–56.

Ussing, H. H., and Zerahn, K., 1951, Active transport of sodium as the source of electric current in the short-circuited isolated frog skin, *Acta Physiol. Scand.* **23:**110–127.

Westergaard, H., and Dietschy, J. M., 1974, Delineation of the dimensions and permeability characteristics of the two major diffusion barriers to passive mucosal uptake in the rabbit intestine, *J. Clin. Invest.* **54:**718–732.

White, J. F., 1977, Alterations in electrophysiology of isolated amphibian small intestine produced by removing the muscle layers, *Biochim. Biophys. Acta* **467:**91–102.

White, J. F., 1982, Intestinal electrogenic HCO_3^- absorption localized to villus epithelium, *Biochim. Biophys. Acta* **687:**343–345.

White, J. F., Ellingsen, D., and Burnup, K., 1984, Electrogenic Cl^- absorption by *Amphiuma* small intestine: Dependence on serosal Na^+ from tracer and Cl^- microelectrode studies, *J. Membr. Biol.* **78:**223–233.

Yamashita, S., Saitoh, H., Nakanishi, K., Masada, M., Nadai, T., and Kimura, T., 1985, Characterization of enhanced intestinal permeability: Electrophysiological study on the effects of diclofenac and ethylenediaminetetraacetic acid, *J. Pharm. Pharmacol.* **37:**512–513.

Yeh, P.-Y., Smith, P. L., and Ellens, H., 1994, Effect of medium-chain glycerides on physiological properties of rabbit intestinal epithelium *in vitro*, *Pharm. Res.* **11:**1148–1153.

Chapter 3

Cultured Intestinal Epithelial Cell Models

Ismael J. Hidalgo

1. INTRODUCTION

In vitro systems such as brush border membrane vesicles (BBMV), basolateral membrane vesicles (BLMV), perfused intestinal loops, stripped intestinal mucosa, and isolated enterocytes have been used to study mucosal drug absorption. Isolated enterocytes should permit the determination of transmembrane transport in the presence of cellular metabolism. However, upon isolation enterocytes lose their polarity and show limited viability (Hartmann *et al.*, 1982). Attempts to develop an *in vitro* system derived from cultured intestinal epithelial cells have found this goal to be extremely difficult. Although intestinal enterocytes have been cultured in suspension, they undergo dedifferentiation when cultured as monolayers (Raul *et al.*, 1978).

The human colon adenocarcinoma cell lines Caco-2, HT-29, and T84 have been widely used to study various intestinal transport processes (Madara *et al.*, 1988; Audus *et al.*, 1990). Because of their high transepithelial electrical resistances (350–1600 $\Omega \cdot cm^2$), T84 cells have been mainly used for studying tight-junction regulation (Madara *et al.*, 1988). HT-29 and Caco-2 cells have had greater application in the study of drug transport and metabolism. Caco-2 cell monolayers do not produce a mucus layer. Thus, the role of the mucus layer in drug absorption has been examined using mucus-secreting HT-29 clones (Lesuffleur *et al.*, 1993). Despite their lack of mucus production, Caco-2 cells are commonly used in drug transport and metabolism studies. These cells undergo spontaneous enterocytic differentiation in culture (Pinto *et al.*, 1983) and have been evaluated as a transport model system of the small intestinal epithelium (Hidalgo *et al.*, 1989; Dix *et al.*, 1990). To validate Caco-2 cell

Ismael J. Hidalgo • Drug Metabolism and Pharmacokinetics (NW12), Rhone-Poulenc Rorer, College-ville, Pennsylvania 19427-0107.

Models for Assessing Drug Absorption and Metabolism, Ronald T. Borchardt *et al.*, eds., Plenum Press, New York, 1996.

monolayers as a transport model system of the small intestinal epithelium, a comparison was made with enterocytes in terms of morphological features, functional expression of marker enzymes (e.g., alkaline phosphatase, sucrase-isomaltase), and permeability properties (Pinto *et al.*, 1983; Hidalgo *et al.*, 1989). This chapter will describe the methodology used in the characterization of Caco-2 cells as a transport model system of the intestinal epithelium. Techniques used to study cellular uptake, transepithelial transport, and drug metabolism, data calculation, and some applications of the model will be described.

2. METHODS

2.1. Materials

Caco-2, HT-29, and T84 cells are derived from human colon adenocarcinoma. They are available from American Type Culture Collection (ATCC, Rockville, MD). Dulbecco's modified Eagle's medium (DMEM), nonessential amino acids (NEAA) solution (100×), L-glutamine (200 mM), trypsin (0.25%)-EDTA (1 mM), and penicillin (10,000 U/ml)-streptomycin (10,000 μg/ml) solution were purchased from Gibco Laboratories (Grand Island, NY). Fetal bovine serum (FBS) was from Hazleton Laboratories (Lenexa, KS). Rat tail collagen (type I) was obtained from Collaborative Research (Bedford, MA). Transwell™ filters, 0.4-μm pore size and 6.5 mm, 12 mm, or 24.5 mm in diameter, and Snapwell™ filters, 0.4-μm pore size and 12 mm in diameter, were from Costar (Cambridge, MA).

2.2. System Establishment and Monitoring

Caco-2 cells have been shown to possess many characteristics of small intestinal enterocytes (Pinto *et al.*, 1983). However, because of their colonic origin the utility of these monolayers for studying drug transport processes encountered in the small intestine should be demonstrated when the system is established. This validation process should include a comparison of the permeability characteristics of Caco-2 cell monolayers with those of the small intestine. For carrier-mediated transport it is important to determine whether the carrier expressed by Caco-2 cells is structurally and/or functionally similar to that found in the small intestinal mucosa. This validation is important because several parameters [e.g., transepithelial electrical resistance (TEER), mannitol fluxes, extent of bile acid transport] have been found to vary between laboratories (Hidalgo *et al.*, 1989; Gochoco *et al.*, 1994; Artursson, 1990; Dix *et al.*, 1990). It is possible that small interlaboratory differences in culture conditions may result in progressive selection of a subpopulation of Caco-2 cells. What follows is a description of the conditions used to establish and validate the model system in various laboratories. Caco-2 cells have been grown on microporous membranes made of nitrocellulose or polycarbonate. Cells grown on both types of filters form mono-layers that can be used to study drug transport. However, nitrocellulose filters have been shown to bind lipophilic compounds and thus may constitute a diffusion barrier for this type of molecules (Artursson, 1990). On the other hand, binding to polycarbonate filters was minimal.

2.2.1. CELL CULTURE

Caco-2 cells were cultured in high (4.5 g/l)-glucose DMEM supplemented with 10% FBS, 1% NEAA, 1% L-glutamine, penicillin (100 U/ml), and streptomycin (100 μg/ml). Cells were grown in T-75 tissue culture flasks under a humidified air–5% CO_2 atmosphere. The culture medium was changed every 2–3 days. Because changes leading to enterocytic differentiation start upon confluence (5–6 days post seeding), it is preferred to subculture the cells before they reach confluence (4–5 days post seeding). Subculture was done as follows: the culture medium was aspirated, the cells were rinsed with calcium- and magnesium-free phosphate-buffered saline (PBS) and then incubated with a thin layer of trypsin (0.25 %)–EDTA (1 mM) at 37°C until they detached (approximately 5 min). The cells were resuspended in complete DMEM and divided into new flasks at a 1:3 split ratio. For uptake/transport experiments, cells were seeded on polycarbonate membranes (Transwell or Snapwell) previously coated with rat tail collagen. Polycarbonate filters were coated with a diluted rat tail collagen solution (1 part of collagen to 3 parts of 60% ethanol). After addition of the collagen solution (70 μl/cm^2), the filters were allowed to dry in the hood for at least 4 hr. Cells were seeded at a density of approximately 60,000 cells/cm^2. When grown on this type of system, Caco-2 cells have access to both the apical (mucosal) and basolateral (serosal) bathing solutions (Fig. 1). This arrangement, which allows the exchange of materials, resembles the situation in the intestinal mucosa *in vivo*. For 24.5-mm-diameter Transwell filters, the media volumes for the apical (inside) and basolateral (outside) bathing solutions were 1.5 and 2.6 ml, respectively. The culture medium was changed 24 hr after seeding to remove cell debris and dead cells. Subsequently, the medium was changed every other day for one week and daily thereafter. Caco-2 cells reached confluence in about 5–6 days post seeding. Following confluence, Caco-2 cells undergo spontaneous enterocytic differentiation characterized by well-developed microvilli, junctional complexes, a tall columnar appearance, and a basophilic nucleus (Pinto *et al.*, 1983; Hidalgo *et al.*, 1989). To validate the utility of Caco-2 cell monolayers as a transport model system of the intestinal epithelium, the system has been characterized in terms of cell polarity and monolayer permeability.

2.2.2. CELL POLARITY

The development of cell polarity can be monitored by measuring the distribution of brush border enzymes. Two brush border enzymes that have been used as markers of cell polarity are alkaline phosphatase and sucrase-isomaltase (Zweibaum *et al.*,

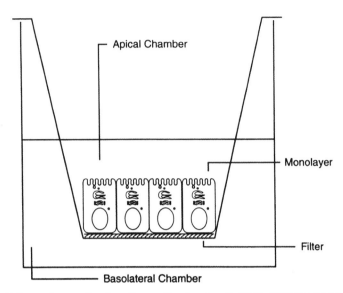

Figure 1. Cell monolayer cultured on Transwell polycarbonate filters. Caco-2 cells are seeded on polycarbonate filters at a density of approximately 60,000 cells/cm^2. Common insert diameters are 6.5, 12, and 24.5 mm. Pore sizes are 0.45 and 3.0 μm. The volume of media used to feed cells grown on 24.5-mm inserts are 1.5 ml in the apical side and 2.6 ml in the basolateral side.

1983). Alkaline phosphatase activity is determined using *p*-nitrophenyl phosphate as substrate (Pinto *et al.*, 1983; Hidalgo *et al.*, 1989). The ultrastructural distribution of alkaline phosphatase activity was examined using transmission electron microscopy (Hidalgo *et al.*, 1989). Results showed that 6 days after seeding, the enzyme was completely restricted to the brush border membrane (Hidalgo *et al.*, 1989). Sucrase-isomaltase (S-I) activity in the brush border membrane and immunofluorescence staining of Caco-2 cells with anti-S-I antibodies also indicate apical localization of the enzyme (Zweibaum *et al.*, 1983). The pattern of specific apical localization of these two enzymes is consistent with cell polarity.

2.2.3. MONOLAYER PERMEABILITY

Caco-2 cell monolayers consist of cells joined by intercellular junctional complexes (tight junctions, intermediate junctions, and spot desmosomes). The presence of tight junctions prevents the lateral diffusion of molecules and provides the monolayers with a measurable transepithelial electrical resistance (TEER). In the absence of tight junctions, drug and ions could quickly diffuse between adjacent cells, and TEER values would be minimal. Two indices of monolayer integrity are (a) TEER and (b) transepithelial fluxes of markers of passive paracellular diffusion. Frequently used paracellular flux markers are [^{3}H]-, or [^{14}C]mannitol and [^{3}H]- or [^{14}C]polyethylene glycol (PEG). The development of tight junctions was monitored using TEER measurements. These measurements can be made using an EVOM Epithelial Voltammeter (World Precision Instruments, New Haven, CT). TEER values were obtained by subtracting resistances of the filter + collagen alone from resistances of the filter + collagen + cells. TEER values were multiplied by the surface area of the filters (4.71 cm^2) and expressed in $\Omega \cdot$cm^2. TEER values of Caco-2 cell monolayers range between 200 and 500 $\Omega \cdot$cm^2 (Hidalgo *et al.*, 1989; Dix *et al.*, 1990).

Mannitol, inulin, lucifer yellow, and PEG 4000 have been used to assess monolayer integrity (Hidalgo *et al.*, 1989; Ranaldi *et al.*, 1992). Mannitol is small (mol. wt. = 182, radius = 41 nm), water-soluble, membrane-impermeant, and non-ionizable and undergoes negligible metabolism. These characteristics make it a good marker of monolayer integrity. The availability of [^{3}H]- or [^{14}C]mannitol makes it possible to use mannitol as an internal marker of monolayer integrity even when the compound of interest is radioactively labeled. We used mannitol (0.5 μCi, ^{3}H or ^{14}C) in both apical-to-basolateral and basolateral-to-apical flux experiments. In experiments in which radioactivity is not desirable, the integrity of the monolayer can be monitored using a fluorescent marker of passive paracellular diffusion (e.g., lucifer yellow). If the radioactive or fluorescent marker interferes with measurement of the compound of interest, the integrity of the monolayers could be assessed at the end of the flux period.

The utility of TEER values and mannitol fluxes in assessing monolayer integrity is illustrated in Fig. 2. In our laboratory, TEER values of Caco-2 cell monolayers increased from 137 $\pm$ 15 $\Omega \cdot$cm^2 at day 9 to 436 $\pm$ 23 $\Omega \cdot$cm^2 at day 15. The associated mannitol fluxes decrease from 0.58 $\pm$ 0.05 %/(hr$\cdot$cm^2) at day 9 to 0.18 $\pm$ 0.015 %/(hr$\cdot$cm^2) at day 14. Both TEER values and mannitol fluxes remained unchanged after day 15 in culture.

2.3. Experimental Protocols

Transport solutions used in uptake and transepithelial transport studies were described in Section 2.1.

2.3.1. UPTAKE EXPERIMENTS

The apical bathing solution consisted of Hanks' balanced salt solution (HBSS) containing 10 mM mannitol and 0.05% BSA, and the basolateral bathing solution consisted of HBSS containing 2 mM glucose plus 8 mM mannitol and 0.05% BSA. The pH of the bathing solutions was usually 7.4. In pH dependence experiments the pH of the bathing solution(s) was adjusted to the desired value using 10 mM MES (pH 5–6.5) or 10 mM HEPES (pH 6.5–7.4). At time zero the compounds were added to the apical (for apical uptake) or basolateral (for basolateral uptake) bathing solution, and

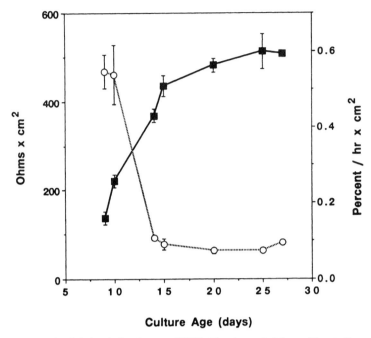

Figure 2. Transepithelial electrical resistances (TEER; ■) and mannitol fluxes (○) as indices of mono-layer integrity. Maximal TEER values and minimal mannitol fluxes are achieved 2 weeks after seeding.

the monolayers were incubated at the appropriate temperature. Following the incuba-tion period, the monolayers were washed four times with ice-cold HBSS. To deter-mine the amount of radioactively labeled compound taken up by the cells, the filter (containing the cells) was cut out, and the cells were dissolved in scintillation cocktail. Unlabeled compounds were extracted using normal procedures for plasma or tissue samples prior to their determination by HPLC. The protein content of the monolayers was determined in each experiment, and uptake rates were expressed in pmol $min^{-1} \cdot (mg\ protein)^{-1}$ or nmol $min^{-1} \cdot (mg\ protein)^{-1}$.

2.3.2. TRANSEPITHELIAL TRANSPORT

Transport experiments were carried out in the same solution used in uptake experiments. Physical integrity of the monolayers was evaluated using TEER and mannitol flux measurements. In our experience mannitol flux is a more sensitive indicator of monolayer damage than TEER measurements. Thus, TEER values were used in addition to and not in place of flux measurements. Tight monolayers are desirable because (a) they exhibit minimal passive paracellular flux, and (b) carefully controlled monolayer integrity should reduce intermonolayer variability. Monolayers with mannitol fluxes greater than $0.6\%/(hr \cdot cm^2)$ and TEER values less than 200

$\Omega \cdot cm^2$ were excluded from transport studies. Transport experiments were carried out with Transwell membranes or in diffusion chambers.

2.3.2a. Transwell Experiments

Transwell polycarbonate filters are available in different sizes (e.g., 6.5, 12, and 24.5 mm). The following description relates to the 24.5-mm system.

Apical-to-Basolateral Transport. Each well in six-well trays received 2.6 ml of basolateral bathing solution. Following preequilibration at the appropriate temperature, inserts containing the monolayers were positioned in the first well of the tray with the basolateral side of the monolayers immersed in the basolateral bathing solution. At time zero, the drug and marker were added to the apical bathing solution (Fig. 1), and the trays were incubated at the temperature of the experiment. At specified times, the inserts were transferred to neighboring wells containing fresh basolateral bathing solution.

Basolateral-to-Apical Transport. Each well in six-well trays contained 2.6 ml of basolateral bathing solution (containing the drugs and/or markers) preequilibrated at the appropriate temperature. At time zero, inserts containing the cell monolayers were placed in the well with the basolateral side of the cells immersed in the basolateral bathing solution. Immediately, 1.5 ml of apical bathing solution preequilibrated at the appropriate temperature was added to the inserts (apical side of the monolayers), and the trays were incubated at the desired temperature. Samples were taken at specified times by removing an aliquot from the apical side and replacing it with an equal volume of drug-free apical bathing solution.

2.3.2b. Transepithelial Transport in Diffusion Chambers

In the absence of stirring, a large unstirred water layer (UWL) exists adjacent to cell monolayers. This UWL can be the rate-limiting barrier for transepithelial transport of lipophilic compounds (Hidalgo *et al.*, 1991). Thus, estimates of transepithelial permeability coefficients or fluxes would reflect the permeability resistance of the UWL rather than resistance of the cell membrane. In addition, the presence of an UWL could result in overestimation of the K_t value associated with active transport (Thomson and Dietschy, 1980). To reduce the effect of the UWL, Transwell trays have been agitated with slide mixers (Artursson, 1990). However, in the absence of standardization the utility of this system is limited.

A side-by-side diffusion apparatus has been developed which uses gas lift to provide stirring (Hidalgo *et al.*, 1991; 1992). The advantage of this system is that it provides stirring without introducing potentially damaging monolayer manipulation. Cell were seeded onto Snapwell filters at the same density used with Transwell filters (i.e., 60,000 cells/cm^2). When the cells were ready (2–3 weeks), the lower part of the

Snapwell insert (containing the monolayer) was detached and mounted in the diffusion apparatus with the help of O-rings. This system allows the adjustment of the stirring rate. The temperature was controlled by using a block heater connected to a recirculating water bath set at the desired temperature. The top of each half-chamber was open. This facilitates drug application and sample withdrawal. The composition of the transport solutions used in this system was the same as described in Section 2.3.1. Monolayer integrity can be assessed using an internal marker of passive paracellular diffusion (e.g., [^{3}H]mannitol) and/or a voltage clamp connected to the diffusion chambers. The volume of each chamber was approximately 5 ml. Samples were taken from the donor and the receiver side prior to addition of the transport compounds. Typical flux experiments lasted 120 min. After addition of the compounds to the donor side, samples (20–100 μl) were taken from the donor chamber at 0, 60, and 120 hr. From the receiver side, 0.5- to 1.0-ml samples were taken at 0, 15, 30, 45, 60, 90, and 120 min. Samples taken from the receiver side were replaced with the same solution. Because of their small volume, samples taken from the donor side were not replaced. The sampling format used resulted in a dilution effect in the receiver chamber. The cumulative amount transported is given by

$$\text{TR}_{\text{cum}} = A_n + \frac{\text{vs}_n}{V_R} \sum_{i=0}^{n-1} A_i \qquad (1)$$

where A_n is the amount of drug measured in sample n, vs_n is the volume of sample n, and V_R is the volume of the receiver chamber.

2.3.2c. Efflux Experiments

Cell monolayers were incubated in the presence of a suitable drug concentration, under conditions described in Section 2.3.1, for 1 hr at 37°C. At the end of the incubation (loading) period, the Transwell inserts containing the cell monolayers were washed (4 times) with ice-cold HBSS and positioned in new wells. The apical and basolateral sides of the monolayers received 1.5 and 2.5 ml of drug-free apical and basolateral bathing solutions, respectively. The bathing solutions were preequilibrated at the temperature at which the efflux was to be determined (e.g., 37 or 4°C). Samples were taken from the apical and basolateral sides at preselected times (e.g., 1, 5, 10, 15, 30, and 60 min). At the end of the efflux period, the filter (containing the monolayers) was cut, and the cells were dissolved as described in Section 2.3.1.

2.4. Calculations of Data

It is often useful to distinguish uptake from transcellular transport. For example, determination of relative rates of uptake and efflux allows one to identify the rate-limiting step of transcellular transport.

2.4.1. CELLULAR UPTAKE

Determination of uptake rates requires that samples be taken shortly after the beginning of the experiment. If samples were taken in the presence of substantial back flux, the associated apparent rate of uptake would reflect only the rate of accumulation (rate of net uptake). The exact duration of the initial uptake phase depends on the characteristics of the compound. Thus, in order to ensure that the correct sampling time for an uptake experiment is chosen, it is often desirable to generate an uptake versus concentration time course. From this curve, sampling times can be chosen that reflect true uptake. In general, the logistics of sampling and assay sensitivity limit the times that can be used for sampling uptake rates.

For active transport, uptake rate can be described by

$$v = \frac{V_t \cdot C}{K_t + C} + K_d \cdot C \qquad (2)$$

where v is the uptake rate [e.g., nmol min^{-1} (mg protein)$^{-1}$], V_t is the maximal uptake rate [e.g., nmol min^{-1} (mg protein)$^{-1}$], K_t is the half-maximal uptake or transport concentration (e.g., mM), C is the concentration of the compound (e.g., mM), and K_d is the coefficient for nonmediated and passive uptake [e.g., nmol min^{-1} (mg protein)$^{-1}$ mM^{-1}]. Computer modeling with a nonlinear least-squares regression analysis program can be used to determine the three model parameters (V_t, K_t, and K_d). Subtraction of the linear portion of the curve (i.e., $K_d \cdot C$) from the curve generated by using Eq. (2) yields the carrier-mediated or saturable component of uptake (Gochoco et al., 1994). When transport is carrier-mediated, it is useful to identify the transport process involved. Determination of transport parameters can be done using Eq. (2). The second term in the equation would be neglected if the uptake is entirely carrier-mediated.

2.4.2. INHIBITION OF UPTAKE

The effect of structural analogs on the carrier-mediated uptake of the compound of interest can provide insight into structural requirements for interaction with the binding site(s). Analogs can be compared in terms of their relative affinities for the binding site(s). An index of the affinity is given by K_i (concentration of inhibitor that doubles the slope of the $1/v$ vs. $1/C$ plot). Although functionally similar, K_i and IC$_{50}$ (concentration of the inhibitor that decreases the uptake of the compound of interest by 50%) are not the same (Segel, 1976). Dixon plots can be used to determine the type of inhibition (i.e., competitive, noncompetitive, or uncompetitive). When the type of inhibition is determined to be competitive, K_i can be estimated using Eq. (3) (Segel, 1976):

$$\frac{1}{v} = \frac{K_t}{V_t \cdot K_i \cdot C}[I] + \frac{1}{V_t}\left(1 + \frac{K_t}{C}\right) \qquad (3)$$

where $[I]$ is the concentration of inhibitor. If V_t and K_t are known, $1/v$ versus $[I]$ curves may be generated for at least two drug concentrations. K_i can be obtained graphically by interpolating the concentration at the intersection point (Fig. 3). The intercept and slope of Eq. (3) can be estimated using linear regression analysis. Dividing the intercept by the slope and rearranging yields Eq. (4), which can be used to calculate K_i.

$$K_i = \frac{(\text{intercept/slope}) \cdot K_t}{K_t + C} \qquad (4)$$

With Caco-2 cells, a good agreement between K_i and IC_{50} values for the inhibition of cephalexin uptake by dipeptides and α-aminocephalosporins was found. Equation (4) is used to calculate K_i when the inhibition process is competitive. When the type of inhibition is not known, a good agreement between K_i [determined using Eq. (4)] and IC_{50} indicates that the inhibition process under investigation is indeed competitive.

2.4.3. TRANSEPITHELIAL TRANSPORT

Transpithelial transport can be expressed in terms of unidirectional fluxes [e.g., pmol/(min·cm^2) or nmol/(hr·cm^2)]. Transepithelial fluxes are proportional to the concentration in the donor chamber. Thus, when transport processes proceed via passive diffusion, permeability coefficient (P_{app}) values represent a convenient way of

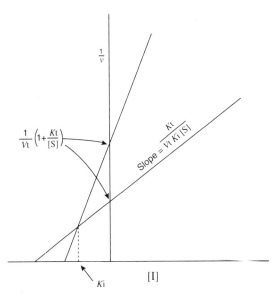

Figure 3.   Dixon plots, showing relevant parameters associated with the slope and intercept. Dixon plots can also indicate whether inhibition is competitive or noncompetitive.

expressing drug transport. P_{app} is obtained by dividing the unidirectional fluxes by the drug concentration in the donor solution:

$$P_{app} = \frac{\Delta Q}{\Delta t \cdot A \cdot C_o} \qquad (5)$$

where ΔQ is the amount transported during the time interval Δt, A is the surface area, and C_o is the initial concentration on the donor side. P_{app} has units of distance/time (e.g., cm/sec, cm/hr). For passive diffusion processes and nonsaturated carrier-mediated transport, the values of P_{app} should be independent of drug concentration. Indeed, a decrease in P_{app} values with increasing drug concentrations indicates that transport is saturable.

2.4.4. INHIBITION OF TRANSPORT

Characterization of carrier-mediated transport often involves demonstration of transport inhibition. In general, inhibition of transepithelial transport is more difficult to show than inhibition of uptake. This is due in part to the fact that transepithelial transport is seldom completely carrier-mediated but often involves some passive transcellular transport. In addition, the tight junctions are not completely imperme-able and may contribute to transepithelial transport. Both passive transcellular trans-port and paracellular transport are not susceptible to inhibition. However, in Caco-2 cell monolayers, the transepithelial transport of cephalexin was shown to be saturable and susceptible to inhibition by peptides and some α-aminocephalosporins, indicat-ing that the majority of the transepithelial transport was mediated by the oligopeptide transporter (Gochoco et al., 1994). Computer modeling using Eq. (2) makes it possible to determine the active component. Identification of the contribution of the active component allows one to determine inhibition of carrier-mediated transport (Gochoco et al., 1994). When most transepithelial transport is carrier-mediated, results from uptake and transepithelial transport inhibition will lead to the same conclusions. For example, the K_t values for uptake and transcellular transport of cephalexin in Caco-2 cells were found to be similar (Gochoco et al., 1994).

3. APPLICATIONS TO ABSORPTION AND METABOLISM STUDIES

3.1. Drug Absorption

3.1.1 ABSORPTION SCREENING

The use of animals for the evaluation of the absorption of new chemical entities is very inefficient. First, developing methods to measure drugs in biological matrices is time-consuming. Second, absorption studies in animals require large amounts of compounds, whereas only small amounts of compound are synthesized during the screening phase of drug discovery. Third, the experiments are too time-consuming. On the other hand, transport studies in Caco-2 cells can be much faster. For example, transport experiments with Caco-2 cell monolayers are normally conducted in buffered biological solutions such as Hanks' balanced salt solution. This makes analytical method development easier. Caco-2 cell transport experiments also require small amounts of compound (a few milligrams).

3.1.2. ABSORPTION MECHANISMS

Caco-2 cells can be used not only to screen molecules for intestinal epithelial transport but also to study mechanisms of drug transport. Most studies on intestinal transport using Caco-2 cell monolayers seek to determine the involvement of specific carriers and provide data for their characterization. For example, Caco-2 cells have been widely used to evaluate carrier-mediated intestinal transporter. They show carrier-mediated transport of large neutral amino acids (Hidalgo and Borchardt, 1990a), glucose (Blais et al., 1987), bile acids (Hidalgo and Borchardt, 1990b), biotin (Ng and Borchardt, 1993), folic acid (Vincent et al., 1985), vitamin B_{12} (Dix et al., 1990), and oligopeptides (Dantzig and Bergin, 1990). The three carriers most commonly investigated with Caco-2 cells are (a) the oligopeptide transporter, (b) the bile acid transporter, and (c) P-glycoprotein. Studies have shown that the K_t value of cephalexin uptake in Caco-2 cells is comparable to that of intestinal BBMV, indicating that the oligopeptide transporter expressed by Caco-2 cells is comparable to that of intestinal mucosa (Yamashita et al., 1984; Gochoco et al., 1994). The apparently low specificity of the oligopeptide transporter suggests the potential for exploiting it to enhance the oral bioavailability of peptidomimetic compounds. The characteristics of bile acid transport in Caco-2 cells also resemble those of the small intestine (Hidalgo and Borchardt, 1990b). These cells have been used to evaluate the potential exploitation of the bile acid carrier to deliver peptide drugs across the intestinal mucosa (Kim et al., 1993). Recent evidence indicates that P-glycoprotein, the expression product of the MDR1 gene, may increase the resistance of the intestinal mucosa to drug absorption (Hunter et al., 1993). The role of P-glycoprotein as an intestinal absorption barrier has yet to be demonstrated in vivo.

3.2. Drug Metabolism

Although Caco-2 cells have been widely used in drug transport studies, their use in drug metabolism studies is less common. They express enzymes found in the brush border membrane such as alkaline phosphatase, aminopeptidases (N, P, and W), dipeptidyl peptidase IV, γ-glutamyl transpeptidase, peptidyl dipeptidase A, and sucrase-isomaltase, cytosolic enzymes such as phenol sulfotransferases, glucuronidase, and glutathione S-transferase, and microsomal enzymes such as cytochrome (CYP) P4501A1 and 1A2 (Pinto *et al.*, 1983; Baranczyk-Kuzma *et al.*, 1991; Boulenc *et al.*, 1992). A recent report described a Caco-2 clone (TC7) which expresses CYP4503A4 and 3A5 (Carriere *et al.*, 1994). Potential identification of additional Caco-2 clones expressing relevant CYP450 enzymes and/or transfection with specific cDNA will increase the application of Caco-2 cells in drug metabolism studies.

3.3. *In Vitro–in Vivo* Correlations

Since one goal of *in vitro* model systems is to predict what happens *in vivo*, it is important to demonstrate *in vitro–in vivo* correlations. Caco-2 cells have been used to rank the permeabilities of series of compounds. Ranking is more difficult when compounds belonging to different classes are combined. An earlier report which examined potential correlations between Caco-2 permeability and absorption found that compounds with permeability coefficients greater than 1.0×10^{-6} cm/sec are likely to be well absorbed (Artursson and Karlsson, 1991). Correlations will be extremely difficult when different classes of molecules are involved. First, the compounds may differ in physicochemical properties such as lipophilicity, molecular volume, hydrogen bonding, solubility, and pK_a. Second, carrier-mediated mechanisms may be involved in the absorption of some compounds whereas others may be passively transported. Third, mucosal or hepatic metabolism may negate differences in intrinsic membrane permeabilities. The extent to which Caco-2 cells mimic the metabolic processes that take place in the intestinal mucosa is not well understood. Caco-2 cells apparently lack some important drug-metabolizing mucosal enzymes. They possess phenol sulfotransferases but lack UDP glucuronyltransferase (Baranczyk-Kuzma *et al.*, 1991). In addition, these cells express low levels of CYP4501A1 and 1A2 but lack CYP4503A4 (Boulenc *et al.*, 1992). The absence of this enzyme limits the application of Caco-2 cells in metabolism studies because CYP4503A4 is involved in the metabolism of numerous drugs (Lown *et al.*, 1994). A recent study described the isolation and characterization of a Caco-2 clone (Caco-2-TC7) which expresses CYP3A (Carriere *et al.*, 1994). Since the expression of the enzymes paralleled the development of differentiation, this Caco-2 clone may be valuable in studying CYP3A regulation. Caco-2 cells transfected with different P450 should constitute a valuable tool to evaluate the role of intestinal P450 in drug transport. They also constitute a useful tool due to their expression of both the permeability and metabolism barriers likely to limit drug absorption. It is also likely that Caco-2 cells will be transfected with relevant cDNA to generate clones useful in studying intestinal regulation of CYP450.

4. ADVANTAGES AND DISADVANTAGES OVER OTHER METHODS

4.1. Advantages

The advantages of Caco-2 cells for drug transport and metabolism studies can be summarized as follows:

1. They can be used to determine both cellular uptake and transepithelial transport.
2. They permit the determination of drug transport in the presence of cellular metabolic reactions which may be important in active drug transport.
3. They contain many drug-metabolizing enzymes absent from membrane preparations.
4. They express cell polarity (a feature absent in BBMV, BLMV, and isolated enterocytes), making it possible to determine directionality of uptake/transport.
5. They remain viable for long periods.
6. They can be used to distinguish luminal disappearance from transepithelial transport. The intestinal loop system is used to determine drug disappearance from the intestinal lumen under the assumption that luminal disappearance is equivalent to drug absorption. However, in some instances drug disappearance exceeds drug transport. Thus, absorption rates predicted from this method overestimate the true absorption (Sugawara *et al.*, 1990).
7. They are of human origin.

4.2. Disadvantages

The disadvantages of Caco-2 cells can be summarized as follows:

1. They lack a mucus layer, which may play a role in drug absorption.
2. They lack the cellular heterogeneity found in the intestinal mucosa (goblet cell, Paneth cells, and undifferentiated crypt cells).
3. They lack some drug-metabolizing enzymes found in the small intestine, such as CYP4503A4. The recent isolation of a Caco-2 clone that expresses CYP3A will help overcome this limitation.
4. Their barrier properties resemble more closely those of colonic epithelium than those of intestinal epithelium (Hidalgo *et al.*, 1989).

REFERENCES

Artursson, P., 1990, Epithelial transport of drugs in cell culture. I: A model for studying the passive diffusion of drugs over intestinal absorptive (Caco-2) cells, *J. Pharm. Sci.* **79:**476–482.

Artursson, P., and Karlsson, J., 1991, Correlation between oral drug absorption in humans and apparent drug permeability coefficients in human intestinal epithelial (Caco-2) cells, *Biochem. Biophys. Res. Commun.* **175:**880–885.

Audus, K. L., Bartel, R. L., Hidalgo, I. J., and Borchardt, R. T., 1990, The use of cultured epithelial and endothelial cells for drug transport and metabolism studies, *Pharm. Res.* **7:**435–451.

Baranczyk-Kuzma, A., Garren, J. A., Hidalgo, I. J., and Borchardt, R. T., 1991, Substrate specificity and some properties of phenol sulfotransferase from human Caco-2 cells, *Life Sci.* **49:**1197–1206.

Blais, A. Bissonnette, P., and Berteloot, A., 1987, Common characteristics for Na+-dependent sugar transport in Caco-2 cells and human fetal colon, *J. Membr. Biol.* **99:**113–125.

Boulenc, X., Bourrie, M., Fabre, J., Roque, C., Joyeux, H., Berger, Y., and Fabre, G., 1992, Regulation of cytochrome P4501A1 gene expression in a human intestinal cell line, Caco-2, *J. Pharmacol. Exp. Ther.* **263:**1471–1478.

Carriere, V., Lesuffleur, T., Barbat, A., Rousset, M., Dussaulx, E., Costet, P., de Waziers, I., Beaune, P., and Zweibaum, A., 1994, Expression of cytochrome P-450 3A in HT29-MTX cells and Caco-2 clone TC7, *FEBS Lett.* **355:**247–250.

Dantzig, A. H., and Bergin, L., 1990, Uptake of the cephalosporin, cephalexin, by a dipeptide transport carrier in the human intestinal cell line, Caco-2, *Biochim. Biophys. Acta* **1027:**211–217.

Dix, C. J., Hassan, I. F., Obray, H. Y., Shah, R., and Wilson, G., 1990, The transport of vitamin B_{12} through polarized monolayers of Caco-2 cells, *Gastroenterology* **98:**1272–1279.

Gochoco, C. H., Ryan, F. M., Miller, J., Smith, P. L., and Hidalgo, I. J., 1994, Uptake and transepithelial transport of the orally absorbed cephalosporin cephalexin, in the human intestinal cell line, Caco-2, *Int. J. Pharm.* **104:**187–202.

Hartmann, F., Owen, R., and Bissell, D. M., 1982, Characterization of isolated epithelial cells from rat small intestine, *Am. J. Physiol.* **242:**G147–G155.

Hidalgo, I. J., and Borchardt, R. T., 1990a, Transport of a large neutral amino acid (phenylalanine) in a human intestinal epithelial cell line: Caco-2, *Biochim. Biophys. Acta* **1035:**25–30.

Hidalgo, I. J., and Borchardt, R. T., 1990b, Transport of bile acids in a human intestinal epithelial cell line, Caco-2, *Biochim. Biophys. Acta* **1035:**97–103.

Hidalgo, I. J., Raub, T. J., and Borchardt, R. T., 1989, Characterization of the human colon carcinoma cell line (Caco-2) as a model system for intestinal epithelial permeability, *Gastroenterology* **96:**736–749.

Hidalgo, I. J., Hillgren, K. M., Grass, G. M., and Borchardt, R. T., 1991, Characterization of the unstirred water layer in Caco-2 cell monolayers using a novel diffusion apparatus, *Pharm. Res.* **8:**222–227.

Hidalgo, I. J., Hillgren, K. M., Grass, G. M., and Borchardt, R. T., 1992, A new side-by-side diffusion cell for studying transport across epithelial cell monolayers, *In Vitro Cell. Dev. Biol.* **28A:**578–580.

Hunter, J., Jepson, M. A., Tsuruo, T., Simmons, N. L., and Hirst, B. H., 1993, Functional expression of P-glycoprotein in apical membranes of human intestinal Caco-2 cells: Kinetics of vinblastine secretion and interactions with modulators, *J. Biol. Chem.* **268:**14991–14997.

Inui, K.-I., Yamamoto, M., and Saito, H., 1992, Transepithelial transport of oral cephalosporins by monolayers of intestinal epithelial cell line Caco-2: Specific transport systems in apical and basolateral membranes, *J. Pharmacol. Exp. Ther.* **261:**195–201.

Kim, D.-C., Harrison, A. W., Ruwart, M. J., Wilkinson, K. F., Fisher, J. F., Hidalgo, I. J., and Borchardt, R. T., 1993, Evaluation of the bile acid transporter in enhancing intestinal permeability to renin-inhibitory peptides, *J. Drug Targeting* **1:**347–359.

Lesuffleur, T., Porchet, N., Aubert, J.-P., Swallow, D, Gum, J. R., Kim, Y. S., Real, F. X., and Zweibaum, A.,

1993, Differential expression of the human mucin genes MUC1 to MUC5 in relation to growth and differentiation of different mucus-secreting HT-29 cell sub populations, *J. Cell Sci.* **106**:771–783.

Lown, K. S., Kolars, J. C., Thummel, K. E., Barnett, J. L., Kunze, K. L., Wrighton, S. A., and Watkins, P. B., 1994, Interpatient heterogeneity in expression of CYP3A4 and CYP3A5 in small bowel. Lack of prediction by the erythromycin breadth test, *Drug Metab. Dispos.* **22**:947–955.

Madara, J. L., Stafford, J., Barenberg, D., and Carlson, S., 1988, Functional coupling of tight junctions and microfilaments in T84 monolayers, *Am. J. Physiol.* **254**:G416–G423.

Ng, K.-Y., and Borchardt, R. T., 1993, Biotin transport in a human intestinal epithelial cell line (Caco-2), *Life Sci.* **53**:1121–1127.

Nicklin, P., Irwin, B., Hassan, I., Williamson, I., and Mackay, M., 1992, Permeable support type influences the transport of compounds across Caco-2 cells, *Int. J. Pharm.* **83**:197–209.

Pinto, M., Robine-Leon, S., Appay, M. D., Kedinger, M., Triadou, N., Dussaulx, E., Lacroix, B., Simon-Assmann, P., Haffen, K., Fogh, J. and Zweibaum, A., 1983, Enterocytic-like differentiation and polarization of the human colon adenocarcinoma cell line Caco-2 in culture, *Biol. Cell.* **47**:323–330.

Ranaldi, G., Islam, K., and Sambuy, Y., 1992, Epithelial cells in culture as a model for the intestinal transport of antimicrobial agents, *Antimicrob. Agents Chemother.* **36**:1374–1381.

Raul, F., Kedinger, M., Simon, P., Grenier, J., and Haffen, K., 1978, Behaviour of isolated rat intestinal cell maintained in suspension or monolayer cultures, *Biol. Cell* **33**:163–168.

Segel, I. H., 1976, *Biochemical Calculation*, Wiley & Sons, New York, p. 252.

Sugawara, M., Saitoh, H., Iseki, K., Miyazaki, K., and Arita, T., 1990, Contribution of passive transport mechanisms to the intestinal absorption of β-lactam antibiotics, *J. Pharm. Pharmacol.* **42**:314–318.

Thomson, A. B. R., and Dietschy, J. M., 1980, Experimental demonstration of the effect of the unstirred water layer on the kinetic constants of the membrane transport of D-glucose in rabbit jejunum, *J. Membr. Biol.* **54**:221–229.

Vincent, M. L., Russell, R. M., and Sasak, V., 1985, Folic acid uptake characteristics of a human colon carcinoma cell line, Caco-2. A newly described cellular model for small intestinal epithelium, *Hum. Nutr. Clin. Nutr.* **39C**:355–360.

Yamashita, S., Yamazaki, Y., Mizuno, M., Masada, M., Nadai, T., Kimura, T., and Sezaki, H., 1984, Further investigations on the transport mechanism of cephalexin and ampicillin across rat jejunum, *J. Pharmacobio-Dyn.* **7**:227–233.

Zweibaum, A., Triadou, N., Kedinger, M., Augeron, C., Robine-Leon, S., Pinto, M., Rousset, M., and Haffen, K., 1983, Sucrase-isomaltase: A marker of foetal and malignant epithelial cells of the human colon, *Int. J. Cancer* **32**:407–412.

Chapter 4

Intestinal Rings and Isolated Intestinal Mucosal Cells

Joseph A. Fix

1. INTRODUCTION

Intestinal rings and isolated intestinal mucosal cells have been employed for over 25 years in the examination of biologic problems in the fields of nutrition (Del Castillo and Muniz, 1991; Fleisher *et al.*, 1989; Gore and Hoinard, 1993; Shaw *et al.*, 1983; Westergaard and Dietschy, 1976), pharmaceutics (Kajii *et al.*, 1985; Meadows and Dressman, 1990; Osiecka *et al.*, 1987; Porter *et al.*, 1985; Tsuji *et al.*, 1986, 1987), cell biology (Weiser, 1973a,b), and metabolism and biochemistry (Grafstrom *et al.*, 1979; Kelley and Chen, 1985; Koster *et al.*, 1984; Sepulveda *et al.*, 1982; Stern, 1966). Of particular interest here is the utility of these relatively simple *in vitro* models for characterizing, within defined limits, the absorptive and metabolic properties of intestinal tissue.

Unlike many absorption models which measure transport of drugs through epithelial cell layers, rings and isolated cells are more accurately defined as uptake or accumulation models of the drug absorption process. These models can be utilized to quantitate the amount or rate of drug accumulation into tissue or cells but not true transcellular transport because passage of drug through the cell or tissue and into a basolateral compartment does not occur. Isolated cells in suspension also lack cell polarity, and therefore absorption is not limited to the apical brush border region.

In spite of some limitations on the utility of intestinal rings and isolated cells in assessing drug absorption, the models do provide important data which are useful in characterizing the overall absorption process for drug candidates.

Joseph A. Fix • Alza Corporation, Palo Alto, California 94304.

Models for Assessing Drug Absorption and Metabolism, Ronald T. Borchardt *et al.*, eds., Plenum Press, New York, 1996.

2. PREPARATION OF EVERTED RINGS OR ISOLATED EPITHELIAL CELLS

Intestinal rings and isolated cells can be prepared from virtually any animal species, but practical considerations for subsequent drug absorption studies generally limit the choice of species for intestinal rings to smaller animals (e.g., mice, rats, guinea pigs, rabbits). In general, animals are fasted for 12–24 hr prior to tissue preparation for both models in order to reduce intestinal washing requirements, which can cause mechanical irritation of the tissue. Food may be allowed prior to ring or cell isolation, if necessary, in the experimental design (i.e., examination of nutritional effects on drug absorption). Most physiologic buffers are suitable for preparation of intestinal rings and cells. Buffer components may be varied to suit individual experimental requirements (e.g., calcium-free medium when measuring calcium-dependent processes). No clear advantage has been identified for any given buffer provided standard physiologic criteria are met, including ionic composition, isotonicity, and sufficient buffering capacity.

2.1. Intestinal Rings

Since the first description (Agar *et al.*, 1954) of the preparation and use of rodent intestinal rings to study amino acid accumulation, the only significant technical change which has occurred is that most investigators now evert the intestinal segment prior to ring preparation. This maximizes access of the investigational drug to the absorptive surface which lines the luminal surface of the intestine. Other modifications have largely been limited to selection of a particular physiologic buffer for washing and storing the isolated tissue. Table I provides a comparison of the original procedure (Agar *et al.*, 1954) and those employed recently by several investigators (Osiecka *et al.*, 1985; Fleisher *et al.*, 1989; Matthews and Burston, 1984; Meadows and Dressman, 1990). Briefly, a segment of intestine is isolated, washed with cold, oxygenated physiologic buffer or saline to remove cellular debris and digestive products, everted over a glass rod, cut into small sections (typically 10–60 mg wet weight), and stored in oxygenated physiologic buffer or culture medium at 4°C. It is important that the tissue remain thoroughly wetted with cold, oxygenated buffer and that physical manipulation, particularly during intestinal eversion on the glass rod, is minimized. Everted rings are generally stable (i.e., retain viability) for up to 30–60 min if maintained in physiologic buffer containing 10 mM glucose or culture medium at 4°C prior to use (Leppert and Fix, 1994).

2.2. Isolated Intestinal Mucosal Cells

Strategies for the isolation of intestinal mucosal cells have been the subject of previous reviews (Hulsmann *et al.*, 1974; Kimmich, 1990). These procedures can

Table I
Comparison of Methods for Preparing Intestinal Rings

Method	Species	Fasted	Intestinal wash	Orientation	Ring size	Storage buffer	Reference
I	Rat	24 hr	Warm saline	Not everted	0.5 cm	Krebs bicarbonate	Agar et al., 1954
II	Rat	16 hr	Cold saline	Everted	30–50 mg	Krebs–Henseleit or Eagle's	Osiecka et al., 1985
III	Rat	12 hr	Buffered saline	Everted	10–30 mg	Same as wash solution	Fleisher et al., 1989
IV	Rat	20 hr	Saline	Everted	2 mm	McIlvaine buffer	Meadows and Dressman, 1990
V	Hamster	—[a]	pH 5 Tris-PO_4	Everted	10–20 mg	Same as wash solution	Matthews and Burston, 1984

[a]Not indicated.

generally be divided into two categories: (i) *ex vivo* treatment of intestinal segments with various combinations of mechanical forces (BreMiller, 1961), chelating agents (Harrison and Webster, 1969; Huang, 1965; Weiser, 1973a,b), and enzymatic treatment (Del Castillo, 1987; Harber *et al.*, 1964) to loosen individual cells from underlying and adjacent cell/tissue connections; and (ii) *in situ* perfusion of the intestinal vasculature with enzyme solutions to dissociate the epithelial cells from the underlying tissues (Hartmann *et al.*, 1982). Since the *in situ* vascular perfusion procedure requires more sophisticated surgical techniques and, at least in our experience (Osiecka *et al.*, 1985), results in a lower cell yield with poorer viability, the *ex vivo* methods will be discussed in this chapter.

Two preparative methods for isolated mucosal cells are presented here (Fig. 1 and Table II). These two methods can afford different cell populations. The Weiser (1973a,b) method utilizes a chelating agent to disrupt cell associations and relies on

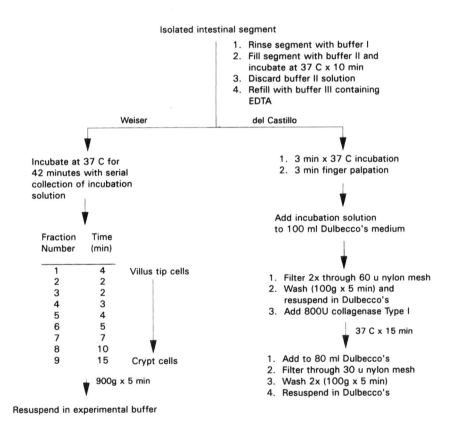

Figure 1. Schematic of the Weiser (1973a) and del Castillo (1987) preparative methods for isolated intestinal cells.

Table II
Wash and Incubation Solutions Used in Weiser and del Castillo Preparations

Solution	Weiser method	del Castillo method
I. Intestinal segment wash solution	0.154 M NaCl with 1 mM dithiothreitol	7 mM K_2SO_4, 44 mM K_2HPO_4, 9 mM $NaHCO_3$, 10 mM HEPES, 180 mM glucose
II. Initial intestinal incubation solution (discarded)	1.5 mM KCl, 96 mM NaCl, 27 mM sodium citrate, 8 mM KH_2PO_4, 5.6 mM Na_2HPO4, pH 7.3	Solution I
III. Second intestinal incubation solution (with suspended cells)	PO_4-buffered saline (calcium and magnesium free), 1.5 mM EDTA, 0.5 mM dithiothreitol	Solution I plus 0.5 mM dithiothreitol and 0.2 mM EDTA

variable incubation times to isolate cells from various segments of the villus-to-crypt axis. Although nine fractions from the Weiser method are indicated in Fig. 1, fractions may be combined to yield suspensions that are largely of villus tip or of crypt origin. The full fractionation into nine separate cell preparations is only of significant utility if the purpose of subsequent experiments is to characterize drug transport as a function of cell differentiation along the villus axis. For most applications in the pharmaceutical field, the absorptive cells of the villus tip are the cells of interest. The del Castillo (1987) modification also utilizes a chelating agent for cell isolation but follows this with enzymatic treatment of the cell suspension to remove damaged cells and cellular debris. This approach provides a heterogeneous cell population (mixture of villus to crypt cells) which exhibits greater initial viability than that observed without enzymatic treatment.

The cell population obtained by either method can be characterized in terms of relative villus-tip and crypt cell content by a variety of methods. Villus cells are particularly rich in alkaline phosphatase (Weiser, 1973a) and sucrase (Dahlquist, 1963) as compared to cells of crypt origin, and these markers can be measured by standard procedures. Likewise, accumulation of glucosamine into acid-precipitable material is also greater in villus-tip cells than in cells of crypt origin. In vivo injection of radiolabeled thymidine prior to cell isolation and its subsequent incorporation into the rapidly dividing, undifferentiated cells of the crypt area can be used to assess the relative purity of a crypt cell preparation (Osiecka et al., 1985).

Results obtained in our laboratory (Osiecka et al., 1985) are consistent with those reported by del Castillo (1987), indicating that final resuspension and storage of isolated cells in oxygenated culture medium (e.g., Dulbecco's or Eagle's medium) at 4°C prior to aliquoting samples for experimental studies provides greater retention of cell viability. Drug accumulation can usually be measured using the same culture medium unless components in the medium are suspected or known to affect the process being examined. In such cases, the medium can be replaced by the appropriate physiologic buffer immediately prior to initiation of uptake studies.

3. DEMONSTRATION OF FUNCTIONAL VIABILITY OF RINGS AND CELLS

The accuracy and reproducibility of transport studies with any *in vitro* model relies on utilizing tissue that displays normal morphological, biochemical, and transport viability. It is also important that viability remain relatively constant throughout the duration of experimental procedures so that results are not adversely influenced by changes which occur as a function of incubation time.

Dye exclusion is the most common and simple approach to determining cellular viability. An aliquot of the final cell suspension containing at least 100 cells for microscopic observation is briefly incubated at 25°C with trypan blue dye (added at an approximate final concentration of 0.1–0.4%). Cells with damaged plasma membranes (i.e., leaky to normally impermeant molecules) will appear blue or purple upon observation by light microscopy. Typically, at least 80% cell viability is considered a minimum, although many investigators require 90–95% viability before cell preparations are deemed acceptable for subsequent use. Dye exclusion staining is applicable only to isolated cells and is not particularly useful for assessing viability of intestinal rings.

Microscopic observation of isolated cells and intestinal rings is necessary to confirm maintenance of normal morphology. Intestinal rings can be placed in Bovin–Dubosque fixative, embedded in paraffin, sectioned to 7-μm thickness, stained with hematoxylin and periodic acid-Schiff reagent (Humason, 1972), and observed by light microscopy (160×). Key observation factors indicative of altered morphology are loss of tissue color, nuclear swelling, and edema of the villi (appearance of larger than normal extracellular spaces). For morphological evaluation of isolated epithelial cells, electron microscopic techniques are necessary. Cells are pelleted by centrifugation and resuspended in Karnovsky's fixative in 0.1 M cacodylate buffer, pH 7.4. After fixing for 4 hr, the cells are washed overnight in the same buffer, postfixed for 2 hr in 1% OsO_4, dehydrated in ethanol, and embedded in Spurr Plastic. Thin sections are stained with uranyl acetate and lead citrate (Glauert, 1975) and observed by electron microscopy (10,000×). Cells should show normal morphology, including intact brush border region and lack of nuclear or mitochondrial swelling.

Although maintenance of morphological integrity is essential, biochemical and/or functional assays of transport are more indicative of true cell viability, including membrane integrity. In choosing which assay(s) to perform, it is important that the assay endpoint is one which will be modified by changes in viability. For example, although metabolism of various substrates can be used to indicate normal cell or tissue functioning, similar metabolic activity and profiles can often be measured in homogenates or subcellular fractions where an intact plasma membrane is not present. In this sense, metabolic assays to determine viability are not particularly useful unless activity is also dependent on an intact plasma membrane which retains its normal barrier and transport properties.

Glucose uptake and metabolism have classically been used to assess both transport and metabolic viability. Cells (10^6/ml) or intestinal rings (20–50 mg) are incubated in Krebs-Henseleit buffer, pH 7.4, at 37°C under an atmosphere of 95% O_2/5% CO_2 in the presence of 1 mM 3-O-methyl-[^{3}H]-D-glucose (3OMG) or 1 mM 1 [^{3}H]-L-glucose. Methods for quantitating accumulation of 3OMG are analogous to those used for measuring drug accumulation and will be discussed in detail later in this chapter. 3OMG is a nonmetabolized sugar which enters the cell via the apical membrane concentrative sodium-dependent sugar transporter (inhibited by 100 μM phlorizin) and exits the cell via the basolateral membrane facilitated diffusional transporter (inhibited by 100 μM phloretin). L-Glucose is not a substrate for the D-glucose-specific sugar transporters, and, therefore, accumulation or transport of L-glucose is indicative of compromised cell integrity. Examples of the response seen in cells and rings exhibiting acceptable viability are shown in Fig. 2, illustrating that L-glucose is only poorly accumulated compared to 3OMG (panel B, cells) and the accumulation of 3OMG is significantly inhibited by the presence of 0.5 mM phlorizin (panel B, cells; panel C, rings). Similar studies substituting phloretin for phlorizin would demonstrate increased cellular accumulation of 3OMG in viable cells (Kimmich, 1990) because phloretin inhibits the basolateral facilitated diffusion transporter responsible for egress of 3OMG from the cells.

A variety of other methods for assessing biochemical and transport viability of intestinal rings and isolated cells are available but will not be discussed here. These procedures are well documented in the literature, and a partial list includes glucose utilization and lactate production (Barker and Summerson, 1941; Stern, 1966), oxygen consumption (Stern, 1966), carbon dioxide production (Kelley and Chen, 1985), nucleotide accumulation (del Castillo, 1987), and amino acid uptake and incorporation into proteins (Weiser, 1973a).

4. EXPERIMENTAL TECHNIQUES FOR DRUG ABSORPTION MEASUREMENTS

Typical drug absorption studies with intestinal rings or isolated cells are described in this section. In the description provided, a simple drug uptake study is outlined. With both everted intestinal rings and isolated cells, various components may be added to the incubation solution to examine particular aspects of a drug absorption process. As examples, known inhibitors of active transport carriers can be included at concentrations 10-fold greater than their K_D to determine whether the drug of interest utilizes that particular carrier. Rings or cells can be preincubated for 10 min

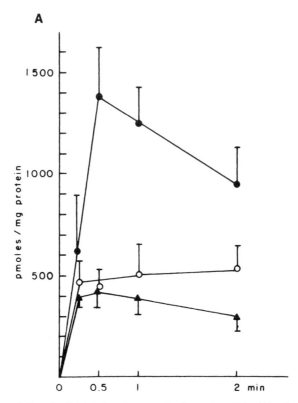

Figure 2.   Accumulation of radiolabeled D-glucose and L-glucose in vesicles (A) ●, 1 mM ³H-D-glucose; ○, 1 mM ³H-D-glucose, 0.5 mM phlorizin; ▲, 1 mM ³H-L-glucose; isolated intestinal cells (B) ●, 1 mM 3-O-methyl³-H-D-glucose; ○, 1 mM 3-O-methyl³-H-D-glucose; ▲, 1 mM ³H-L-glucose, and everted intestinal rings (C) ●, 1 mM 3-O-methyl-³H-D-glucose; ○, 1 mM 3-O-methyl-³H-D-glucose, 0.5 phlorizin. Results are means ± SD for *n* = 3 determinations. [Reproduced with permission from Osiecka *et al.* (1985).]

with 5 μM ouabain to determine whether drug accumulation is a sodium-dependent process. Ionic dependencies can be ascertained by varying ionic composition of the incubation medium (provided that isotonicity is maintained).

4.1.   Intestinal Rings

Everted intestinal rings (40–60 mg) are removed from cold storage buffer within 30 min of preparation and placed in a 12 mm × 75 mm glass culture tube containing 1 ml of 95% O_2/5% CO_2-saturated Krebs–Henseleit buffer containing selected concentrations (typically in the range of 0.1–10.0 mM) of the test drug with or without trace quantities (0.1 μCi) of ³H- or ¹⁴C-labeled drug. The use of radiolabeled substrates for

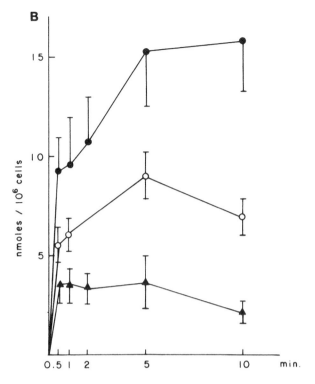

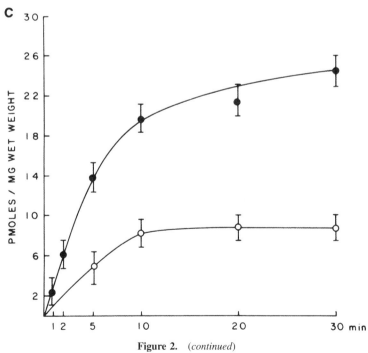

Figure 2. (*continued*)

uptake experiments is preferred since quantitation of drug uptake is greatly simplified compared to extraction and chemical analysis (e.g., HPLC methods). Additionally, because the total amount of drug accumulated in a 10-min incubation is generally small (e.g., less than 5% of that in the incubation solution), chemical methods often lack sufficient sensitivity. Incubations are performed at 37°C and 4°C with mild shaking for a maximum of 10 min. Previous studies have shown significant damage to everted rings if they are incubated at 37°C for times in excess of 20 min (Osiecka *et al.*, 1985). Rings can be removed from the incubation solution at earlier time points (e.g., 1, 2, 5, and 10 min) to establish a temporal profile of drug accumulation. For 37°C transport experiments, rings are preequilibrated to 37°C for 5 min immediately prior to being placed in the uptake solution, which is also at 37°C. Uptake is terminated by removing each ring from the incubation solution and quickly rinsing three times in ice-cold Krebs–Henseleit buffer and blotting dry with filter paper.

Processing of intestinal rings to permit quantitation of drug content depends, to a certain extent, on whether radioisotopic or chemical assays are being performed. For radioactive measurements, three general approaches are feasible: (i) homogenization of tissue, (ii) tissue combustion, and (iii) tissue solubilization.

Homogenization of intestinal rings with a variety of mechanical devices can be used with subsequent liquid scintillation counting of aliquots from the sample. Care should be exercised, and proper controls instituted, in correcting for possible quenching or fluorescence in the biologic sample which may alter counting efficiency.

Tissue combustion, utilizing an instrument such as the Packard model 306 Tissue Oxidizer, provides the most reproducible data from radioisotopic experiments. In this procedure, the entire ring (40–60 mg) is processed in the sample oxidizer, resulting in combustion of the radiolabeled substrate to radiolabeled CO_2 or H_2O (depending on the radioisotope employed) with nearly 100% counting efficiency and little if any quenching or fluorescence.

Tissue solubilization for radioactive materials can also be utilized although this approach is less efficient. In general, the ring is placed in a minimum volume of solubilizing agent [e.g., 1 N HCl or perchloric acid, 6 N KOH, or commercially available tissue solubilizing agents such as Scintigest (Fisher)] and incubated for 12–24 hr at ambient temperature to ensure complete digestion of the biologic tissue. Samples obtained from this procedure often possess significant coloration, which must be quenched (e.g., by hydrogen peroxide treatment) prior to scintillation counting.

When nonradioactive drugs are used in intestinal ring studies, assay of drug content obviously depends on chemical analysis. Of the methods described above for measurement of radioactivity, only tissue combustion is unacceptable for use if chemical analysis is to be performed. In the case of HPLC analysis, the general procedures for tissue homogenization or tissue solubilization can be utilized provided the composition of the final phase (e.g., physiologic buffer with homogenization or strong acid/base with tissue solubilization) is compatible with the HPLC procedure being utilized. Some effort will undoubtedly have to be expended in extracting the drug from the biologic medium and preparing it for HPLC analysis. It is not the intent in this chapter to provide a detailed discussion of various HPLC or other analytical procedures. In many cases, methods which are suitable for extraction and analysis of drug from biologic fluid are also amenable to use with homogenized or solubilized tissue preparations.

Since everted rings include a significant amount of nonepithelial tissue, estimations of nonspecific binding and extracellular fluid are required. Standard techniques (Rosenberg *et al.*, 1962) employing impermeant markers, such as radiolabeled inulin, can be used to determine the fraction of accumulated drug that is trapped in extracellular fluid.

One example of the data which may be obtained from everted intestinal ring studies is shown in Fig. 3. The relative uptakes of the four compounds (propranolol > salicylate > cimetidine > PEG 4000) are consistent with known *in vivo* absorptions of these compounds.

4.2. Isolated Intestinal Mucosal Cells

Aliquots (0.9 ml) of isolated intestinal cells (at least 10^6 cells/ml) are placed in ice-cold 12 mm × 75 mm glass culture tubes and maintained on ice until initiation of uptake studies. Prior to initiation of uptake studies which will be performed at 37°C, culture tubes are transferred to a shaking water bath at 37°C for 5 min. Drug uptake is initiated by adding 100 μl of drug solution (10-fold concentrated) to the cell suspension. Ideally, this drug concentrate should utilize the same buffer as the incubation solution. Incubations may be conducted for up to 60 min at 37°C or 4°C without significant damage to isolated cells, although in many cases, particularly active transport systems, the initial rates of uptake may be more informative. Incubation tubes should be maintained in an atmosphere of O_2/CO_2 and provided with sufficient mixing to ensure a uniform suspension of cells. For very short incubation times (e.g., less than 10 min), capping the incubation tubes should be sufficient for maintaining oxygenation of the buffer. For longer incubation times, the use of a manifold gas distribution apparatus is recommended.

Termination of drug uptake experiments in isolated cell preparations generally involves either rapid filtration or centrifugation. Direct centrifugation of cell suspensions at $300 × g$ for 3 min will provide a soft pellet from which the supernatant may be aspirated. Time is critical with this termination step because the loose cell pellet will retain contact with the supernatant drug solution and a certain amount of drug-containing fluid will be trapped as extracellular fluid in the pellet. The amount of drug nonspecifically trapped in the extracellular fluid of the cell pellet can be estimated as described for intestinal rings.

A modified centrifugal termination of isolated cell suspension experiments alleviates some of the concerns associated with direct centrifugation. Small aliquots

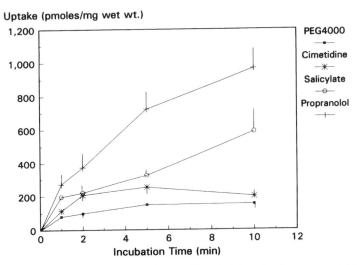

Figure 3. Accumulation of radiolabeled drug in everted intestinal rings. Results are means ± SD for $n = 4$ determinations. All drugs were added at a final concentration of 1 mM.

(50–100 μl) of the incubation solution can be layered onto a 50-μl "cushion" in the bottom of a 400-μl microcentrifuge tube. Some practice is required to ensure that the interface between the two liquids is not broken during the layering process. The cushion can be either 12% sucrose with 2.5% bovine serum albumin (Osiecka *et al.*, 1985) or a 3:2 v/v mixture of di-*n*-butyl phthalate/di-*n*-nonyl phthalate. This preparation is then centrifuged at 13,000 × *g* for 20–30 sec. With this adaptation, the cells will pellet below the sucrose/albumin or oil layer and effectively be washed free of extracellular fluid or loose nonspecifically adsorbed drug as they pass through the layer. This results in a cleaner cell pellet which can be lysed, solubilized, or resuspended for analysis of drug content.

Rapid filtration is another common method used to terminate drug uptake studies with isolated cell suspensions. Since this method affords very rapid separation of cells from the incubation medium, it is particularly useful for initial uptake rate studies. Aliquots of the incubation mixture are removed and quickly added to Whatman GF/C glass microfiber filters on a filter manifold under pressure. The samples are filtered under vacuum (approximately 80 kPa pressure) and washed 2–3 times with cold buffer. The filters can then be removed and placed directly in scintillation cocktail for radioactive determination. When nonradiolabeled drugs are used, filters can be placed in distilled water and sonicated to lyse cells and release the drug content. Detergents (e.g., Triton X-100) can also be used to solubilize cells retained on the filters prior to drug determination.

With either termination procedure (centrifugation or filtration) for isolated intestinal cells, control experiments must be performed to verify that the separation procedure itself does not cause cell lysis and loss of drug content. This is a particular concern for the filtration method, where the use of an excessive pressure to facilitate filtration can cause physical disruption of the cells and subsequent loss of drug in the filtrate. Cells can be resuspended from a centrifugation pellet or gently rinsed from a filter with cold physiologic buffer and examined microscopically. The presence of significant cellular debris may be indicative of cell damage which might compromise the validity of results. A more exacting method prior to conducting drug transport studies is to validate the isolation procedures using a well-absorbed radiolabeled marker (e.g., 3-O-methyl-[^{3}H]glucose). In this case, a series of identical culture tubes are prepared and incubated with a known concentration of radiolabeled 3OMG. Isolation and termination parameters can then be varied (e.g., centrifugation times vs. speeds and filtration pressures vs. cell number) to identify those conditions which provide the optimal results in terms of drug retention.

5. ADVANTAGES, LIMITATIONS, AND POTENTIAL APPLICATIONS OF RINGS AND CELLS IN QUANTITATING DRUG TRANSPORT

The most obvious advantage of using everted intestinal rings for drug accumulation studies is the inherent simplicity of the system. Only inexpensive, common laboratory equipment is required, and investigators can become comfortable with the procedure with only a few attempts. Few systems offer the potential for obtaining relevant data on drug accumulation with so little technical expertise being required. The isolation and experimental procedures for intestinal cells are technically more difficult than those needed for rings and do require some surgical expertise as well as specialized laboratory equipment (e.g., centrifuges, filtering manifolds, etc.). The time required to optimize these procedures also is significantly greater than that needed for rings, especially because of the time required to become proficient at techniques which result in acceptable cell viability.

An additional advantage of both the ring and cell models is the ability to carefully control experimental conditions. Components may be added to or deleted from the incubation buffer to test particular parameters which may affect the drug transport process. As mentioned previously, active transport systems can be evaluated by inclusion of specific inhibitors of known carrier systems (e.g., amino acid, bile salt, vitamin). Ionic influences on drug absorption can also be evaluated by varying buffer composition. This ability to control the experimental conditions affords the opportunity to design studies which probe the mechanistic aspects of drug absorption. This type of information is not readily available from *in vivo* studies and can assist in understanding the absorption characteristics of drugs with various structural features.

Intestinal rings afford an added advantage in being reasonably resistant to modifications in the incubation buffer. Studies have shown that the pH of the incubation solution may be adjusted from pH 5.5 to pH 8.5 without significant damage to intestinal rings (Leppert and Fix, 1994). Low concentrations of co-solvents (e.g., up to 10% DMSO or ethanol) may also be used to improve drug solubility.

The ring and cell models each have one unique disadvantage which must be recognized in order to properly evaluate absorption data. Everted rings are small segments of the intestinal tissue in which the "cut" ends of the segment may constitute a significant portion of the total tissue mass. These are areas where nonspecific drug adsorption or absorption may occur. The use of impermeant markers to estimate this nonspecific absorption, which is unrelated to transport across the intact epithelium, can be used to correct for this possible effect. With isolated intestinal cells, the loss of cell polarity in the isolation procedure is the major disadvantage. The apical brush border region of epithelial cells is the primary pathway for *in vivo* drug absorption. However, when cell suspensions are prepared, the entire cell surface becomes available for drug absorption. Therefore, it is not possible to strictly determine whether drug accumulation in isolated epithelial cells is occurring from the apical or from the basolateral direction. Care should also be exercised in assuming that previously localized active transport systems (i.e., systems known to occur only in apical or basolateral membrane domains *in vivo*) have remained as such in an isolated cell suspension (Albers and Moore, 1994). The physical and biological parameters that control distribution of membrane carriers may change once cell-to-cell contacts are lost.

Both intestinal rings and isolated cell suspensions are characterized by relatively low drug accumulation, primarily due to limited intracellular volumes. Because of this, inadequate sensitivity in chemical analysis of drug content can be a limiting factor. Where possible, the use of radiolabeled substrates offers a significant advantage in both uptake models because it allows reproducible quantitation, with adequate sensitivity, to be achieved.

Everted rings or isolated cells have proven to be useful models for evaluating several aspects of drug transport, provided that drug accumulation is adjusted for nonspecific adsorption and drug contamination in extracellular fluid. Perhaps the most meaningful data obtainable from isolated cell and everted ring experiments are relative comparisons of drug accumulation. Certainly, carrier-mediated transport can be determined using substrate inhibition of radiolabeled drug uptake. Both models are also useful for providing a relative ranking of the permeabilities of compounds possessing various physicochemical properties (Leppert and Fix, 1994). Given the inherent simplicity of both *in vitro* models, isolated intestinal cells and everted rings may best serve for initial screening of drug absorption and to identify factors which can be utilized to modify drug absorption.

REFERENCES

Agar, W. T., Hird, F. J. R., and Sidhu, G. S., 1954, The uptake of amino acids by the intestine, *Biochim. Biophys. Acta* **14**:80–84.

Albers, T., and Moore, R., 1994, Isolation temperatures affect distribution of polarized membrane proteins in isolated intestinal epithelial cells, *Gastroenterology* **106:**A218.

Barker, S. B., and Summerson, W. H., 1941, The colorimetric determination of lactic acid in biological material, *J. Biol. Chem.* **138:**535–554.

BreMiller, R. A., 1961, Attempt to separate cells of the gastric mucosa, *Gastroenterology* **40:**798–802.

Dahlquist, A., 1961, *Methods Enzymol.* **8:**584–591.

Del Castillo, J. R., 1987, The use of hyperosmolar, intracellular-like solutions for the isolation of epithelial cells from guinea-pig small intestine, *Biochim. Biophys. Acta* **901:**201–208.

Del Castillo, J. R., and Muniz, R., 1991, Neutral amino acid transport by isolated small intestinal cells from guinea pigs, *Am. J. Physiol.* **261:**G1030–G1036.

Fleisher, D., Sheth, N., Griffin, H., McFadden, M., and Aspacher, G., 1989, Nutrient influences on rat intestinal phenytoin uptake, *Pharm. Res.* **6:**332–337.

Glauert, A. M. (ed.), 1975, *Practical Methods in Electron Microscopy*, North-Holland, Amsterdam.

Gore, J., and Hoinard, C., 1993, Linolenic acid transport in hamster intestinal cells is carrier-mediated, *J. Nutr.* **123:**66–73.

Grafstrom, R., Moldeus, P., Andersson, B., and Orrenius, S., 1979, Xenobiotic metabolism by isolated rat small intestinal cells, *Med. Biol.* **57:**287–293.

Harber, D. S., Stern, B. K., and Reilly, R. W., 1964, Removal and dissociation of epithelial cells from the rodent gastrointestinal tract, *Nature* **203:**319–320.

Harrison, D. D., and Webster, H. L., 1969, The preparation of isolated intestinal crypt cells, *Exp. Cell Res.* **55:**257–260.

Hartmann, F., Owen, R., and Bissell, D. M., 1982, Characterization of isolated epithelial cells from rat small intestine, *Am. J. Physiol.* **242:**G147–G155.

Huang, K. C., 1965, Uptake of L-tyrosine and 3-O-methylglucose by isolated intestinal epithelial cells, *Life Sci.* **4:**1201–1206.

Hulsmann, W. C., Van den Berg, J. W. O., and De Jonge, H. R., 1974, *Methods Enzym.* **32:**665–673.

Humason, G. L. (ed.), 1972, *Animal Tissue Techniques*, W. H. Freeman and Company, San Francisco.

Kajii, H., Horie, T., Hayashi, M., and Awazu, S., 1985, Fluorescence study on the interaction of salicylate with rat small intestinal epithelial cells: Possible mechanism for the promoting effects of salicylate on drug absorption *in vivo*, *Life Sci.* **37:**523–530.

Kelley, M. J., and Chen, T. S., 1985, Action of 5-thio-D-glucose on D-glucose metabolism: Possible mechanism for diabetogenic effect, *J. Pharmacol. Exp. Ther.* **232:**760–763.

Kimmich, G. A., 1990, *Methods Enzymol.* **192:**324–340.

Koster, A. S., Borm, P. J. A., Dohmen, M. R., and Noordhoek, J., 1984, Localization of biotransformational enzymes along the crypt–villus axis of the rat intestine. Evaluation of two cell isolation procedures, *Cell Biochem. Function* **2:**95–101.

Leppert, P. S., and Fix, J. A., 1994, Use of everted intestinal rings for *in vitro* examination of oral absorption potential, *J. Pharm. Sci.* **83:**976–981.

Matthews, D. M., and Burston, D., 1984, Uptake of a series of neutral dipeptides including L-alanyl-L-alanine, glycylglycine and glycylsarcosine by hamster jejunum *in vitro*, *Clin. Sci.* **67:**541–549.

Meadows, K. C., and Dressman, J. B., 1990, Mechanism of acyclovir uptake in rat jejunum, *Pharm. Res.* **7:**299–303.

Osiecka, I., Porter, P. A., Borchardt, R. T., Fix, J. A., and Gardner, C. R., 1985, *In vitro* drug absorption models. I. Brush border membrane vesicles, isolated mucosal cells and everted intestinal rings: Characterization and salicylate accumulation, *Pharm. Res.* **6:**284–293.

Osiecka, I., Cortese, M., Porter, P. A., Borchardt, R. T., Fix, J. A., and Gardner, C. R., 1987, Intestinal absorption of α-methyldopa: *In vivo* mechanistic studies in rat small intestinal segments, *J. Pharmacol. Exp. Ther.* **242:**443–449.

Porter, P. A., Osiecka, I., Borchardt, R. T., Fix, J. A., Frost, L., and Gardner, C., 1985, *In vitro* drug absorption models. II. Salicylate, cefoxitin, α-methyldopa and theophylline uptake in cells and rings: Correlation with *in vivo* bioavailability, *Pharm. Res.* **6:**293–298.

Rosenberg, L., Downing, S., and Segal, L., 1962, Extracellular space estimation in rat kidney slices using ^{14}C-saccharides and phlorizin, *Am. J. Physiol.* **202**:800–804.

Sepulveda, F. V., Burton, K. A., and Brown, P. D., 1982, Relation between sodium-coupled amino acid and sugar transport and sodium/potassium pump activity in isolated intestinal epithelial cells, *J. Cell. Physiol.* **111**:303–308.

Shaw, R. D., Li, B. U. K., Hamilton, J. W., Shug, A. L., and Olsen, W. A., 1983, Carnitine transport in rat small intestine, *Am. J. Physiol.* **245**:G376–G381.

Stern, B. K., 1966, Some biochemical properties of suspensions of intestinal epithelial cells, *Gastroenterology* **51**:855–867.

Tsuji, A., Hirooka, H., Tamai, I., and Terasaki, T., 1986, Evidence for a carrier-mediated transport system in the small intestine available for FK089, a new cephalosporin antibiotic without an amino group, *J. Antibiot.* **34**:1592–1597.

Tsuji, A., Hirooka, H., Terasaki, T., Tamai, I., and Nakashima, E., 1987, Saturable uptake of cefixime, a new oral cephalosporin without an α-amino group, by the rat intestine, *J. Pharm. Pharmacol.* **39**:272–277.

Weiser, M. M., 1973a, Intestinal epithelial cell surface membrane glycoprotein synthesis. I. An indicator of cellular differentiation, *J. Biol. Chem.* **248**:2536–2541.

Weiser, M. M., 1973b, Intestinal epithelial cell surface membrane glycoprotein synthesis. II. Glycosyltransferases and endogenous acceptors of the undifferentiated cell surface membrane, *J. Biol. Chem.* **248**:2542–2548.

Westergaard, H., and Dietschy, J. M., 1976, The mechanism whereby bile acid micelles increase the rate of fatty acid and cholesterol uptake into the intestinal mucosal cell, *J. Clin. Invest.* **58**:97–108.

Chapter 5

Models of Drug Absorption *in Situ* and in Conscious Animals

Robin Griffiths, Ann Lewis, and Phillip Jeffrey

1. INTRODUCTION

A variety of techniques have been used to bridge the gap between overtly *in vitro* models of drug absorption and studies in an animal population. These vary from the simplest isolated gut loop methods, in which depletion of drug from the lumen is monitored, to sophisticated systems in which the physiological variables such as blood flow, gut content, and gut function are either directly controlled or are held constant. The feature common to these experiments is that the gut remains *in situ* in the anesthetized animal so that the normal function is perturbed as little as possible. With use of the appropriate preparation, it is possible to examine the functionally intact intestine with access to both luminal and serosal sides.

However, data generated from isolated perfused gut loops *in situ* (or *in vitro*) do not always accurately reflect the situation in the intact whole animal. There are many potentially confounding variables *in vivo*. For example, splanchnic blood flow is naturally variable and is decreased under anesthesia. Also, in the conscious animal there is a time-dependent aspect of drug presentation to the absorptive surface throughout the length of the gut which involves the drug experiencing different environmental conditions [pH, mucus complement, varying gut wall metabolic enzyme concentrations (Hartiala, 1973)], and indeed different functional anatomy [proportion of mucosal tissue, surface area (Robinson *et al.*, 1977)].

When absorption is studied in the whole animal, it is necessary to be able to

Robin Griffiths, Ann Lewis, and Phillip Jeffrey • SmithKline Beecham Pharmaceuticals, DMPK, The Frythe, Welwyn, Herts AL6 9AR, United Kingdom.

Models for Assessing Drug Absorption and Metabolism, Ronald T. Borchardt *et al.*, eds., Plenum Press, New York, 1996.

differentiate between absorption (drug availability) to the hepatic portal blood and to the blood of the systemic circulation, in order to quantify the contributions of malabsorption *per se* and first-pass elimination in the gut wall and the liver. To this end, a number of chronic cannulation procedures have been developed, allowing drug delivery to, and blood sampling from, central and peripheral veins.

2. *IN SITU* ABSORPTION MODELS

A wide variety of isolated gut loop techniques are used, primarily in rodents, in the study of drug absorption and/or metabolism. The various techniques can be classified as follows.

2.1. Cannulation of the Lumen Only

2.1.1. STATIC METHOD

The static method is often referred to as the "Doluisio method," after the work of Doluisio *et al.* (1969). It involves simple cannulation of a segment of the gut lumen of the anesthetized rat; the blood and nervous supply to the gut are left intact as far as possible. Usually, a syringe is attached to cannulas at either end of the gut segment in order for repeated samples of the luminal contents to be taken for assay. The technique has the advantage of great simplicity and can give good results, especially when care is taken to compensate for water flux. However, "absorption" is necessarily measured only as the disappearance of drug from the gut lumen, and it is often difficult to distinguish between binding to the gut wall, metabolic degradation, and precipitation of drug in the segment.

2.1.2. SINGLE-PASS AND CONTINUOUS LOOP PERFUSION METHODS

The static method has been extended by several authors to include single-pass perfusion of the lumen. For example, Lewis and Fordtran (1975) investigated the effects of flow rate, surface area, permeability, and intraluminal pressure on glucose, mannitol, and urea absorption in the rat ileum. Recirculating perfusion of the lumen has also been used to study these rate-limiting factors (Higuchi *et al.*, 1981).

Yorgey *et al.* (1986) modified the preparation to include both portal and jugular vein blood sampling, allowing for a more complete pharmacokinetic analysis of the absorption and presystemic metabolism of haloperidol, tolmetin sodium, and fenoctimine sulfate.

2.2. Cannulation of the Lumen with Blood Replacement

A more completely definitive experiment is possible if the blood supply to and from the segment of gut is artificially controlled. The venous drainage of a small intestinal loop can be collected via a single mesenteric vein and continually replaced with fresh heparinized whole rat blood which is constantly infused from a reservoir via the saphenous vein or appropriate mesenteric artery (Windmueller and Spaeth, 1981). This "autoperfusion" method using whole fresh rat blood ensures that the homeostasis of the gut tissue is maintained and that the experimental conditions remain constant. As samples are available from both the serosal and luminal sides of the gut, the rates of drug absorption (calculated from the rate of appearance of drug in the blood) and metabolism can be determined. A similar technique was employed by Blanchard *et al.* (1989) to study carbenoxolone absorption.

The effects of different methods of lumen perfusion (closed loop, single-pass, recirculating, and oscillating perfusion) on theophylline availability to the systemic circulation have been investigated by Schurgers *et al.* (1986) using rat donor blood infused via the jugular vein. These techniques suffer from the disadvantage of only being suitable for relatively small gut segments (approximately 10 cm), since the gut loop size is limited by the single mesenteric vein drainage and the need for large supplies of fresh whole rat blood.

2.3. Cannulation of the Lumen and Vascular Bed

This group of techniques can be divided into two procedures:

1. The lumen and vascular bed are cannulated, and the gut segment is displaced and maintained in an organ bath.
2. The lumen and vascular bed are cannulated, and the gut is left *in situ.*

In both preparations the vascular bed is cannulated via the superior mesenteric artery for vascular perfusate supply and via the hepatic portal vein for vascular perfusate drainage. Some examples of the perfusions, types of vascular perfusates, and applications are summarized in Table I.

The success of vascularly perfused intestinal preparations is dependent upon maintaining a permanent and sufficient oxygen supply to the mucosal cells. Preparations without suitable oxygen carrier in the vascular perfusate will not maintain their functional and structural integrity. The simplest solution is the use of donor rat blood, but this approach requires several rats to be exsanguinated as blood donors. Also, the blood may not be metabolically inert and may therefore complicate metabolism studies.

Table I

Some Examples of the Application of Isolated Perfused Rat Gut Loops
in Situ and *in Vivo* and the Types of Vascular Perfusate Used

Perfusate	Type of perfusion[a]	Drug investigated	Reference
Donor rat blood	OB	—[b]	Windmueller *et al.*, 1970
	OB	Antipyrine, urea, salicylic acid	Ochsenfahrt, 1979
	OB	Paracetamol, salicylamide	Sakai *et al.*, 1980
	IS	Carbenoxolone	Blanchard *et al.*, 1989
Outdated human	IS	Paracetamol	Pang *et al.*, 1986
erythrocytes	IS	Enalapril	Pang *et al.*, 1985
	IS	—[b]	Hirayama *et al.*, 1989
Bovine erythrocytes	IS	—[b]	Hanson and Parsons, 1976
	IS	Buprenorphine	Castle *et al.*, 1985
	IS	—[b]	Nicholls *et al.*, 1983
Perfluorocarbon	OB	1-Naphthol	De Vries *et al.*, 1989a,b
emulsion (FC-43)	OB	Theophylline	De Vries *et al.*, 1989c
	OB	Ethoxyresorufin, 1-naphthol	Hartmann *et al.*, 1984
	OB	Antipyrine, salicylic acid	Takahashi *et al.*, 1988
	IS	β-Lactam antibiotics	Miyazaki *et al.*, 1986

[a]OB, *in vitro* perfusion, the lumen and vascular bed are cannulated, and the gut is removed and placed in an organ bath; IS, the lumen and vascular bed are cannulated, and the gut is left *in situ*.
[b]Methodological paper; no specific drugs were investigated.

Physiological saline (Krebs and Henseleit, 1932) containing albumin and either washed human or bovine erythrocytes to improve oxygen transport capacity is a simple, easy and cheap alternative to donor rat blood. However, despite the proven advantages of the system (Table I), several workers have experienced problems with it (Hartmann *et al.*, 1984; Takahashi *et al.*, 1988; De Vries *et al.*, 1989b), such as erythrocyte aggregation causing interruption of blood flow, hemolysis, and an uneven distribution of oxygen-carrying erythrocytes in different regions of the microvasculature. Hypersecretion, hypermotility, water flux, and low vasculature resistance are other complications arising from the use of erythrocyte-containing preparations, but these can be avoided by addition of dexamethasone and noradrenaline to the vascular perfusate (Windmueller *et al.*, 1970) or by the optimization of vascular perfusate albumin concentration and the use of a lumen distension pressure (Castle *et al.*, 1985).

The perfluorocarbon perfluorotributylamine (FC-34), emulsified with the pluronic polyol Pluronic F-68 to form an FC-43 emulsion, has been used as an alternative to erythrocyte-based vascular perfusates for isolated perfused rat gut loops (Table I) as well as for maintaining "bloodless" rats *in vivo* (Geyer, 1975). Perfluorobutylamine has a small particle size, < 6 μm, is chemically inert, has a linear oxygen dissociation curve, and is therefore an ideal oxygen carrier (Hartmann *et al.*, 1984). The use of this type of oxygen carrier does not require the addition of noradrenaline (used to prevent hypermotility and hypersecretion) to the vascular perfusate (De Vries *et al.*, 1989b). However, care must be taken in preparing the emulsion. The fluorocarbon is dispersed by sonication in the presence of the polyol, and this procedure must be done at low temperature (0–5°C) with thorough gassing of the reagents with CO_2 prior to and during sonication. This process provides an inert atmosphere, facilitates emulsification, and prevents the formation of fluoride ions which could contaminate the vascular perfusate (Geyer, 1975).

2.4. Simultaneous Perfusion of the Rat Small Intestine and Liver

The rat intestine and liver are arranged serially; arterial blood enters the small intestine via the superior mesenteric artery and leaves via the hepatic portal vein, which, together with the hepatic artery, perfuses the liver. The anatomical placement of these organs is such that simultaneous perfusion of both organs, with sampling via the portal vein and the collection of bile, enables the contribution of both the liver and the intestine to the overall elimination of a drug to be assessed in the same preparation. Further modification of such a preparation would also enable enterohepatic circulation to be investigated. Perfusion of the entire rat small intestine (duodenum, jejunum, and ileum) in series with the liver (Fig. 1) has been used to investigate the absorption and metabolism of [^{14}C]enalapril (Pang *et al.*, 1985). Combined small intestine/liver perfusion was performed in recirculating mode using a vascular perfusate containing outdated human erythrocytes, at a flow rate of 10 ml/min; the liver was perfused via the portal vein. A more physiologically realistic method, involving dual perfusion of the liver via the hepatic artery (2.5 ml/min) and the hepatic portal vein (7.5 ml/min), was developed by Hirayama *et al.* (1989) and used in studies of the first-pass metabolism of salicylamide (Xu *et al.*, 1989). Although this preparation represents the blood supply *in vivo*, the method requires cannulation of the hepatic artery as well as the superior mesenteric artery. Cannulation of the hepatic artery is via the celiac plexus, which has three branches—the left gastric artery (supplying the stomach), the splenic artery, which has branches to the stomach and pancreas, and the hepatic artery, which has branches to the stomach and duodenum (Greene, 1963). Extreme care is therefore needed to ensure occlusion of all these branches; failure to do so will result in an underperfusion of the liver and an overperfusion of the intestine.

2.5. Assessment of the Viability of Perfusion Systems

In any perfusion system it is essential to maintain the organ or tissue in a viable state to ensure accurate and reproducible results. Ideally, to fully investigate drug absorption and/or metabolism in perfused gut loops, the preparation should provide

A

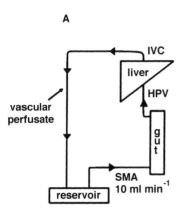

B

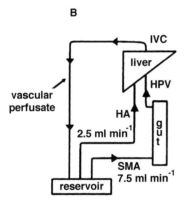

Figure 1. Schematic illustration of recirculating small intestine–liver perfusions. In preparation A the liver is perfused via the hepatic portal vein only (Pang *et al.*, 1985). In preparation B the liver is perfused via the hepatic artery and the hepatic portal vein (Hirayama *et al.*, 1989). Abbreviations: IVC, Inferior vena cava; HPV, hepatic portal vein; HA, hepatic artery; SMA, superior mesenteric artery.

the opportunity to examine the functionally intact intestinal mucosa with access to the luminal, vascular, and serosal sides, without the interference of uncontrolled neuronal and hormonal effects, metabolic products of other organs, or cellular components of the vascular perfusate (e.g., plasma esterases).

The isolated perfused gut loop should fulfill the following criteria: (i) structural integrity as assessed by light and transmission electron microscopy; (ii) maintenance of an intact vascular and microvascular bed; (iii) absence of arrhythmic contractions; (iv) absence of significant secretion of water and electrolytes into the lumen; and (v) maintenance of aerobic metabolism (i.e., as reflected by lactate/pyruvate ratio).

Using donor rat blood as the vascular perfusate, Sakai *et al.* (1980) maintained viability for up to 2 hr as indicated by vascular perfusate pressure, tissue glucose and oxygen consumption, lack of Evans blue absorption by the jejunum, and histological examination of the jejunum after perfusion. Windmueller *et al.* (1970) maintained viability for up to 5 hr by adding noradrenaline and dexamethasone to the vascular perfusate of donor rat blood. Viability was assessed by tissue oxygen consumption and motility, water transport, lymph flow, and electron microscopic examination of the jejunum at the end of the perfusion. Castle *et al.* (1985), using washed bovine erythrocytes as vascular perfusate, assessed viability on the basis of the parameters of oxygen consumption, glucose utilization, dry weight:wet weight ratios, vascular perfusate flow rate, and net water flux as well as by histological examination of the jejunum after perfusion using light microscopy. They found that the preparation was viable for 60 min. Nicholls *et al.* (1983), using a similar perfusate, maintained viability for 45 min based on oxygen consumption and glucose utilization.

Hartmann *et al.* (1984) and De Vries *et al.* (1989a), using an FC-43 emulsion as vascular perfusate, validated their perfused rat gut preparations according to the criteria of rate of glucose utilization and lactate production, lactate/pyruvate ratio, oxygen utilization, and perfusion pressure. The preparation was considered to be viable for 3 hr. In contrast, Miyazaki *et al.* (1986), using the same vascular perfusate and the competitive inhibition of L-phenylalanine absorption by L-methionine, the transport of L-phenylalanine against a concentration gradient, and assessment of jejunal morphology using scanning electron microscopy, observed that their preparation was valid for only 60 min.

A combined small intestine/liver preparation was fully validated for up to 2 hr by Hirayama *et al.* (1989) using [^{14}C]glucose absorption (against a concentration gradient), lack of [^{3}H]-PEG 4000 and Evans blue absorption into the small intestine during perfusion, constant perfusion pressure, bile flow, hemoglobin concentration, and evidence of glucose utilization by the intestine and production by the liver.

3. ABSORPTION ASSESSMENT IN CONSCIOUS ANIMALS

The final measure of "absorption" in the whole animal is the availability of orally (or intragut) administered drug to the systemic circulation. However, this pragmatic measure alone carries little information as to the sequential mechanisms involved in the success or failure of the drug formulation. In order to quantify the contributions of malabsorption, lymphatic absorption, or first-pass elimination to oral bioavailability in the conscious animal, it is necessary to be able to deliver drug directly to the gut, the hepatic portal system, and the peripheral vasculature. In addition, blood samples should be available from the portal blood as well as systemically, and lymph samples should be available from the mesenteric lymph flow. These procedures involve the use of cannulae chronically implanted in conscious animals: the most useful cannulations are to the vena cava (via the femoral vein), jugular vein, hepatic portal vein, and duodenum. The vena cava cannula is used for intravenous (i.v.) drug delivery, the jugular cannula for blood sampling, and the portal cannula for delivery or sampling, depending on the nature of the study.

As these preparations are chronic (with the exception of lymphatic cannulation), and usually involve studies of crossover design, it is essential that the physiological status of the animal is maintained constant. The principal difficulty in this regard is local inflammation around the site of implantation of the cannula, perhaps giving rise to a frank phlebitis. This may give rise to cannula blockage or thrombus formation. However, a much less obvious consequence can be a large increase in acute-phase proteins in the blood. Yasuhara *et al.* (1985) have shown that the increases in plasma α_1-acid glycoprotein resulting from cannula-induced phlebitis were sufficient to dramatically alter the pharmacokinetics of propranolol. The cannula designs and procedures listed below were specifically designed to avoid inflammation, and these methods have been shown to have no significant effect on propranolol kinetics or plasma acute phase proteins.

3.1. Surgical Techniques

3.1.1. ANIMAL CARE

Surgery in all species is carried out under general anesthesia (Table II). In the dog and rabbit, surgical implantation of cannulae is conducted using sterile techniques. Although less stringent procedures are possible for rodent surgery, it is necessary to sterilize all cannulae in advance and to minimize the risk of infection by soaking all instruments in antiseptic. Immediately before surgery, an analgesic (Table II) is administered, and post surgery antibiotic (Table II) is given. In those procedures which involve laparotomy in the rodent species (or any surgical procedure in the guinea pig), a 5% (w/v) solution of dextrose in water is administered over a period of 48 hr after surgery via the hepatic portal vein or jugular vein in order to supplement the animal's diet during recovery. Anticoagulants should be avoided while the peritoneal wound is healing.

3.1.2. CANNULA INSERTION

The cannulae were constructed from polyethylene and silastic tubing (Tables III and IV). All cannulae are filled with sterile saline (0.9% w/v) prior to insertion into the vessel. Following implantation, each cannula is either externalized at the nape of the neck (rat, mouse, gerbil, guinea pig) by means of a trocar or connected to a vascular access port implanted subcutaneously in the flank of the animal (dog, rabbit, monkey). The rodent species are placed in jackets which support a protective metal tether through which the cannulae are passed. The end of the tether is anchored by means of a swivel in order to give the animal free movement around the cage (Fig. 3).

Table II
Surgical Implantation of Cannulae in Various Species:
Anesthetics, Analgesics, and Antibiotics Administered

Species	Procedure[a]	Anesthetic	Analgesic (dose)[b]	Antibiotic (dose)[c,d]
Rat	iv	Halothane/O_2 or isoflurane/O_2	Zenecarp (0.1 ml)	Penbritin (15 mg/100 g, im)
	ipv, id	Halothane/O_2 or isoflurane/O_2	Zenecarp (0.1 ml)	Penbritin (15 mg/100 g, im, ip)
Mouse	iv	Tribromoethanol	Zenecarp (0.01 ml)	Penbritin (2.5 mg/25 g, im)
	ipv, id	Tribromoethanol	Zenecarp (0.01 ml)	Penbritin (2.5 mg/25 g, im, ip)
Gerbil	iv	Isoflurane/O_2	Zenecarp (0.01 ml)	Penbritin (15 mg/100 g, im)
	ipv, id	Isoflurane/O_2	Zenecarp (0.01 ml)	Penbritin (15 mg/100 g, im, ip)
Guinea pig	iv, ipv	Halothane or isoflurane	Zenecarp (0.1 ml)	Tribrissen 24% (0.2 ml/kg, sc)
Rabbit	iv, ipv	Hypnorm/midazolam/ isoflurane/O_2[e]	Zenecarp (0.25 ml)	Tribrissen 24% (0.2 ml/kg, sc, 3 days)
Dog	iv, ipv, id	Halothane/NO/O_2	Temgesic (0.5 ml)/ Zenecarp (1.0 ml/12.5 kg)	Tribrissen 24% (1.0 ml/8 kg, iv and po, 3 days)
Monkey	iv, ipv	Isoflurane/O_2	Banamine	Tribrissen 24% (0.2 ml/kg, sc, 3 days)

[a]Abbreviations: iv, Intravenous; ipv, intra-hepatic portal vein; id, intraduodenal.
[b]Zenecarp, 5% carprofen in benzyl alcohol; Banamine, flunixin meglutamine salt.
[c]Penbritin, ampicillin sodium BP; Tribrissen, 24% sulfadiazine and trimethoprim BP (Vet).
[d]Abbreviations: im, Intramuscular; ip, intraperitoneal; sc, subcutaneous; po, oral.
[e]Ventilated.

When not in use, the cannulas are filled with sterile heparin solution [100 international units (IU)/ml] and sealed. The vascular access ports are filled with sterile heparin solution (500 IU/ml). All cannulas are flushed at least once every 2 days to maintain patency, and the vascular access ports are flushed weekly.

3.1.3. FEMORAL VEIN/VENA CAVA CANNULATION (RAT, MOUSE, GERBIL, RABBIT, MONKEY)

An incision is made in the inner thigh in order to expose the femoral vein. The vein is then cleared of tissue and ligated. Gentle tension is applied to the vein using the ligature, and a small hole is cut in the top of the vein so that a cannula can be inserted and pushed up so that the tip enters the vena cava. The cannula is then tied in position

Table III
Surgical Implantation of Cannulae: Equipment Specifications and Suppliers

Equipment[a]	Code	Size	Supplier
Polyethylene cannula	a	0.28 mm i.d., 0.61 mm o.d.	Portex Ltd., Hythe, Kent, UK
Polyethylene cannula	b	0.4 mm i.d., 0.8 mm o.d.	Portex Ltd., Hythe, Kent, UK
Polyethylene low-density cannula	c	0.2 mm i.d., 0.3 mm o.d.	Advanced Polymers, Salem, MA
Silastic cannula	d	0.020 in. i.d., 0.037 in. o.d.	Dow Corning Corp., Medical Products, Midland, MI
Silastic cannula	e	0.012 in. i.d., 0.025 in o.d.	Dow Corning Corp., Medical Products, Midland, MI
VAP Dog (HPV)		Model GPV 5FR 21″	Norfolk Medical, Skokie, Illinois
VAP Dog (Duodenal)		Model GPV 9FR 14″	Norfolk Medical, Skokie, IL
VAP Monkey (HPV)		Model SLA	Norfolk Medical, Skokie, IL
VAP Monkey (femoral)		Model GPV	Norfolk Medical, Skokie, IL
VAP Monkey (duodenal)		Model GPV	Norfolk Medical, Skokie, IL
VAP Rat/Rabbit (femoral, HPV)		Model SLA	Norfolk Medical, Skokie, IL
Rigid duodenal cannula			SmithKline Beecham Research Engineering Dept.
Animal jackets			Harvard Apparatus Ltd., Edenbridge, Kent, UK
Tethers and swivels			Harvard Apparatus Ltd., Edenbridge, Kent, UK

[a]Abbreviations: VAP, vascular access port HPV, hepatic portal vein.

using the ligature, and two further ligatures are tied around the vein and cannula. The patency of the cannula is checked by drawing blood back down the cannula. The cannula is then externalized, and the leg wound closed with sutures.

3.1.4. JUGULAR VEIN CANNULATION (RAT, MOUSE, GERBIL, GUINEA PIG)

An incision is made in the neck slightly to the right of the midline, and, using blunt dissection, the right external jugular vein is exposed and cleared of tissue. Two ligatures are placed around the vein. One is tied to occlude the jugular vein anteriorly, and gentle tension is applied to this ligature. The second ligature is loosely tied around the vein toward the heart, leaving ca. 1 cm of exposed vein. A small hole is made in the side of the vein with iris scissors, and the vein wall is held open with watchmaker forceps to enable a cannula to be inserted into the vein toward the heart. It is important that the cannula is positioned so that it does not enter the vena cava, as there is a danger that an i.v. infusion dose administered via the femoral vein would be sampled in its first pass. The loose ligature is then gently tied around the vein, fastening the cannula.

Table IV
Cannula Construction

Species	Cannula	Tubing[a]
Rat	Femoral	95 cm of **a** marked 7.5 cm from beveled end
	Jugular	72 cm of **b** and 2.25 cm of **d**, beveled slightly
	Hepatic portal	Cannula constructed in two parts, joined during surgery; part 1: 0.9 cm of **e** connected to 1 cm of **a**; part 2: 14 cm of **e** connected to 85 cm of **a**
	Duodenal	100 cm of **b** and 2.25 cm of **d**
	Mesenteric lymph duct	95 cm of **a**
Mouse	Femoral	54 cm of **c**
	Jugular	0.75 cm of **e** joined to 54 cm of **a**
	Hepatic portal	54 cm of **c**
	Duodenal	0.75 cm of **e** joined to 54 cm of **a**
Gerbil	Femoral	54 cm of **c**
	Jugular	0.75 cm of **e** joined to 54 cm of **a**
	Hepatic portal	54 cm of **c**
	Duodenal	0.75 cm of **e** joined to 54 cm of **a**
Guinea pig	Jugular	100 cm of **b** and 2.25 cm of **d**, beveled slightly
Rabbit	Femoral	VAP model SLA 4FR
	Hepatic portal	VAP model SLA 2FR
Dog	Hepatic portal	VAP model GPV 5FR
	Duodenal	VAP model GPV 9FR
Monkey	Femoral	VAP model GPV 5FR
	Hepatic portal	SLA model GPV 3.5FR
	Duodenal	VAP model GPV 7FR

[a]For explanation of codes (**a**–**e**), see Table III.

The occlusion ligature is tied firmly around the vein, and a third ligature is inserted between the other two ligatures and again firmly tied. Patency of the cannula is checked by withdrawal of blood, and the untied end of the cannula is externalized at the nape of the neck. The wound is then closed with sutures.

An alternative to femoral vein cannulation is to use both left and right external jugular veins for drug administration and sampling. This is particularly useful in the guinea pig and mouse.

3.1.5. HEPATIC PORTAL VEIN CANNULATION (RAT, MOUSE, GERBIL, GUINEA PIG)

A laparotomy is performed and the hepatic portal vein is exposed. A ligature is placed in the connective tissue at the base of the vein, and a cannula is inserted directly into the vein using a short piece of stiff wire inside the cannula that protrudes slightly

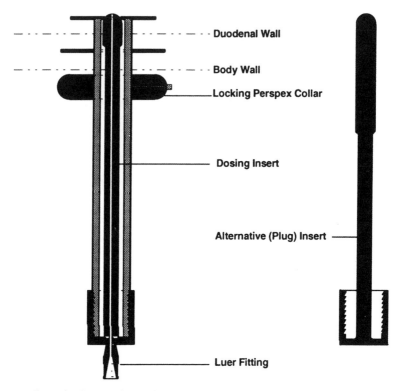

Figure 2. Design of the rigid duodenal cannula for implantation into the dog.

to provide a piercing point. The wire is removed, and the cannula is connected to an
extension cannula, which is secured in place with the ligature. An incision is made in
the body wall close to the laparotomy, and the untied end of the cannula is passed
through the body wall, leaving a small loop of cannula inside the peritoneum to allow
for body movement, and then externalized as above. The cannula is secured by a
ligature around the hole in the body wall. The body wall and outer laparotomy wound
are then closed with sutures.

3.1.6. HEPATIC PORTAL VEIN CANNULATION (DOG, RABBIT, MONKEY)

A laparotomy is performed and a loop of the small intestine is externalized. A
suitable mesenteric vein (i.e., affecting as short a length of gut as possible) is cleared
of surrounding tissue. A small hole is made in the vein, and a cannula is inserted. The
position of the tip of the cannula may be adjusted depending on whether the cannula is
intended for dose administration or blood sampling. For drug input, the cannula ought

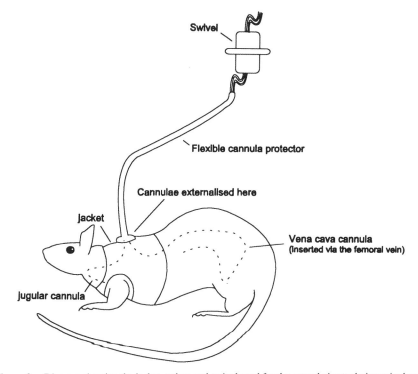

Figure 3.   Diagram showing the jacket, tether, and swivel used for the cannulation techniques in the rat.

to be as far from the liver as possible, to allow complete mixing of the dose with the blood before entering the liver. For blood sampling, the cannula ought to be as close to the liver as possible in order to ensure sampling of the entire mesenteric, splenic, and gastric outputs. The untied end of the cannula is then passed through the body wall using a trocar, leaving a small loop of cannula inside the peritoneum, and externalized via a vascular access port implanted subcutaneously in the animal's flank. In the dog the vascular access port is implanted subcutaneously before cannulation of the vein. The body wall and outer laparotomy wound are then closed with sutures.

3.1.7. DUODENAL CANNULATION (RAT, MOUSE, GERBIL, GUINEA PIG)

A laparotomy is performed and the first loop of the duodenum is exposed. A small hole is made approximately 1 cm from the pyloric sphincter, and the silastic end of the cannula is inserted. A ligature is placed around the hole and cannula and tied so as to secure the cannula. A second ligature is then placed around the hole and cannula and secured. An incision is made in the body wall close to the laparotomy, and the distal end of the cannula is passed through the body wall, leaving a small loop of cannula inside the peritoneum, and then externalized as above. The cannula is secured by a ligature around the hole in the body wall. The body wall and outer laparotomy wound are then closed with sutures.

3.1.8.   DUODENAL CANNULATION USING A VASCULAR ACCESS PORT (DOG, MONKEY)

A laparotomy is performed and the duodenal loop of the small intestine is externalized. A small hole is made in the duodenum, and a cannula is inserted (ca. 5 cm). The cannula is secured in position by means of purse string sutures around the hole and cannula. The distal end of the cannula is then passed through the body wall using a trocar, leaving a small loop of cannula inside the peritoneum, and externalized via a vascular access port implanted subcutaneously in the animal's flank. In the dog the vascular access port is implanted subcutaneously before cannulation of the duodenum. The body wall and outer laparotomy wound are closed with sutures.

3.1.9.   DUODENAL CANNULATION USING A RIGID CANNULA (DOG)

A laparotomy is performed and the duodenal loop of the small intestine is externalized. A small hole is made in the duodenum, and a titanium cannula (Fig. 2) is inserted. The cannula is secured in position by means of sutures, and the body wall and peritoneal wound are closed around the shaft of the titanium cannula.

3.1.10.   MESENTERIC LYMPH DUCT CANNULATION (RAT)

Approximately 15 min prior to anesthesia, the rat may be given cream or oil by gavage in order to aid the visualization of the lymphatic duct. A laparotomy is then performed, and the small intestine is moved aside to expose the ligament of Treitz and the mesenteric lymph duct (which can be clearly seen using a dissecting microscope). A trocar is then inserted dorsoventrally past the spinal column and through the body wall in line with the mesenteric lymph duct so that a cannula can be inserted through the trocar to lie close to the lymph duct. The trocar is removed and the cannula is filled with heparin solution. A fine suture is placed under the lymph duct, taking care not to puncture the duct or the adjacent blood vessels. A small hole is made in the wall of the duct, and the cannula tip is inserted ca. 0.5 cm into the duct. Once a flow of lymph is established under gravity, the cannula is secured in place with the previously inserted suture, and a second suture is then tied around the vessel and cannula in a convenient position. The lymph duct can sometimes be divided into two branches, and care should be taken to ensure that if one branch is cannulated, the other is occluded to ensure total lymph collection. (In calculating the relative importance of lymphatic absorption, it is important to have a complete collection of lymph as only then can the total mass of drug input by this route be estimated and compared to the total drug absorbed.) The cannula is secured by a ligature around the hole in the body wall, and the untied end of the cannula is then passed underneath the skin and externalized at the nape of the neck as above. The skin at the site of trocar entry is sutured. The body wall and outer laparotomy wound are then closed with sutures, and the rat is returned to its cage. To maintain a constant lymph flow, the end of the cannula must lie below the rat so that the lymph can drain under gravity.

3.2. DATA ANALYSIS IN *IN VIVO* EXPERIMENTS

After oral (or intraduodenal) administration, the overall bioavailability of a drug, that is, the fraction of dose reaching the systemic circulation (F_{oral}), is normally calculated as:

$$F_{oral} = \frac{AUC_{po}}{AUC_{iv}} \cdot \frac{dose_{iv}}{dose_{po}}$$

where AUC is the area under the drug concentration (plasma, blood)–time curve from zero to infinity, and the subscripts po and iv designate oral (or intraduodenal) administration and intravenous administration, respectively.

However,

$$F_{oral} = (1 - f_G) \cdot (1 - f_H) \cdot (1 - f_{abs})$$

where, after oral administration, f_{abs} is the fraction of drug malabsorbed (not leaving the gut), and f_G and f_H are the fractions of drug cleared by the gut wall and liver, respectively. If a drug is administered to animals by the different routes implicit in the equation, then assuming that equal doses were given by each route and that the drug obeys linear kinetics:

$$f_G = 1 - \frac{AUC_{po}}{AUC_{ihpv}}$$

$$f_H = 1 - \frac{AUV_{ihpv}}{AUC_{iv}}$$

where the subscript ihpv designates intra-hepatic portal vein administration.

It should be noted that the relation

$$F_H = \frac{AUV_{ihpv}}{AUC_{iv}}$$

represents the bioavailability after intra-portal vein administration and therefore depicts the maximum availability of an oral (or intraduodenal) formulation given that

100% of the dose is absorbed from the gut and is metabolically stable during the passage through the gut wall.

These multiple input experiments can either be carried out in crossover fashion or as switched experiments (Griffiths and Lewis, 1996) in which the comparator route administration (usually a constant-rate i.v. infusion) is started as soon as input from the initial route (e.g., a constant-rate ihpv infusion) is complete.

It should be noted that the above treatment assumes linear kinetics and defines 100% bioavailability as that produced following i.v. administration. This is the usual comparator; however, it could be less than that which would be produced from intraarterial dosing, if the drug underwent a significant first-pass elimination through the lungs.

4. COMPARISON OF METHODS USED TO STUDY GASTROINTESTINAL ABSORPTION

Isolated gut loops represent undisrupted tissues with relatively undisturbed morphology. Compared to isolated cells, these preparations preserve many *in vivo* features. The use of isolated perfused gut loops enables absorption processes to be investigated without interference from gastric emptying, gastrointestinal motility, bile acids, or hormones and provides flexible, viable experimental conditions. However, although perfusion studies allow sophisticated questions to be asked, the preparations are not simple, and considerable resources are required to set up, run, and validate such studies. In our experience, they are best reserved for the answering of specific questions when a problem has been encountered in *in vivo* experiments.

No single technique can provide all the answers, and the choice of technique is therefore very much dependent on the nature of the research.

REFERENCES

Blanchard, J., Tang, L. M., and Earle, M. E., 1989, Reevaluation of the absorption of carbenoxolone using an *in situ* rat intestinal technique, *J. Pharm. Sci.* **79:**411–414.

Castle, S. J., Tucker, G. T., Woods, H. F., Underwood, J. C. E., Nicholson, C. M., Havler, M. E., Lewis, C. J., Flockhart, I. R., and Lloyd-Jones, G., 1985, Assessment of an *in situ* rat intestine preparation with perfused vascular bed for studying the absorption and first-pass metabolism of drugs, *J. Pharmacol. Methods* **14:**255–274.

De Vries, M. H., Hofman, G. A., Koster, A. Sj., and Noordhoek, J., 1989a, Systemic intestinal metabolism of 1-naphthol. A study in the isolated perfused rat small intestine, *Drug Metab. Dispos.* **17:**573–578.

De Vries, M. H., Hofman, G. A., Koster, A. Sj., and Noordhoek, J., 1989b, Absorption and presystemic glucoronidation of 1-naphthol in the vascularly fluorocarbon emulsion perfused rat small intestine. The influence of 1-naphthol concentration, perfusate flow and noradrenaline, *Naunyn-Schmiedeberg's Arch. Pharmacol.* **340:**239–245.

De Vries, M. H., Rademaker, C. M. A., Geerlings, C., Van Dijk, A., and Noordoek, J., 1989c, Pharmacokinetic modelling on the effect on the intestinal secretion of theophylline, using the isolated vascularly perfused rat small intestine, *J. Pharm. Pharmacol.* **41:**528–533.

Doluisio, J. T., Billups, N. F., Dittert, L. W., Sugita, E. T., and Swintosky, J. V., 1969, Drug absorption I: An *in situ* rat gut technique yielding realistic absorption techniques, *J. Pharm. Sci.* **58:**1196–1200.

Geyer, R. P., 1975, "Bloodless" rats through the use of artificial blood substitutes, *Fed. Proc.* **34:**1499–1505.

Greene, E. C., 1963, Anatomy of the rat, in: *Transactions of the American Philosophical Society*, New Series, Vol. 27, Hafner Publishing Company, New York, pp. 198–200.

Griffiths, R., and Lewis, V. A., 1996, in preparation.

Hanson, P. J., and Parsons, D. S., 1976, The utilization of glucose and production of lactate by *in vitro* preparations of rat small intestine: Effects of vascular perfusion, *J. Physiol.* **255:**775–795.

Hartiala, K., 1973, Metabolism of hormones, drugs and other substances by the gut, *Physiol. Rev.* **53:**496–534.

Hartmann, F., Vieillard-Baron, D., and Heinrich, R., 1984, Isolated perfusion of the small intestine using perfluorotributylamine as artificial oxygen carrier, *Adv. Exp. Med. Biol.* **180:**711–720.

Higuchi, W. I., Ho, N. F. H., Park, J. Y., and Komiya, I., 1981, Rate-limiting steps and factors in drug absorption, in: *Drug Absorption Proceedings of the Edinburgh International Conference* (L. F. Prescott and W. S. Nimmo, eds.), Adis Press, Balgowlah, Australia, pp. 35–60.

Hirayama, H., Xu, X., and Pang, K. S., 1989, Viability of the vascularly perfused, recirculating rat intestine and intestine-liver preparations, *Am. J. Physiol.* **257:**249–258.

Krebs, H. A., and Henseleit, K., 1932, Untersuchungen ber die Harnstoffbildung im Tierkrper, *Hoppe-Seyler's Z. Physiol. Chem.* **210:**33–66.

Lewis, L. D., and Fordtran, J. S., 1975, Effect of perfusion rate on absorption, surface area, unstirred water layer thickness, permeability and intraluminal pressure in the rat ileum *in vivo*, *Gastroenterology* **68:**1509–1516.

Miyazaki, K., Sunada, K., Iseki, K., and Arita, T., 1986, Simultaneous vascular and luminal perfusion of rat small intestine, *Chem. Pharm. Bull.* **34:**3830–3835.

Nicholls, T. J., Leese, H. J., and Bronk, J. R., 1983, Transport and metabolism of glucose by rat small intestine, *Biochem. J.* **212:**183–187.

Ochsenfahrt, H., 1979, The relevance of blood flow for the absorption of drugs in the vascularly perfused intestine of the rat, *Naunyn-Schmiedeberg's Arch. Pharmacol.* **306:**105–112.

Pang, K. S., Cherry, W. F., and Ulm, E. H., 1985, Disposition of enalapril in the perfused rat intestine-liver preparation: Absorption, metabolism and first-pass effect, *J. Pharmacol. Exp. Ther.* **233:**788–795.

Pang, K. S., Yuen, V., Fayz, S., Kopple, J. N., and Mulder, G. J., 1986, Absorption and metabolism of acetaminophen by the *in situ* perfused rat small intestine preparation, *Drug Metab. Dispos.* **14:**102–111.

Robinson, J. W. L., Menge, H., Sepulveda, F. A., and Mirkovitch, V., 1977, Functional and structural characteristics of the jejunum and ileum in the dog and the rat, *Digestion* **15:**188–189.

Sakai, S., Akima, M., Hinohara, Y., Sasaki, M., and Niki, R., 1980, Vascularly perfused rat small intestine: A research model for drug absorption, *Jpn. J. Pharmacol.* **30:**231–241.

Schurgers, N., Bijdendijk, J., Tukker, J. T., and Crommelin, D. J. A., 1986, Comparison of four experimental techniques for studying drug absorption kinetics in the anesthetized rat *in situ*, *J. Pharm. Sci.* **75:**117–119.

Takahashi, H., Nishikawa, M., Hayashi, M., and Awazu, S., 1988, The use of a perfluorocarbon emulsion as a vascular perfusate in drug absorption, *J. Pharm. Pharmacol.* **40:**252–257.

Windmueller, H. G., and Spaeth, A. E., 1981, Vascular autoperfusion of rat small intestine *in situ*, *Methods Enzymol.* **77:**120–129.

Windmueller, H. G., Spaeth, A. E., and Ganote, C. E., 1970, Vascular perfusion of isolated rat gut; norepinephrine and glucocorticoid requirement, *Am. J. Physiol.* **218:**197–204.

Xu, X., Hirayama, H., and Pang, K. S., 1989, First-pass metabolism of salicylamide. Studies in the once-through vascularly perfused rat intestine–liver preparation, *Drug. Metab. Dispos.* **17:**556–563.

Yasuhara, M., Fujiwara, J., Kitade, S., Katayama, H., Okumura, K., and Hori, R., 1985, Effect of altered plasma protein binding on pharmacokinetics and pharmacodynamics of propranolol in rats after surgery: Role of alpha-1-acid glycoprotein, *J. Pharmacol. Exp. Ther.* **235:**513–520.

Yorgey, K. A., Pritchard, J. F., Renzi, N. L., and Dvorchik, B. H., 1986, Evaluation of drug absorption and presystemic metabolism using an *in situ* intestinal preparation, *J. Pharm. Sci.* **75:**869–872.

Chapter 6

Model Systems for Intestinal Lymphatic Transport Studies

Christopher J. H. Porter
and William N. Charman

1. INTRODUCTION

Transport via the intestinal lymphatic system has been shown to contribute to the absorption of a number of highly lipophilic xenobiotics (Yeung and von Saigent, 1972; Noguchi *et al.*, 1985; Fukui *et al.*, 1989; Ichihashi *et al.*, 1991a). Although intestinal lymphatic drug transport leads directly to an increase in oral bioavailability, it also confers other potential advantages such as avoidance of hepatic first-pass metabolism, direct targeting to the associated lymphoid tissue, and indirect targeting to specific sites such as those associated with low-density lipoprotein receptors and lymphocytes (Bijsterbosch and van Berkel, 1990; Charman and Stella, 1991).

The transport of lipophilic compounds via the intestinal lymphatics generally occurs in tandem with lipoprotein biosynthesis, and consequently a common approach for enhancing lymphatic drug transport is the coadministration of appropriate lipids (Charman, 1992). Lipophilic compounds that are transported lymphatically are primarily associated with the triglyceride core of the chylomicron fraction of lymph.

Notwithstanding the various effects of fatty acid chain length and lipid class on lipoprotein flux, Charman and Stella (1986a) described a simple approach for estimating the likely maximum contribution of lymphatic transport to the oral bioavailability of a candidate drug. The simple "ball-park estimate," which is the product of the

---

Christopher J. H. Porter and William N. Charman • Department of Pharmaceutics, Victorian College of Pharmacy, Monash University, Parkville, Victoria 3052, Australia.

Models for Assessing Drug Absorption and Metabolism, Ronald T. Borchardt *et al.*, eds., Plenum Press, New York, 1996.

triglyceride solubility of the compound and the mass of lipoprotein-based lipid appearing in intestinal lymph, assumes that the candidate drug has a high partition coefficient (e.g., log $P > 5$). Therefore, before undertaking the complicated experimental procedures required to determine lymphatic drug transport, it is prudent to realistically assess the potential for lymphatic transport by examination of the physicochemical properties of the candidate drug. It is important to note that if the putative site of action of the drug is within the lymphatic system, then the absolute amount of drug transported into the intestinal lymph need not be substantial to exert the desired pharmacological effect. For example, Takada *et al.* (1986) suggested that the pharmacodynamic endpoints of cyclosporin therapy may be better correlated with drug concentration in the lymph rather than concentration in plasma.

Although there have been a number of animal models described in the literature for estimating intestinal lymphatic drug transport (e.g., different sites of cannulation, different species, anesthetized or conscious studies), the laboratory rat is generally the preferred model system. This chapter examines the methodology associated with performing lymphatic transport studies in the rat (and in particular the anesthetized rat) and then briefly describes the methodological and formulation-related factors which impact upon the design and interpretation of intestinal lymphatic transport studies.

2. METHODS

Lymphatic transport studies performed in the anesthetized rat are robust, relatively inexpensive, and straightforward with respect to drug administration and blood sampling. The method employs a triple-cannulated rat such that the mesenteric lymph duct, jugular vein, and duodenum are accessed. The extent of intestinal lymphatic drug transport can be affected by various formulation and experimental factors, and the influence of these different factors is discussed in Section 3. The experimental techniques described below are presented in the order in which they are normally performed.

2.1. Materials

Heparin solutions: 5 units/ml in normal saline (for soaking jugular vein cannula and as a venous flush solution) and 200 units/ml in normal saline (for soaking lymphatic cannulas).

Anesthetic: 60 mg/ml sodium pentobarbitone.

Lymph collection tubes: 5-ml blood collection tubes containing 7.5 mg of EDTA and 100 µl of normal saline.

Blood collection tubes: 1.5 ml Eppendorf tubes containing 20 µl of 200 units/ml heparin solution.

Surgical equipment: A typical set of surgical instruments would include 15-cm dissecting scissors, 12-cm microscissors, 11.5-cm smooth and serrated curved micro-forceps, 11.5-cm curved and straight jeweler's forceps, and 10-cm straight (blunt) microforceps. Syringe infusion pumps are used to control the rate of the duodenal infusion. If required, a second infusion pump may be connected to the duodenal infusion line to administer the dose. The body temperature of the anesthetized rats is maintained at 37°C on a thermostatically controlled warming pad. Ideally, cannulation of the mesenteric lymph duct is performed with the aid of a low-power (50×) dissecting microscope.

Mesenteric lymph duct cannula: 20-cm length of polyethylene tubing (0.5 mm i.d., 0.8 mm o.d.; Dural Plastics, New South Wales, Australia) with a 45° bevel. A 1- to 2-mm-thick disk of silastic tubing, with an internal diameter similar to the external diameter of the polyethylene tubing, is placed around the cannula approximately 3 mm behind the bevel to act as an anchor and reference point for the cannula. The cannula is presoaked overnight in 200-units/ml heparin solution before surgery.

Jugular vein cannula: 20-cm length of polyethylene tubing (0.58 mm i.d., 0.965 mm o.d., PE 50; Clay Adams, Parsippany, NJ) with a blunted 45° bevel. Blunting the end of the bevel decreases the chance of inadvertently pushing the cannula through the wall of the jugular vein. A mark is placed on the cannula 3.5 cm from the bevel to indicate the distance to insert the cannula for it to reach the right atrium of the heart.

Duodenal/peritoneal cannula: 10-cm length of PE 50 tubing (with a 45° bevel at one end) which is fashioned into a U-shape with the aid of gentle heating.

Tracheal tubes: 3-cm length of polyethylene tube which is conical in shape such that the approximate internal/external diameters of the smaller and larger ends of the cannula are 2 mm/3 mm and 4 mm/6 mm, respectively.

2.2. Animal Handling and Preparation

The ideal weight range for male Sprague-Dawley rats undergoing mesenteric lymph cannulation is 275–300 g. Rats weighing more than 300 g can be difficult to cannulate owing to the presence of excess fat in the peritoneal cavity. Surgery is typically performed in the morning of the study day on rats that have been fasted overnight (water available *ad libitum*) in wire bottom cages (to prevent coprophagy). As the rats are unlikely to have eaten during the day prior to the overnight fast, the effective fasting period would equate to 24 hr.

On the morning of the experiment, anesthesia is induced (and then maintained) with intraperitoneal sodium pentobarbitone (50 mg/kg every 2 hr), and the abdominal region of the rat is shaved. The tracheotomy is normally performed first to avoid accumulation of fluid in the airways, which is followed by the abdominal surgery and the jugular vein cannulation. Once the operator becomes proficient with the procedures, two rats can be prepared for experimentation within a 2-hr surgical period.

2.3. Surgical Procedures

2.3.1. TRACHEOTOMY

Rats continue to salivate under anesthesia. Although this does not present problems for surgical interventions of short duration (2–4 hr), it can lead to breathing difficulties and eventual asphyxiation if left unchecked during longer procedures. Anticholinergic agents such as atropine can be used to decrease fluid accumulation in the anesthetized rat. However, these agents interfere with normal digestive/motility patterns, and consequently a tracheotomy is the preferred approach for ensuring patency of the airways during the experimental procedures. A 5 mm × 5 mm hole is cut in the skin above the trachea midway between the pectoral muscles and the chin. The layers of muscle covering the trachea are gently separated with curved micro-forceps to expose the trachea. A pair of curved forceps is inserted under the trachea, and a 10-cm length of 3-0 silk passed underneath and loosely tied around the trachea. A small incision is made in the top of the trachea, and the tracheal tube inserted approximately 1.5 cm. The tube is tied in place with the wide end exposed to enable drainage of excess tracheal secretions, and the trachea is realigned to its original position.

2.3.2. JUGULAR VEIN CANNULATION

Cannulation of the jugular vein in the anesthetized rat is a relatively simple procedure as the cannula can be externalized at the point of entry into the jugular vein. The rat is placed on its back with its head toward the operator. A 1- to 2-cm incision is made in the skin along a straight line above the right jugular vein from the clavicle to a point laterally displaced about 1 cm from the center line at approximately the level of the right ear. The muscle and fat surrounding the jugular vein are dissected away, and the portion of the external jugular vein caudal to the bifurcation into the right anterior facial and right posterior facial veins is isolated. Curved smooth forceps are then inserted underneath the vein, and two 10-cm lengths of 5-0 silk are passed through the legs of the forceps underneath the vein. The vein is tied off just caudal to the bifurcation using one piece of silk (which becomes the rostral tie) and then placed under tension using a small pair of artery forceps clamped onto the tie. The caudal tie is then loosely tied around the vein (which will eventually anchor the cannula). A small incision is made in the anterior surface of the vein, and one point of a pair of straight jeweler's forceps is inserted approximately 1 cm. The jugular vein cannula (attached to a 5-ml syringe filled with 5-units/ml heparin solution) is threaded into the vein using the forceps as a guide. The cannula is gently worked into the vein until the mark 3.5 cm from the end of the cannula is over the entry point into the vein. The exact distance of this point from the end of the cannula will vary according to animal size and species (which would be determined by dissection). Care must be taken while working the cannula down the vein to avoid puncturing the wall of the vessel. Of paramount importance is the tension applied to the rostral tie, which prevents the cannula "dragging" the vein during insertion. If the cannula does not insert smoothly (i.e., it stops or bounces back), this often indicates that it has passed into a branching vein or has become jammed in a valve. In these situations, the cannula should be pulled back and then gently reinserted. Raising the chest of the rat by holding the skin covering the chest can prevent the cannula from passing into branched veins during insertion. In addition, twisting the cannula during insertion can facilitate passage through venous valves. Once the cannula has been placed correctly, the tension on the rostral tie is released, the patency of the cannula is verified, and the cannula is sutured into place using both ties.

2.3.3. MESENTERIC LYMPH DUCT CANNULATION

Many operators choose to predose animals with lipid prior to attempting cannulation of the mesenteric lymph duct as this aids identification and visualization of the lymphatics. However, we typically perform lymph duct cannulations on fasted rats in accord with our established experimental protocol (see Section 2.4). It is recommended that rats be predosed with 0.5 ml of peanut oil (or equivalent) while the operator becomes familiar with the surgical techniques. Once confidence has been attained in cannulating the mesenteric lymph duct in the predosed rat, the operator may readily switch to working with fasted rats.

Prior to abdominal surgery, an area on the right side of the animal, from the sternum to the flank along the line of the diaphragm and stretching about 3 cm caudally, is shaved. The rat is placed on its back with its head to the left of the operator and its tail to the right (i.e., 90° removed from the position used for cannulation of the jugular vein). This position is adopted because the mesenteric lymph duct runs laterally across the midline, and most operators prefer to perform cannulations via an up-and-down (north/south) movement as opposed to a crosswise (east/west) movement. Access to the mesenteric lymph duct is improved by bridging the rat over a 10-ml syringe and taping the right foreleg onto the operating bench on the left side of the body. This twists and lifts the body such that the right lateral side of the animal is maximally exposed.

An incision is made through the abdominal muscle from a position 3- to 4-mm caudal to the xiphoid process of the sternum and extending along the line of the rib cage to the flank. Upon opening the animal, the operator should be able to see the lower lobes of the liver, the right kidney, and the small intestine. The small intestine is then gently pushed across the midline to the left side of the animal to maximally expose the blood vessels and lymph duct (Fig. 1). The mesenteric lymph duct runs alongside the mesenteric artery, which itself runs perpendicularly to the inferior vena cava at approximately the level of the right kidney. The area surrounding the mesenteric lymph duct and mesenteric artery is usually encapsulated in a number of

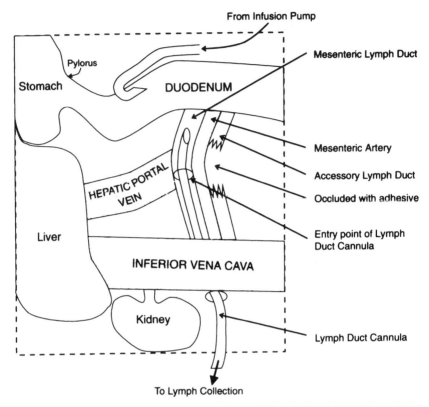

Figure 1. Schematic diagram depicting placement of mesenteric lymphatic and duodenal cannulas in the anesthetized rat preparation. The drawing is not to scale.

fine, clear membranes. These must be removed before attempting to cannulate the lymph duct; otherwise, the cannula may be inadvertently placed between layers of membrane instead of within the duct. The membranes are removed by gently taking hold of part of the membrane in the area between the vena cava and the lymph duct with nonserrated forceps and then gently pulling the membrane toward the centerline of the rat, thereby peeling the membrane from the vessels. Care should be taken to avoid taking hold of the membranes directly over the lymph duct since it is easy to simultaneously grasp both the membrane and lymph duct, thereby ripping the lymph duct and ruining the preparation. Clearing the membranes above the lymph duct is both the most difficult part of the surgery and the most important. Although it is tempting to save time by only partially "clearing" the membranes from above the lymph duct, this inevitably leads to problems in piercing the duct and positioning the cannula.

Once the surface of the duct has been cleared, the cannula is routed underneath the inferior vena cava so that it is positioned for insertion into the duct. This is achieved by gently passing a pair of blunt-nosed forceps under the right kidney and vena cava and surfacing just below the lymph duct. The cannula [attached to a 1-ml syringe containing heparin (200 units/ml)] is then fed between the legs of the forceps. Once the forceps are removed, this leaves the cannula running under the vena cava and in the same direction as the duct. The mesenteric lymph duct, rather than running in a line exactly perpendicular to the torso, often bends slightly toward the tail end of the animal. In these situations, it is wise for the operator to manipulate the cannula such that it also bends in a similar direction. Since the tubing used for these cannulations is generally supplied on a roll, the cannulas are often naturally bent one way or the other, and it may just be a case of making sure the curve is in the right direction. Alternatively, the cannula may be rolled around a pencil or a battery to induce a slight bend. Once the surface above the cannulation point has been cleared and the cannula sited correctly, the lymph duct is cannulated and any accessory lymph ducts (commonly running down the other side of the mesenteric artery) are occluded. Routinely, a small incision is first made in the mesenteric lymph duct with the microscissors, the accessory lymph duct(s) is then cut, and the cannula is finally inserted through the incision in the duct. The procedures are best performed in this order as incision of the mesenteric duct is most straightforward while there is fluid pressure in the duct (which is removed as soon as an incision is made in either the mesenteric or accessory ducts). Additionally, it is preferable to disrupt the accessory duct before actually inserting the mesenteric cannula.

Occlusion of the cannula is the most common source of cannulation failure. The mesenteric lymph duct has little inherent structure of its own, and it can easily be drawn over the end of the cannula. Consequently, time must be spent coordinating the angle and position of both the cannula and the bevel to maximize the efficiency of the cannulation. The patency of the cannulation is checked by removing the syringe from the end and observing for flow of lymph. If there is no lymph flow, it needs to be determined whether the cannula has been incorrectly placed (e.g., in a membrane) or has become occluded after having been correctly placed. Once the success of the cannulation has been verified, a drop of cyanoacrylate adhesive is placed over the entry point of the cannula into the duct to seal the system. Another drop of cyanoacrylate adhesive is placed over the area where the accessory duct was cut, thereby causing all lymph draining the small intestine to flow through the mesenteric lymph duct (Fig. 1). The peritoneal cavity is then flushed with normal saline to clear any debris and to complete polymerization of the cyanoacrylate adhesive.

During the surgical procedures, care should be taken to stop bleeding within the peritoneal cavity because a proportion of this can drain into the mesenteric lymphatics. Although red blood cells can be separated from the mesenteric lymph by mild centrifugation, the presence of blood may increase the chance of clot formation within the cannula.

2.3.4. DUODENAL AND PERITONEAL CANNULATION

The duodenum is cannulated approximately 1 cm below the pylorus by piercing the lumen with an 18G needle and following it with the cannula, which is secured with cyanoacrylate adhesive (Fig. 1). The U-shaped cannula allows for administration of rehydration solution (1.4 ml/hr) and drug formulations in the direction of intestinal flow. After duodenal cannulation, the abdomen is gently repositioned to realign the intestines, and the abdominal wall is closed with 3-0 silk suture using individual knots to facilitate closing around the individual cannulas. Additionally, a U-shaped cannula is threaded into the peritoneal cavity between suture points to provide for easy intraperitoneal administration of anesthetic. The skin is then sealed with cyano-acrylate adhesive.

2.4. General Experimental Protocol and Animal Monitoring

Scheme 1 depicts a typical experimental protocol. In the period immediately following lymphatic cannulation, the patency of the lymphatic cannula should be continually checked (against clot formation) since flow may be as low as 200–300 μl/hr during the 2- to 3-hr recovery/rehydration period. Normal saline is infused intraduodenally during this period at a rate of 1.4 ml/hr. During the dosing period, the saline infusion is either stopped and the drug infused in its place (in which case the dose is made up to volume with normal saline to deliver 1.4 ml/hr) or, for small dose volumes, the dose is "piggy-backed" into the saline infusion line via a T-piece connector. At the completion of the dosing period, the normal saline infusion is resumed for the duration of the experiment. At the conclusion of the experiment, the rats are sacrificed by an overdose of intravenous pentobarbitone, and the integrity of the cannulas is verified by dissection.

2.5. Lymph Collection and Blood Sampling

Lymph is collected at hourly intervals into chilled 5-ml blood collection tubes containing 7.5 mg of EDTA dissolved in 100 μl of normal saline. The EDTA acts as an anticoagulant and a protease inhibitor by chelating metal cofactors. Additional protease inhibitors such as 2 mM phenylmethylsulfonyl fluoride (PMSF), aprotinin at 20 trypsin inhibitory units/ml, and leupeptin (1 μg/ml) may also be added. Lipase/lipid transferase can be inhibited by the addition of 1 mM Ellman's reagent [5,5′-dithiobis(2-nitrobenzoic acid)]. Oxidation can be suppressed by the use of low temperature and the addition of 0.02% glutathione. If required, a bacteriostatic agent such as sodium azide may be used. The strategy governing the addition of specific inhibitors to the lymph collection tubes is dictated by the data required from the

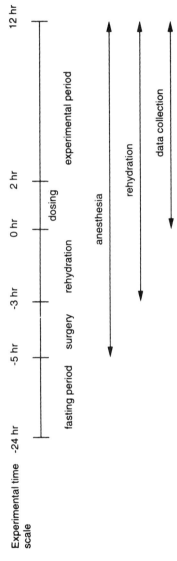

Scheme 1. Depiction of the timing of fasting, surgical, recovery, and experimental procedures involved in the triple-cannulated anesthetized rat model for studying intestinal lymphatic transport.

sample. For example, an anticoagulant is probably the only additive required if total drug transport is being assessed, whereas more comprehensive preservation strategies are required if the structural characteristics of the different lipoprotein subclasses are under study. Although lymph is stable at 4°C for several days, it should be processed as soon as possible.

Blood samples are withdrawn from the jugular vein as required, and the plasma is separated and then frozen. Depending on the number and volume of blood samples, the blood volume may be replaced with either saline, blank plasma from a donor rat, or reconstituted red blood cells collected from the experimental rat (collected after separation of plasma for analysis and then mixed with blank plasma from a donor). The choice of technique depends on the total volume of blood removed from the animal over the experimental period and the potential effects on drug binding and metabolism that may occur with a decrease in hematocrit.

2.6. Drug and Triglyceride Analysis

The analysis of lymph samples offers a number of analytical opportunities to comprehensively map the drug transport process. Firstly, lymph concentrations of drug can be quantitatively determined using either HPLC-based or radioanalytical techniques. As fistulation of the mesenteric lymph duct essentially collects all lymph draining the small intestine, the absolute quantity of drug transported is simply calculated by multiplication of the concentration of drug in lymph by the corresponding volume of lymph produced (assessed gravimetrically) during each collection period.

As the lymphatic transport of lipophilic drugs is associated with lipoprotein biosynthesis, an estimate of the mesenteric flux of triglyceride lipid is an important parameter. The triglyceride content of mesenteric lymph comprises both endogenous and exogenous components (Shiau *et al.*, 1985). Although the relative contribution of each lipid source to total lipid transport is most accurately determined using radiolabeled exogenous lipid, a simple strategy for estimating endogenous lipid turnover involves collection and analysis of lymph lipid from rats receiving a blank (normal saline) infusion. Triglyceride concentrations in lymph are readily determined using automated clinical chemistry analyzers. Employing the experimental procedure described in Scheme 1, the fasted triglyceride output (based on C18 triglyceride) in anesthetized rats receiving an infusion of normal saline was found to be 2.67 ± 0.35 mg/hr. The mass of exogenous lipid transport in subsequent experiments can then be estimated by difference from the total measured triglyceride transport. Although this approach for determining exogenous lipid transport is limited by the inability to perform crossover experiments, our experience has been that the data are accurate (as assessed by near-quantitative recovery of exogenous lipid loads) and reproducible.

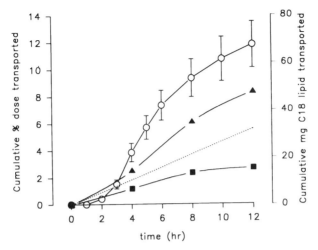

Figure 2. Cumulative lymphatic transport of a model lipophilic drug (○) and triglyceride lipid as a function of time in the anesthetized rat preparation. Data are presented as means ± SE ($n = 6$). Anesthetized rats were intraduodenally administered 2 mg of a model lipophilic compound dissolved in 50 μl of lipid (2:1 oleic acid:monoolein) formulated as an oil-in-water emulsion. The closed symbols represent the cumulative transport of triglyceride lipid, and the dashed line depicts transport of endogenous triglyceride (blank lymph) determined in separate rats (see Section 2.6). Total triglyceride transport (▲) represents endogenous and exogenous components, and exogenous lipid transport (■, determined as the difference between total and endogenous lipid transport) essentially represents transport of formulation lipid.

For example, the contribution of endogenous and exogenous lipid to total mesenteric lymph triglyceride transport in the anesthetized rat model is presented in Fig. 2. Additionally, the lymphatic transport profile of a highly lipophilic drug is included in Fig. 2 to demonstrate the relationship between drug and triglyceride lipid transport.

Although these studies are directed toward quantifying the extent of lymphatic drug transport, it is important to determine the extent of absorption occurring via the portal blood in the context of the oral bioavailability of the drug. It is reasonable to assume that systemic plasma concentrations of drug in the lymph-fistulated rat reflect absorption of drug via the portal blood. Therefore, the contribution of portal blood absorption to bioavailability in the lymph-fistulated rat can be determined by conducting parallel experiments in sham-operated rats where the drug is administered intravenously and comparing the relative areas under the plasma concentration–time profiles.

Fractionation of lymph into the various lipoprotein subclasses (chylomicrons, VLDL, LDL, and HDL) provides useful data for characterizing the transport process. The review by Raub *et al.* (1992) provides an excellent description of the methods used in the isolation and characterization of lymph lipoprotein subclasses.

2.7.   Alternative Animal Models

2.7.1.   CONSCIOUS RAT MODEL

The surgical techniques utilized in the conscious rat model are the same as described for the anesthetized model, except that the lymph and jugular vein cannulas are tunneled under the skin to exit the animal at the back of the neck, where they are connected to a saddle/swivel leash arrangement to allow continuous infusion and sampling (Raub *et al.*, 1992). In this case, the jugular line is used for both saline rehydration (1–2 ml/hr) and blood sampling. The protocol of Raub *et al.* (1992) describes a 3-day recovery period between jugular vein surgery and lymphatic cannulation and a 2-day recovery period after abdominal surgery. In the conscious model, rats are orally dosed and rehydrated intravenously, negating the requirement for an intraduodenal line.

A more simple conscious rat model can be employed if cannulation of the jugular vein is omitted in terms of blood sampling (although blood could still be sampled from the tail vein or the optic plexus). Noguchi *et al.* (1985) described a method in which the mesenteric lymph cannula was externalized through the abdominal wall and lymph was collected into a small bottle secured in place by a jacket. The jacket allowed for free and unrestricted movement and was fitted around the front legs of the animal. The jacket extended approximately three-quarters of the way down the abdomen and was secured by ties along the back. The collection bottle contained 0.5 ml of heparin (200 units/ml) into which the end of the cannula was placed to prevent clotting. From a timing standpoint, mesenteric cannulations were performed on the day prior to dosing, after which the rats were given a 24-hr recovery period (fasting with access to water *ad libitum*). A methodological advantage of this approach was that surgery was performed using nonfasted rats, thereby aiding visualization of the lymphatics.

2.7.2.   OTHER LYMPHATIC TRANSPORT MODELS

The dog has been used to study lymphatic transport (Rajpal and Kirkpatrick, 1972; Raub *et al.*, 1992). The thoracic duct, rather than the mesenteric duct, was cannulated. The external jugular vein was ligated above and below the join with the thoracic duct, and the cannula was sutured into that section of the jugular vein. Thoracic lymph flows into the cannula via the pouch/reservoir that is created by ligation of the external jugular vein. Although the procedure is not an actual thoracic duct cannulation, the inherent advantages are that the preparation is more robust than direct cannulation of the thoracic duct and lymph samples can be obtained without performing a thoracotomy.

Methodology using an anesthetized pig has been described which enabled the simultaneous collection of mesenteric lymph, hepatic portal blood, and systemic blood (White *et al.*, 1991). Although the reported technique only described approaches for taking samples of mesenteric lymph (and not its complete collection), it may be possible to modify the technique to collect all mesenteric lymph, thereby enabling drug transport to be quantitatively assessed.

3. METHODOLOGICAL DIFFERENCES IN TRANSPORT STUDIES

Drug transport via the intestinal lymphatics is the culmination of a number of steps which include absorption via the enterocyte, association with the products of lipid digestion, secretion into mesenteric lymph, and transport via thoracic lymph into the systemic circulation. Different animal and surgical models impact on the efficiency of lymphatic transport, and the following sections highlight some of the major differences. Awareness of how these methodological differences can influence lymphatic transport is important when interpreting and assessing lymphatic transport data.

3.1. Mesenteric versus Thoracic Lymph Duct Cannulation

Lymph can be collected from either the mesenteric or thoracic duct. Although an orally administered drug directly gains access to lymphatic fluid after absorption via the enterocyte, it can also indirectly gain access to peripheral lymph by equilibration from systemic blood (Fig. 3). Therefore, collection of thoracic lymph can overestimate the actual intestinal lymphatic transport because the thoracic duct collects lymph from the small intestine as well as hepatic and peripheral sources. For example, Noguchi *et al.* (1985) demonstrated that 32.3 ± 2.6% of an orally administered dose of DDT (dissolved in oleic acid) was recovered in thoracic lymph, whereas only 21.9 ± 2.3% was recovered in mesenteric lymph. The additional amount of drug recovered in the thoracic lymph reflected the contribution of drug equilibration between systemic plasma and peripheral lymph. Therefore, a mesenteric lymph model should be used for an accurate assessment of lymphatic transport associated with the small intestine.

3.2. Fasting and Hydration Effects

The duration of the period of fasting prior to commencing lymphatic transport studies can markedly affect the extent of drug transport. Charman *et al.* (1986) demonstrated that the intestinal lymphatic transport of DDT was increased twofold when the period of fasting prior to drug administration was increased from 2 to 48 hr. This effect was most likely due to the mobilization of endogenous lipoproteins due to the extended period of fasting. The extent of hydration prior to experimentation can

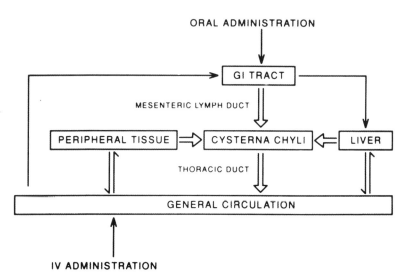

Figure 3. Schematic representation describing the different lymphatic duct cannulation sites and the potential for equilibration of drugs between the general circulation and the peripheral lymph.

also affect the drug transport profile as it influences the rate of appearance of lipoproteins in lymph after administration of exogenous lipid (Tso *et al.*, 1985). Although the timing of fasting, hydration, and dosing periods may affect the absolute extent of drug transport in a particular study, the methodological differences are usually constant across a series of experiments. Therefore, problems are only encountered when comparing transport data collected under different experimental protocols.

3.3. Anesthetized versus Conscious Models

The influence of anesthesia on lymphatic transport in the rat is difficult to assess as oral dosing is employed in the conscious model whereas anesthetized rats are dosed intraduodenally. Consequently, it is not possible to separate the relative effects of anesthesia from the increased gastric processing inherent in orally dosed animals. Recent results from this laboratory have examined this matter with regard to the lymphatic transport of a highly lipophilic model compound (Porter *et al.*, 1993). It was found that lymphatic drug transport after intraduodenal administration of a mixed micellar formulation to anesthetized rats was the same as that after oral administration of the same formulation to conscious rats. In contrast, lymphatic transport of the drug was less after intraduodenal administration of a peanut oil solution to anesthetized rats compared with oral administration of the same formulation to conscious rats (Fig. 4).

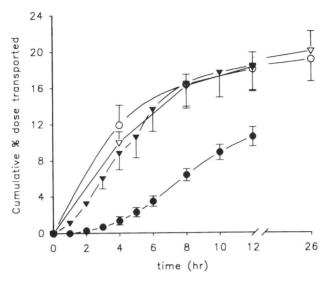

Figure 4. Cumulative percent dose of drug (mean ± SE, $n \geqslant 4$) collected in intestinal lymph as a function of time for four different combinations of lipid vehicle and animal model. All formulations contained 2 mg of a model lipophilic compound dissolved in 50 μl of lipid (2:1 oleic acid:monoolein). The experimental groups were an orally dosed (conscious rat) micellar lipid formulation (▽), an orally dosed (conscious rat) lipid solution (○), an intraduodenally dosed (anesthetized rat) micellar lipid formulation (▼), and an intraduodenally dosed (anesthetized rat) lipid solution (●).

These data suggest that the degree of formulation dispersion impacts on the extent of lymphatic transport in the intraduodenally dosed anesthetized model, where preduodenal emulsification does not occur. Notwithstanding the formulation dependencies associated with the anesthetized rat, the model has the advantage of greater experimental control combined with the ability to mechanistically probe the inherent ability of the small intestine to lymphatically transport compounds without the complication of secondary gastric effects associated with oral administration.

3.4. Choice of Coadministered Lipid

The requirement for the coadministration of lipid to optimize lymphatic drug transport has been well established (Palin *et al.*, 1982; Palin and Wilson, 1984; Ichihashi *et al.*, 1991b; Charman, 1992). It is also known that long-chain fatty acids (or their triglyceride equivalents) are essential for chylomicron formation (Charman, 1992). In the anesthetized rat model, long-chain fatty acids (or combinations of a fatty acid and a monoglyceride) facilitate lymphatic transport relative to an equivalent triglyceride, which must be digested prior to absorption (Charman and Stella, 1986b).

Charman and Stella (1986b) also examined the effect of different lipid dose volumes on the lymphatic transport of DDT. Increasing the dose volume of lipid from 50 to 200 μl did not affect the extent of lymphatic transport, although the lag time for appearance of DDT in the lymph was decreased with the lower volume of administered lipid. Similar results have been reported with benzo[a]pyrene (Laher *et al.*, 1984). From consideration of the effects of lipid class and lipid volume on lymphatic transport, we now routinely dose a candidate drug in 50 μl of a 2:1 molar ratio of oleic acid/ monoolein mixture when using the anesthetized rat model described in Scheme 1.

3.5. Scaling Rat Lymphatic Transport Data to Higher Species

Extrapolation of formulation-effect data to lymphatic transport profiles in species other than the rat is difficult. The secretion of bile, and the subsequent formation of mixed micelles of bile salts and the products of lipid digestion, is a prerequisite for the absorption of long-chain fatty acids required for the stimulation of lymphatic transport. In the rat, bile flow is continuous and independent of food intake whereas in higher species, food/lipid is required to stimulate the numerous events that lead to the digestion and absorption of lipids. Therefore, results obtained in the fasted rat, where a small quantity of formulation lipid can be processed by the constant stream of bile, may not be mirrored in higher species, where a mass of lipid (larger than commonly used in oral formulations) may be required to stimulate bile production and the related digestive events. Some of these limitations may be addressed by utilizing a dog model, which is more representative of the human situation. The small blood volume of the rat limits the number and volume of blood samples that can be taken, and this impacts on the required sensitivity of the analytical procedures. Although these limitations can be overcome by moving to a larger animal model, the cost and level of surgical support required to perform such studies is often prohibitive. Therefore, the most practical approach to assess the likely lymphatic transport of a series of compounds is to use the rat model and, if required, progress to a more advanced model such as the dog.

4. APPLICATION TO ABSORPTION AND METABOLISM STUDIES

Drug transport via the mesenteric lymphatics can have a considerable impact on the absorptive and metabolic profile of the drug relative to absorption via the portal blood. The time scale of lymphatic transport is slower than that for portal blood absorption owing to the complex sequence of events inherent in lymphatic transport. Therefore, the plasma profile of a drug absorbed via the portal blood as well as transported via the intestinal lymphatics would typically be broad, reflecting the slow input of lipoproteins (and associated drug) to the systemic circulation. Lymphatic transport may also result in the appearance of double peaks in plasma profiles, although this can arise through gastric emptying and/or resolubilization effects leading to portal blood absorption (Charman *et al.*, 1993).

Drugs which reach the systemic circulation via the lymphatic system avoid the first-pass metabolic processes associated with absorption via the portal blood. This can lead to changes in the proportion of metabolite relative to parent compound if the extent of drug absorption via the portal blood and intestinal lymphatic transport changes in response to the administered formulation. A candidate drug must be extremely lipophilic for lymphatic transport to be a major contributor to oral bioavailability, and consequently the use of lipophilic prodrugs can be a useful strategy to facilitate the passage of some compounds into the lymphatics. This strategy becomes particularly attractive for compounds whose site of action is located within the lymphatic system. Recent work with mepitiostane, a highly lipophilic prodrug of an antitumor agent (epitiostanol), has demonstrated the utility of this approach (Ichihashi *et al.*, 1991a,b).

In conclusion, it is important to note that there are many examples in the literature where authors have suggested (although not confirmed) that intestinal lymphatic transport may contribute to the oral bioavailability of a drug. Through application of the methods described in this chapter, it is possible to unambiguously establish the contribution of lymphatic transport to oral bioavailability. In addition to such studies establishing the contribution of lymphatic transport to oral bioavailability, the data are necessary to subsequently guide rational formulation development studies for lipophilic drugs.

REFERENCES

Bijsterbosch, M. K., and van Berkel, T. J. C., 1990, Native and modified lipoproteins as drug delivery systems, *Adv. Drug Deliv. Rev.* **5:**231–251.

Charman, W. N., 1992, Lipid vehicle and formulation effects on intestinal lymphatic transport, in: *Lymphatic Transport of Drugs* (W. N. Charman and V. J. Stella, eds.), CRC Press, Boca Raton, Florida, pp. 113–179.

Charman, W. N., and Stella, V. J., 1986a, Estimating the maximum potential for intestinal lymphatic transport of lipophilic drug molecules, *Int. J. Pharm.* **34:**175–178.

Charman, W. N., and Stella, V. J., 1986b, Effects of lipid vehicle class and lipid vehicle volume on the intestinal lymphatic transport of DDT, *Int. J. Pharm.* **33:**165–172.

Charman, W. N., and Stella, V. J., 1991, Transport of lipophilic molecules by the intestinal lymphatic system, *Adv. Drug Deliv. Rev.* **7:**1–14.

Charman, W. N., Noguchi, T., and Stella, V. J., 1986, An experimental system designed to study the *in situ* intestinal lymphatic transport of lipophilic drugs in anesthetized rats, *Int. J. Pharm.* **33:**155–164.

Charman, W. N., Rogge, M. C., Boddy, A. W., Barr, W. H., and Berger, B. M., 1993, Absorption of danazol after administration to different sites of the gastrointestinal tract and the relationship to single- and double-peak phenomena in the plasma profiles, *J. Clin. Pharmacol.* **33:**1207–1213.

Fukui, E., Kurohara, H., Kageyu, A., Kurosaki, Y., Nakayama, T., and Kimura, T., 1989, Enhancing effect of medium chain triglyceride on intestinal absorption of *d*-α-tocopherol acetate from lecithin-dispersed preparations in the rat, *J. Pharmacobio-Dyn.* **12:**80–86.

Ichihashi, T., Kinoshita, H., and Yamada, H., 1991a, Absorption and disposition of epithiosteroids in rats (2): Avoidance of first pass metabolism of mepitiostane by lymphatic absorption, *Xenbiotica* **21:** 873–880.

Ichihashi, T., Kinoshita, H., Takagishi, Y., and Yamada, H., 1991b, Effect of oily vehicles on absorption of mepitiostane by the lymphatic system in rats, *J. Pharm. Pharmacol.* **44:**560–564.

Laher, J. M., Rigler, M. W., Vetter, R. D., Barrowman, J. A., and Patton, J. S., 1984, Similar bioavailability and lymphatic transport of benzo(a)pyrene when administered to rats in different amounts of dietary fat, *J. Lipid. Res.* **25:**1337–1342.

Noguchi, T., Charman, W. N., and Stella, V. J., 1985, Lymphatic appearance of DDT in thoracic or mesenteric lymph duct cannulated rats, *Int. J. Pharm.* **24:**185–192.

Palin, K. J., and Wilson, C. G., 1984, The effect of different oils on the absorption of probucol in the rat, *J. Pharm. Pharmacol.* **36:**641–643.

Palin, K. J., Wilson, C. G., Davis S. S., and Phillips, A. J., 1982, The effect of oils on the lymphatic absorption of DDT, *J. Pharm. Pharmacol.* **34:**707–710.

Porter, C. J. H., Charman, S. A., and Charman, W. N., 1993, Influence of anesthetized or conscious rat models on the lymphatic transport of a highly lipophilic compound, *Pharm. Res.* **10:**S209 (abstract).

Rajpal, S. G., and Kirkpatrick, J. R., 1972, Creation of a thoracic duct fistula: An improved technique, *J. Surgi. Res.* **13:**260–264.

Raub, T. J., Douglas, S. L., Melchior, G. W., Charman, W. N., and Morozowich, W., 1992, Methodologies for assessing intestinal lymphatic transport, in: *Lymphatic Transport of Drugs* (W. N. Charman and V. J. Stella, eds.), CRC Press, Boca Raton, Florida, pp. 63–111.

Shiau, Y.-F., Popper, D. A., Reed, M., Umstetter, C., Capuzzi, D., and Levine, G. M., 1985, Intestinal lipoproteins are derived from both endogenous and exogenous sources, *Am. J. Physiol.* **248:** G164–G169.

Takada, K., Yoshimura, H., Yoshikawa, H., Muranishi, S., Yasumuru, T., and Oka, T., 1986, Enhanced selective lymphatic delivery of cyclosporin A by solubilisers and intensified immunosuppressive activity against mice skin allograft, *Pharm. Res.* **3:**48–51.

Tso, P., Pitts, V., and Granger, D. N., 1985, Role of lymph flow in chylomicron transport, *Am. J. Physiol.* **249:**G21–G28.

White, D. G., Storey, M. J., and Barnwell, S. G., 1991, An experimental model for studying the effects of a novel lymphatic drug delivery system for propranolol, *Int. J. Pharm.* **69:**169–174.

Yeung, D. L., and von Saigent, M. J., 1972, Absorption of retinol and retinyl esters via the lymph and the portal vein in the rat, *Can. J. Physiol. Pharmacol.* **50:**753–760.

Chapter 7

Buccal Tissues and Cell Culture

Elizabeth Quadros, James P. Cassidy, and Harry Leipold

1. INTRODUCTION

The buccal mucosa may be an alternative route of administration for selected compounds that cannot be delivered using conventional oral dosage forms, because they undergo either extensive first-pass metabolism or degradation in the gastrointestinal tract. The buccal route has several advantages for long-term controlled drug delivery. The oral mucosa is readily accessible for placement and removal of a delivery device, is well supplied with both vascular and lymphatic drainage, and avoids both hepatic first-pass metabolism and presystemic metabolism in the gastrointestinal tract. Additionally, the buccal mucosa is considerably more permeable than the skin, an accepted route for controlled drug delivery, and thus this alternative route would expand the number of compounds that could be delivered in therapeutic doses. Furthermore, the time lag through buccal mucosa is considerably shorter than that seen though skin. Unidirectional delivery of the drug to the mucosa from a device with an impermeable backing reduces drug loss due to swallowing. The development of a small, thin flexible device that causes minimal disruption to normal activities such as eating, drinking, and talking is the ultimate aim of this area of drug delivery research. As part of developing such a delivery system, the degree of drug permeation through the buccal mucosa must be determined. Initial *in vitro* studies to measure steady-state drug flux and time lag and to evaluate different delivery systems can be performed in modified Ussing chambers using buccal mucosa isolated from an animal model.

Elizabeth Quadros and James P. Cassidy • Ciba Pharmaceuticals, Summit, New Jersey 07901.
Harry Leipold • Emisphere Technologies, Inc., Hawthorne, New York 10532.

Models for Assessing Drug Absorption and Metabolism, Ronald T. Borchardt *et al.*, eds., Plenum Press, New York, 1996.

Permeation, metabolism, and toxicity can be assessed *in vitro* using a recently developed buccal cell culture system that allows the generation of multiple cultures from a small amount of starting tissue. Pharmacokinetic parameters, metabolism, and bioavailability can be evaluated *in vivo* using drug delivery systems in the dog model, which has been selected based on the similarity between canine and human buccal mucosa.

2. METHODS

2.1. Modified Ussing Chambers

2.1.1. MATERIALS

Transport medium: Calcium- and magnesium-free Earle's balanced salt solution (EBSS), 15 mM HEPES, 10 mM BES, 10 mM TES, 100 U penicillin/ml, and 100 μg streptomycin/ml, pH 7.4.

Krebs–Henseleit buffer: 118 mM NaCl, 4.75 mM KCl, 1.2 mM KH_2PO_4, 25 mM $NaHCO_3$, 2.4 mM $MgSO_4$ and 2.5 mM $CaCl_2$ containing 10 mM glucose. The pH is maintained at 7.4 by bubbling with 95% O_2/5% CO_2. The individual stock solutions may be prepared at 10× concentration and stored at 4°C for several weeks, but the working buffer should be made fresh daily.

2.1.2. SYSTEM ESTABLISHMENT AND MONITORING

Canine buccal mucosa most closely resembles that of humans, based on morphology and permeability properties (Ebert *et al.*, 1987; Quadros *et al.*, 1991a; Cassidy *et al.*, 1993a,b), and is therefore our species of choice (Quadros *et al.*, 1991b). However, the rabbit may be more readily accessible to many laboratories and is suitable for preliminary studies. The nonkeratinized mucosa in this species is located posterior to the diastema between the incisor and molar teeth behind a region of keratinized mucosa. The buccal mucosa in the dog is nonkeratinized. Rabbits are sacrificed by carbon dioxide inhalation, and dogs by anesthetization with an intravenous injection of sodium pentobarbital and subsequent exsanguination. The nonkeratinized buccal mucosa is removed and placed in Krebs–Henseleit buffer on ice. If tissue cannot be mounted in Ussing chambers within 30 min, it may be stored in transport medium on ice. Buccal mucosa is fairly robust compared to intestinal tissues, and we have used it up to 4 hr after removal from a dog without any loss of barrier properties. The underlying muscle is removed by careful dissection while keeping the tissue moist with buffer. This is more readily accomplished in the dog since the connective tissue is looser, whereas the attachment of the connective tissue and muscle to the epithelium is much tighter in the rabbit. The epithelial tissue is then mounted in modified Ussing chambers with an exposed surface area of 0.64 or 1 cm^2 (WPI, Sarasota, FL). Buffer (10 ml) is added to each half-chamber, and the temperature at the tissue surface is maintained at 37°C by water-jacketing. Gas lift with 95% O_2/5% CO_2 is used to circulate the buffer and maintain the pH. Oxygen may be used as the gas phase if other buffers are used, for example, to vary the pH. Transepithelial potential difference (p.d.) and short-circuit current (I_{sc}) are measured by salt bridges of 2% agar in Krebs–Henseleit buffer in contact with silver/silver chloride electrodes (WPI). The bridges for measuring p.d. are placed close to the surface of the tissue, and bridges are placed at a distance from the tissue to allow the passage of a current to clamp the p.d. at zero and to measure the I_{sc}. The electrodes are connected to a voltage/current clamp (DVC-1000, WPI) via a preamplifier. Any offset between the electrodes and the fluid resistance of the buffer is compensated for before the tissue is mounted in the chamber. The experiments are performed with the tissue unclamped, which more closely mimics the physiological state, except for intermittent brief clamping to allow the measurement of the I_{sc}. The transepithelial resistance may be calculated using Ohm's law:

$$V = IR \qquad (1)$$

where R is the resistance ($\Omega \cdot cm^2$), V is the potential difference (mV), and I is the current ($\mu A/cm^2$). Conductance (G) is the reciprocal of the resistance. The electrophysiological parameters are recorded every 15 to 30 min throughout the experiment to assess tissue viability, and they remain stable for at least 6 hr in dog and rabbit buccal tissue (Quadros et al., 1991b).

2.1.3.   EXPERIMENTAL PROTOCOL

After an equilibration period of 30 min–1 hr to allow stabilization of the electrophysiological parameters, the buffer solutions are drained from the chambers and replaced with the test drug on the donor side (generally the mucosal side) and buffer in the receiver compartment. Samples (generally 0.5–1 ml) are taken from the receiver side for several hours, and the fluid removed is replaced with an equal volume of buffer. At the end of the experimental period, both the donor and receptor fluids may be collected for further analysis. The tissue may be fixed in the chamber using 10% buffered formalin, pH 7, and processed for histological assessment.

Buccal drug delivery systems may also be evaluated in Ussing chambers. Nonwoven Hill Top chambers (Hill Top Labs, Cincinnati, OH) are removed from their adhesive backing, loaded with drug solution (220 μl for a 1-cm^2 system), and applied to the mucosa after equilibration of the tissue in Krebs–Henseleit buffer. These systems have a backing material that prevents fluid loss by evaporation. Buccal permeation of buprenorphine was identical from free solution and from solution applied to Hill Top chambers, validating the use of these systems (Cassidy et al., 1993b). Much smaller amounts of drug are required for application on Hill Top chambers, which is an important consideration when drug supply is limited or the drug is expensive. For those systems that have no backing, Parafilm® or another appropriate backing may be applied to prevent fluid evaporation. The residual drug in the system at the end of the study may be extracted and analyzed. The disadvantage of using these systems is that electrophysiological parameters cannot be monitored while the system is in place.

2.1.4.   CALCULATIONS

The samples are assayed for drug content by an appropriate analytical method, including HPLC, radioimmunoassay, or radioisotopic measurement. The cumulative amount of drug permeated is plotted against time (Fig. 1), and the steady-state flux, J_{ss}, is calculated by linear regression of the linear portion of the curve at time points greater than twice the time lag. The time lag is obtained by extrapolation of the regression line to the abscissa. The apparent permeability coefficient, P, is given by

$$P = \frac{C_r V}{A t C_d} \qquad (2)$$

where C_r is the drug concentration in the receiver solution, V is the volume of the receiver solution, A is the area of tissue exposed, t is time, and C_d is the drug concentration in the donor solution.

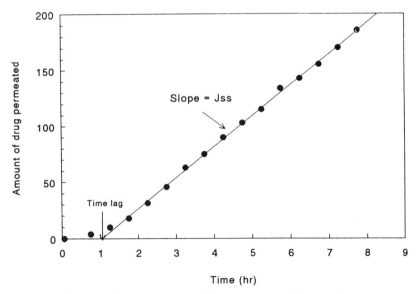

Figure 1.   Cumulative amount of drug absorbed plotted versus time.

2.2. Buccal Cell Culture

2.2.1. MATERIALS

Transport medium: see Section 2.1.1.

Primary growth medium: MEM with Earle's salts and nonessential amino acids, 300 μg L-glutamine/ml, 10% fetal bovine serum (FBS), 25 mM HEPES, 0.5% dimethyl sulfoxide (DMSO), 10^{-9} M cholera toxin, 10 U penicillin/ml, 10 μg streptomycin/ml, 2.5 μg amphotericin B/ml.

Culture medium: MEM with Earle's salts and nonessential amino acids, 300 μg L-glutamine/ml, 10% FBS, 25 mM HEPES, 10^{-9} M cholera toxin, 10 ng epidermal growth factor (EGF)/ml, 10 U penicillin/ml, 10 μg streptomycin/ml, and 50 μg gentamicin/ml.

Flux medium: Culture medium without EGF and cholera toxin.

2.2.2. SYSTEM ESTABLISHMENT AND MONITORING

The culture procedure is based on a modification of that reported by Wilkinson *et al.* (1987). Canine buccal tissue is excised from beagles of either sex after sacrifice by anesthetization with intravenous sodium pentobarbital and subsequent exsanguination. Tissue is transported to the laboratory on ice in transport medium. The excised tissue is rinsed and trimmed free of underlying muscle, a process that is generally completed within 4 hr of tissue collection. The epithelial layers are separated from the connective tissue after overnight incubation at 4°C in primary growth medium containing 10 mg dispase/ml (Boehringer Mannheim, Indianapolis, IN). Epithelial sheets are placed in transport medium containing 0.25% trypsin and 5 mM EDTA (Sigma Chemical Co., St. Louis, MO), cut into small pieces, and stirred gently at room temperature for 45 min. Cells are dispersed by pipetting, centrifuged at 4°C and 50 × *g*, resuspended in primary growth medium, and plated in either 60-mm culture dishes or 75-cm² culture flasks (Falcon, Fisher Scientific, Springfield, NJ) at a density of $0.75 \times 10^5 - 1 \times 10^5$ cells/cm². Cultures are maintained in an incubator at 37°C with 5% CO_2 and 95% humidity. The medium is replaced twice weekly with culture medium. When the primary cells reach confluence, they are passaged at a split ratio of 1:3 onto Anocell™ 25 tissue culture inserts (3.37 cm²) in 6-well plates. The medium of first-passage cells is replaced twice weekly with culture medium. One week after confluence is reached, the transepithelial resistance and potential difference across each culture are measured using an Epithelial Voltohmmeter with STX electrodes (WPI, Sarasota, FL). Once these parameters stabilize, generally 3–5 weeks post confluence, flux studies are performed. During the establishment of these cell cultures, the fluxes of horseradish peroxidase (HRP) and CGS 16617, a small hydrophilic molecule, were monitored at weekly intervals. The fluxes fell and stabilized at a similar time as the resistance and potential difference became stable (Fig. 2; Leipold

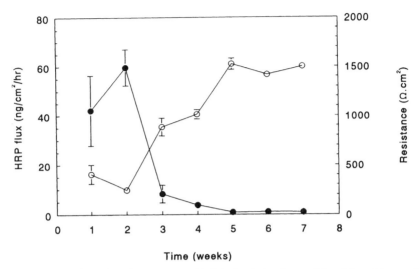

Figure 2. Effect of time in culture on transepithelial electrical resistance (○) and flux of horseradish peroxidase (●).

and Quadros, 1991). Since it is simpler to monitor electrophysiological parameters as a measure of barrier function, this approach was used in further studies.

Cells can also be stored in liquid nitrogen, thawed, and placed in culture for flux and toxicity studies. When primary cultures grown in 75-cm² flasks reach confluence, they are rinsed with calcium- and magnesium-free EBSS and treated with trypsin/EDTA to release them. FBS is added to give a final concentration of 20%, and the cells are centrifuged at 50 × g for 10 min. The cells are washed twice with MEM and resuspended in MEM with 20% FBS and 10% DMSO (1 ml per flask). The cell suspension in 1-ml aliquots is transferred to cryogenic storage vials. The vials are placed in a Styrofoam-insulated box at −70°C for 2 hr for slow cooling and vials are then transferred to liquid nitrogen for storage.

To reestablish the cells in culture, the vials are thawed rapidly in a 37°C water bath with agitation, and the contents of each vial are transferred to a 75-cm² flask. At confluence the cells are passaged at a split ratio of 1:3 into 75-cm² flasks. The next passage is either onto filter inserts in 6-well plates or directly into 96-well plates.

2.2.3. EXPERIMENTAL PROTOCOL

After stabilization of the barrier properties, flux studies are performed in either flux medium or EBSS containing 25 mM Tris. The latter medium was selected for its simplicity and lack of factors, such as proteins, that may bind the test compound or interfere with its analysis. Donor and receiver chambers are rinsed once, and 2 ml of drug solution is added to the donor side and 2 ml of solution to the receiver side of the chamber. Cultures are incubated at 37°C with 5% CO_2 and 95% humidity on a rotating platform (Lab-line) set at 100 rpm. Samples (generally 200–500 μl) are collected from the receiver side at intervals up to 4 hr and replaced with an equal volume of receiver solution. A modification of the above method is necessary for rapidly permeating compounds when sink conditions are not maintained in the receiver solution. The inserts with the donor solution are lifted out of the wells at frequent intervals (e.g., 10 min) and are transferred to plates with fresh receiver solution. At the end of the experiment, the transepithelial resistance and potential difference across each culture are measured.

Cellular toxicity of the drug under study or putative absorption enhancers may be assessed in the same cultures used for transport studies. A variety of markers, such as lactate dehydrogenase, arachidonic acid metabolites, and chromium-51, have been used to assess cellular and tissue damage. Neutral red is taken up by the lysosomes, and cellular damage decreases its uptake. The assay has been used in several cell types, is simple and reproducible, and, in fibroblasts, correlates well with the Draize eye irritancy test *in vivo* (Borenfreund and Puerner, 1985). At the end of flux studies, the donor and receiver solutions are removed, and the cells are washed with buffer and incubated with neutral red solution (50 μg/ml) for 2 hr. The wells are rinsed twice, and the dye is extracted by the addition of 50% ethanol/1% acetic acid for at least 20 min at room temperature. The absorbance is read at 540 nm. Alternatively, toxicity studies may be performed independently of drug permeation studies on cells cultured in 96-well plates (Leipold and Quadros, 1993).

2.2.4.   CALCULATIONS

The steady-state flux, time lag, and permeability coefficients are calculated as described in Section 2.1.4.

2.3.   *In Vivo* Dog Model

2.3.1.   EXPERIMENTAL PROCEDURE

Beagles (7–14 kg) are fasted overnight but are allowed water *ad libitum* until the time of experimentation. A 22-g Abbocath® (Abbott Hospitals, Inc., North Chicago, IL) is inserted into the cephalic vein, checked for patency, and flushed with sterile heparinized saline (40 U/ml). The dog is anesthetized with sodium pentobarbital (25 mg/kg), and additional doses are administered as necessary to maintain light anesthesia. Cannula patency is maintained with an intravenous drip of sterile lactated Ringer solution (Abbott Hospitals, Inc.) at a flow rate of 1 ml/min. A blood sample (3–5 ml) is drawn into a heparinized Monoject® syringe (Sarstedt, Newton, NC), and the fluid volume is replaced with heparinized saline. Plasma is obtained by centrifugation at $2000 \times g$ for 10 min and stored for later analysis.

Absorption of a drug from a buccal system is compared to either an intravenous bolus injection or infusion administered through a second catheter in the saphenous vein. Plasma samples are obtained over a time period appropriate for the pharmacokinetics of the compound of interest. The buccal device is applied to the oral mucosa and covered by a Surlyn® membrane held in place by peripheral dental adhesive (Super Polygrip, Dentco Inc., Jersey City, NJ). The mouth is held open by a standard canine dental clamp, and the tongue is held back by wrapping with moistened gauze. The device is left in place for up to 4 hr, and blood samples are taken during and after the application. The position of the device is checked intermittently, and the mucosa is carefully inspected after removal of the system. The residual drug in the system is extracted for analysis.

2.3.2. CALCULATIONS

The flux of drug across the buccal mucosa at steady state is given by

$$\text{Flux} = \frac{C_{ss}\text{Cl}}{A} \tag{3}$$

where C_{ss} is the plasma concentration at steady state, Cl is the clearance, and A is the area of the device. The plasma concentration at steady state is obtained by linear regression of the linear portion of the cumulative AUC (area under the plasma concentration versus time curve) versus time curve. The intercept on the abscissa yields the time lag to steady state. The clearance of the drug is obtained by standard pharmacokinetic analysis of the intravenous data by dividing the dose of the drug by the AUC. It is assumed that the clearance of the drug is unchanged by the route of administration.

The bioavailability of the drug absorbed by the buccal route may be calculated as follows:

$$F_{\text{bucc}} = \frac{\text{AUC}_{\text{bucc}}}{\text{AUC}_{\text{iv}}} \cdot \frac{\text{Dose}_{\text{iv}}}{\text{Dose}_{\text{bucc}}} \tag{4}$$

where F_{bucc} is the fraction absorbed by the buccal route, AUC_{bucc} is the area under the curve after buccal dosing, $\text{Dose}_{\text{bucc}}$ is the buccal drug dose (amount loaded—amount recovered), Dose_{iv} is the intravenous dose of drug, and AUC_{iv} is the area under the curve after intravenous dosing.

3. APPLICATIONS TO ABSORPTION AND METABOLISM

The Ussing chamber has been used for many years, initially to study ion fluxes (Ussing and Zerahn, 1951) and more recently to measure drug flux across isolated tissues. It provides a completely controlled environment in terms of temperature, oxygen tension, buffer, and drug concentration and allows measurement of the permeation of the drug across a known surface area of isolated buccal mucosa. Both donor and receiver solutions may be sampled at selected intervals to determine both permeation of drug through the tissue and its metabolism (if any). It is therefore ideal for preliminary feasibility studies or the evaluation of several structurally related compounds that may be produced in the drug discovery process. The judicious use of absorption studies at an early stage of drug development may avoid much frustration later on in the process. The effects of putative absorption enhancers—both on the flux of the drug and on the viability of the tissue (as measured by electrophysiology or flux of a model compound) and its ability to recover from exposure to the agent—may also be measured in this system.

Screening of drugs for their permeation through buccal mucosa and tissue metabolism may be done more rapidly using cultured cells. Toxicity of the drugs themselves or potential absorption enhancers may be assessed in the same cultures in which flux studies are performed, or separately on cells grown in 96-well plates. The use of colorimetric assays, such as neutral red, or fluorometric assays and reading on automatic plate readers simplify many of these procedures.

Both buccal absorption of a compound from a delivery device and its metabolism in an intact animal can be assessed in the *in vivo* dog model. Buccal bioavailability and steady-state flux can be calculated by comparing the plasma levels of the drug after buccal administration to those obtained after intravenous administration. The size of delivery system required to deliver the desired plasma levels of drug may then be calculated. The dose can be calculated by residual analysis of the system.

4. ADVANTAGES AND DISADVANTAGES COMPARED TO OTHER METHODS

The advantages of the Ussing chamber method lie in the ability to study drug flux across the tissue of interest and metabolism by that tissue alone. Preliminary screening of prototype buccal delivery systems may also be performed in this model. A potential disadvantage is the limited amount of tissue available per animal, particularly in the case of the rabbit, which has sufficient tissue for only two chambers. The barrier properties of the tissue can be monitored using electrophysiological measurements and permeation of a standard marker such as mannitol, if desired. Underlying muscle and connective tissue may remain despite attempts to remove them and may complicate flux studies. It is unlikely that they present a significant permeability barrier (Squier and Hall, 1985), but tissue binding and metabolism of drug may occur. Good correlation has been shown between *in vitro* and *in vivo* fluxes from nonwoven and hydrogel systems.

The development of the buccal cell culture system allows the amplification of cells from a small piece of tissue, and the greater simplicity of the system allows more experimental data to be gathered. Cell culture may also be applied to the growth of human buccal cells. We have demonstrated that cells stored frozen in liquid nitrogen retain their original permeability properties, allowing even greater expansion of the original tissue. As with isolated buccal mucosa, the transepithelial electrical resistance and potential difference may be monitored. Clearly, cell culture may suffer from the disadvantage that the cells are grown predominantly as monolayers and may not retain the same barrier properties as the intact tissue, which is a stratified, squamous epithelium. Conflicting reports exist in the literature about the location of the permeability barrier in intact tissue. De Vries (1991) reported that the barrier for beta blockers is in the basal layer, whereas Harris and Robinson (1992) reported that the membrane-coating granules in the stratum granulosum provide the major barrier. Buccal drug delivery devices cannot be assessed in the cell culture system described above, although the potential irritating effect of individual soluble components could be assessed. However, multilayered buccal cell cultures may be developed by growing cells at the air–liquid interface. This may be useful in the assessment of drug delivery systems *in vitro.*

The use of the dog *in vivo* model is particularly suitable for the later stages in the development of a compound for buccal delivery. It requires technical expertise and facilities with appropriate veterinarian and technical support. Its clear advantages are that the studies are performed in an intact animal and that the dog appears to be a good model for man for the limited number of compounds (diclofenac sodium and buprenorphine) examined thus far. *In vivo* models are important to assess metabolism of a compound that frequently occurs at sites remote from the absorptive surface.

REFERENCES

Borenfreund, E., and Puerner, J. A., 1985, Toxicity determined *in vitro* by morphological alterations and neutral red, *Toxicol. Lett.* **24:**119–124.

Cassidy, J., Berner, B., Chan, K., John, V., Toon, S., Holt, B., and Rowland, M., 1993a, Human transbuccal absorption of diclofenac from a prototype hydrogel delivery device, *Pharm. Res.* **10:**126–129.

Cassidy, J. P., Landzert, N. M., and Quadros, E., 1993b, Controlled delivery of buprenorphine, *J. Controlled Release* **25:**21–29.

De Vries, M. E., 1991, Buccal Drug Absorption and Development of Mucoadhesive Polymer Systems, Ph.D. Thesis, Leiden University, pp. 56–68.

Ebert, C. D., John, V. A., Beall, P. T., and Rosenzweig, K. A., 1987, Transbuccal absorption of diclofenac sodium in a dog model, in: *Controlled-Release Technology*, ACS Symposium Series, No. 348 (P. I. Lee and W. R. Good, eds.), American Chemical Society, Washington, D.C., pp. 310–321.

Harris, D., and Robinson, J. R., 1992, Drug delivery via the mucous membranes of the oral cavity, *J. Pharm. Sci.* **81:**1–10.

Leipold, H., and Quadros, E., 1991, Permeability of canine buccal keratinocytes in culture to CGS 16617 and horseradish peroxidase, *Pharm. Res.* **8:**S199.

Leipold, H., and Quadros, E., 1993, Bile salt toxicity in cultures canine keratinocytes, *Pharm. Res.* **10:**S286.

Quadros, E., Cassidy, J., Tipnis, V., Livingston, T., and Langley, S., 1991a, Controlled buccal delivery of buprenorphine in man, *Pharm. Res.* **8:**S156.

Quadros, E., Cassidy, J., Gniecko, K., and LeRoy, S., 1991b, Buccal and colonic absorption of CGS 16617, a novel ACE inhibitor, *J. Controlled Release* **19**:77–86.

Squier, C. A., and Hall, B. K., 1985, *In vitro* permeability of porcine oral mucosa after epithelial separation, stripping and hydration, *Arch. Oral Biol.* **30**:485–491.

Ussing, H. H., and Zerahn, K., 1951, Active transport of sodium as the source of electric current in the short-circuited isolated frog skin, *Acta Physiol. Scand.* **23**:110–127.

Wilkinson, J. E., Smith, C., Suter, M., and Lewis, R. M., 1987, Long-term cultivation of canine keratinocytes, *J. Invest. Dermatol.* **88**:202–206.

Chapter 8

Isolated Hepatocytes

M. Vore, Y. Liu, and T. C. Ganguly

1. INTRODUCTION

Transport across the basolateral and canalicular domains of the hepatocyte plasma membrane represents two important but very distinct processes essential for the movement of drugs or endogenous compounds from the plasma into the hepatocyte and from the hepatocyte into bile. This chapter will cover transport in isolated rat hepatocytes as a method that is very useful and practical for characterizing transport across the basolateral domain. The isolated perfused rat liver has also been used extensively to characterize transport from plasma to liver; this method is covered in Chapter 10. Cultured hepatocytes have also been used to study the mechanisms of transport of substrates into the hepatocyte; methods for preparation of cultured hepatocytes are covered in Chapter 9.

Suspensions of isolated rat hepatocytes have been used extensively to characterize the uptake of substrates across the basolateral domain of the hepatocyte (Schwarz and Greim, 1981; Klaassen and Watkins, 1984). Isolated hepatocyte suspensions permit analysis of multiple samples over short time periods (e.g., 15-sec intervals) so that initial velocities and kinetic parameters for transport can be estimated. Variables related to binding to plasma proteins and liver blood flow are eliminated. The investigator is also able to manipulate the extracellular medium in order to determine if ion gradients, for example, an out $>$ in Na^+ gradient, are essential for uptake into the cell. The high yield of cells also permits determination of a relatively large number of data points from a single rat liver. Isolated hepatocytes are also used extensively for metabolism studies, although this application will not be discussed here.

M. Vore, Y. Liu, and T. C. Ganguly • Graduate Center for Toxicology, University of Kentucky, Lexington, Kentucky 40503.

Models for Assessing Drug Absorption and Metabolism, Ronald T. Borchardt *et al.*, eds., Plenum Press, New York, 1996.

2. METHODS

2.1. Isolation of Cells

In Chapter 9, LeCluyse *et al.* have detailed the surgical procedures and perfusion methods for the isolation of cells from the rat liver, so that these will not be repeated here. The only difference in the method that we have used is the removal of the liver from the animal and collagenase perfusion of the isolated liver in a temperature-controlled chamber (Brock and Vore, 1984; Moldéus *et al.*, 1978). We have used this method for transport studies in freshly isolated hepatocytes where it is not necessary to maintain absolutely sterile conditions. We have found, however, that sterilization of all perfusion buffers increases yield and viability of the hepatocytes. Although it is difficult to definitively assess the efficacy of a good enzyme batch, in our hands type II collagenase obtained from Worthington has consistently yielded intact hepatocytes. Under these conditions, the liver is perfused with the collagenase buffer (70 mg/100 ml Ca^{2+}-free perfusion buffer) and is then removed to a beaker containing 50 ml of calcium-free and collagenase-free perfusion buffer at 37°C. The liver is gently dispersed with blunt forceps to tease the hepatocytes from the liver capsule, and the cell suspension is filtered through 240 μm of mesh nylon into a 250-ml round-bottomed flask, which is rotated at the lowest speed on a Brinkmann Instruments rotor-evaporator at 37°C under 95% O_2/5% CO_2 atmosphere for 20 min. (We have found that it is usually not worthwhile to attempt to extract hepatocytes from poorly perfused liver lobes.) The cells are then gently centrifuged at $50 \times g$ for 90 sec at room temperature. The supernatant is gently aspirated and discarded, and the cellular pellet is washed three times with an ice-cold wash buffer consisting of 137 mM NaCl, 5.2 mM KCl, 0.9 mM $MgSO_4$, 0.12 mM $CaCl_2$, and 3 mM Na_2HPO_4. The final cellular pellet is resuspended in an incubation buffer consisting of the wash buffer containing 10 mM Tris-HCl (pH 7.4). If the effect of ions (e.g., Na^+ or Cl^-) on transport is to be determined, then the initial cellular pellet is divided into two portions, and the cells in each portion are washed and resuspended in the appropriate final incubation buffer. Viability is determined by trypan blue exclusion as described in Chapter 9. We routinely obtain viability of about 95%, with no need for use of Percoll gradients to remove nonviable cells.

2.2. Experimental Protocols for Uptake

Uptake into hepatocytes is determined by incubating hepatocytes with radio-labeled (about 240 nCi) substrate and unlabeled substrate in a total volume of 4 ml. It is essential to establish the linearity of uptake with respect to protein (or number of cells); we have found that uptake is linear for bile acids and other organic anions in the range of 1.0–2.0 mg of cellular protein/ml of incubation buffer. A total volume of 4 ml of incubation buffer permits consistent and easy removal of four or five 0.2-ml aliquots at short time intervals for determination of uptake into the cellular pellet. An orbital shaking incubator is used to minimize cell lysis during incubation. We have found that use of a small (25 ml) Erlenmeyer flask, which is heated and the center pushed up with a glass rod, prevents the formation of a concentrated pool of cells at the center of the flask. The cells (in 3.9 ml of incubation buffer) are preincubated at 37°C under a stream of 95% O_2/5% CO_2 for 5 min, and then 0.1 ml of substrate is added at time zero. Use of vehicle other than incubation buffer should be accompanied by studies demonstrating that the vehicle does not decrease viability of cells. Timed samples (0.2 ml) are removed with an automatic pipettor at timed intervals and placed in a 0.4-ml polyethylene microfuge tube containing 3 M KOH (0.05 ml) under a 0.1-ml layer of silicone oil. Silicone oil of density 1.05 g/ml is combined with 0.883-g/ml mineral oil, to give a final density of 1.02 g/ml. The samples are centrifuged *immediately* for about 10 sec in a tabletop microcentrifuge which attains *g* values of 10,000 within 1–2 sec. Upon centrifugation, the cells, together with a small volume of adherent fluid, pass through the oil into the KOH. A visible layer of cells *above* the silicone oil layer indicates that either the correct silicone oil density has not been obtained or the cells are not viable. The cells are allowed to sit overnight to allow dissolution of the cellular pellet in the KOH. The amount of substrate taken into cells is determined by cutting the microfuge tube at the silicone oil–KOH interface and placing the tip containing the cellular pellet into a scintillation vial and assaying for radioactivity. (We use a large dog nail trimmer to cut the tubes.) Radioactivity in the cell-free supernatant may also be determined. Adherent fluid volume and cellular water volume are determined by incubating cells with [carboxyl-^{14}C]dextran and [^{3}H]-H_2O, respectively (Baur *et al.*, 1975). An aliquot of the medium in each incubation flask is assayed directly for protein concentration at the end of the uptake experiment.

2.3. Calculations of Data

Knowledge of the specific activity (nCi/nmol) of the substrate, substrate concentration, protein concentration, cell viability, and uptake in 4–5 samples over the linear range permits calculation of the slope of the regression line to determine the rate of uptake as nanomoles per minute per milligram of protein. Measurement of uptake at 4–5 times permits discarding of one time sample that is clearly in error without loss of the entire estimate. Correlation coefficients of 0.97 or greater should be routinely obtained. If possible, it is desirable to determine each uptake rate in duplicate (i.e., using a separate flask for each determination).

2.4. Comments

1. Preliminary experiments should determine the time course of uptake of the substrate so that subsequent measures are made while uptake is in the linear range. For substrates that are taken up actively, such as taurocholate, linearity extends for only 90 sec. In this case, four, and preferably five, time points should be sampled within 90 sec, requiring sampling every 15–20 sec, in order to obtain a valid estimate of initial rates. This rapid sampling schedule requires practice as well as two or three microcentrifuges. Thus, the 15-, 30-, 45-, 60-, and 75-sec samples are spun in centrifuges 1, 2, 3, 1, and 2, respectively. Slower rates of uptake permit a more leisurely sampling schedule.

2. We have not found it necessary to determine the protein concentration in each timed sample. A rapid swirling of the cells in the flask immediately before each timed sample and before measuring an aliquot for protein ensures an adequately uniform distribution of cells in all samples. The pushed-up center of the Erlenmeyer flask is important for enhancing a uniform distribution of cells.

3. The entire transport experiment should be completed within 2–3 hr of isolation of the cells so that cell viability is uniform throughout the experiment. Viability should be determined in the stock of cells at the end of the experiment; a loss of 1–2% over 2–3 hours is acceptable. The average of the initial and the final viability of the cells is used in the calculation of initial uptake rates.

4. It is important to determine if significant metabolism of substrate occurs within the time period of measurement of uptake. Metabolism of substrate taken up by the hepatocyte will increase the apparent rate of uptake by decreasing the intracellular concentration of substrate, enhancing the out $>$ in gradient of substrate and thus facilitating diffusion. Studies characterizing the uptake of L-alanine utilize aminooxyacetate and DL-cycloserine to inhibit alanine metabolism and permit accurate estimation of rates of uptake (Teo and Vore, 1990).

5. The K_m and V_{max} for uptake can be readily determined by using a series of substrate concentrations. It is also possible to investigate energy requirements by adding metabolic inhibitors, ion requirements (e.g., substitution of choline for Na^+ in the incubation buffer), and the effects of potential competitive inhibitors on initial uptake rates. An experienced investigator can complete 40 uptake determinations from a single liver in 2–3 hr.

6. The buffer/water which adheres to the surface of the hepatocyte and theoretically contains substrate will pass through the silicone oil with the cells upon centrifugation. In order to correct for the overestimated total radioactivity in the pellet, the adherent fluid volume is determined. This is accomplished by incubating hepatocytes (1.5–2.5 mg of cellular protein/ml) with the poorly permeable [carboxyl-^{14}C]dextran (50 nCi/ml) at 37°C for 10 min. The cells are pelleted as before (200-μl aliquot), and radioactivity is determined in the supernatant (S) and pellet (P).

Correction for the adherent fluid volume is then accomplished by the following equation:

Adherent fluid volume (nCi/ml) =
nCi/ml of pellet − [(dpm of S/dpm of P) × nCi/ml of cell-free supernatant]

7. Cellular water volume (ml/mg protein) is similarly determined by incubating cells with [^{3}H]-H$_2$O (50 nCi/ml) for 10 min and determining the radioactivity in the supernatant (S) and pellet (P) following centrifugation of an aliquot (200 ml) of the cell suspension:

Cellular water volume (ml/mg protein) =
(dpm of P/nCi/ml of cell-free supernatant)/mg protein in 0.2 ml of aliquot

3. ADVANTAGES AND DISADVANTAGES OVER OTHER METHODS

The major advantages of isolated hepatocytes for assessing the role of the liver in first-pass absorption and metabolism of drugs are that (i) multiple experiments can be carried out with cells from one liver and (ii) the ability to control the extracellular milieu allows the investigator to explore mechanisms of transport. Thus, one can determine if uptake is due to passive diffusion or active transport or is coupled to uptake of ions. While extrapolations can be made to assess uptake by the whole liver, this is probably best done in the isolated perfused liver, where compounds excreted in bile are in fact eliminated from the system (assuming the bile duct is cannulated). In hepatocytes, excretion in bile represents efflux into the extracellular milieu, where substrate can be taken back up into the hepatocyte.

Isolated hepatocytes are relatively inexpensive to prepare in that the equipment required is not highly specialized and the procedure is not labor intensive. One well-trained individual can carry out uptake experiments on two livers in one well-organized day. Thus, it is possible to study a control and experimental animal, for example, each day using the same buffers, collagenase preparations, etc. The methods can readily be adapted to characterize metabolism by maintaining a 95% O$_2$/5% CO$_2$ atmosphere when longer times are used (e.g., 5–60 min). Again, the ability to analyze multiple samples from one liver and the ability to add metabolic inhibitors and control the atmosphere (e.g., the use of CO or N$_2$) makes this approach suited for mechanistic studies.

REFERENCES

Baur, H., Kaspereck, S., and Pfaf, E., 1975, Criteria of viability of isolated hepatocytes, *Hoppe-Seyler's Z. Physiol. Chem.* **357**:827–838.

Brock, W. J., and Vore, M., 1984, Characterization of uptake of steroid glucuronides into isolated male and female rat hepatocytes, *J. Pharmacol. Exp. Ther.* **229:**175–181.

Klaassen, C. D., and Watkins, J. B., III, 1984, Mechanisms of bile formation, hepatic uptake and biliary excretion, *Pharmacol. Rev.* **36:**1–67.

Moldéus, P., Högberg, J., and Orrenius, S., 1978, Isolation and use of liver cells, *Meth. Enzymol.* **52:**60–71.

Schwarz, L. R., and Greim, H., 1981, Isolated hepatocytes: An analytical tool in hepatotoxicology, in: *Frontiers in Liver Diseases* (P. D. Berk and T. C. Chalmers, eds.), Neuherberg, Germany.

Teo, S., and Vore, M., 1990, Mirex exposure inhibits the uptake of estradiol 17β(β-D-glucuronide), taurocholate and L-alanine into isolated rat hepatocytes, *Toxicol. Appl. Pharmacol.* **104:**411–420.

Chapter 9

Cultured Rat Hepatocytes

Edward L. LeCluyse, Peter L. Bullock,
Andrew Parkinson, and Jerome H. Hochman

1. INTRODUCTION

The use of *in vitro* and *in vivo* systems to evaluate hepatic drug uptake and metabolism, cytochrome P450 induction, drug interactions affecting hepatic metabolism, hepatotoxicity, and cholestasis is an essential part of the drug development process (Tavoloni and Boyer, 1980; Powis *et al.*, 1989; Bertrams and Ziegler, 1991; Jurima-Romet and Huang, 1992; Komai *et al.*, 1992; Jurima-Romet and Huang, 1993). Primary hepatocyte culture is one of many techniques used to address these issues. Although primary hepatocytes maintained under conventional culture conditions have been broadly used to study drug metabolism and hepatotoxicity, the rapid loss of liver-specific functions and the failure of cultured hepatocytes to reestablish normal bile canaliculi (cell polarity, cell architecture) have limited their application.

Modifications to conventional culture conditions have resulted in dramatic improvements in the maintenance of hepatic function and longevity of hepatocyte cultures (Maher, 1988). Addition of exogenous chemicals (2% dimethyl sulfoxide, 3 mM phenobarbital, or 25 mM nicotinamide) to the culture medium (Paine *et al.*, 1979; Isom *et al.*, 1985; Miyazaki *et al.*, 1985), co-culture with various epithelial or mesenchymal cells (Guguen-Guillouzo *et al.*, 1983; Goulet *et al.*, 1988; Kuri-Harcuch and Mendoza-Figueroa, 1989; Donato *et al.*, 1990), and the use of complex extracellu-

Edward L. LeCluyse • INTERx Research/Merck Research Laboratories, Lawrence, Kansas 66047 and the Department of Pharmacology, Toxicology, and Therapeutics, University of Kansas Medical School, Kansas City, Kansas 66160. *Peter L. Bullock and Andrew Parkinson* • Department of Pharmacology, Toxicology, and Therapeutics, University of Kansas Medical School, Kansas City, Kansas 66160. *Jerome H. Hochman* • INTERx Research/Merck Research Laboratories, Lawrence, Kansas 66047.

Models for Assessing Drug Absorption and Metabolism, Ronald T. Borchardt *et al.*, eds., Plenum Press, New York, 1996.

lar matrix substrata (rat liver biomatrix, or Matrigel) (Rojkind *et al.*, 1980; Bissell *et al.*, 1987) have all been shown to prolong the usable lifetime of hepatocytes. Each of these modifications is subject to functional and logistical limitations. For example, in the case of co-cultures, the presence of multiple cell types can complicate the analysis of drug extraction and metabolism. Similarly, addition of high concentrations of exogenous chemical agents can lead to altered drug metabolism due to induction of, or competition for, drug-metabolizing pathways.

In this chapter we will discuss a relatively new model for maintaining hepatocytes in culture in which liver-specific functions are maintained by establishing conditions that mimic the native extracellular matrix geometry. Dunn *et al.* (1989, 1991) demonstrated that overlaying cultured hepatocytes with a top layer of gelled collagen prolongs their viability and preserves liver-specific protein synthesis. Further studies showed that hepatocytes maintained in this matrix "sandwich" configuration also reestablish a structurally and functionally normal bile canalicular network and show better maintenance of drug uptake and enzyme-induction potential (Sidhu *et al.*, 1993; Musat *et al.*, 1993; LeCluyse *et al.*, 1994). The retention of these hepatic functions and the relative simplicity of this culture system suggest that matrix-sandwiched hepatocytes will have considerable utility for short- and long-term enzyme induction and toxicity studies.

2. METHODS

The methods outlined in this section are limited to those determined to be the most applicable for initiating and maintaining primary cultures of rat hepatocytes. Details regarding the perfusion of rat liver for the isolation of hepatocytes are described elsewhere (see Section 7). The basic methods adopted by our laboratories for establishing hepatocyte cultures are essentially modifications of those developed by Dich and Grunnet (1989) and Berry *et al.* (1991). In our experience, long-term maintenance of liver-specific properties is primarily affected by the medium and extracellular matrix; thus, a major emphasis will be placed on describing these culture conditions. For extensive discussions regarding nearly all aspects of rat hepatocyte isolation and monolayer culture, the reader is referred to the work of Berry *et al.* (1991) and Alpini *et al.* (1994).

2.1. Culture Media and Supplements

2.1.1. BASAL MEDIA

A number of commercially available culture media have been successfully employed for culturing rat hepatocytes, including Dulbecco's modified Eagle's medium, Liebovitz L-15 medium, Waymouth 752/1 medium, Ham's F-12 medium, and modified Williams' medium E. Medium should be purchased or prepared without the pH indicator dye phenol red, especially when glucuronidation pathways are under investigation (Driscoll *et al.*, 1982). In our laboratories, Williams' medium E or a 1:1 mixture of Dulbecco's modified Eagle's and Ham's F-12 media have been used with satisfactory results. We have also employed modified Chee's medium (Waxman *et al.*, 1990) and Hepatocyte Culture Medium (Dich and Grunnet, 1989), which contain atypically high concentrations of some media components, particularly amino acids. Inasmuch as Hepatocyte Culture Medium is not commercially available and must be prepared from stock reagents, effects due to this medium will be referred to only when they differ from those of modified Chee's medium. The advantages and/or disadvantages of using these "enriched" versus conventional media will be discussed later.

All buffers and media should be prepared with type I reagent-grade water (18 MΩ·cm). After dissolution of the basic powder formulation, including sodium bicarbonate as recommended by the supplier, the media should be adjusted to pH 7.4 with NaOH or HCl depending on the medium formulation. The following components must also be added to modified Chee's medium before adjusting the pH: 580 mg glutamine/l, 168 mg arginine/l, and 10 mg thymidine/l. After the pH has been adjusted, the medium should be supplemented with 10 ml/l of a mixture of antibiotics and antimycotics (100 μg penicillin/ml, 100 μg streptomycin/ml, 25 μg Fungizone/ml) (JRH Biosciences or Gibco) and then filter-sterilized through a 0.2-μm cellulose acetate membrane filter (Corning). All media containers should be stored at 0–4°C and protected from light if not used immediately. Certain amino acids (e.g., tryptophan) are susceptible to photooxidation upon prolonged exposure to light, which can subsequently alter the cytochrome P450 activity in hepatocyte cultures (Kocarek *et al.*, 1993a).

2.1.2. MEDIA SUPPLEMENTS

Dexamethasone can be prepared in an appropriate solvent such as DMSO or ethanol as a 10,000× stock solution. Because the solution in DMSO is self-sterilizing, 0.5–1.0-ml aliquots can be directly distributed to 2-ml polyethylene vials and stored at −20°C. Samples should not be refrozen after use, and fresh stocks should be prepared on a weekly basis. Premixed insulin, transferrin, and selenium (ITS) are available as a solution (Collaborative Research) or lyophilized powder (Sigma) which can then be added directly to medium. A complex of bovine serum albumin (BSA) and linoleic acid, which is important for regulation of intracellular lipid levels, can be prepared by dissolving 5 g of fatty-acid-free BSA in 90 ml of 0.15 M NaCl and adding 50 mg of linoleic acid methyl ester. The volume is adjusted to 100 ml and distributed to sterile 15-ml centrifuge tubes as 5- to 10-ml aliquots, which can then be stored at −20°C. Alternatively, BSA/linoleic acid complex (Sigma) can be obtained as a lyophilized powder that is reconstituted in sterile water just before use. ITS+ (Collaborative

Research) contains a complex of BSA and linoleic acid in addition to insulin, transferrin, and selenium and can be used to supplement serum-free media.

2.1.3. COMPLETE MEDIA FOR HEPATOCYTE ISOLATION AND CULTURE

Fully supplemented medium is used for resuspending and washing cells during the isolation procedure as well as for maintaining cultures. Either Williams' medium E, a 1:1 mixture of Dulbecco's modified Eagle's and Ham's F-12 media, modified Chee's medium, or Hepatocyte Culture Medium are suitable depending on the purpose of the investigation (see Section 4.1). Supplemented medium can be prepared a day in advance with 5–10% fetal calf serum, glutamine (2 mM), ascorbic acid (50 μg/ml), insulin [5 μg/ml (0.25 units/ml)], dexamethasone (0.04–0.4 μg/ml), transferrin (5 μg/ml), and selenium (5 ng/ml). Williams' medium E is also supplemented with 10 mM HEPES. For experiments requiring serum-free medium, the fetal calf serum should be replaced with 5 ml of BSA/linoleic acid complex (1.0 mg/ml final concentration).

After addition of supplements, the medium should be filtered with a low-protein-binding cellulose acetate membrane (0.2 μm) to ensure sterility (Corning). Alternatively, small aliquots may be preincubated at 37°C and checked for contamination prior to use. Generally, one liter of medium containing fetal calf serum is required for the preparation and initial plating of hepatocytes from one adult rat liver. Another 500 ml of serum-containing or serum-free medium is also required following cell attachment. Prolonged storage ($>$2–3 days) of hormone-supplemented media is not generally recommended.

2.1.4. PREPARATION OF CULTURE DISHES

Typically, 40–50 large dishes (100 mm, Costar) or 120–150 small dishes (60 mm, Nunc LUX or Permanox) are required to accommodate hepatocytes from one adult rat liver. Culture dishes are coated with extracellular matrix material to enhance cell attachment and survival. Extracellular matrix components such as collagen type I, collagen type IV, Matrigel, laminin, and fibronectin have all been successfully used as attachment substrata. In our laboratories, culture dishes are precoated with collagen type I in either a gelled or ungelled state at least 1 day prior to hepatocyte isolation. The effects of the biophysical state of the collagen substratum on hepatocyte monolayers will be discussed in a later section.

Commercially available collagen type I is usually prepared from rat tail tendons or bovine dermis in HCl or acetic acid and stored at 4°C. The obtain a rigid, ungelled collagen film for cell attachment, 4–5 drops (200–250 μl) of an acid collagen solution [3–4 mg/ml (Vitrogen®)] is dispensed with a sterile pipet into culture dishes. With a sterile rubber or Teflon policeman, the collagen is spread evenly over the entire surface of the plate, care being taken to ensure that no "dry" spots remain. Alternatively, a collagen stock solution (Vitrogen®) can be diluted to a final concentration of 100 μg/ml with a sterile, aqueous solution of morphocarbodiimide (130 μg/ml) and 2-ml aliquots dispensed into 60-mm dishes (Waxman *et al.*, 1990). Treated dishes are then stored at 37°C in a humidified incubator overnight. Just before use, residual collagen is aspirated and replaced with fresh medium for 30–60 min to neutralize any residual acid or dishes can be rinsed twice with sterile phosphate buffered saline. To obtain a gelled collagen substratum, neutralized collagen type I [e.g., 8:1:1 (v/v/v) collagen (3–4 mg/ml), 10× Dulbecco's modified Eagle's medium (filtered), 0.1 N NaOH] is prepared on ice and spread onto Petri dishes as described above. Freshly coated dishes are then placed at 37°C in a humidified incubator for >45 min to allow the matrix material to gel. Fresh medium is added to the dishes, which are then stored at 37°C in a humidified chamber until utilized. Just before cell isolation, the medium is aspirated from the precoated culture dishes. Precoated dishes can be stored for prolonged periods but should be kept at 4°C, particularly to avoid dehydration of gelled substrata.

2.2. Hepatocyte Isolation and Primary Cell Culture

For our studies, hepatocytes are isolated from rat liver by a modification of the three-step collagenase perfusion method described by Quistorff *et al.* (1989). Detailed descriptions of the perfusion methods utilizing either a bench-top perfusion system or a self-contained compact perfusion unit (M/X Perfuser II) are outlined in Section 7. However, many variations of the collagenase-perfusion techniques developed by Berry and Friend (1969) and Seglen (1976) have been employed successfully to isolate rat hepatocytes for subsequent cultivation.

Following collagenase perfusion, the digested liver is carefully removed and placed into a sterile, covered crystallization dish and transported to a sterile hood, where 35 ml of medium kept at room temperature and supplemented with 5% fetal calf serum and hormones is immediately added. The hepatocytes are dispersed by tearing open Glisson's capsule (outer membrane) with the aid of two sterile forceps and gently shaking the liver until most of the cells are released into the medium. After assembling the filter unit (see Section 7), the cell suspension is then filtered through the 100-mesh nylon net (Spectrum) into a 250-ml beaker. The liver cells should not be forced through the filter; instead, the filter on the rubber ring should be moved slowly up and down until the cell suspension drains completely. Afterward, another 35 ml of medium is added to the crystallization dish, which is gently swirled to release any remaining cells from the liver remnant, and filtered as before. If the perfusion and cell preparation have been successful up to this point, only the vascular tree of the liver will remain on the filter.

The cell suspension is divided equally between two 50-ml sterile conical centrifuge tubes and centrifuged at $50 \times g$ for 2 min at room temperature. The supernatant fractions are discarded, and the cell pellets are gently resuspended in 35–40 ml of medium by inverting the tubes several times. Alternatively, the pellets can be resuspended by carefully drawing the medium up and down several times with a wide-bore 25-ml pipet. The cell suspension is centrifuged as before. The supernatant fraction is aspirated, and sufficient medium is added to the cell pellets to attain a final volume of 25 ml. An equal volume of 90% isotonic Percoll [1:9 (v/v) 10× PBS:Percoll] (Pharmacia) is added to the suspension, which is mixed well by inverting the tube and centrifuged at $70–150 \times g$ for 5 min at room temperature (it may be necessary to vary the g-force somewhat depending on the age and strain of the animals). Compromised hepatocytes and remaining nonparenchymal cells are located at the top of the Percoll gradient (Kreamer *et al.*, 1986). The supernatant fraction is aspirated, and the cell pellets are resuspended in a combined volume of 35–40 ml of medium and transferred into one 50-ml centrifuge tube. The cells are washed once again by centrifuging at $50 \times g$ for 2 min. As an alternative to Percoll separation, parenchymal cells may be enriched by centrifuging the isolated cells three times at low speed in the absence of Percoll (Quistorff *et al.*, 1989). The final cell pellet is resuspended gently in 35–40 ml of medium. The cells should be dispensed into dishes as soon as possible to prevent anaerobic damage.

Cell number and viability can be calculated by diluting an aliquot of the cell suspension 1:9 (v/v) with phosphate-buffered saline, pH 7.4, containing 0.04% trypan blue and counting with a hemocytometer. The nuclei of damaged cells will stain blue when viewed under brightfield optics. Cells should appear spherical without surface "blebs." Viability should be >90% when cells are isolated by Percoll centrifugation. Values lower than this usually lead to poor cell attachment. The cell concentration is adjusted to $1.5 \times 10^6–1.8 \times 10^6$ cells/ml, and 6-ml aliquots are dispersed into each 100-mm precoated dish. If 60-mm dishes are used, the cell suspension is further diluted to 1.0×10^6 cells/ml, and 3-ml aliquots are added to each culture dish. (As a simple alternative to the use of a hemocytometer to calculate cell numbers, a suitable cell density can be obtained by diluting the final pellet to ~45–50 times the packed cell volume with fresh medium.) The vessel containing the isolated hepatocytes should be frequently swirled during the course of plating cells to keep them suspended and aerated; otherwise, hepatocytes settle rapidly.

The dishes are placed into an incubator (5–10% CO_2, 95% humidity at 37°C) and gently swirled in a "figure 8" pattern to maintain a uniform monolayer of cells on the dish bottom. (Swirling the dishes in a circular motion usually results in concentration of the cells at the center and/or edge of the dishes.) Hepatocytes usually are allowed to attach to the substratum for 1–3 hr. Afterward, culture dishes are gently swirled, and the medium is aspirated to remove any unattached cells and loose debris. Monolayers are overlaid with fresh, warm medium containing supplements as applicable (see Section 5). The medium should be changed on a daily basis for the first few days in culture. Depending on the medium, the interval between changes can be prolonged to

2–3 days (Dich and Grunnet, 1989). To expedite the plating and feeding procedures, dishes may be kept on removable trays, thereby allowing multiple dishes to be processed at one time. If several dishes are aspirated at a time, care should be taken to leave cultures without medium for no longer than 3–4 min.

2.3. Overlay of Cell Cultures with Extracellular Matrix

2.3.1. COLLAGEN OVERLAY

After cell attachment, a neutralized collagen solution is prepared on ice [e.g., 8.0 ml of collagen type I (3–4 mg/ml), 1.0 ml of 10× Dulbecco's modified Eagle's medium, 1.0 ml of 0.1 N NaOH]. Medium from culture dishes to be overlaid is first thoroughly aspirated, particularly around the edge of the dishes. Neutralized collagen solution is added to each dish (0.25 ml/60 mm, 0.5 ml/100 mm), and the dish is then briefly tilted and rotated to spread collagen solution uniformly over the monolayer. The dishes are returned to the incubator for 45–60 min to allow the collagen to gel. Afterward, 3 or 6 ml of fresh medium is added back to the cultures, care being taken not to dislodge the top collagen layer. Successful "sandwiching" has been attained with several brands and sources of collagen type I. The best results have been obtained with collagen stocks at ⩾3 mg/ml, although reasonable gels have been obtained at half that concentration. However, when low collagen concentrations are used, the top gel has a greater tendency to be unstable and/or detach from the cells.

2.3.2. MATRIGEL OVERLAY

A stock solution of Matrigel (Collaborative Research) at a concentration of 5 mg/ml is prepared on ice by first thawing the supplier's product at 4°C and then diluting with sterile ice-cold 150 mM NaCl and storing in 5-ml aliquots at −20°C. Matrigel solutions > 10 mg/ml are very viscous and gel easily upon warming. Therefore, care should be taken to keep all stock solutions of Matrigel as cold as possible when handling and to perform all pipetting steps with ice-cold sterile pipettes. Just before use, the Matrigel stock solution is slowly thawed at 4°C, diluted 20-fold with ice-cold medium to a final concentration of ~250 μg/ml. After cell attachment, the medium is aspirated from culture dishes, and 3 ml (60-mm plates) or 6 ml (100-mm plates) of medium/Matrigel mixture is overlaid onto dishes with sterile pipets precooled to −20°C. Matrigel-treated cultures are allowed to incubate overnight, and the medium is changed every 24–48 hr. This procedure produces a thin coat of matrix that gels at 37°C and attaches to the upper surface of the hepatocyte monolayer (Caron, 1990; Sidhu *et al.*, 1993). A one-time application yields essentially the same results as those obtained after daily additions of Matrigel (Sidhu *et al.*, 1993).

3. PROPERTIES OF PRIMARY CULTURES OF RAT HEPATOCYTES

3.1. Evaluation of Monolayer Integrity

The biochemical and morphological integrity of hepatocyte cultures can and should be assessed by several criteria [membrane permeability, ATP levels, lactate dehydrogenase (LDH) release, etc.; Alpini *et al.*, 1994]. The simplest methods involve light microscopic examination of hepatocytes after exposure to colored or fluorescent dyes, such as trypan blue or propidium iodide, which are excluded from cells with intact plasma membranes. Cultures should be inspected by light microscopy on a routine basis to ensure that preparations are consistent and that no abnormal or unexpected toxicity has occurred. Hepatocytes should maintain their normal cuboidal appearance with a uniform cytoplasm, one or two centrally located nuclei, and well-delineated borders. In addition, cells should be relatively free of autophagic and lipid vesicle formation.

3.2. General Morphological Properties of Sandwiched Hepatocytes

Over the initial 24–48 hr, cells plated at high density onto rigid ungelled collagen type I with an overlay of collagen or Matrigel will spread and flatten to some degree but remain in chords or trabeculae (Fig. 1A). On the other hand, cells plated onto gelled collagen type I with an extracellular matrix overlay will remain in compact chords with few signs of spreading (Fig. 1B). With time, hepatocytes on either substratum show signs of additional spreading although those on gelled collagen retain more of their original morphological characteristics (Fig. 1C,D). Without the presence of an extracellular matrix overlay, cultured hepatocytes generally exhibit signs of extensive spreading and gross deterioration within 1 week (Dunn *et al.*, 1991). The viability of hepatocyte cultures as well as the preservation of normal cell morphology is greatly enhanced by the addition of an extracellular matrix overlay (Dunn *et al.*, 1991; Musat *et al.*, 1993; Sidhu *et al.*, 1993; LeCluyse *et al.*, 1994). In our experience, the useful lifetime of hepatocyte cultures can be extended to at least 2–3 weeks with the proper combination of matrix and medium conditions.

3.3. Reestablishment of Structural and Functional Bile Canaliculi

Initial signs of the formation of a bile canalicular network are apparent during the initial 24 hr after overlaying of cultures with extracellular matrix. The complete development of the bile canalicular network is characterized by the presence of a translucent band around the periphery of nearly all cells (e.g., Fig. 1D). Additional maturation occurs over the course of the next several days and appears to involve the refining and narrowing of the channels. These structures are similar to native bile canaliculi by several structural and functional criteria (Musat *et al.*, 1993; LeCluyse *et al.*, 1994). The uniformity, rate, and extent of bile canalicular network formation are somewhat dependent on three factors: (1) the thickness of the cell monolayer (cell shape), (2) the presence of serum and dexamethasone in the medium, and (3) the timing of the extracellular matrix overlay following cell adhesion to the dishes. Hepatocyte monolayers appear to require at least 24–48 hr in culture to establish elaborate, continuous bile canalicular networks. Similarly, reestablishment of the secretory function of bile canalicular networks is observed in sandwiched hepatocytes only after 3–4 days in culture (LeCluyse *et al.*, 1994).

3.4. Use of Hepatocyte Cultures for *in Vitro* Studies

For some studies, primary cultures of rat hepatocytes can be used immediately after cell attachment. Historically, hepatocyte cultures were typically used within several days of isolation because of the inherent limitations of conventional culture methods (Berry *et al.*, 1991). With the improvements in culture technology as outlined in this chapter, studies utilizing hepatocyte monolayers can be performed over several days or weeks with minor qualifications. For instance, a period of at least 24–48 hr appears to be necessary for cells to repair damage related to the isolation procedures and to allow cells to "adapt" to the culture environment. During this transition period, a rapid loss of most constitutive cytochrome P450 activity is observed even under the best culture conditions obtainable (Kocarek *et al.*, 1993b). Furthermore, hepatocyte cultures appear to be refractory to certain enzyme inducers during the first 24–48 hr after isolation (Schuetz *et al.*, 1984; Sinclair *et al.*, 1990). A deterioration of monolayer integrity and liver-specific function can also occur in cultures of hepatocytes within the first several days despite an extracellular matrix overlay if adequate medium conditions are not present. Conversely, normal differentiation of the plasma membrane and development of bile canalicular networks will not generally occur without the proper matrix conditions. Therefore, any particular application may be greatly affected by the media and/or matrix conditions employed during the course of hepatocyte culture.

4. EFFECTS OF CULTURE CONDITIONS ON LIVER-SPECIFIC FUNCTION

4.1. Media Effects

Serum has been used routinely as a component for the preparation of fully supplemented media since the earliest attempts to cultivate rat hepatocytes (Bissell,

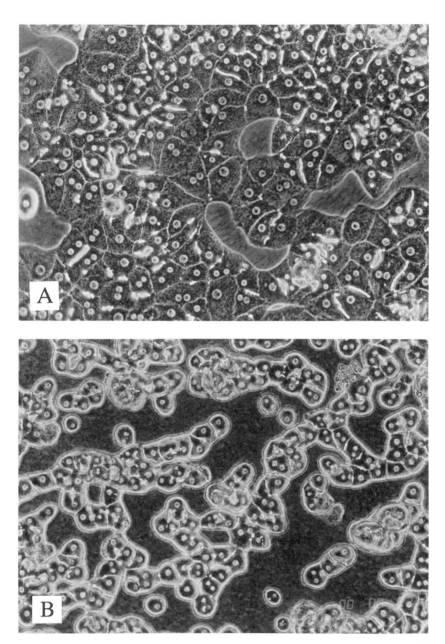

Figure 1.   Morphology of primary cultures of collagen-sandwiched rat hepatocytes maintained on either a rigid (A, C) or gelled (B, D) substratum of collagen type I. Cultures were examined and photographed on day 1 (A, B) and day 14 (C, D). Note differences in substratum-induced cell shape and the retention of general morphological features over time by cultures maintained on gelled collagen (D). Bile canaliculi (bc) can be observed as translucent bands around individual cells.

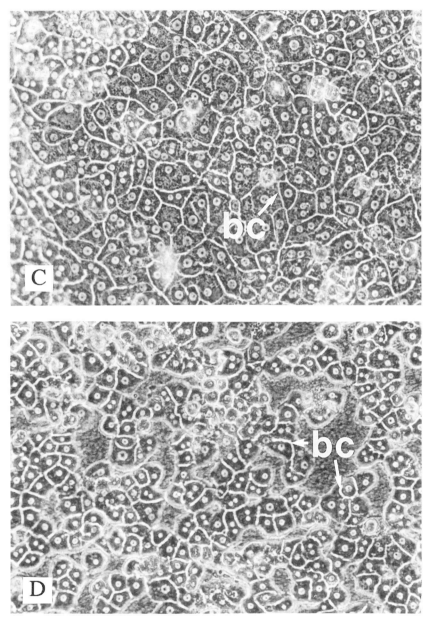

Figure 1. (*continued*)

1973; Bonney, 1974). The presence of serum in tissue culture media has been reported to improve cell attachment, survival, and morphology (Williams *et al.*, 1977; Ichihara *et al.*, 1986). However, serum generally is believed to promote growth and have a dedifferentiating effect on hepatocytes by decreasing the levels of liver-specific mRNA while increasing the levels of common or nonspecific mRNA (Clayton and Darnell, 1983; Enat *et al.*, 1984; Jefferson *et al.*, 1984). In addition, serum-containing medium appears to favor attachment and proliferation of non-parenchymal cells (e.g., bile-duct epithelial, Kupffer, and Ito cells) as well as inhibit the induction of cyto-chrome P450 activity by phenobarbital under conventional culture conditions (Enat *et al.*, 1984; Jefferson *et al.*, 1984; Waxman *et al.*, 1990; Kocarek *et al.*, 1993a). In our experience, the presence of serum during the first 24–48 hr of culture enhances overall cell morphology, including the formation of bile canalicular networks. How-ever, prolonged exposure to serum (>2–3 days) promotes the loss of cytochrome P450 activity and inducibility as well as the eventual deterioration of monolayers. Inasmuch as the chemical composition of serum is still relatively unknown and there can be significant lot-to-lot variations, serum should generally be avoided whenever possible for long-term maintenance of hepatocytes.

There is a general consensus that glucocorticoids markedly improve the attach-ment, survival, morphology, and overall performance of hepatocytes seeded on simple substrata (e.g., collagen) (Laishes and Williams, 1976; Yamada *et al.*, 1980). As suggested by the effects of dexamethasone (a synthetic glucocorticoid) on the overall pattern of hepatocyte protein synthesis (Colbert *et al.*, 1985), glucocorticoids directly influence a wide range of activities in culture, in general favoring better preservation of tissue-specific functions including albumin synthesis (Guguen-Guillouzo *et al.*, 1983; Jefferson *et al.*, 1985; Lescoat *et al.*, 1985; Reid *et al.*, 1986). In cultured rat hepatocytes dexamethasone has been found to increase extracellular matrix secretion (e.g., fibronectin), promote an ordered arrangement of the cytoskeleton, enhance gap junction expression and function, support cytochrome P450 activity, and curtail the decrease in protein synthesis observed in hepatocytes during the initial 24 hr in culture (Marceau *et al.*, 1986; Forster *et al.*, 1986; Kwiatkowski *et al.*, 1994; Ren *et al.*, 1994; Arterburn *et al.*, 1995). The formation of elaborate networks of bile canalicular networks is also enhanced in the presence of dexamethasone, especially in conjunc-tion with an overlay of extracellular matrix (Lambiotte *et al.*, 1973; LeCluyse *et al.*, 1994). Conversely, glucocorticoids down-regulate the expression of P-glycoprotein, nitric oxide synthase, and collagen type I in cultured hepatocytes (Jefferson *et al.*, 1985; Fardel *et al.*, 1993; Geller *et al.*, 1993; Chieli *et al.*, 1994).

Low levels of dexamethasone (25–100 nM) are apparently sufficient for the long-term preservation of hepatocyte monolayers (Dich *et al.*, 1988; Berry *et al.*, 1991) as well as for the maintenance of their responsiveness to P450 inducers (Mathis *et al.*, 1989; Kocarek *et al.*, 1994; Sidhu *et al.*, 1995). Higher levels of dexamethasone (1 μM) improve overall cell morphology but can induce the synthesis of certain P450 enzymes through a nonclassical glucocorticoid response pathway (Schuetz and Guzelian, 1984; Vind *et al.*, 1989).

Insulin is considered necessary for the long-term survival of cultured hepatocytes as well as for the preservation of many liver-specific functions and is therefore specified in virtually all hepatocyte culture medium formulations. Early studies reported that insulin improved the survival and attachment of adult hepatocytes (Chapman *et al.*, 1973; Laishes and Williams, 1976). It has also been found to enhance amino acid transport, protein synthesis (including albumin), glycogenesis, and lipogenesis while inhibiting protein degradation and potentiating inhibition of RNA degradation by amino acids (Ballard *et al.*, 1980; Schwarze *et al.*, 1982; Guguen-Guillouzo and Guillouzo, 1983; Flaim *et al.*, 1985; Balavoine *et al.*, 1993; Dahn *et al.*, 1993). Kimball *et al.* (1995) reported that insulin, when used in combination with dexamethasone and glucagon, maintained constant levels of albumin synthesis and cellular RNA for 8 days. In our experience, elimination of either dexamethasone or insulin from the culture medium has a detrimental effect on the viability and integrity of the cell monolayers when maintained beyond 3–4 days. However, cultures of primary rat hepatocytes maintained on Matrigel-coated dishes in medium supplemented with insulin alone retain good inducibility of cytochrome P450 enzymes (Schuetz *et al.*, 1988; Lindblad *et al.*, 1991; Kocarek *et al.*, 1993a,b).

The choice of medium for maintaining hepatocyte cultures will depend on the proposed applications. A 1:1 mixture of Dulbecco's modified Eagle's medium and Ham's F-12 containing 5% fetal calf serum, insulin, and 1.0 μM dexamethasone is sufficient for the maintenance of good monolayer morphology and formation of bile canalicular networks and for performing short-term (<7 days) studies on biliary transport (see Section 5.1). For examining P450 enzyme induction, serum-free media such as Dulbecco's modified Eagle's medium/Ham's F-12, Waymouth 752, and Williams' medium E are commonly used in combination with an appropriate extracellular matrix overlay. The use of modified Chee's medium and Hepatocyte Culture Medium, which contain amino acid concentrations that are on average 5–10 times higher than those in most conventional media, results in enhanced inducibility of certain P450 enzymes compared to conventional medium formulations, such as Dulbecco's modified Eagle's medium (Waxman *et al.*, 1990; Sidhu *et al.*, 1993). In addition, both media have striking effects on hepatocyte survival and morphology (Sidhu *et al.*, 1993; Jauregui *et al.*, 1986; Arterburn *et al.*, 1995).

Enriched media probably improve the performance and survival of hepatocyte monolayers because of the high amino acid content. High concentrations of certain amino acids (e.g., leucine, proline, phenylalanine) have been shown to inhibit the rate of autophagic protein degradation while stabilizing certain levels of mRNA as well as the activity of some liver-specific enzymes (Seglen *et al.*, 1980; Hutson *et al.*, 1987; Balavoine *et al.*, 1993). Our results have shown that modified Chee's medium supports the production of albumin and carboxylesterases as well as the induction response of P450 enzymes (see Section 5.2) better than conventional media (Fig. 2) (Yan *et al.*, 1995). Although Williams' medium E supports the highest CYP2B induction response, enriched media such as modified Chee's medium also enhance both monolayer and cell morphology and improve the yield of microsomal material. Prior to extensive use, however, enriched media should be carefully evaluated as to their suitability for particular applications.

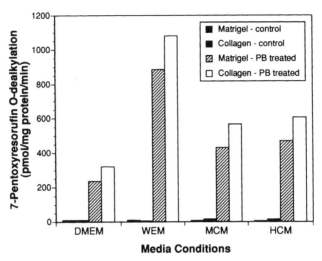

Figure 2.   Effects of media and overlay conditions on the induction of 7-pentoxyresorufin O-dealkylation (CYP2B) by phenobarbital in cultured rat hepatocytes. Isolated rat hepatocytes were seeded on collagen, overlaid with Matrigel or collagen, and cultured in serum-free media (Dulbecco's modified Eagle's medium [DMEM], Williams' E medium [WEM], modified Chee's medium [MCM], Hepatocyte Culture Medium [HCM]). Cultures were left untreated for 3 days followed by treatment with 100 μM phenobarbital (PB) for an additional 3 days. Cells were harvested and homogenized in 50 mM Tris-HCl, pH 7.4, 150 mM KCl, 2 mM EDTA. Microsomes were then prepared and analyzed for 7-pentoxyresorufin O-dealkylation, a marker of CYP2B activity.

4.2.   Matrix Effects

Several different approaches have been developed in an effort to preserve hepatic function by manipulating the extracellular matrix. The preservation of liver-specific functions, including cytochrome P450 expression, and the suppression of common genes have been reported in hepatocyte cultures maintained on Matrigel-coated dishes (Ben-Ze'ev *et al.*, 1988; Schuetz *et al.*, 1988; Bucher *et al.*, 1990). An alternative technique which involves overlaying the hepatocyte cultures with an additional layer of extracellular matrix has also resulted in striking improvements in hepatocyte morphology and liver-specific gene expression (Caron, 1990; Dunn *et al.*, 1991; Musat *et al.*, 1993; Sidhu *et al.*, 1993; LeCluyse *et al.*, 1994). Although each of these approaches has represented significant progress, they differ quantitatively and qualitatively in the specific liver functions they support. For our studies, we have chosen to use biologically relevant matrix components in a "sandwich" configuration in an attempt to more closely model the native architecture of the hepatocyte environment. In addition to producing dramatic effects on the maintenance of gene expression (Dunn *et al.*, 1991), the matrix configuration greatly enhances the viability and morphology of hepatocyte cultures as well as the formation of functional bile canalicular networks (Musat *et al.*, 1993; LeCluyse *et al.*, 1994). Sandwiched cultures generally exhibit more normal bile acid transport characteristics and superior cytochrome P450 inducibility compared with those maintained under conventional culture conditions. The influence of the biophysical state (gelled vs. rigid) and the geometry (sandwiched vs. unsandwiched) of the extracellular matrix on the induction of several different cytochrome P450 enzymes is shown in Fig. 3. The optimal matrix configuration is partially dependent on the medium employed and the particular enzyme(s) examined (compare induction of CYP1A by β-naphthoflavone to induction of CYP2B by phenobarbital). The use of modified Chee's medium improves the CYP2B and CYP3A induction response in sandwiched cultures maintained on a rigid substratum as well as in unsandwiched cultures on a gelled substratum (Fig. 3A,B and E,F). Similarly, Sidhu *et al.* (1994) found that the composition of the substratum is not important for optimal induction of CYP2B by phenobarbital when hepatocytes are maintained with an extracellular matrix overlay and an appropriate medium. On the other hand, the induction of CYP1A and 2A by β-naphthoflavone is dependent to a much greater extent on the matrix environment than on the medium formulation (Fig. 3C,D, and G,H). Our studies have shown that the type of extracellular matrix material used for hepatocyte overlay apparently is not critical for optimal performance of hepatocyte cultures. For instance, no major differences have been found in the activity and phenobarbital inducibility of P450 enzymes in hepatocyte monolayers whether overlaid with Matrigel or collagen type I (Fig. 2).

5. APPLICATIONS TO DRUG DEVELOPMENT AND METABOLISM

5.1. Biliary Secretion

Elaborate networks of bile canaliculi in matrix-overlaid hepatocyte monolayers represent a structurally separate compartment for the secretion of drug metabolites. Sandwiched hepatocytes also reestablish the normal polarized distribution of several different classes of canalicular transport systems. The multispecific organic anion transporter (MOAT), P-glycoprotein [associated with multidrug resistance (MDR)], and bile acid transporter are all functionally active in the canalicular membrane as indicated by the vectorical secretion of marker compounds into the lumen of the bile canalicular networks (Fig. 4). Thus, it is conceivable that many issues involving the regulation of biliary activity, such as the mechanisms of intrahepatic cholestasis and the rate and extent of secretion of xenobiotics, could be more easily addressed with this *in vitro* model system.

The use of sandwiched hepatocytes in conjunction with marker compounds (see Fig. 4) could potentially serve as both a structural and a functional model with which to determine the involvement of specific canalicular carrier systems in the biliary excretion of new drug candidates. Similarly, the potency of inhibitors to affect

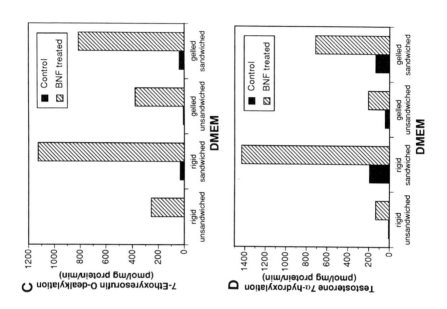

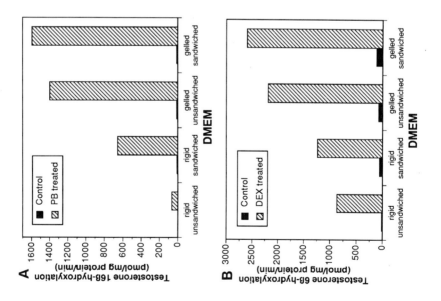

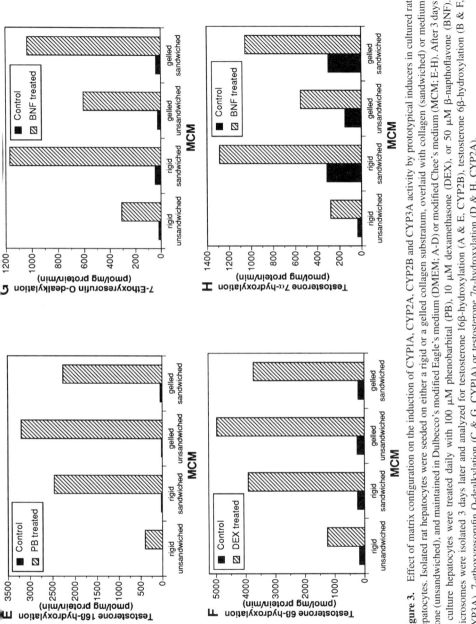

Figure 3. Effect of matrix configuration on the induction of CYP1A, CYP2A, CYP2B and CYP3A activity by prototypical inducers in cultured rat hepatocytes. Isolated rat hepatocytes were seeded on either a rigid or a gelled collagen substratum, overlaid with collagen (sandwiched) or medium alone (unsandwiched), and maintained in Dulbecco's modified Eagle's medium (DMEM; A-D) or modified Chee's medium (MCM; E-H). After 3 days in culture hepatocytes were treated daily with 100 μM phenobarbital (PB), 10 μM dexamethasone (DEX), or 50 μM β-napthoflavone (BNF). Microsomes were isolated 3 days later and analyzed for testosterone 16β-hydroxylation (A & E, CYP2B), testosterone 6β-hydroxylation (B & F, CYP3A), 7-ethoxyresorufin O-dealkylation (C & G, CYP1A) or testosterone 7α-hydroxylation (D & H, CYP2A).

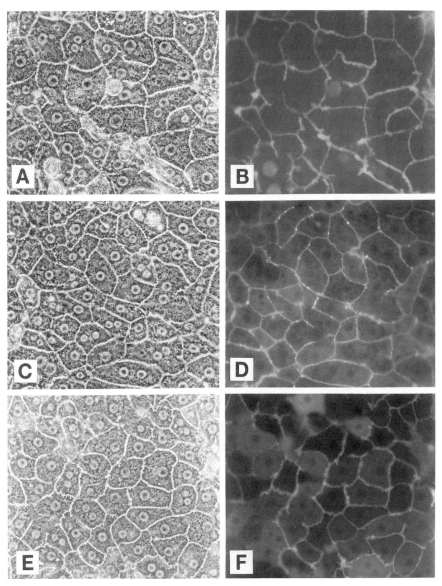

Figure 4.   Corresponding phase-contrast and fluorescent images of sandwiched rat hepatocytes cultured for 5–7 days in serum-containing Dulbecco's modified Eagle's medium/Hams' F-12 supplemented with 1.0 μM dexamethasone, illustrating the secretion of various model compounds into bile canalicular networks. Hepatocyte cultures were treated with either carboxyfluorescein diacetate (A, B), rhodamine (C, D), or fluorescein-taurocholate (E, F) as substrates for the multispecific organic anion transporter (Oude Elferink *et al.*, 1993), P-glycoprotein (Chiele *et al.*, 1994), and bile acid transporter (Watanabe *et al.*, 1991), respectively. Intense fluorescence is primarily localized to structures corresponding to the bile canaliculi.

specific canalicular transporters could be examined under more controlled conditions. Alternatively, cultures may be used to study the effects of new drug candidates on the morphology of the bile canalicular networks as an indicator of choleretic or cholestatic potential. In our studies, the structural and functional effects exhibited in sandwiched cultures of hepatocytes after treatment with model cholestatic agents, such as phalloidin and cytochalasin D, were similar to those observed *in vivo* (Phillips *et al.*, 1975; Oda and Phillips, 1977; Elias *et al.*, 1980; LeCluyse *et al.*, 1996).

5.2. Microsomal Enzyme Induction

5.2.1. CYTOCHROME P450

Microsomal cytochrome P450 (CYP) enzymes are major monooxygenases involved in liver phase I metabolism. Members of the CYP1, CYP2, and CYP3 families are the most catalytically active P450 enzymes in rat hepatic drug metabolism, but marked species differences exist in their function and activity (substrate specificity). Many of the P450 enzymes can be induced by drugs at therapeutic concentrations, and induction of these enzymes can change the rate and pattern of drug metabolism. There are five major classes of P450 enzyme inducers, represented by β-naphthoflavone, phenobarbital, dexamethasone, ethanol, and clofibric acid, which primarily induce P450 enzymes belonging to the CYP1A, CYP2B, CYP3A, CYP2E, and CYP4A subfamilies, respectively (Parkinson, 1996). Induction of cytochrome P450 can be an important cause of drug–drug interactions, hence, regulatory agencies may request that new drugs be tested for their potential to induce P450 enzymes. The testing process typically involves treating rats, mice, dogs, or monkeys *in vivo*, followed by the preparation of liver microsomes for analysis of P450 enzyme activity *in vitro*. With few exceptions (Diaz *et al.*, 1990), this *ex vivo* approach cannot be used to test drugs as P450 enzyme inducers in humans. Therefore, hepatocyte cultures can make a significant contribution to testing new drugs as P450 enzyme inducers.

Sandwiched hepatocytes are particularly useful in screening new drug candidates for their ability to induce P450 enzymes because they retain their ability to respond to enzyme inducers for two or more weeks. When rat hepatocytes are seeded on collagen, overlaid with Matrigel, and cultured for up to 10 days, they respond to 3 days of treatment with β-naphthoflavone (50 μM), phenobarbital (100 μM), and dexamethasone (10 μM) with a marked induction of CYP1A, CYP2B, and CYP3A enzymes, respectively. The degree of P450 induction is comparable (within a factor of 2–3) to that observed following *in vivo* treatment of rats with these prototypical inducers. Consequently, primary cultures of rat hepatocytes can potentially be used to screen new drug candidates for their ability to induce cytochrome P450 enzymes. However, there are important considerations which must be kept in mind when employing cultured hepatocytes for drug screening. First, we have observed that induction of CYP2B enzymes occurs at concentrations of phenobarbital ranging from 10 to 250 μM. At higher concentrations (500–1500 μM), induction of CYP2B enzymes decreases, whereas induction of CYP1A and CYP3A increases. Therefore, it is important to test new drug candidates over a range of concentrations. It is also important that drug candidates be tested *in vitro* at concentrations that are comparable to those achieved *in vivo*, and at concentrations that do not result in cellular toxicity.

The induction of cytochrome P450 by some agents is largely due to their metabolites, not the parent compound. The enzyme-inducing potential of such chemicals would likely be underestimated in primary cultures of rat hepatocytes, particularly if these metabolites are formed by the action of gastric acid or by intestinal microflora. The enzyme-inducing effects of some drug candidates are an impediment to their development because of concerns over liver or thyroid tumor formation in chronic toxicity tests. In this case, primary cultures of rat hepatocytes are ideally suited to screening backup compounds, provided the leading drug candidate also causes P450 induction *in vitro*. However, it would be prudent to verify that backup compounds testing negative *in vitro* also fail to induce P450 enzymes *in vivo*. The enzyme-inducing effects of some drug candidates resides predominantly in one enantiomer (Grossman *et al.*, 1992). Primary cultures of rat hepatocytes provide an excellent means to examine the enzyme-inducing effects of drug enantiomers, which may be available in low amounts. Primary cultures of hepatocytes also are well suited for examining species differences in P450 induction and are particularly useful for studying the induction of cytochrome P450 in human hepatocytes (Diaz *et al.*, 1990; Morel *et al.*, 1990; Pichard *et al.*, 1990; Curi-Pedrosa *et al.*, 1994).

As was stated in Section 4, the choice of medium and matrix can have profound effects on the performance of hepatocyte monolayers, and such is the case with P450 enzyme induction. The induction of immunoreactive CYP2B and related enzyme activities is highly dependent on medium formulation (Fig. 2) (Sidhu *et al.*, 1993). We have also observed that primary cultures of rat hepatocytes cultured in Chee's medium secrete hydrolase S, a serum carboxylesterase, whereas hepatocytes cultured in Williams' medium E do not support this liver-specific function (Yan *et al.*, 1995). The age of the cultures before inducers are introduced, the relative potency of inducers within each class, the final concentration of inducers in culture medium, and the duration of exposure to inducers also have profound effects on the induction of P450 enzymes in cultured hepatocytes.

Drug induction of phase I metabolism may, in many cases, be attributed to the increased expression of a particular P450 subfamily, which can easily be ascertained by measuring the metabolism of P450-specific substrates. The activity of CYP1A and CYP2B enzymes can be determined by measuring the O-dealkylation of 7-ethoxy- and 7-pentoxyresorufin, respectively, as determined by the fluorometric method of Burke *et al.* (1985). The activity of CYP2B and CYP3A enzymes may be determined by measuring the rates of testosterone 16β- and 6β-hydroxylation, respectively, in microsomes isolated from cultured hepatocytes or in intact cultures (e.g., Vind *et al.*,

1989; Wortelboer *et al.*, 1990). The various pathways of testosterone hydroxylation catalyzed by rat P450 enzymes can then be determined by reversed-phase HPLC, essentially according to the procedure described by Wood *et al.* (1983), as modified by Sonderfan *et al.* (1987). Detailed methods describing the use of hepatocyte cultures for examining cytochrome P450 regulation are also given elsewhere (Waterman and Johnson, 1991; Li *et al.*, 1991).

5.2.2. PHASE II ENZYMES

Hepatic enzymes that catalyze phase II drug metabolism include microsomal and cytosolic transferases that conjugate many drugs and endogenous compounds with normal cellular constituents such as glucuronic acid, glutathione, and sulfate. Several studies suggest that activities of phase II enzymes are better preserved in culture than those of the corresponding phase I enzymes (Rogiers and Vercruysse, 1993). However, there are other reports that describe a loss of both phase I and phase II enzymes in cultured hepatocytes (Niemann *et al.*, 1991).

The UDP-glucuronosyltransferases (UDP-GT) are a family of microsomal enzymes, many of which are inducible by the same drugs and xenobiotics that induce cytochrome P450. In rats, the UDP-GT enzymes inducible by phenobarbital, β-naphthoflavone, dexamethasone, and clofibric acid preferentially glucuronidate 1-naphthol, chloramphenicol, digitoxigenin monodigitoxoside, and bilirubin, respectively (Watkins *et al.*, 1982). UDP-GT activity has generally been reported to be well maintained for short culture periods (<1 week) (Donato *et al.*, 1991); however, individual subfamilies may be better preserved than others (e.g., 3-methylcholanthrene- versus phenobarbital-inducible) (Niemann *et al.*, 1991). Phenol red glucoronidation levels have been examined in long-term cultures of rat hepatocytes maintained in three different media (modified Chee's, Williams' E, and Waymouth's) by Jauregui *et al.* (1986). Modified Chee's medium showed the greatest capacity to sustain UDP-GT activity for prolonged periods (28 days) compared to Williams' E (7 days) and Waymouth's (2 days).

Inasmuch as the various isoforms are inducible by exogenous components, consideration must be given as to whether or not measurable activity is due to constitutive or induced expression (Section 5.2.1). The UDP-GT activity of hepatocyte cultures can be determined with a modification of the methods of Driscoll *et al.* (1982) and Lilienblum *et al.* (1982).

Four gene families make up the glutathione S-transferases (GST) found in cytosol and microsomal fractions, although GST activity is 5–40 times higher in the cytosolic fraction than in the microsomal fraction. These enzymes conjugate reduced glutathione (glycine–α-glutamic acid–cysteine) (GSH) with electrophilic compounds and in this way detoxify reactive intermediates produced by P450 enzymes during phase I metabolism. For example, cytochrome P450 converts acetaminophen to a reactive metabolite, *N*-acetylbenzoquinoneimine, that is conjugated with GSH

(Sipes and Gandolfi, 1991). The activity and inducibility of several classes of GST can be maintained to some degree in monolayers of rat hepatocytes cultured under appropriate conditions (Donato *et al.*, 1990; Rogiers *et al.*, 1990b; Vandenberghe *et al.*, 1991; Dwivedi *et al.*, 1993). GST expression in co-cultured hepatocytes is maintained at 50% or better of that observed in freshly isolated cells (Donato *et al.*, 1991; Vandenberghe *et al.*, 1992). However, expression of the fetal isoform, GST 7 (π), is also observed under most culture conditions. In general, the degree to which individual GST enzymes are expressed over time is largely dependent on the media and matrix conditions (Rogiers *et al.*, 1990a; Donato *et al.*, 1991; Vandenberghe *et al.*, 1988, 1991, 1992). Inducibility of all classes of GST enzymes (GST 1/2, 3/4, 7) by phenobarbital is observed in both conventional cultures of hepatocytes and in co-cultures (Vandenberghe *et al.*, 1991). Methods for determining GST expression and activity have been described by Dwivedi *et al.* (1993) and Habig *et al.* (1974).

In mammalian liver, cytosolic sulfotransferases (ST) constitute a family of enzymes that catalyze the conjugation of drugs with sulfate from phosphoadenosine-5'-phsophosulfate (PAPS). Compounds that undergo sulfation are often first hydroxylated by cytochrome P450 enzymes during phase I metabolism (e.g., hydroxysteroids and bile salts). This phase II pathway is easily saturated owing to depletion of the cofactor, PAPS, which is synthesized from cysteine. Sulfotransferase activity is often difficult to detect in primary cultures of hepatocytes because of the low availability of cysteine. Hepatic sulfotransferases are subject to both chemical and hormonal regulation *in vivo* (Liu *et al.*, 1994). Therefore, constitutive activity can be difficult to detect in primary cultures of hepatocytes, possibly due to the lack of hormone regulation and low availability of cysteine. However, a number of investigators have reported sulfotransferase activity in cultures of rat hepatocytes maintained under various culture conditions (Kirkpatrick and Belsaas, 1985; Sweeny and Reinke, 1988; Kane *et al.*, 1991; Galle *et al.*, 1989; Schrenk *et al.*, 1991; Utesch and Oesch, 1992a,b).

Acetaminophen sulfation, which is catalyzed by a phenol sulfotransferase, was shown to be better maintained in 4-day-old cultures on Matrigel compared to those on simple collagen (Kane *et al.*, 1991). Likewise, phenol sulfotransferase activity with 2-naphthol as substrate decreased to about 20% of initial activity in hepatocytes cultured on gelled collagen, while the sulfotransferase activity was maintained at about 50% after 7 days in co-cultured hepatocytes (Utesch and Oesch, 1992a). It should be noted, however, that the medium contained relatively high levels of dexamethasone (1 μM) which has been shown to induce ST1A1 expression both *in vivo* and *in vitro* (Liu *et al.*, 1994, 1996). Liu *et al.* (1996) characterized the mRNA levels of six different sulfotransferase isoforms in primary cultures of both male and female rat hepatocytes maintained under various culture conditions. The expression of all sulfotransferase enzymes with the exception of phenol sulfotransferase (ST1A1) declined to less than 20% of the initial values within the first 24 hours regardless of the matrix or media conditions. By contrast, ST1A1 mRNA levels remained at >30%

of initial values after 4 days even in the absence of dexamethasone. In the presence of 0.1 μM dexamethasone, ST1A1 mRNA at day 4 was induced to levels that were >100% of day zero values in cultures maintained on Matrigel with modified Chee's medium. Methods for the determination of sulfotransferase activity in cultured hepatocytes have been described by several investigators (Grant and Hawksworth, 1986; Arand *et al.*, 1987; Kane *et al.*, 1991).

5.3. Drug Metabolism

As stated previously, rat hepatocytes typically lose constitutive P450 activity in the initial 24–48 hr of culture even though other components of the P450-mediated monooxygenase system, cytochrome P450 reductase and cytochrome b_5, are relatively well maintained (Akrawi *et al.*, 1993). The extent to which individual P450 enzymes are expressed in cultured hepatocytes depends greatly on the medium and matrix conditions (Utesch *et al.*, 1991; Kocarek *et al.*, 1993b; Donato *et al.*, 1994). Many of the early studies performed with hepatocyte cultures measured cytochrome P450 content by the method of Omura and Sato (1964), which does not distinguish between individual P450 isoforms. This can be an important factor in the interpretation of results in that some P450 enzymes are inducible by various chemicals including supplements that have been used for maintenance of cell cultures. Therefore, many of the culture conditions routinely used for maintaining hepatocytes, especially those which seemingly "maintain" total cytochrome P450 activity, must be scrutinized in light of their effects on the regulation of individual P450 enzymes.

More recently, a considerable effort has been made to study the regulation of the individual P450 enzymes during short- and long-term cultivation of adult rat hepatocytes (Kocarek *et al.*, 1993b, 1994, 1995; Sidhu *et al.*, 1993, 1994; Schuetz *et al.*, 1988, 1990; Li *et al.*, 1991; Utesch *et al.*, 1991; Rogiers and Vercruysse, 1993; Donato *et al.*, 1994). When individual P450 enzymes are carefully examined in cultured rat hepatocytes with specific cDNA or antibody probes, it is readily apparent that a dramatic alteration in cytochrome P450 enzyme profiles takes place during the first 24–48 hours. For instance, Kocarek *et al.* (1993b) examined the mRNA expression of 10 different P450 enzymes or subfamilies over a 5-day period on a Matrigel substratum. Their results showed that most P450 transcription ceases after the isolation of hepatocytes from intact liver. After continued incubations, three patterns of expression were observed depending on the specific P450 enzymes. Some of the enzymes re-express themselves in tissue-specific form after 2–4 days while others remain unexpressed, and still others were observed to exhibit a "ping-pong" form of expression. Related studies have shown similar alterations in specific isoforms of both phase I and phase II drug-metabolizing enzymes (Rogiers and Vercruysse, 1993; Utesch *et al.*, 1991; Donato *et al.*, 1994).

One must also bear in mind that significant sex-related differences exist in the expression of certain P450 enzymes in mature rats (Zaphiropoulos *et al.*, 1989; Bullock *et al.*, 1991). Furthermore, in the absence of growth hormone, the expression of some sex-specific P450 enzymes (e.g., CYP2C11) is initially lost and minimally restored during cultivation of rat hepatocytes. These differences can be important to the application of rat hepatocyte cultures for phase I metabolism studies because they affect the constitutive expression of prominent drug-metabolizing enzymes. Until the hormonal factors that control the expression of drug-metabolizing enzymes are better understood, cultured hepatocytes cannot possess the metabolic capability of hepatocytes *in vivo*. Therefore, whereas long-term cultures of rat hepatocytes have proven to be an excellent model for measuring cytochrome P450 induction, they currently do not provide an appropriate *in vitro* system for investigating the cytochrome P450-dependent metabolism and toxicity of drugs.

6. ADVANTAGES AND DISADVANTAGES OF CULTURED HEPATOCYTES

One of the major obstacles to evaluating the use of hepatocyte cultures for pharmaceutical applications is the numerous hormonal, media, and substrate conditions that have been described in the literature for preserving liver-specific functions. No comprehensive comparison of culture conditions with pharmacologically and toxicologically relevant endpoints has thus far been reported. Nonetheless, many recent investigations have tried to focus on the more specific effects of the culture environment on gene regulation (e.g., Rana *et al.*, 1994). From the growing body of evidence it has become clear that three important factors in maintaining liver-specific function in primary cultures of hepatocytes are matrix geometry, cell–cell contacts, and media composition (soluble components). It is very likely that the hepatic extracellular matrix and the large number of soluble factors in the plasma and interstitial fluid are equally important in regulating hepatocyte gene expression and cell function *in vivo*. Clearly, it is difficult to duplicate exactly the dynamic environment of the systemic and portal blood flow (exemplified by the constant changes in the levels of nutrients and hormonal factors) within the confines of a static culture environment.

The utility of cultured hepatocytes must also be considered in light of the architecture and function of the liver as a whole. There are a number of metabolic differences between periportal and perivenous hepatocytes in the mammalian liver resulting from zonal differences in the activity of several enzymes, and possibly from morphological differences as well (Smith and Wills, 1981; Thurman *et al.*, 1986; Ugele *et al.*, 1991; Gebhardt, 1992). There is also evidence that differences in the expression of certain inducible P450 enzymes exist along the liver acinus of the rat (Wojcik *et al.*, 1988; Bars *et al.*, 1989). This metabolic heterogeneity is thought to be a function of the location in the microcirculation and may be related to inherent gradients of oxygen, hormones, metabolites, and matrix composition (Probst and Jungermann, 1983; Wolfe and Jungermann, 1985; Reid *et al.*, 1992). Cultures of hepatocytes isolated by standard collagenase perfusion techniques are usually an assortment of cells from all zones comprising the liver lobule. Therefore, any patterns in the metabolism or inductive response of a particular drug attributable to the architecture and microcirculation of the intact liver may not be entirely reflected *in vitro*. Moreover, the use of a Percoll gradient may further exacerbate this situation by selecting for specific subpopulations of cells (Kreamer *et al.*, 1986).

With these limitations in mind, primary cultures of well-differentiated hepatocytes offer a valuable system for the examination of many issues relevant to drug development and discovery. Hepatocyte cultures represent the only *in vitro* model for long-term studies in a well-defined environment. Thus, they allow extended studies of drug–drug interactions on enzyme induction whereas other *in vitro* model systems (e.g., liver slices, cell suspensions) are limited by the short time during which hepatocytes under these conditions retain acceptable viability and liver-specific gene expression. A large number of cells are obtained from a single adult rat, thus reducing the number of laboratory animals required for drug testing. Addition of test solutions to cell culture vessels is relatively simple and requires less compound for fulfilling dosing regimens. The use of uncomplicated media or buffers affords easy preparation of samples for routine analysis.

The mechanism(s) involved in enzyme induction and species differences can potentially be identified more easily in hepatocyte cultures (Burger *et al.*, 1990, 1992; Schuetz *et al.*, 1990; Sidhu *et al.*, 1994). Another advantage of using sandwiched hepatocyte cultures is for determining drug-induced hepatotoxicity such as that resulting in intrahepatic cholestasis. In addition, drugs suspected of being extracted by the liver via an active transport process (e.g., bile acid carrier) may be more readily studied with cultured hepatocytes. Lastly, the isolated effects of individual xenobiotics (such as tumor promoters) on specific cellular pathways can be determined under more controlled conditions compared with performing similar experiments *in vivo*.

As a final note, no one set of culture conditions completely preserves or restores the normal structural and functional properties of hepatocytes as they are expressed *in vivo*, although certain combinations appear to be ideal for restoring or expressing specific aspects of liver function. For example, hepatocytes maintained in serum-free modified Chee's medium with a Matrigel overlay maintain relatively high levels of cytochrome P450 induction, whereas hepatocytes maintained in a collagen-sandwich configuration with media containing fetal calf serum and moderate levels of dexamethasone exhibit more normal tissue architecture, including the formation of bile canalicular networks. Therefore, a specific hepatic function or process may be stabilized under one particular set of culture conditions while being diminished or lost in another. It is appropriate then to consider that the media and matrix conditions may need to be "customized" to the particular application(s) of interest.

7. APPENDIX

The three-step collagenase perfusion method routinely employed in our laboratories for the isolation of rat hepatocytes is essentially derived from the two-step method developed by Berry and Friend (1969) and Seglen (1976) as modified by Quistorff *et al.* (1989). The isolation procedures will be discussed with reference to (1) using standard laboratory equipment and glassware, making it amenable to almost any facility equipped to perform routine cell culture, and (2) using a commercially available self-contained perfusion unit (M/X Perfuser II). For the reader's consideration, high yields of rat hepatocytes have also been successfully prepared by EDTA dissociation alone (Berry *et al.*, 1983; Wang *et al.*, 1985; Meredith, 1988). However, this method has currently not gained widespread use despite reports of superior cell viability, monolayer morphology, and retention of many liver-specific functions relative to hepatocytes prepared by collagenase perfusion techniques. More recently, Utesch *et al.* (1991) reported that the expression of individual P450 isoenzymes was independent of the isolation method. Additional methods for the preparation and use of cultured hepatocytes specifically for examining P450 regulation have been described by Li *et al.* (1991).

7.1. Materials

7.1.1. ANIMALS

Adult male rats weighing about 150–300 g are typically used for hepatocyte isolation. However, there are significant strain- and sex-related differences in hepatic metabolism (Zaphiropoulos *et al.*, 1989; Bullock *et al.*, 1991). Therefore, the choice of sex and strain may be an important consideration when studies on phase I metabolism are performed.

7.1.2. PERFUSION BUFFERS

Ca^{2+}- and Mg^{2+}-free buffer for perfusion step 1 (P1 buffer): 118 mM NaCl, 4.7 mM KCl, 1.2 mM KH_2PO_4, 25 mM $NaHCO_2$, 0.5 mM EGTA, and 5.5 mM glucose. The pH is adjusted to 7.4 using HCl or NaOH, and the buffer is filter-sterilized and stored at 4°C.

Buffer for perfusion step 2 (P2 buffer): Same as P1 buffer without EGTA, plus 2.0 mM $CaCl_2$, 1.2 mM $MgSO_2$, and 0.03% collagenase (150 mg/500 ml).

Buffer for perfusion step 3 (P3 buffer): Same as P2 but without collagenase.

Collagenase should be added to the appropriate buffer just before each perfusion. The digestion properties of collagenase of a particular type and from a particular source will vary immensely depending on the ratios of contaminating proteases in the individual lots. Therefore, investigators should determine which titration, brand, and lot numbers yield the best results for their particular purposes. Collagenase from the manufacturer should be divided into working aliquots (e.g., 150 mg) and kept desiccated at 4°C.

7.1.3. EQUIPMENT

7.1.3a. Perfusion System

The M/X Perfuser II (MX International, Aurora, CO) with infusion of carbogen (95% O_2/5% CO_2) is a self-contained perfusion system routinely used in our laboratory for performing rat liver perfusion. Prior to use, the perfusion system and all tubing should be rinsed with plenty of 70% ethanol. Alternatively, a peristaltic pump (Gilson Minipulse) capable of generating variable flow rates of 10–40 ml/min may be used in combination with a standard thermostated water bath and a regulated supply of carbogen or oxygen.

7.1.3b. Catheter

A double cannula [16-gauge × 5.1 cm or 18-gauge × 3.2 cm Teflon intravenous (i.v.) catheter (Jelco™, Critikon)] is convenient and easy to use. A 24- to 27-in. length of polyethylene tubing for cannulation of the superior vena cava and recirculation of perfusate is needed for use with the M/X Perfuser II system.

7.1.3c. Cell Filtration System

A simple yet effective filtration device consists of a 250-ml beaker, an inverted Buchner funnel rubber gasket, and a nylon net [100 mesh (160 μm); Spectrum Scientific)] (Quistorff et al., 1989). The outer edge of the rubber gasket usually requires some milling before an adequate fit is obtained. Prior to use, equipment should be sterilized.

7.1.3d. Centrifuge

A conventional laboratory low-speed centrifuge is required that is equipped with a swing-out rotor and is capable of reproducibly generating low g-values ($\sim 50 \times g$).

7.1.3e. Surgical Instruments and Glassware for M/X Perfuser II

Two curved, fine-tipped forceps, 1 medium, toothed forceps, 1 pair of scissors (must be able to cut through skin and ribs), 2 pairs of hemostats, and 1 small (10-cm diameter) crystallization dish are needed for the preparation and subsequent removal of the liver. Prior to use, all instruments and glassware should be sterilized.

Surgical Tray for Benchtop Perfusion Method.   The following items are assembled and autoclaved in a stainless steel tray (20 cm × 30 cm × 3 cm deep): a test tube rack, four 1-ml serological pipets; scissors, hemostats, and forceps as listed above; 4 lengths of autoclavable PVC tubing (3 mm i.d., 6 mm o.d.—3 20-cm pieces and 1 45-cm piece; and 3 three-way nylon stopcocks.

7.2. Procedures for Hepatocyte Isolation

7.2.1. PREPERFUSION PREPARATION: METHOD A

The M/X Perfuser unit should be switched on, and the temperature of the tank chambers brought to 39–40°C. P2 buffer is prepared under sterile conditions by adding an aliquot of collagenase (~150 mg) to 500 ml of P3 buffer and allowing it to dissolve completely. One 500-ml bottle each of perfusion buffers (P1, P2, and P3), two 500-ml bottles of medium supplemented with 5% fetal calf serum, ITS, or supplemented with ITS+ and 0.1 μM dexamethasone (serum free) (see Section 4.1) are placed into a 37°C water bath. Isotonic Percoll is prepared by adding 5 ml of sterile 10× PBS to 45 ml of Percoll (for 2 gradients). Four pieces of suture (3 pieces of 4-0 surgical silk and 1 piece of #2 silk) are required for tying ligatures. After warming perfusion buffers, 500 ml of P1 buffer is added to tank #1 of the M/X Perfuser units, and 500 ml of P2 buffer is added to tank #2. The air is then displaced from all lines and the bubble trap by slowly pumping perfusion buffer through tubing. Removing all air is essential because the passage of a bubble into the perfused liver will block flow and prevent adequate digestion of the tissue. Oxygenation of perfusion tanks is then initiated. P3 buffer is kept in a water bath at 37°C until needed.

7.2.2. PREPERFUSION PREPARATION: METHOD B

Sterile bottles of all perfusion buffers and media are placed in a water bath at 40°C as in method A. A 1-ml serological pipet attached to regulated carbogen or oxygen is placed into the P1 buffer, and a low flow of gas is begun (~5 bubbles/sec). The PVC tubing is then assembled with stopcocks (Fig. 5). When the perfusion buffers are warm, P2 buffer is prepared by adding collagenase to a bottle of P3 buffer as described in method A. The P2 buffer is returned to the water bath along with the P1 and P3 buffers, and a 1-ml serological pipet is placed into each bottle as shown in Fig. 5. After the peristaltic pump is added to the system, the tubing is then primed with the corresponding buffers. After priming the tubing, stopcock S3 should be open to P2 (closed to P3), and stopcock S2 should be open to P1 (closed to P2). This configuration

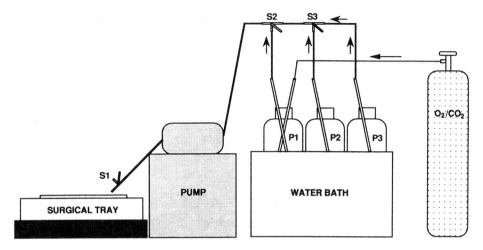

Figure 5 Schematic diagram of the bench-top rat liver perfusion system. S, stopcock; P, perfusion buffer.

allows the perfusion to begin with P1. It is advisable to incorporate a simple bubble trap somewhere along the infusion line to help prevent the accidental passage of air into the liver.

7.2.3. HEPATOCYTE ISOLATION

The rat is anesthetized with an intraperitoneal injection of pentobarbital (50–60 mg/kg). After a surgical plane of anesthesia is achieved, the rat is placed onto the platter of the M/X perfusion apparatus or onto the test tube rack situated inside the stainless steel tray. The tail and forelimbs are secured with masking tape, and the abdomen is thoroughly washed with 70% ethanol. The skin is first cut with a midline incision from pubis to sternum followed by a similar incision in the abdominal wall, care being taken not to enter the thoracic cavity (Fig. 6A). The midline incision is then extended laterally to the left at both ends about 1.5–2.0 cm (following the rib margin from the sternum), and the elongated flap is reflected away from the abdominal cavity. A single, curving incision from the pubic end of the midline incision to the right lateral base of the rib cage is made, care being taken to avoid the thoracic cavity, and the long flap is reflected away from the abdominal cavity. Good sterile technique should be practiced during all steps involving access to the open body cavity. Using a sterile PBS-soaked gauze, the intestines are moved out of the abdominal cavity to the animal's left side so that the portal vein and the inferior vena cava can be visualized. Hemostats may be used, if necessary, to hold the duodenum and upper jejunum to one side for easier access to the portal vein. Prior to cannulation of the portal vein, the left liver lobe may be held to one side with a PBS-soaked gauze. (Care should be taken

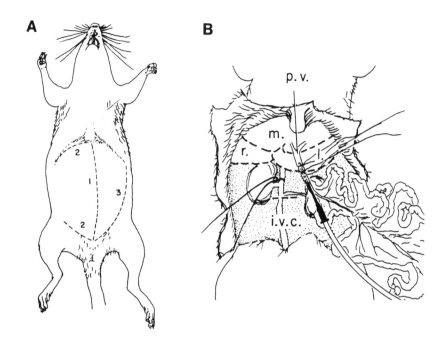

Figure 6.   (A) Diagram illustrating the sequence (1–3) and location of abdominal incisions prior to liver perfusion. (B) Diagrammatic representation of the location and configuration of ligatures and cannula for performing liver perfusion. In the figure, the stomach is not shown and the liver lobes are represented as dashed lines to allow easier visualization of the catheter and ligatures. Ligatures are placed just above right kidney (1) and above insertion point of catheter (2). l., Left lobe; m., median lobe; r., right lobe; p.v., portal vein; i.v.c., inferior vena cava; — — — —, incision point for initial buffer effusion. [Adapted from Greene (1963).]

whenever handling the lobes of the liver since bruises occur easily and subsequently affect the quality of the perfusion.) Two ligatures are loosely placed around the portal vein (ca. 5 mm from the bifurcation to the different lobes) while another (#2 silk) is placed around the inferior vena cava above the right kidney (Fig. 6B). (The portal vein and surrounding viscera should be kept moist at all times with warm sterile PBS.) Buffer flow is initiated at slow speed (~ 2 ml/min). The catheter is carefully inserted into the portal vein. The metal needle guide is removed, and the cannula gently pushed forward so that it will be securely in the vein. As soon as retrograde bleeding is observed, the ligatures around the cannula are tightened, the perfusion tubing is connected to the back of the cannula, and the inferior vena cava is cut below the right kidney (this will be the exit point for the perfusate). The perfusion is then started with P1 buffer by slowly increasing buffer flow to 35–40 ml/min.

The thoracic cavity is cut open, and the ventral portion of the rib cage is cut away to give easy access to the heart. A ligature is loosely placed around the superior vena cava, and a small hole is cut in the side of the right atrium. A cannula (polyethylene tubing) is then inserted through the right atrium into the superior vena cava, and the ligature firmly tightened. The other end of the polyethylene cannula is placed into a waste bottle, and the ligature around the inferior vena cava is tightened (this will cause the perfusate to drain out the cannula in the superior vena cava). The liver should have a light tan color and be homogeneously bleached without spots of unperfused areas. Flow through the return tubing should be even and without interruption. If the lobes of the liver begin to inflate, the return tubing should be checked to ensure that it is not blocked or crimped. The perfusion with P1 buffer should be continued for ~10 min to sufficiently remove interstitial calcium. (Inefficient calcium removal will result in the improper separation of the hepatocytes, and, consequently, cell yields will be poor.) The perfusate should then be switched to P2 buffer, and the perfusion speed reduced to 20–30 ml/min. For perfusions performed with the M/X Perfuser II, the collagenase solution can easily be recirculated by placing the polyethylene tubing from the superior vena cava into the input port on the top of the lid of tank #2. With a small sterile hose connected to a sink aspirator, the remaining P1 buffer from tank #1 is removed and replaced with 250 ml of P3 buffer. The collagenase perfusion is continued for 10–15 min depending upon the size and appearance of the liver. Initially, the lobes of the liver become somewhat enlarged, and may become "blistered" after 10–15 min of collagenase digestion. Furthermore, the buffer flow through the return tubing begins to slow down to a drip as the perfusate starts to leak out through the liver surface. The liver is then flushed with P3 buffer for ~2–4 min at 35–40 ml/min. For perfusions utilizing a benchtop component system, P1 buffer is oxygenated until half the volume remains, and then the pipet is moved to the P2 buffer. When perfusion with P1 is complete, stopcock S2 is moved to close P1, making P2 available (Fig. 5). P2 is oxygenated in the same way as P1, and when perfusion with P2 is complete, stopcock S3 is moved to close P2, thereby opening P3. Waste perfusate is allowed to drain into the stainless steel pan.

When the perfusion is completed, the liver is extremely fragile with very little structure and should not be directly grasped. The digested liver can be removed by first grasping the wall of the thoracic cavity just anterior to the liver with toothed forceps and lifting slightly. The superior vena cava and other adhesions around the top of the liver are then gently cut. The inferior vena cava is then grasped at the point of ligation, and the vessels below the forceps as well as all remaining adhesions are cut while gently lifting the liver out of the abdominal cavity. (Care should be taken not to cut into the small intestine or stomach when removing adjoining adhesions.) The liver can then be processed for cell culture (Section 2.2) or for studies utilizing cell suspensions (Chapter 10).

ACKNOWLEDGMENTS

P.L.B. and A.P. were supported by grants from the Procter & Gamble Company (University Animal Alternatives Research Program) and from the National Institutes of Health (GM37044).

REFERENCES

Akrawi, M., Rogiers, V., Vandenberghe, Y., Palmer, C., Vercruysse, A., Shephard, E. A., and Phillips, I. R., 1993, Maintenance and induction in co-cultured rat hepatocytes of components of the cytochrome P450-mediated monooxygenase, *Biochem. Pharmacol.* **45:**1583–1591.

Alpini, G., Phillips, J. O., Vroman, B., and LaRusso, N. F., 1994, Recent advances in the isolation of liver cells, *Hepatology* **20:**494–514.

Arand, M., Robertson, L. W., and Oesch, F., 1987, A fluorometric assay for quantitating phenol sulfotransferase activities in homogenates of cells and tissues, *Anal. Biochem.* **163:**546–551.

Arterburn, L. M., Zurlo, J., Yager, J. D., Overton, R. M., and Heifetz, A. H., 1995, A morphological study of differentiated hepatocytes *in vitro*, *Hepatology* **22:**175–187.

Balavoine, S., Feldmann, G., and Lardeux, B., 1993, Regulation of RNA degradation in cultured rat hepatocytes: Effects of specific amino acids and insulin, *J. Cell. Physiol.* **156:**56–62.

Ballard, F. J., Wong, S. S., Knowles, S. E., Partridge, N. C., Martin, T. J., Wood, C. M., and Gunn, J. M., 1980, Insulin inhibition of protein degradation in cell monolayers, *J. Cell Physiol.* **105:**335–346.

Bars, R., Mitchell, A., Wolf, C., and Elcombe, C., 1989, Induction of cytochrome P-450 in cultured rat hepatocytes, *Biochem. J.* **262:**151–158.

Ben-Ze'ev, A., Robinson, G. S., Bucher, N. L., and Farmer, S. R., 1988, Cell–cell and cell–matrix interactions differentially regulate the expression of hepatic and cytoskeletal genes in primary cultures of rat hepatocytes, *Proc. Natl. Acad. Sci. USA.* **85:**2161–2165.

Berry, M. N., and Friend, D. S., 1969, High yield preparation of isolated rat liver parenchymal cells, *J. Cell Biol.* **43:**506–520.

Berry, M. N., Farrington, C., Gay, S., Grivell, A. R., and Wallace, P. G., 1983, Preparation of isolated hepatocytes in good yield without enzymatic digestion, in: *Isolation, Characterization, and Use of Hepatocytes* (R. A. Harris and N. W. Cornell, eds.), Elsevier, New York, pp. 7–10.

Berry, M. N., Edwards, A. M., and Barritt, G. J., 1991, *Isolated Hepatocytes: Preparation, Properties and Applications*, Elsevier, New York.

Bertrams, A., and Ziegler, K., 1991, Hepatocellular uptake of peptides by bile acid transporters: Relationship of carrier-mediated transport of linear peptides with renin-inhibiting activity to multispecific bile acid carriers, *Biochim. Biophys. Acta* **1091:**337–348.

Bissell, D. M., Hammaker, L. E., and Meyer, U. A., 1973, Parenchymal cells from adult rat liver in nonproliferating monolayer culture. I. Functional studies, *J. Cell Biol.* **59:**722–734.

Bissell, D. M., Arenson, D. M., Maher, J. J., and Rold, F. J., 1987, Support of cultured hepatocytes by a laminin-rich gel, *J. Clin. Invest.* **79:**801–812.

Bonney, R. J., Becker, J. E., Walker, P. R., and Potter, V. R., 1974, Primary monolayer cultures of adult rat liver parenchymal cells suitable for study of the regulation of enzyme synthesis, *In Vitro* **9:**399–413.

Bucher, N. R., Robinson, G. S., and Farmer, S. R., 1990, Effects of extracellular matrix on hepatocyte growth and gene expression: Implications for hepatic regeneration and the repair of liver injury, *Semin. Liver Dis.* **10**(1):11–19.

Bullock, P., Gemzik, B., Johnson, D., Thomas, P., and Parkinson, A., 1991, Evidence from dwarf rats that growth hormone may not regulate the sexual differentiation of liver cytochrome P450 enzymes and steroid 5α-reductase, *Proc. Natl. Acad. Sci. USA.* **88:**5227–5231.

Burger, H. J., Schuetz, E. G., Schuetz, J. D., and Guzelian, P. S., 1990, Divergent effects of cycloheximide on the induction of class II and class III cytochrome P450 mRNAs in cultures of adult rat hepatocytes, *Arch. Biochem. Biophys.* **281:**204–211.

Burger, H. J., Schuetz, E. G., Schuetz, J. D., and Guzelian, P. S., 1992, Paradoxical transcriptional activation of rat liver cytochrome P-450 3A1 by dexamethasone and the antiglucocorticoid pregnenolone 16α-carbonitrile: Analysis by transient transfection into primary monolayer cultures of adult rat hepatocytes, *Proc. Natl. Acad. Sci. USA.* **89:**2145–2149.

Burke, M., Thompson, S., Elcombe, C., Halpert, J., Haaparanta, T., and Mayer, R., 1985, Ethoxy-, pentoxy-, and benzyloxyphenoxazones and homologues: A series of substrates to distinguish between different induced cytochromes P-450, *Biochem. Pharmacol.* **34**:3337–3345.

Caron, J. M., 1990, Induction of albumin gene transcription in hepatocytes by extracellular matrix proteins, *Mol. Cell. Biol.* **10**(3)**:**1239–1243.

Chapman, G. S., Jones, A. L., Meyer, U. A., and Bissell, D. M., 1973, Parenchymal cells from adult rat liver in nonproliferating monolayer culture. II. Ultrastructural studies, *J. Cell Biol.* **59**:735–747.

Chieli, E., Santoni-Ruguiu, E., Cervelli, F., Sabbatini, A., Petrini, M., Romiti, N., Paolicchi, A., and Tongiani, R., 1994, Differential modulation of P-glycoprotein expression by dexamethasone and 3-methylcholanthrene in rat hepatocyte primary cultures, *Carcinogenesis* **15**(2)**:**335–341.

Clayton, D. F., and Darnell, J. E., 1983, Changes in liver specific compared to common gene transcription during primary culture of mouse hepatocytes, *Mol. Cell. Biol.* **3**:1552–1561.

Colbert, R. A., Amatruda, J. M., and Young, D. A., 1985, The hepatic glucocorticoid domain: Evidence for early and late hormone-mediated changes in the synthesis of individual protein gene products, *Biochim. Biophys. Acta* **826**:49–66.

Curi-Pedrosa, R., Daujat, M., Pichard, L., Ourlin, J. C., Clair, P., Gervot, L., Lesca, P., Domergue, J., Joyeux, H., Fourtanier, G., and Maurel, P., 1994, Omeprazole and lansoprazole are mixed inducers of CYP1A and CYP3A in human hepatocytes in primary culture, *J. Pharmacol. Exp. Ther.* **269**:384–392.

Dahn, M. S., Hsu, C. J., Lange, M. P., Kimball, S. R., and Jefferson, L. S., 1993, Factors affecting secretory protein production in primary cultures of rat hepatocytes, *Proc. Soc. Exper. Biol. Med.* **203**:38–44.

Diaz, D., Fabre, I., Daujat, M., Saint Aubert, B., Bories, P., Michel, H., and Maurel, P., 1990, Omeprazole is an aryl hydrocarbon-like inducer of human hepatic cytochrome P450, *Gastroenterology* **99**:737–747.

Dich, J., and Grunnet, N., 1989, Primary cultures of rat hepatocytes, in: *Methods in Molecular Biology, Vol. 5: Animal Cell Culture* (J. W. Pollard and J. M. Walker, eds.), Humana Press, Clifton, New Jersey, pp. 161–176.

Dich, J., Vind, C., and Grunnet, N., 1988, Long-term culture of hepatocytes: Effect of hormones on enzyme activities and metabolic capacity, *Hepatology* **8**:39–45.

Donato, M. T., Gomez-Lechon, M. J., and Castell, J. V., 1990, Drug metabolizing enzymes in rat hepatocytes co-cultured with cell lines, *In Vitro Cell. Dev. Biol.* **26**:1057–1062.

Donato, M. T., Castell, J. V., and Gomez-Lechon, M. J., 1991, Co-cultures of hepatocytes with epithelial-like cell lines: Expression of drug-biotransformation activities by hepatocytes, *Cell Biol. Toxicol.* **7**:1–14.

Donato, M. T., Castell, J. V., and Gómez-Lechón, M. J., 1994, Cytochrome P450 activities in pure and co-cultured rat hepatocytes. Effects of model inducers, *In Vitro Cell. Dev. Biol.* **30A**:825–832.

Driscoll, J. L., Hayner, N. T., Williams-Holland, R., Spies-Karotkin, G., Galletti, P. M., and Jauregui, H. O., 1982, Phenolsulfonphthalein (phenol red) metabolism in primary monolayer cultures of adult rat hepatocytes, *In Vitro* **18**(10)**:**835–842.

Dunn, J. C. Y., Yarmush, M. L., Kowbe, H. G., and Tompkins, R. G., 1989, Hepatocyte function and extracellular matrix geometry: Long-term culture in a sandwich configuration, *FASEB J.* **3**:174–177.

Dunn, J. C. Y., Tompkins, R. G., and Yarmush, M. L., 1991, Long-term *in vitro* function of adult hepatocytes in a collagen sandwich configuration, *Biotechnol. Prog.* **7**:237–245.

Dwivedi, R., Primiano, T., and Novake, R., 1993, Xenobiotic-mediated expression of hepatic glutathione-S-transferase genes in primary rat hepatocyte culture, *Biochim. Biophys. Acta* **1174**:43–53.

Elias, E., Hruban, Z., Wade, J. B., and Boyer, J. L., 1980, Phalloidin-induced cholestasis: A microfilament-mediated change in junctional complex permeability, *Proc. Natl. Acad. Sci. USA.* **77**:2229–2233.

Enat, R., Jefferson, D. M., Ruiz-Opaza, N., Gatmaitan, Z., Leinwand, L. A., and Reid, L. M., 1984, Hepatocyte proliferation *in vitro*: Its dependence on the use of serum-free hormonally defined medium and substrata of extracellular matrix, *Proc. Natl. Acad. Sci. USA.* **81**:1411–1415.

Fardel, O., Lecureur, V., and Guillouzo, A., 1993, Regulation by dexamethasone of P-glycoprotein expression in cultured rat hepatocytes, *FEBS Lett.* **327**(2)**:**189–193.

Flaim, K. E., Hutson, S. M., Lloyd, C. E., Taylor, J. M., Shiman, R., and Jefferson, L. S., 1985, Direct effect of insulin on albumin gene expression in primary cultures of rat hepatocytes, *Am. J. Physiol.* **249**:E447–E453.

Forster, U., Luippold, G., and Schwarz, L. R., 1986, Induction of monooxygenase and UDP-glucoronosyl-transferase activities in primary cultures of rat hepatocytes, *Drug Metab. Dispos.* **14**(3):353–360.

Galle, P. R., Theilmann, L., Raedsch, R., Rudolph, G., Kommerell, B., and Stiehl, A., 1989, Taurine and glycine conjugation and sulfation of lithocholate in primary hepatocyte cultures, *Biochim. Biophys. Acta* **1003**:250–253.

Gebhardt, R., 1992, Metabolic zonation of the liver: Regulation and implications for liver function, *Pharmacol. Ther.* **53**:275–354.

Geller, D. A., Nussler, A. K., Di Silvio, M., Lowenstein, C. Z. J., Shapiro, R. A., Wang, S. C., Simmons, R. L., and Billiar, T. R., 1993, Cytokines, endotoxin, and glucocorticoids regulate the expression of inducible nitric oxide synthase in hepatocytes, *Proc. Natl. Acad. Sci. USA.* **90**:552–526.

Goulet, F., Normand, C., and Morin, O., 1988, Cellular interactions promote tissue-specific function, biomatrix deposition, and junctional communication of primary cultured hepatocytes, *Hepatology* **8**:1010–1018.

Grant, M., and Hawksworth, G., 1986, The activity of UDP-glucuronosyltransferase, sulphotransferase and glutathione-S-transferase in primary cultures of rat hepatocytes, *Biochem. Pharmacol.* **35**:2979–2982.

Grant, M. H., Melvin, M. A. L., Shaw, P., Melvin, W. T., and Burke, M. D., 1985, Studies on the maintenance of cytochromes P-450 and b5, monooxygenases and cytochrome reductases in primary cultures of rat hepatocytes, *FEBS Lett.* **190**:99–103.

Greene, E. C., 1963, *Anatomy of the Rat*, Hafner Press, New York.

Grossman, S. J., DeLuca, J. G., Zamboni, R. J., Keenan, K. P., Patrick, D. H., Herold, E. G., van Zwieten, M. J., and Zacchei, A. G., 1992, Enantioselective induction of peroxisomal proliferation in CD-1 mice by leukotriene antagonists, *Toxicol. Appl. Pharmacol.* **116**:217–224.

Guguen-Guillouzo, C., and Guillouzo, A., 1983, Modulation of functional activities in cultured rat hepatocytes, *Mol. Cell. Biochem.* **53/54**:35–56.

Guguen-Guillouzo, C., Clement, B., Baffet, G., Beaumont, C., Morel-Chany, E., Glaise, D., and Guillouzo, A., 1983, Maintenance and reversibility of active albumin secretion by adult rat hepatocytes co-cultured with another liver epithelial cell type, *Exp. Cell Res.* **143**:47–54.

Habig, W. H., Pabst, M. J., and Jakoby, W. B., 1974, Glutathione-S-transferases: The first enzymatic step in mercapturic acid formation, *J. Biol. Chem.* **249**:7130–7139.

Hutson, S. M., Stinton-Fischer, C., Shiman, R., and Jefferson, L. S., 1987, Regulation of albumin synthesis by hormones and amino acids in primary cultures of rat hepatocytes, *Am. J. Physiol.* **252**:E291–E298.

Ichihara, A., Nakamura, T., Noda, C., and Tanaka, K., 1986, Control of enzyme expression deduced from studies on primary cultures of hepatocytes, in: *Research in "Isolated and Cultured Hepatocytes"* (A. Guillouzo and C. Guguen-Guillouzo, eds.), John Libbey, London, pp. 187–207.

Isom, H. C., Secott, T., Georgoff, I., Woodworth, C., and Mummaw, J., 1985, Maintenance of differentiated rat hepatocytes in primary culture, *Proc. Natl. Acad. Sci. USA.* **86**:7432–7436.

Jauregui, H. O., McMillan, P. N., Driscoll, J., and Naik, S., 1986, Attachment and long-term survival of adult rat hepatocytes in primary culture: Comparison of different substrate and tissue culture media formulations, *In Vitro Cell. Dev. Biol.* **22**:13–22.

Jefferson, D., Clayton, D., Darnell, J., and Reid, L., 1984, Posttranscriptional modulation of gene expression in cultured rat hepatocytes, *Mol. Cell. Biol.* **4**:1929–1934.

Jefferson, D. M., Reid, L. M., Giambrone, M.-A., Shafritz, D. A., and Zern, M. A., 1985, Effects of dexamethasone on albumin and collagen gene expression in primary cultures of adult rat hepatocytes, *Hepatology* **5**(1):14–20.

Jurima-Romet, M., and Huang, H. S., 1992, Enalapril hepatotoxicity in the rat. Effects of modulators of cytochrome P450 and glutathione, *Biochem. Pharmacol.* **44**:1803–1810.

Jurima-Romet, M., and Huang, H. S., 1993, Comparative cytotoxicity of angiotensin-converting enzyme inhibitors in cultured rat hepatocytes, *Biochem. Pharmacol.* **46**:2163–2170.

Kane, R., Tector, J., Brems, J., Li, A., and Kaminski, D., 1991, Sulfation and glucuronidation of acetamino-phen by cultured hepatocytes reproducing *in vivo* sex-differences in conjugation on Matrigel and type I collagen, *In Vitro Cell. Dev. Biol.* **27A**:943–960.

Kimball, S. R., Horetsky, R. L., and Jefferson, L. S., 1995, Hormonal regulation of albumin gene expression in primary cultures of hepatocytes, *Am. J. Physiol.* **268**(31)**:**E6–E14.

Kirkpatrick, R. B., and Belsaas, R. A., 1985, Formation and secretion of glycolithocholate-3-sulfate in primary hepatocyte cultures, *J. Lipid Res.* **26:**1431–1437.

Kocarek, T. A., Schuetz, E. G., and Guzelian, P. S., 1993a, Transient induction of cytochrome P450 1A1 mRNA by culture medium component in primary cultures of adult rat hepatocytes, *In Vitro Cell. Dev. Biol.* **29A:**62–66.

Kocarek, T. A., Schuetz, E. G., and Guzelian, P. S., 1993b, Expression of multiple forms of cytochrome P450 mRNAs in primary cultures of rat hepatocytes maintained on Matrigel, *Mol. Pharmacol.* **43:**328–334.

Kocarek, T. A., Schuetz, E. G., and Guzelian, P. S., 1994, Biphasic regulation of cytochrome P450 2B1/2 mRNA expression by dexamethasone in primary cultures of adult rat hepatocytes maintained on matrigel, *Biochem. Pharmacol.* **48**(9)**:**1815–1822.

Kocarek, T. A., Schuetz, E. G., Strom, S. C., Fisher, R. A., and Guzelian, P. S., 1995, Comparative analysis of cytochrome P4503A induction in primary cultures of rat, rabbit, and human hepatocytes, *Drug Metab. Dispos.* **23**(3)**:**415–421.

Komai, T., Shigehara, E., Tokui, T., Koga, T., Ishigami, M., Kuroiwa, C., and Horiuchi, S., 1992, Carrier-mediated uptake of pravastatin by rat hepatocytes in primary culture, *Biochem. Pharmacol.* **43:** 667–670.

Kreamer, B. L., Staecker, J. L., Sawada, N., Sattler, G. L., Hsia, M. T. S., and Pitot, H. C., 1986, Use of a low-speed, iso-density Percoll centrifugation method to increase the viability of isolated rat hepatocyte preparations, *In Vitro* **22**(4)**:**201–211.

Kuri-Harcuch, W., and Mendoza-Figueroa, T., 1989, Cultivation of adult rat hepatocytes on 3T3 cells: Expression of various liver differentiated functions, *Differentiation* **41**(2)**:**148–157.

Kwiatkowski, A. P., Baker, T. K., and Klaunig, J. E., 1994, Comparison of glucocorticoid-mediated changes in the expression and function of rat hepatocyte gap junctional proteins, *Carcinogenesis* **15**(8)**:**1753–1757.

Laishes, B. A., and Williams, G. M., 1976, Conditions affecting primary cell cultures of functional adult rat hepatocytes. II. Dexamethasone enhanced longevity and maintenance of morphology, *In Vitro* **12:** 821–832.

Lambiotte, M., Vorbrodt, A., and Benedetti, E. L., 1973, Expression of differentiation of rat foetal hepatocytes in cellular culture under the action of glucocorticoids: Appearance of bile canaliculi, *Cell Differentiation* **2:**43–53.

LeCluyse, E. L., Audus, K. L., and Hochman, J. H., 1994, Formation of extensive canalicular networks by rat hepatocytes cultured in collagen-sandwich configuration, *Am. J. Physiol.* **266** (*Cell Physiol.* **35**)**:** C1764–C1774.

LeCluyse, E. L., Audus, K. L., and Hochman, J. H., 1996, Role of the cytoskeleton in the regeneration and maintenance of bile canalicular networks in collagen sandwiched hepatocytes, *Exp. Cell Res.*, in press.

Lescoat, G., Clement, T. B., Guillouzo, A., and Guguen-Guillouzo, C., 1985, Modulation of fetal and neonatal rat hepatocyte functional activity by glucocorticoids in co-culture, *Cell Differ.* **16:**259–268.

Li, D., Schuetz, E. G., and Guzelian, P. S., 1991, Hepatocyte culture in the study of P450 regulation, *Methods Enzymol.* **206:**335–345.

Lilienblum, W., Walli, A. K., and Bock, K. W., 1982, Differential induction of rat liver microsomal UDP-glucuronosyltransferase activities by various inducing agents, *Biochem. Pharmacol.* **31:**907–913.

Lindblad, W. J., Schuetz, E. G., Redford, K. S., and Guzelian, P. S., 1991, Hepatocellular phenotype *in vitro* is influenced by biophysical features of the collagenous substratum, *Hepatology* **13:**282–288.

Liu, L., Liu, Y. P., and Klaassen, C. D., 1994, Effect of steroids on rat liver sulfotransferase activities. Thirty-third Annual Meeting of the Society of Toxicology, *Toxicologist* **14**(1)**:**342.

Liu, L., LeCluyse, E., and Klaassen, C. D., 1996, Sulfotransferase gene expression in primary cultures of rat hepatocytes, *Biochem. Pharmacol.*, in press.

Maher, J. J., 1988, Primary hepatocyte culture: Is it home away from home?, *Hepatology* **8:**1162–1166.

Marceau, N., Baribault, H., Germain L., and Noel, M., 1986, *Research in "Isolated and Cultured*

Hepatocytes" (A. Guillouzo and C. Guguen-Guillouzo, eds.), John Libbey Eurotext Ltd., Inserm, London, p. 39.

Mathis, J. M., Houser, W. H., Bresnick, E., Cidlowski, J. A., Hines, R. N., Prough, R. A., and Simpson, E. R., 1989, Glucocorticoid regulation of the rat cytochrome P450c (P450IA1) gene: Receptor binding within intron I, *Arch. Biochem. Biophys.* **269**(1):93–105.

Meredith, M. J., 1988, Rat hepatocytes prepared without collagenase: Prolonged retention of differentiated characteristics in culture, *Cell Biol. Toxicol.* **4**(4):405–425.

Miyazaki, M., Handa, Y., Oda, M., and Sato, J., 1985, Long term survival of functional hepatocytes from adult rat in the presence of phenobarbital in primary culture, *Exp. Cell Res.* **159**:176–190.

Morel, F., Beaune, P. H., Ratanasavanh, D., Flinois, J.-P., Yang, C.-S., Guengerich, F. P., and Guillouzo, A., 1990, Expression of cytochrome P-450 enzymes in cultured human hepatocytes, *Eur. J. Biochem.* **191**: 437–444.

Morin, O., and Normand, C., 1986, Long-term maintenance of hepatocyte functional activity in co-culture: Requirements for sinusoidal endothelial cells and dexamethasone, *J. Cell Physiol.* **129**:103–110.

Musat, A. I., Sattler, C., Sattler, G. L., and Pitot, H. C., 1993, Re-establishment of cell polarity of hepatocytes in primary culture, *Hepatology* **18**:198–205.

Niemann, C., Gauthier, J.-C., Richert, L., Ivanov, M.-A., Melcion, C., and Cordier, A., 1991, Rat adult hepatocytes in primary pure and mixed monolayer culture, *Biochem. Pharmacol.* **42**:373–379.

Oda, M., and Phillips, M. J., 1977, Bile canalicular membrane pathology in cytochalasin B-induced cholestasis, *Lab. Invest.* **37**(4):350–356.

Omura, T., and Sato, R., 1964, The carbon monoxide-binding pigment of liver microsomes. I. Evidence for its hemoprotein nature, *J. Biol. Chem.* **239**:2370–2378.

Oude Elferink, R. P. J., Bakker, C. T. M., Roelofsen, H., Middelkoop, E., Ottenhoff, R., Heijn, M., and Jansen, P. L. M., 1993, Accumulation of organic anion in intracellular vesicles of cultured rat hepatocytes is mediated by the canalicular multispecific organic anion transporter, *Hepatology* **17**:434–444.

Paine, A. J., Lesley, J. W., and Legg, R. F., 1979, Apparent maintenance of cytochrome P450 by nicotinamide in primary cultures of rat hepatocytes, *Life Sci.* **24**:2185–2192.

Parkinson, A., 1996, Biotransformation of xenobiotics, in: *Casarett and Doull's Toxicology, The Basic Science of Poisons*, fifth edition, (C. D. Klaassen, ed.), McGraw-Hill, New York, pp. 113–186.

Phillips, M. J., Oda, M., Mak, E., Fisher, M. M., and Jeejeebhoy, K. N., 1975, Microfilament dysfunction as a possible cause of intrahepatic cholestasis, *Gastroenterology* **69**:48–58.

Pichard, L., Fabre, I., Fabre, G., Domergue, J., Saint-Aubert, B., Mourad, G., and Maurel, P., 1990, Cyclosporin A drug interactions: Screening for inducers and inhibitors of cytochrome P-450 (cyclosporin A oxidase) in primary cultures of human hepatocytes and in liver microsomes, *Drug Metab. Dispos.* **18**:595–606.

Powis, G., Melder, D. D., and Wilke, T. J., 1989, Human and dog, but not rat, isolated hepatocytes have decreased foreign compound-metabolizing activity compared to liver slices, *Drug Metab. Dispos.* **17**: 526–531.

Probst, I., and Jungermann, K., 1983, The glucagon–insulin antagonism and glucagon–dexamethasone synergism in the induction of PEP-carboxy kinase in cultured rat hepatocytes, *Hoppe-Seylers Z. Physiol. Chem.* **364**:1739–1746.

Quistorff, B., Dich, J., and Grunnet, N., 1989, Preparation of isolated rat liver hepatocytes, in: *Methods in Molecular Biology, Vol. 5: Animal Cell Culture* (J. W. Pollard and J. M. Walker, eds.), Humana Press, Clifton, New Jersey, pp. 151–160.

Rana, B., Mischoulon, D., Xie, Y., Bucher, N. L. R., and Farmer, S. R., 1994, Cell-extracellular matrix interactions can regulate the switch between growth and differentiation in rat hepatocytes: Reciprocal expression of C/EBPα and immediate-early growth response transcription factors, *Mol. Cell. Biol.* **14**:5858–5869.

Reid, L. M., Narita, M., Fujita, M., Murray, Z., Liverpool, C., and Rosenberg, L., 1986, Matrix and hormonal regulation of differentiation in liver cultures, in: *Research in "Isolated and Cultured*

Hepatocytes" (A. Guillouzo and C. Guguen-Guillouzo, eds.), John Libbey Eurotext, Inserm, London, pp. 225–258.

Reid, L. M., Fiorino, A. S., Sigal, S. H., Brill, S., and Holst, P. A., 1992, Extracellular matrix gradients in the space of Disse: Relevance to liver biology, *Hepatology* **15:**1198–1203.

Ren, P., de Feijter, A. W., Paul, D. L., and Ruch, R. J., 1994, Enhancement of liver cell gap junction protein expression by glucocorticoids, *Carcinogenesis* **15**(9)**:**1807–1813.

Rogiers, V., and Vercruysse, A., 1993, Rat hepatocyte cultures and co-cultures in biotransformation studies of xenobiotics, *Toxicology* **82:**193–208.

Rogiers, V., Vandenberghe, Y., Callaerts, A., Sonck, W., and Vercruysee, A., 1990a, Effects of dimethyl-sulphoxide on phase I and II biotransformation in cultured rat hepatocytes, *Toxic. In Vitro* **4:**439–442.

Rogiers, V., Vandenberghe, Y., Callaerts, A., Verleye, G., Cornet, M., Mertens, D., Sonck, W., and Vercruysse, A., 1990b, Phase I and phase II xenobiotic biotransformation in cultures and co-cultures of adult rat hepatocytes, *Biochem. Pharmacol.* **40:**1701–1706.

Rojkind, M., Gatmaitan, Z., Mackensen, S., Giambrone, M.-A., Ponce, P., and Ried, L. M., 1980, Connective tissue biomatrix: Its isolation and utilization for long term cultures of normal rat hepatocytes, *J. Cell. Biol.* **87:**255–263.

Schrenk, D., Eisenmann-Tappe, I., Gebhardt, R., Mayer, D., El Mouelhi, M., Rohrdanz, E., Munzel, P., and Bock, K. W., 1991, Drug metabolizing enzyme activities in rat liver epithelial cell lines, hepatocytes and bile duct cells, *Biochem. Pharmacol.* **41:**1751–1757.

Schuetz, E. G., and Guzelian, P. S., 1984, Induction of cytochrome P-450 by glucocorticoids in rat liver. II. Evidence that glucocorticoids regulate induction of cytochrome P-450 by a nonclassical receptor mechanism, *J. Biol. Chem.* **259:**2007–2012.

Schuetz, E. G., Wrighton, S. A., Barwick, J. L., and Guzelian, P. S., 1984, Induction of cytochrome P-450 by glucocorticoids in rat liver. I. Evidence that glucocorticoids and pregnenolone 16α-carbonitrile regulate *de novo* synthesis of a common form of cytochrome P-450 in cultures of adult rat hepatocytes and in the liver *in vivo*, *J. Biol. Chem.* **259:**1999–2006.

Schuetz, E. G., Li, D., Omiecinski, C. J., Muller-Eberhard, U., Kleinmann, H. K., Elswick, B., and Guzelian, P. S., 1988, Regulation of gene expression in adult rat hepatocytes cultured on a basement membrane matrix, *J. Cell Physiol.* **134:**309–323.

Schuetz, E. G., Schuetz, J. D., May, B, and Guzelian, P. S., 1990, Regulation of cytochrome P-450b-e and P-450p gene expression by growth hormone in adult rat hepatocytes cultured on a reconstituted basement membrane, *J. Biol. Chem.* **265:**1188–1192.

Schwarze, P. E., Solheim, A. E., and Seglen, P. O., 1982, Amino acid and energy requirements for rat hepatocytes in primary culture, *In Vitro* **18:**43–54.

Seglen, P. O., 1976, Preparation of isolated rat liver cells, in: *Methods in Cell Biology*, Vol. 19 (D. M. Prescott, ed.), Academic Press, New York, pp. 29–83.

Seglen, P. O., Gordon, P. B., and Poli, A., 1980, Amino acid inhibition of autophagic/lysosomal pathway of protein degradation in isolated rat hepatocytes, *Biochim. Biophys. Acta* **630:**103–118.

Sidhu, J. S., and Omiecinski, C. J., 1995, Modulation of xenobiotic-inducible cytochrome P450 gene expression by dexamethasone in primary rat hepatocytes, *Pharmacogenetics* **5:**24–36.

Sidhu, J. S., Farin, F. M., and Omiecinski, C. J., 1993, Influence of extracellular matrix overlay on phenobarbital-mediated induction of CYP2B1, 2B2, and 3A1 genes in primary adult rat hepatocyte culture, *Arch. Biochem. Biophys.* **30:**103–113.

Sidhu, J. S., Farin, F. M., Kavanagh, T. J., and Omiecinski, C. J., 1994, Effect of tissue-culture substratum and extracellular matrix overlay on liver-selective and xenobiotic inducible gene expression in primary rat hepatocytes, *In Vitro Toxicol.* **7**(3)**:**225–242.

Sinclair, P. R., Bement, W. J., Haugen, S. A., Sinclair, J. F., and Guzelian, P. S., 1990, Induction of cytochrome P-450 and 5-aminolevulinate synthase activities in cultured rat hepatocytes, *Cancer Res.* **50:**5219–5224.

Sipes, I. G., and Gandolfi, A. J., 1991, Biotransformation of toxicants, in: *Casarett and Doull's Toxicology*, 4th ed. (M. O. Amdur, J. Doull, and C. D. Klaassen, eds.), Pergamon Press, New York, p. 108.

Smith, M. T., and Wills, E. D., 1981, Effects of dietary lipid and phenobarbitone on the distribution of cytochrome P-450 in the liver studied by quantitative histochemistry, *FEBS Lett.* **127**:33–36.

Sonderfan, A., Arlotto, M., Dutton, D., McMillen, S., and Parkinson, A., 1987, Regulation of testosterone hydroxylation by rat liver microsomal cytochrome P-450, *Arch. Biochem. Biophys.* **255**:27–41.

Sweeny, D. J., and Reinke, L. A., 1988, Sulfation of acetaminophen in isolated rat hepatocytes. Relationship to sulfate ion concentrations and intracellular levels of 3′-phosphoadenosine-5′-phosphosulfate, *Drug. Metab. Dispos. Biol. Fate. Chem.* **16**:712–715.

Tavoloni, N., and Boyer, J. L., 1980, Relationships between hepatic metabolism of chlorpromazine and cholestatic effects in the isolated perfused rat liver, *J. Pharmacol. Exp. Ther.* **214**:269–274.

Thurman, R. G., Kaufman, F. C., and Jungermann, K. (eds.), 1986, *Regulation of Hepatic Metabolism. Inter- and Intracellular Compartmentation*, Plenum Press, New York.

Ugele, B., Kempen, J. M., Gebhardt, R., Meijer, P., Burger, H.-J., and Princen, H. M. G., 1991, Heterogeneity of rat liver parenchyma in cholesterol 7α-hydroxylase and bile acid synthesis, *Biochem. J.* **276**:73–77.

Utesch, D., and Oesch, F., 1992a, Dependency of the *in vitro* stabilization of differentiated functions in liver parenchymal cells upon the type of cell line used for co-culture, *In Vitro Cell. Dev. Biol.* **28**:193–198.

Utesch, D., and Oesch, F., 1992b, Phenol sulfotransferase activity in rat liver parenchymal cells cultured on collagen gels, *Drug Metab. Dispos.* **20**:614–615.

Utesch, D., Molitor, E., Platt, K.-L., and Oesch, F., 1991, Differential stabilization of cytochrome P-450 isoenzymes in primary cultures of adult rat liver parenchymal cells, *In Vitro Cell. Dev. Biol.* **27A:** 858–863.

Vandenberghe, Y., Ratanasavanh, D., Glaise, D., and Guillouzo, A, 1988, Influence of medium composition and culture conditions on glutathione S-transferase activity in adult rat hepatocytes during culture, *In Vitro Cell. Dev. Biol.* **24**:281–288.

Vandenberghe, Y., Morel, F., Foriers, A., Ketterer, B., Vercruysse, A., Guillouzo, A., and Rogiers, V., 1989, Effect of phenobarbital on the expression of glutathione S-transferase isoenzymes in cultured rat hepatocytes, *FEBS Lett.* **251**:59–64.

Vandenberghe, Y., Tee, L., Morel, F., Rogiers, V., Guillouzo, A., and Yeoh, G., 1991, Regulation of glutathione S-transferase gene expression by phenobarbital in cultured adult rat hepatocytes, *FEBS Lett.* **284**:103–108.

Vandenberghe, Y., Tee, L., Rogiers, V., and Yeoh, G., 1992, Transcriptional- and post-transcriptional-dependent regulation of glutathione S-transferase expression in rat hepatocytes as a function of culture conditions, *FEBS Lett.* **313**:155–159.

Vind, C., Dich, J., and Grunnet, N., 1989, Effects of cytochrome P450-inducing agents on the monooxygenation of testosterone in long-term cultures of hepatocytes from male and female rats, *Arch. Biochem. Biophys.* **275**:140–150.

Wang, S.-R., Renaud, G., Infante, J., Catala, D., and Infante, R., 1985, Isolation of rat hepatocytes with EDTA and their metabolic functions in primary culture, *In Vitro Cell. Dev. Biol.* **21**:526–530.

Watanabe, N., Tsukada, N., Smith, C. R., and Phillips, M. J., 1991, Motility of bile canaliculi in the living animal: Implications for bile flow, *J. Cell Biol.* **113**:1069–1080.

Waterman, M. R., and Johnson, E. F. (eds.), 1991, Cytochrome P450, in: *Methods in Enzymology*, Vol. 206, Academic Press, New York.

Watkins, J. B., Gregus, Z., Thompson, T. N., and Klaassen, C. D., 1982, Induction studies on the functional heterogeneity of rat liver UDP-glucuronosyl-transferases, *Toxicol. Appl. Pharmacol.* **64**:439–446.

Waxman, D. J., Morrissey, J. J., Naik, S., and Jauregui, H. O., 1990, Phenobarbital induction of cytochromes P450: High-level long-term responsiveness of primary rat hepatocyte cultures to drug induction, and glucocorticoid dependence of the phenobarbital response, *Biochem. J.* **271**:113–119.

Williams, G. M., Bermudez, E., and Scaramuzzino, D., 1977, Rat hepatocyte primary cell cultures. III. Improved dissociation and attachment techniques and the enhancement of survival by culture medium, *In Vitro* **13**:809–817.

Wojcik, E., Dvorak, C., Chianale, J., Traber, P. G., Keren, D., and Gumucio, J., 1988, Demonstration by *in situ* hybridization of the zonal modulation of rat liver cytochrome P-45b and P-450e gene expression after phenobarbital, *J. Clin. Invest.* **82:**658–666.

Wolfe, D., and Jungermann, K., 1985, Long-term effects of physiological oxygen concentrations on glycolysis and gluconeogenesis in hepatocyte culture, *Eur. J. Biochem.* **151:**299–303.

Wood, A., Ryan, D., Thomas, P., and Levin, W., 1983, Regio- and stereoselective metabolism of two C$_{19}$ steroids by five highly purified and reconstituted rat hepatic cytochrome P-450 isozymes, *J. Biol. Chem.* **258:**8839–8847.

Wortelboer, H. M., de Kruif, C. A., van Iersel, A. A. J., Falke, H. E., Noordhoek, J., and Blaauboer, B. J., 1990, The isoenzyme pattern of cytochrome P450 in rat hepatocytes in primary culture, comparing different enzyme activities in microsomal incubations and in intact monolayers, *Biochem. Pharmacol.* **40:**2525–2534.

Yamada, S., Otto, P. S., Kennedy, D. L., and Whayne, T. F., Jr., 1980, The effects of dexamethasone on metabolic activity of hepatocytes in primary monolayer culture, *In Vitro* **16**(7)**:**559–570.

Yan, B., Yang, D., Bullock, P., and Parkinson, A., 1995, Rat serum carboxylesterase: Cloning, expression, regulation, and evidence of secretion from liver, *J. Biol Chem.* **270:**19128–19134.

Zaphiropoulos, P. G., Mode, A., Norstedt, G., and Gustafsson, J. A., 1989, Regulation of sexual differentiation in drug and steroid metabolism, *Trends Pharmacol. Sci.* **10**(4)**:**149–153.

Chapter 10

Isolated Perfused Liver

Kim L. R. Brouwer and Ronald G. Thurman

1. INTRODUCTION

The isolated perfused liver is a useful intact organ model for examining the hepatobiliary disposition of drugs without the complication of many factors that are difficult to control *in vivo* such as neuronal and hormonal influences on hepatic metabolism, as well as absorption, distribution, metabolism, and excretion by nonhepatic routes. The intact perfused organ preserves hepatic architecture, cell polarity, and bile flow, in contrast to *in vitro* models like liver slices, hepatocytes, microsomes, and liver plasma membrane vesicles.

The history of liver perfusion dates back to the mid-1800s, when Claude Bernard (1855) first described the conversion of glycogen to glucose in livers perfused with tap water. Numerous improvements in the apparatus and technique, including perfusion with blood and incorporation of a lung into the circuit to improve oxygenation, were made in the late 1800s (Asp, 1873; von Frey and Gruber, 1885; Jacobj, 1890). Further advances in the technique were made when Trowell (1942) studied urea synthesis in isolated rat livers perfused with oxygenated saline and when Lupton (1947) demonstrated the effects of warfarin in the isolated rat liver perfused with citrated rat blood.

In the early 1950s, Miller and colleagues at the University of Rochester initiated landmark studies using blood-perfused isolated rat livers to demonstrate the role of the liver in plasma protein synthesis (Miller *et al.*, 1951) and in the biologic effects of insulin (Haft and Miller, 1958), glucagon, and cortisol (Miller, 1965). However, this

Kim L. R. Brouwer • Division of Pharmaceutics, School of Pharmacy, University of North Carolina, Chapel Hill, North Carolina 27599. *Ronald G. Thurman* • Laboratory of Hepatobiology and Toxicology, Department of Pharmacology, University of North Carolina, Chapel Hill, North Carolina 27599.

Models for Assessing Drug Absorption and Metabolism, Ronald T. Borchardt *et al.*, eds., Plenum Press, New York, 1996.

technique was not accepted widely by biochemists until its utility was demonstrated by recognized authorities such as Sir Hans Krebs (Hems *et al.*, 1966) and Henry Lardy (Veneziale *et al.*, 1967). Concurrently, German scientists at the University of Munich (Scholz and Bücher, 1965) developed a liver perfusion system quite different from the one used by Miller and colleagues. This hemoglobin-free perfusion technique, first developed by Bücher and his students, Scholz and Brauser (Scholz and Bücher, 1965), and further refined by Thurman and Sies, did not quench optical signals to the same degree as blood-containing perfusate and was preferable to Miller's technique for obtaining direct physical measurements via spectroscopy and fluorescence.

There has been long-standing debate between the Rochester and Munich schools concerning the benefits and limitations of these two different methods of liver perfusion. Despite differences in perfusate composition and flow rate, the basic approach to liver perfusion is similar in both techniques, and important contributions to the understanding of hepatobiliary function and the disposition of endogenous and exogenous substrates and metabolites have been made by investigators using either system. The general technique of isolated rat liver perfusion has been reviewed previously (Miller, 1973b; Meijer *et al.*, 1981; Gores *et al.*, 1986). This chapter will compare and contrast the Miller and Munich type systems with specific reference to practical considerations and applications. Differences between these systems should be considered carefully in study design, as one approach may be more suitable than the other, depending on the questions to be addressed in specific experiments.

During the last 30 years, the perfused liver has been used extensively to study metabolic regulation. It has become increasingly apparent that preservation of hepatic architecture, cell polarity, and bile flow may be critical in data interpretation. In addition, the role of nonparenchymal (e.g., Kupffer, Ito, and endothelial) cells in metabolic regulation and cell-to-cell interactions recently has received significant attention (Ballet and Thurman, 1991). These considerations have led to a resurgence of interest in the use of whole-liver perfusion for studying hepatic drug disposition and metabolism. In addition, the perfused liver is being used with increased frequency to examine enzyme localization, regulation of bile flow, factors that influence the hepatobiliary disposition of xenobiotics, and drug toxicity in different regions of the liver lobule.

Many different species have served as liver donors for perfusion studies, including the monkey, calf, sheep, pig, dog, cat, rabbit, guinea pig, hamster, and mouse. Owing to limitations of oxygen delivery at practical flow rates, the hemoglobin-free model usually is limited to organs of less than 25 g (e.g., from rat, mouse, hamster, guinea pig). The rat is used most commonly in liver perfusion studies, in part because it requires minimal surgical manipulations owing to its convenient size. Historically, the rat also has been the rodent of choice in most *in vivo* and *in vitro* drug metabolism studies, particularly in the drug development process. Furthermore, the rat is a convenient species for studying the effects of experimentally-induced liver disease (e.g., alcoholic liver injury) and drug-induced alterations in hepatic function.

2. METHODS

Livers may be perfused *in situ* or in an isolated, *ex situ* fashion. *In situ* perfusion may be complicated by perfusate loss to extrahepatic organ systems, and difficulty may be encountered in maintaining the carcass at physiologic temperatures. If the carcass is left in the perfusion chamber for several hours, autolysis will occur, and toxins and bacteria from the abdominal cavity may contaminate the liver, perfusate, and apparatus. *Ex situ* perfusion, which requires isolation of the liver from the carcass and placement onto a perfusion platform, facilitates temperature control and eliminates the other complications mentioned above; with proper surgical technique, bacterial contamination is obviated.

2.1. Perfusion Apparatus

2.1.1. CLOSED "MILLER TYPE" SYSTEM

The perfusion apparatus based on the Miller system consists of a temperature-controlled, humidified perfusion chamber containing a platform for the liver and a reservoir (Fig. 1). A Plexiglas box or desiccator (approximately 46 cm × 46 cm × 46

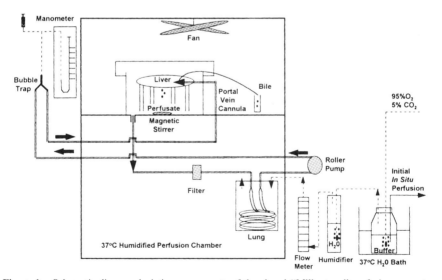

Figure 1. Schematic diagram depicting components of the closed "Miller type" perfusion apparatus. Solid lines with arrows depict perfusate or buffer flow while dashed lines indicate gas flow.

cm; Liberty Industries, Inc.) with a shelf approximately 23 cm from the bottom of the box may be adapted for use as the perfusion chamber. Silicone electrical heating tape (1.27 cm × 122 cm; L-03111-40, Cole-Parmer) may be mounted with mending plates around the inside of the chamber, but not on the door; one strip should be mounted midway between the bottom of the box and the shelf and a second strip between the shelf, and the top of the box. A direct dialing Thermistemp temperature controller (YSI model 63RC) should be mounted on the exterior of the box and connected directly to the heating tape through a small hole drilled in the box. A small fan (~10 cm; 273-241C, Archer) mounted on the inside top of the chamber will circulate air sufficiently to maintain a constant temperature throughout the chamber. Humidity may be maintained with several open beakers containing water. The temperature of the liver should be monitored continuously with a flat surface temperature probe (15-176-48, YSI) placed between two lobes of the liver; the probe should be connected to an indicating-type temperature controller (YSI model 73A). In order to maintain the liver and perfusate temperature at 37°C, the temperature of the box must be kept at ~45°C. The reservoir (~200 ml; 100 mm high × 65 mm wide) containing the removable liver platform (75 mm × 60 mm) may be constructed from Plexiglas and can reside on the shelf as indicated in Fig. 1. The liver platform should be constructed with a hole (~6-mm diameter) in the center and several surrounding smaller holes (~2-mm diameter), to allow perfusate to drip from the platform into the reservoir. A lightweight plastic cover should be placed over the top of the reservoir during perfusion to minimize evaporative loss. A small stir bar should be placed in the reservoir to ensure constant mixing of the perfusate. The magnetic stirrer may be located on the bottom of the chamber, directly below the reservoir. A peristaltic or pulsating perfusion pump (Masterflex pump model 7523-10; size 16 silicone tubing, Masterflex) and pump head (Masterflex model 7016-20) are required to pump perfusate at a constant rate through the system.

The "Hamilton lung" (Hamilton *et al.*, 1974) is used for oxygenating hemoglobin-containing perfusate. It consists of a specimen jar (~500-ml capacity) with four ports in the lid (gas inlet, gas outlet, perfusate inlet, and perfusate outlet) and 4.6 m of silastic tubing (0.058 in. i.d., 0.077 in. o.d.; T5715-6, Baxter). In our experience, oxygenation is accomplished most readily by diverting perfusate inside the lung via miniature polypropylene "tee" fittings (model 6365-90, Cole-Parmer) through two 2.3-m lengths of silastic tubing. The 95% O_2/5% CO_2 gas mixture should be warmed to 37°C by bubbling through a 2-l flask of Krebs–Henseleit bicarbonate buffer (maintained at 37°C in a water bath) and humidified by bubbling through water via a gas dispersion tube (L-06614-25, Cole-Parmer). Gas flow should be maintained at ~70–80 psi via a flow meter (L-03295-22, Cole-Parmer).

Latex tubing (amber natural ⅛ in. i.d. × ¹⁄₃₂ in. wall; Baxter) may be used to circulate perfusate through the system. Before entering the lung, perfusate should be filtered through a syringe filter holder (25 mm; L-02928-20, Cole-Parmer) to remove blood clots and/or debris. Prior to entering the liver, perfusate should pass through an inverted glass Y tube mounted on the side of the chamber, approximately level with the liver platform, facilitating removal of air bubbles. The level of the perfusate should be maintained midway up the stem of the Y tube, which is connected via latex tubing to a T tube mounted on the top of the perfusion chamber. One arm of the T tube should be connected to a 10-ml syringe to allow fine adjustment of the perfusate level in the Y tube. The other arm should be connected to a manometer gauge (L-00905-00, Cole-Parmer) to allow continuous monitoring of inflow perfusion pressure.

Perfusate pH should be monitored continuously. The pH of the perfusion medium is 7.4 initially and should be maintained in the physiologic range by periodic addition of a few drops of a saturated solution of sodium bicarbonate.

2.1.2. OPEN "MUNICH TYPE" SYSTEM

An alternative system for perfusing livers without the use of blood products, based on the approach first developed by the Munich school, is the open perfusion system (Fig. 2). It is comprised of the following components: a constant-temperature recirculating water bath (L-01228-00, Cole-Parmer), a Masterflex L/S digital flow monitoring drive pump (L-07523-00, Cole-Parmer), Masterflex standard pump heads (tubing size 14, LEXAN polycarbonate housing, stainless steel rotor; L-07014-21, Cole-Parmer), multiple pump head mounting hardware (L-07013-05, Cole-Parmer) with Masterflex L/S thin-wall tubing (silicone for size 14 pump head, L-064411-14, Cole-Parmer), double-jacketed tubing consisting of clear plastic tubing ($\frac{5}{16}$ in. i.d. $\times$ $\frac{7}{16}$ in. o.d., T6010-4; $\frac{1}{8}$ in. i.d. $\times$ $\frac{1}{4}$ in. o.d., T6010-10; $\frac{3}{32}$ in. i.d. $\times$ $\frac{5}{32}$ in. o.d.,

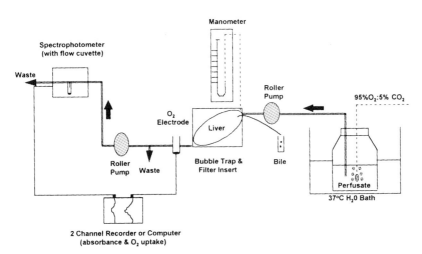

Figure 2.   Schematic diagram depicting components of the open "Munich type" perfusion apparatus. Solid lines with arrows depict buffer flow while dashed lines indicate gas flow.

T6010-1X; Baxter Scientific) covering intramedic polyethylene tubing (Baxter Scientific), and a perfusion block with a bubble trap (contact Dr. Thurman).

The cannula tubing used is intramedic polyethylene tubing (Baxter Scientific). Clark type oxygen electrodes modified by Thurman (Instech Laboratories Inc., Plymouth Meeting, PA) with a Teflon membrane kit (L-05522-00, Cole-Parmer) are placed in the outflow location on the perfusion block and connected to a dual-channel differential oxygen amplifier (Instech) with an electrode cable (Instech). Data can be recorded with a dual-channel chart recorder (L-08373-20, Cole-Parmer) or an on-line computer via a data acquisition board (L-08302-00, Cole-Parmer) and terminal panel (L-08303-20, Cole-Parmer) if the latter are compatible with available software.

Oxygenation of perfusate is achieved by bubbling 95% O_2/5% CO_2 into hemoglobin-free perfusate. PyrexPlus poly(vinyl chloride)-coated aspirator bottles (1 liter, B7580-1LS; 2 liter, B7580-2LS; Baxter Scientific) used in conjunction with gas dispersion tubes (G2010-2; Baxter Scientific) warm and oxygenate buffer prior to delivery by the perfusion pump. Multiple aspiration bottles for the delivery of solutions containing different substrates to the perfused liver can be controlled with three-way stopcocks (S8966-2, Baxter Scientific).

2.1.3. SYSTEM MAINTENANCE

It is important to warm the perfusion system to 45°C prior to use to maintain the perfusate temperature at 37°C. Saline should be circulated through the system and discarded to remove particulate matter and residual fluid before addition of perfusate to the reservoir. After completion of liver perfusion and removal of the liver from the platform, residual perfusate in the system should be discarded. The system should be cleaned thoroughly by perfusing first with hot water and then flushing several times with distilled water. Ethanol or other organic solvents should be avoided because even residual amounts remaining after the cleaning procedure, which may represent millimole quantities of the solvent, are known to affect hepatic function. If the perfusate contains hemoglobin, tubing should be changed frequently (after 4–6 liver perfusions of ~2.5-hr duration) to avoid extensive accumulation of protein in the tubing. This is particularly important in the lung, where protein accumulation can result in inadequate perfusate oxygenation and increased inflow perfusion pressure. In contrast, frequent tubing changes are unnecessary in the Munich type perfusion system; tubing may last for extended periods of time (~4 months) since buffer is oxygenated directly with a gas dispersion tube.

A pilot study should be conducted in the perfusion system before initiating studies with a new substrate in order to assess substrate stability in the perfusion medium in the absence of a liver and to determine the extent of loss or binding of substrate to the tubing and apparatus. In all cases, the tubing should be discarded after each experiment if the substrate accumulates extensively in tubing, as is the case for lipophilic toxins.

2.2. Perfusate Composition and Flow Rate

2.2.1. GENERAL COMPONENTS

The bicarbonate-buffered saline solution originally described by Krebs and Henseleit (1932), often referred to as Krebs–Henseleit bicarbonate buffer, containing 118 mM NaCl, 5.0 mM KCl, 1.1 mM $MgSO_4$, 1.2 mM KH_2PO_4, 2.5 mM $CaCl_2$, and 25 mM $NaHCO_3$, is used most commonly. Glucose (1% w/v) may be added to serve as the energy source, although endogenous hepatic glycogen or fatty acids have been shown to be a sufficient source of energy. Typically, we prepare the buffer solution in Millipore-filtered water containing all ingredients except $CaCl_2$ and $NaHCO_3$. A stock solution is prepared by adding the energy source [e.g., glucose (10 g)] and $NaHCO_3$ (in 25 ml of water) to 500 ml of buffer solution and bubbling this solution with 95% O_2/5% CO_2 for 10 min. After addition of $CaCl_2$ (in 10 ml of water), which is added last to avoid precipitation of calcium as the phosphate salt, the stock solution should be diluted to a final volume of 1 l with buffer solution. If necessary, the pH should be adjusted to 7.4 with NaOH. After filtration, the stock solution may be stored for one week in the refrigerator. Alternatively, more concentrated stock solutions may be refrigerated and fresh perfusate prepared on the day of the experiment. Some investigators increase the phosphate concentration to 2 mM based on a report by Sestoft and Kristensen (1979) that it is more physiologic for the rat and improves the energy status of the isolated liver.

2.2.2. OXYGEN-CARRYING CAPACITY

2.2.2a. Red Blood Cell-Containing Perfusion Media

A variety of perfusates containing heparinized whole blood from rats, washed red blood cells from cow, sheep, or rabbit, or outdated human cells diluted with buffer solution and containing various additives have been employed in liver perfusion studies (Brauer et al., 1951; Miller et al., 1951; Hems et al., 1966; Miller, 1973a,b). Defibrinated blood requires special processing by high-speed centrifugation to remove the buffy coat and clear the defibrinated plasma of microaggregates of platelets and fibrin (Miller et al., 1964). Fresh blood from donor rats should be heparinized with ~50–100 units/ml of blood (Miller, 1973b). Heparin is essential even if clotting factors have been removed from the perfusate because the functional liver produces and secretes fibrinogen and prothrombin, as well as Factors V, VII, and X. In the absence of heparin, clotting will occur in the perfusion system (Miller, 1973a). To remove any gross clots, the heparinized blood should be filtered through a sterile 8 cm x 8 cm surgical gauze sponge moistened with perfusate solution placed on a funnel support. Blood remaining on the gauze sponge can be rinsed with a small volume of perfusate solution. Liver perfusions have been conducted successfully with heparinized rat whole blood diluted from 67% (Miller, 1973b) to 20% (Brouwer and Vore, 1985) with buffer solutions. Washed red blood cells should be diluted to a hematocrit of 15–20% (Meijer *et al.*, 1981). Dilution is required to prevent obstruction of sinusoidal flow due to aggregated erythrocytes. The oxygen-carrying capacity of red blood cells enables perfusion of livers at physiologic flow rates [~2 ml min^{-1} (g liver)$^{-1}$; Roth and Rubin, 1976a; Fiserova-Bergerova and Hughes, 1983]. Although Riedel *et al.* (1983) reported that a hematocrit of 20% provides optimal oxygenation at physiologic perfusion pressures, mean oxygen consumption in a 20% heparinized whole blood-containing medium (16 ml of rat donor blood in a total perfusate volume of 80 ml) was approximately 1.4 μmol min^{-1} (g liver)$^{-1}$ (Brouwer and Vore, 1985), consistent with reports by other investigators using isolated perfused liver systems (Mihaly *et al.*, 1982; Riedel *et al.*, 1983; Jones *et al.*, 1984) and slightly lower than values [1.6–1.8 μmol min^{-1} (g liver)$^{-1}$] reported by Thurman and Scholz (1969). Oxygen consumption values *in vivo* in rats range from 1.4 to 2 μmol min^{-1} (g liver)$^{-1}$ (Mitzkat and Meyer, 1973; Yoshihara *et al.*, 1988).

2.2.2b.   Hemoglobin-Free Perfusion Media

Krebs–Henseleit bicarbonate buffer (pH 7.4, 37°C) can be saturated directly with a 95% O_2/5% CO_2 mixture with glass gas aspirators designed for nonrecirculating perfusion systems (Scholz and Bücher, 1965). The omission of hemoglobin allows direct oxygenation, eliminating the need for a lung apparatus. Furthermore, effluent perfusate will not contain interfering substances such as erythrocytes which limit spectrophotometric or fluorometric analysis of metabolic function (gluconeogenesis, glycolysis, urea production) or drug metabolites (Thurman and Scholz, 1969; Sies, 1978). The absence of erythrocytes also simplifies the complex task of monitoring oxygen consumption by the liver. Normal livers remain viable for at least 2 hr and consume oxygen at the rate of 1.2–2.0 μmol min^{-1} (g liver)$^{-1}$ at flow rates of 4 ml min^{-1} (g liver)$^{-1}$.

Fluorocarbons also have been used to increase oxygen-carrying capacity and maintain metabolic function of perfused livers (Goodman *et al.*, 1973). Fluorocarbons may alter hepatobiliary function and hepatic disposition of substrates and are not recommended for routine use in liver perfusions.

2.2.3.   ADDITIVES

Maintenance of oncotic pressure is important for hepatic function. As the oncotic pressure of the perfusate decreases, cytosolic enzymes are released into the perfusate, suggesting decreased viability of the organ (Rosini *et al.*, 1976). Impaired fatty acid synthesis has been noted with the use of albumin-free perfusion media (Brunengraber *et al.*, 1981). However, the necessity of maintaining oncotic pressure during short-term perfusions by the addition of agents such as bovine serum albumin is debatable. The addition of albumin to hemoglobin-free perfusion media is not an absolute requirement (Sies, 1978) whereas up to 4% bovine serum albumin is recommended in red blood cell-containing perfusates (Meijer *et al.*, 1981). Albumin concentration in rat blood is ~3.16 g/dl (Guarino *et al.*, 1973). We do not add additional albumin to perfusate containing 20% rat blood, as this perfusate contains ~0.75 albumin/dl in addition to smaller percentages of other oncotic agents.

Although endogenous hepatic glycogen or fatty acids may be a sufficient energy source, glucose (0.3–1% w/v) also may be added to the perfusate. Plasma expanders such as 3% dextran (Pang and Gillette, 1978) or polyvinylpyrrolidone, gelatin hydrolysates, or sucrose may be suitable in specific experimental designs but are not necessary on a routine basis.

In the rat, ~40% of canalicular bile secretion is attributed to bile acid-dependent flow (Klaassen, 1971). Bile flow deteriorates with time if physiologic concentrations of bile acids are not maintained in the perfusate. Furthermore, bile acids may influence hepatic extraction of certain ligands, including asialoglycoproteins (Russel *et al.*, 1983). Based on the total bile acid concentration (50–170 μM) in portal blood of rats (Carey, 1982) and portal vein flow of 1.0–1.6 ml min^{-1} (g liver)$^{-1}$ (Roth and Rubin, 1976a; Fiserova-Bergerova and Hughes, 1983), at least 30 μmol sodium taurocholate/hr may be needed to maintain bile flow. Meijer *et al.* (1981) recommend the use of 15 μmol sodium taurocholate/hr (dissolved in saline and infused at 0.9 ml/ hr). Relatively constant bile flow has been maintained during 2-hr perfusions with 30 μmol taurocholate/hr infused at 2 ml/hr in hemoglobin-containing recirculating perfusate (Studenberg and Brouwer, 1992); 50 μM taurocholate is sufficient to maintain bile flow in the Munich type perfusion system (Kari *et al.*, 1985).

Other additives, including amino acids, hormones (e.g., insulin, cortisol), glucagon, and ^{14}C- or ^{3}H-labeled substrates, may be included in the perfusion medium (John and Miller, 1969b) or infused directly into the portal vein. In hemoglobin-containing perfusates where the perfusate volume is small (~80 ml for the closed system), the volume of additives should be minimized to avoid dilution of erythrocytes. Furthermore, consideration should be given to the influence of additives on perfusate pH. These issues are not a concern in the hemoglobin-free perfusion system because the total volume of perfusate is large (~5 liters for a 2-hr perfusion in the open system).

2.3. Surgical Procedures

An abbreviated description of the operative procedure is given in the following sections. A more detailed description of the operative procedure, including excellent figures, is provided by Miller (1973b).

2.3.1. SURGICAL INSTRUMENTS AND SUPPLIES

Surgical instruments: One toothed 15-cm tissue forceps; two medium, fine-tipped forceps; one straight/blunt, heavy duty, 13-cm scissors; one straight/straight, fine-tipped, 11-mm scissors; one sharp/sharp, curved iris, 5.7 cm scissors; two curved hemostats.

Supplies: Sterile gauze sponges (5 cm × 5 cm), Q-tips, polyethylene (PE-10) bile duct cannula (~18 cm long and slightly beveled at one end), silk 3-0 suture (at least four, ~18-cm ties), portal vein cannula connected to intravenous infusion tubing. A portal vein cannula may be fashioned by cutting the hub from a 16G needle, filing smooth at the cut end, and filing smooth around the beveled edge of the other end; two grooves may be filed ~2 and 5 mm from the beveled tip so that the ligatures can be tied securely to the cannula. If the perfusate contains blood, a 30-ml syringe with an 18G needle prefilled with ~100 units heparin/ml of rat blood is needed.

2.3.2. BLOOD DONORS

Once sufficient anesthesia is achieved with the agent of choice, the abdominal cavity is opened as described by LeCluyse *et al.* in the Appendix of Chapter 9. After the intestines are displaced laterally with a gauze pad, the inferior vena cava is exposed with Q-tips. An 18G needle attached to a 30-ml syringe containing ~100 units heparin/ml of rat blood is inserted into the vessel (beveled side up), and blood is withdrawn slowly. A 400-g rat yields ~16 ml of blood. Alternatively, cardiac puncture with a heparinized needle and syringe can be performed to obtain blood.

2.3.3. BILE DUCT CANNULATION

Rats (~200–250 g) utilized as liver donors are anesthetized prior to cannulation of the bile duct and portal vein. The choice of anesthetic depends on the nature of the experiment. Urethane (1 g/kg i.p.) often is selected because it does not alter bile flow (Watkins *et al.*, 1984). Although the use of diethyl ether, methoxyflurane, and sodium pentobarbital anesthesia in isolated liver perfusion studies does not appear to influence the overall rate and extent of lidocaine clearance (Ngo *et al.*, 1995), these agents should be used with caution in drug metabolism studies. The effects of diethyl ether on hepatic concentrations of UDP-glucuronic acid and drug metabolism are well documented (Watkins *et al.*, 1984). Although barbiturates decrease oxygen uptake, these anesthetic agents are washed out during surgery (within 1–2 min) and are used routinely with the open perfusion method (Scholz *et al.*, 1966). In addition to the choice of an anesthetic agent, the age, gender, and fasted versus fed state of the blood and liver donors should be considered in the experimental design.

The rat is prepared for surgery as described above for blood donors. The upper duodenum (bright pink segment of intestine immediately after the stomach) is lifted up and away from the liver to expose the portal vein and adjacent bile duct. One ligature should be placed around the bile duct, approximately midway between the liver and duodenum, and tied securely, causing distension of the duct. The second tie is placed loosely ~5 mm proximal to the first tie. Gentle traction is applied to the two ligatures to straighten the bile duct after it has been freed from tissue, fat, and omentum adhering between the two ties. A small cut (~¼ the diameter of the bile duct) is made in the ventral surface of the duct with iris scissors, and a beveled PE-10 cannula (held by forceps with the bevel facing up) is inserted into the bile duct and advanced ~15 mm, ideally to the juncture at which the bile canaliculi from each lobe pool into the common bile duct. Although the bile duct is remarkably resilient, care should be taken to avoid puncturing it with the beveled tip of the cannula. Once the bile cannula is positioned properly, it is tied into the bile duct with the proximal ligature. Bile should flow freely from the cannula once this ligature has been tightened. Occasionally, a small blood clot, tissue, or debris may occlude the cannula and prevent flow; gentle suction on the exteriorized end of the cannula with a 30G needle attached to a 1-ml syringe usually is sufficient to clear the cannula. Finally, the distal ligature is tied around the bile duct cannula to minimize accidental dislodging of the cannula during liver isolation and manipulation onto the perfusion platform. In the presence of adequate bile acids, bile should flow at a rate of ~1 μl min^{-1} (g liver)$^{-1}$ in the rat (Boyer and Klatskin, 1970).

2.3.4. LIVER ISOLATION

After cannulation of the bile duct, two ligatures are placed loosely around the portal vein, one in the natural opening above the superior pancreaticoduodenal vein (~5 mm below the bifurcation to the different lobes) and the second ligature ~5 mm below the superior pancreaticoduodenal vein. Care should be taken to avoid occluding portal vein blood flow by pulling on the ligatures or nicking the portal vein during placement of the ties. Unlike the bile duct, the ventral surface of the portal vein is relatively free of adherent tissue and fat, and does not need to be cleaned prior to cannulation. Once 37°C Krebs–Henseleit buffer, oxygenated with 95% O_2/5% CO_2, is flowing at the desired initial flow rate [~2 ml min^{-1} (g liver)$^{-1}$] through the double-jacketed infusion tubing (used to minimize O_2 loss) connected to the portal vein cannula, and all air bubbles have been cleared from the infusion line and cannula, gentle traction is applied to the two ligatures to straighten the portal vein. A small cut (~¼ the diameter of the vein) is made immediately in the ventral surface of the vein with the iris scissors, and the cannula (bevel facing up) is inserted into the portal vein and advanced ~3–5 mm. The cannula should not be advanced beyond the juncture of the portal vein to the individual lobes. While maintaining gentle traction on the distal tie to keep the cannula from slipping out of the vein, the proximal ligature is secured over the vein at the upper groove on the cannula. The inferior vena cava is immediately cut below the right kidney to avoid an increase in pressure in the liver, and the distal ligature is secured over the vein at the lower groove on the cannula. At this point, the suprahepatic inferior vena cava is cannulated as described by LeCluyse *et al.* in the Appendix of Chapter 9 so that effluent concentrations of perfusate can be sampled directly to quantitate oxygen and/or substrate concentrations. In experimental designs where perfusate effluent does not need to be measured directly, this vein may be transected rapidly after securing the distal ligature to allow outflow of perfusate. Cannulation of the portal vein may be facilitated by holding the cannula at a 45° angle relative to the vein until the beveled tip is inserted into the vessel; the cannula should be straightened parallel to the vessel before advancing. When the cannula is positioned properly in the portal vein, the liver will blanch to the light tan color of oxidized cytochromes *b* and *c*.

The liver is removed from the carcass as quickly as possible, care being taken to avoid twisting the portal vein cannula and/or occluding the outflow. First, adhesions and ligaments of the stomach and duodenum are cut as they are pulled carefully up and away from the small lobes of the liver. Particular care must be taken around the area of the bile duct cannula. In an effort to minimize bacterial contamination, transecting or perforating the esophagus, stomach, or intestines should be avoided. Instead, the left hemidiaphragm may be cut from the lateral costal edge to the esophagus. The rib cage is elevated slightly while allowing the liver to fall forward freely, and the tissue that attaches the liver to the diaphragm is transected. The diaphragm may be used to stabilize the suprahepatic vena cava cannula. If the vena cava has not been cannulated, a clean cut across the vena cava should be made at the surface of the liver immediately before it passes through the diaphragm. Loose tissue (especially residual diaphragm) that could occlude perfusate outflow from the liver should be removed. The palm of the left hand is cupped and the fingers are inserted downward into the cavity behind the liver. The lobes of the liver are positioned in the cupped palm just as they were in the body; care should be taken to avoid occluding perfusate inflow or outflow. Remaining adhesions are cut between the carcass and the fingers of the left hand. The infusion tubing, with buffer flowing through it, is disconnected carefully, and the liver is placed gently on the perfusion platform. The lobes of the liver should be arranged as they were positioned in the body at the time of cannulation, and the portal and biliary cannulas should be clearly visible and not twisted. The superior vena cava cannula, if present, should be positioned down through a central hole in the liver platform; otherwise, the severed vena cava will drip effluent perfusate directly through this hole into the reservoir. The circulating perfusate is connected via the portal vein cannula, and the resulting pressure monitored. If the perfusate contains blood, the color of the liver will change rapidly from light tan to reddish brown. In the Munich type system, the liver is perfused continuously throughout the experiment with Krebs–Henseleit buffer at a flow rate of ~4 ml min^{-1} (g liver)$^{-1}$ [after initial perfusion at ~2 ml min^{-1} (g liver)$^{-1}$], and there is no need to disconnect and reconnect flow through the portal vein cannula. The suprahepatic vena cava cannula is held above the liver with a small micromanipulator or clamp. With either method, the inflow portal pressure should not exceed 13–14 cm water. If the pressure is excessive, the outflow may be occluded and it may be necessary to reposition or discard the liver. Once the liver is positioned and perfusion has begun, the flat surface temperature probe is placed between two lobes of the liver, the bile cannula is positioned in a collection tube, and the liver and reservoir are covered to minimize evaporation of perfusate. To maintain a viable preparation, liver isolation should not exceed 10 min, and, with practice, the procedure takes approximately 5–6 min. After perfusion, the liver is removed from the apparatus, nonhepatic tissue is excised, and the liver is blotted and weighed.

2.4. Viability Assessments

Perfusion of the liver as described above should yield a viable organ for hepatic uptake, metabolism, and excretion studies for ~2–3 hr. Although prolonged perfusions for 8–12 hr have been conducted (John and Miller, 1969a; Bartosek et al., 1973), glucose and lipid synthesis are constant for only ~2 hr. The liver is a complex organ system with a variety of regulatory, metabolic, storage, and secretory functions that deteriorate at varying rates; no single test will predict total hepatic function reliably. Thus, numerous measures of viability are employed to assess the functional capacity of the perfused liver.

2.4.1. GENERAL ORGAN FUNCTION

The gross appearance of the liver is an important measure of viability. If the procedure has been conducted properly, the liver should be uniform in color, with no white spots (due to air emboli) or dark splotches (due to nonhomogeneous perfusion, trapped blood, or gross damage) on the surface of the liver. The liver should not appear swollen; perfusate should flow uniformly out of the suprahepatic vena cava cannula or drip freely from the platform.

Inflow perfusion pressure should approximate normal portal pressure (11–14 cm water; 8–10 mm Hg) when perfusing with hemoglobin-containing media (Brauer et al., 1956; Meijer et al., 1981). In the hemoglobin-free system, inflow perfusion pressure is ~10 cm water, although each system will vary slightly. If liver perfusion is conducted at insufficient pressures, nonhomogeneous distribution of perfusate will occur. Conversely, if perfusion pressures are too high, the size of sinusoidal fenestrations may increase, and large particles (e.g., chylomicrons) that normally would be excluded may gain access to the space of Disse (Fraser et al., 1980). Inflow perfusion pressure should remain relatively constant, increasing not more than 1 cm of water per hour, unless vasoactive agents are being investigated. An increase in portal perfusate pressure under conditions in which the flow rate is held constant suggests increased hepatic resistance and is an indicator of decreased viability.

Baseline bile flow after cannulation of the bile duct should be ~1 ml min^{-1} (g liver)$^{-1}$ (Boyer and Klatskin, 1970) and will decrease gradually by ~15% if taurocholate is infused. In the absence of bile acid addition, bile flow may decrease by 30–40% over a 2-hr perfusion period (Meijer *et al.*, 1981).

In a viable liver with recirculating perfusion, perfusate pH will decrease gradually (~0.1 pH unit/30 min) from 7.4 as perfusion continues. The perfusate pH should be maintained at ~7.4 by periodic addition of saturated sodium bicarbonate, as needed, to the perfusate reservoir. Accumulation of nonvolatile acids when perfusate is recirculated (Meijer *et al.*, 1981) is not a problem with single-pass perfusion.

Oxygen consumption is a critical determinant of organ viability, particularly for the isolated perfused liver. Biotransformation of many substrates in the liver requires molecular oxygen. Inflow and outflow pO_2 values often are measured as an index of oxygen availability in isolated perfused liver systems. In the hemoglobin-free perfusion system, rates of oxygen uptake by the liver can be monitored directly with a Clark type oxygen electrode in the outflow. For each experiment, calibration of the electrode must be performed with gas mixtures (0%, 21%, and 95% O_2). Oxygen consumption by the perfused liver (rate expressed as μmoles per minute per gram of liver) is calculated as the product of the perfusate flow and the difference between the inflow and outflow oxygen concentration and is expressed per gram of wet liver weight.

If the perfusate contains hemoglobin, total oxygen content is the sum of the oxygen dissolved in perfusate and oxygen bound to hemoglobin (Weibel, 1984). The amount of dissolved oxygen is linearly related to pO_2 (0.003 ml/100 ml of blood per mm Hg pO_2). The oxygen bound to hemoglobin is dependent on the hemoglobin concentration (15.6 g hemoglobin/100 ml of rat blood) and the oxygen saturation (% Sat.) of hemoglobin, which is a nonlinear function of pO_2 (1.34 ml of O_2/g of 100% saturated hemoglobin). Thus, oxygen content of the perfusion medium may be calculated (Ganong, 1983) as

$$
\begin{aligned}
\text{ml of } O_2/\text{ml of perfusate} = &\ [(0.003 \text{ ml of } O_2/100 \text{ ml of blood per mm Hg } pO_2) \\
&\times \text{mm Hg } pO_2] + [0.209 \text{ ml of } O_2/100 \text{ ml of rat blood} \\
&\times (\text{ml of rat blood/total ml of perfusate}) \times (\% \text{ Sat./100})]
\end{aligned}
$$

where 1 ml of O_2 is equivalent to 39.3 μmol of O_2 at 37°C.

In a perfusion medium that does not contain hemoglobin, pO_2 is a valid measure of oxygen delivery. In contrast, inflow and outflow pO_2 values in themselves will not be valid indicators of oxygen delivery or consumption when perfusate contains hemoglobin because the oxygen content of a blood-containing perfusion medium depends both on pO_2 and the hemoglobin content (Brouwer and Vore, 1985). The inflow and outflow pO_2 of the perfusate and the % Sat. of hemoglobin in the perfusate may be measured periodically with a blood gas analyzer. Samples for blood gas analysis must not be exposed to atmospheric oxygen and should be kept on ice prior to analysis.

Oxygen consumption *in vivo* in rats ranges from 1.4 to 2.5 μmol min^{-1} (g liver)$^{-1}$ (Mitzkat and Meyer, 1973; Yoshihara *et al.*, 1988). Maximal oxygen consumption in isolated perfused liver systems ranges from 1.4 to 2.5 μmol min^{-1} (g liver)$^{-1}$

(Thurman and Scholz, 1973; Mihaly *et al.*, 1982; Riedel *et al.*, 1983; Jones *et al.*, 1984; Brouwer and Vore, 1985), depending on substrate additions. In a viable liver, oxygen consumption should remain relatively constant. The importance of maintaining adequate oxygen delivery during drug metabolism studies to ensure constant oxygen consumption in the isolated liver cannot be overemphasized. Hexobarbital metabolism was inhibited progressively as oxygen consumption was decreased below 3.7 μmol min^{-1} (g liver)$^{-1}$ (Roth and Rubin, 1976b). Antipyrine clearance was linearly related to oxygen consumption in isolated perfused rat livers; when oxygen consumption was reduced to the point that the flow rate or hemoglobin content of the perfusion medium was the rate-limiting step in oxygen delivery, the hepatic clearance of this low-extraction-ratio compound actually became flow-dependent (Brouwer and Vore, 1985).

Potassium concentrations can be measured either in the inflow perfusate or in the reservoir by use of an ion-selective microelectrode. A rapid increase in perfusate potassium concentration suggests decreased viability of liver cells with release of this predominantly intracellular ion into the perfusion medium.

The concentrations of hepatic enzymes (lactate dehydrogenase, transaminases, alkaline phosphatase) leaking into perfusate frequently are monitored as measures of liver viability (Bergmeyer, 1988; Bradford *et al.*, 1986). Hyperoxia may result in the release of lysosomal enzymes (e.g., acid phosphatase).

Uptake of trypan blue may be used to assess viability by dye exclusion in specific regions of the liver lobule (Belinsky *et al.*, 1984a; Bradford *et al.*, 1986). This technique involves infusion of trypan blue into livers at the end of the experiment. After removal of excess dye, livers are perfused with paraformaldehyde and embedded in paraffin or plastic, and sections are stained with the cytoplasmic stain eosin. Trypan blue can be identified readily in the nuclei of damaged cells.

Alternatively, the integrity of liver cells and organelles can be assessed retrospectively by electron microscopy, although these procedures require specialized expertise and are not performed routinely. Swollen and distended sinusoids, absence of microvilli on the hepatocyte surface, cytoplasmic vacuolization, and mitochondrial swelling are indicative of hypoxic injury (Schmucker and Curtis, 1974; Schmucker *et al.*, 1975; Lemasters *et al.*, 1981).

2.4.2. SPECIFIC HEPATIC FUNCTIONS

Other measures of hepatic viability, although not performed routinely, include assessment of the pyridine nucleotide oxidation–reduction status of the cytosol or mitochondria by measuring the ratios of lactate to pyruvate or β-hydroxybutyrate to acetoacetate, respectively (Krebs, 1966; Lloyd *et al.*, 1973). Oxygenation also can be assessed by measuring tissue levels of ADP/ATP, but this is labor-intensive compared to measurement of O_2 consumption via electrodes (Anundi *et al.*, 1987). Specific tests of metabolic performance, such as gluconeogenesis or ketogenesis from lactate and fatty acids, respectively (Sherrill and Dietschy, 1972; Scholz *et al.*, 1973; Thurman and Scholz, 1973), or ureagenesis from ammonia (Häussinger, 1983; Takei *et al.*, 1990) also have been measured. In addition, the hepatic clearance, transcellular transport, metabolism (e.g., conjugation), and biliary excretion of compounds such as bile acids or other substrates may provide useful measures of liver viability.

2.5. Experimental Protocols and Data Collection and Analysis

The isolated perfused liver preparation may be selected for a variety of experimental purposes. Liver perfusion can be used to examine hepatic metabolic function or hepatic response to endogenous or exogenous compounds. Alternatively, substrate disposition may be evaluated quantitatively. Examination of the pharmacokinetic disposition of substrates in the isolated organ system represents a powerful tool for elucidation of many phenomena, including drug–drug interactions and the influence of physiologic alterations (e.g., aging or disease) on xenobiotic disposition.

Samples of perfusate (typically from the reservoir in recirculating systems and from perfusate inflow and outflow in the open system) are collected periodically throughout the experiment for quantitation of substrate and/or derived metabolites. Bile usually is collected continuously throughout the experiment, over fixed time intervals, and the volume is determined gravimetrically (assuming a specific gravity of 1.0). The mass of substrate and/or derived metabolite(s) is quantitated in each bile sample, and the data are plotted as cumulative mass excreted in bile versus time or as biliary excretion rate versus time at the midpoint of each collection interval.

2.5.1. SINGLE-PASS PERFUSION

In nonrecirculating (single-pass, open) perfusion systems, hemoglobin-free oxygenated perfusate is pumped through the liver only once at a constant flow rate (Q). In order to maintain adequate oxygen delivery, flow rates are 2–3 times higher than under physiologic conditions. With this experimental design, the steady-state hepatic extraction ratio of substrate can be assessed directly, and the rates of metabolite formation can be calculated as the sum of the rates of metabolite efflux in perfusate and bile (Yu *et al.*, 1982). The inflow (in) and outflow (out) perfusate are sampled continuously via flow-through detection; alternatively, samples are collected at periodic intervals and analyzed to determine the perfusate concentrations (C) of substrate. Although many investigators calculate rates of substrate or product taken up or released, data also may be expressed as extraction and clearance. The hepatic extraction (E_H) and hepatic clearance (Cl_H) of substrate are calculated as:

$$E_H = (C_{in} - C_{out})/C_{in}$$
$$Cl_H = Q \times E_H$$

Nonrecirculating perfusion requires large volumes of perfusate and therefore may not be practical for blood-containing perfusate or when the supply of substrate or other perfusate additives is limited. A distinct advantage of nonrecirculating systems is that the influent perfusion medium is kept constant; metabolites produced by the liver are removed from the system and do not recirculate. Thus, steady-state conditions can be achieved readily, and substrate and derived metabolite disposition, as well as the response of the organ, can be examined at different dose levels in a single preparation; experiments can be designed so that each liver serves as its own control (Ballet and Thurman, 1991). Composition of the perfusion medium is manipulated easily, and different metabolic conditions may be studied in the same liver. If the hepatic extraction of a compound is low [e.g., antipyrine (Pang and Rowland, 1977b); high concentrations of alcohols (20–30 mM; Bradford *et al.*, 1993)], nonrecirculating systems may not be suitable for examining hepatic clearance because the difference between inflow and outflow concentrations may be within assay variability.

2.5.2. RECIRCULATING PERFUSION

In recirculating systems, a relatively small volume (80–100 ml) of blood-containing perfusate is reoxygenated and recirculated through the liver at a constant flow rate (Q) that approximates liver blood flow *in vivo*. With this experimental design, the Cl_H of substrate is estimated from the dose introduced into the reservoir and the total area under the substrate concentration versus time curve (AUC) in the reservoir. The AUC may be calculated by the trapezoidal method and extrapolated to infinite time with the terminal elimination rate constant (Gibaldi and Perrier, 1982). Accurate estimation of the AUC requires characterization of the concentration–time profile over a minimum of 2–3 half-lives of the substrate in question. E_H is calculated indirectly from Cl_H:

$$Cl_H = Dose/AUC$$
$$E_H = Cl_H/Q$$

If the dose is introduced into the reservoir and sampling occurs from the reservoir, the clearance calculated is hepatic clearance. Alternatively, if sampling occurs immediately after the organ (e.g., from the vena cava cannula), or if the dose is introduced directly into the portal vein (regardless of the sampling site), intrinsic hepatic clearance (a measure of maximal hepatocellular activity in removing substrate from the perfusion medium) is calculated, assuming the well-stirred model of hepatic drug disposition (Pang and Rowland, 1977a,b).

The majority of hepatic biotransformation products formed *in vivo* traverse the sinusoidal membrane and ultimately are excreted by the kidneys. In the recirculating isolated perfused liver, biliary excretion is the only route of metabolite elimination. Therefore, metabolite usually accumulates in perfusate; accumulation may be more extensive if the sinusoidal membrane represents a diffusional barrier for translocation of metabolite from perfusate back into the hepatocyte (e.g., Studenberg and Brouwer, 1992). Such accumulation may be advantageous in mass-balance determinations of metabolite formation. In addition, accumulation of derived metabolite in the perfusate may allow kinetic evaluation of subsequent hepatic uptake of the metabolite. However, the potential for drug–metabolite interactions, either in binding, transport, or metabolism, may be magnified in the recirculating perfusion system as compared to the single-pass system or *in vivo*. In addition, lactate also accumulates during perfusion in recirculating systems and may result in significantly lower rates of glucose biosynthesis relative to single-pass systems (Williamson *et al.*, 1969; Thurman and Scholz, 1973).

2.5.3. RETROGRADE PERFUSION

Normal flow through the perfused liver is from the periportal to the pericentral region (anterograde direction); reversed or retrograde perfusion is a useful tool in examining the heterogeneous distribution of enzyme systems in the liver (Pang and Terrell, 1981; Kashiwagi *et al.*, 1982). Localization of metabolic events such as drug metabolism and oxygen uptake in specific zones of the liver lobule can be analyzed with micro light guides and miniature oxygen electrodes placed directly on periportal and pericentral regions of the liver (Ballet and Thurman, 1991). For example, oxygen uptake is 2–3 times greater in periportal than pericentral regions; when the direction of flow is reversed, the rate of oxygen uptake reverses even though mitochondria in periportal areas have larger cristae (Matsumura *et al.*, 1986).

2.6. Comparison of Techniques

As discussed, a variety of perfusion fluids have been used by researchers, including heparinized or defibrinated whole blood diluted with a buffer solution and supplemented with glucose, amino acids, albumin, vitamins, and/or antibiotics or semisynthetic media with washed erythrocytes of human or bovine origin. These fluids allow adequate tissue oxygenation at relatively low flow rates and may be adapted to either circulating or nonrecirculating systems. All fluids containing red blood cells are prone to progressive hemolysis (Schmucker *et al.*, 1975), deterioration of mixed-function oxidation, interference by hemoglobin with absorption measurements in the perfusate or intact organ, interference with fluorescence from the liver surface (Scholz *et al.*, 1969), and utilization of substrates and production of metabolites by red cells (Goodman *et al.*, 1973). The glycolytic capacity of red blood cells may influence perfusion conditions. Such shortcomings have caused many laboratories to select hemoglobin-free perfusion fluids consisting of osmotically balanced and buffered electrolyte solutions. To compensate for the decreased oxygen-carrying capacity of these fluids relative to that of blood, flow rates are elevated about 2- to 3-fold over physiologic values to provide adequate oxygenation of the tissue. Similar rates of oxygen uptake have been noted in rat livers perfused with blood (Brauser *et al.*, 1972) and hemoglobin-free bicarbonate buffer (Thurman and Scholz, 1969). Practical considerations and specific applications often dictate whether or not the perfusion media should contain red blood cells. The presence of normal constituents of blood, including serum proteins and lipids, as well as the enhanced oxygen-carrying capacity of hemoglobin, permitting the use of physiologic flow rates, may be important in some experimental designs. Obvious disadvantages of hemoglobin-containing media include requirements for a source of blood or red blood cells, increased technical complexity, the inability to control the complex composition of the medium, and the presence of vasoconstrictive or other endogenous substances originating from the blood donor. Perfusion with hemoglobin-free medium may allow greater flexibility in both experimental design and sample collection.

3. APPLICATIONS OF THE ISOLATED PERFUSED LIVER

3.1. General Applications

The principal advantage of the isolated perfused liver system is the ability to allow examination of metabolic activity, physiologic status, and/or pharmacologic response of the liver in the absence of extrahepatic influences. As outlined in Table I, this preparation has been used extensively to study the biochemical regulation of hepatic metabolism, hepatic synthetic function, and mechanisms of bile formation and secretion. The utility of this system in examining the influence of physiologic (e.g., hepatic flow, oxygen delivery, disease states) and pharmacologic (e.g., metabolic inhibitors) variables on hepatic extraction of substrates (e.g., drugs, proteins, peptides) and derived metabolites has been documented. Liver perfusion has been a useful method for probing functional heterogeneity in different zones of the liver lobule, including the heterogeneous distribution of hepatic drug-metabolizing enzymes.

Specialized techniques such as quantitative histochemical (Kauffman and Matschinsky, 1986) and ultramicrobiochemical (Conway *et al.*, 1987) measurements have been used to examine the influence of model compounds on metabolic pathways and to study key enzymes (e.g., glucuronyltransferase, arylsulfatase) involved in drug metabolism and toxicity in sublobular zones of the perfused liver. Micro light guides placed on specific sublobular regions of the liver surface provide a noninvasive method for determining local rates of mixed-function oxidation in periportal and pericentral regions of the perfused liver (Ji *et al.*, 1981; Lemasters *et al.*, 1986), and oxygen tension and rates of oxygen uptake may be measured in distinct regions of the perfused liver lobule with miniature oxygen electrodes (Matsumura and Thurman, 1983). Localized metabolic rates can be quantitated based on changes in regional oxygen uptake (Thurman *et al.*, 1986; Ballet and Thurman, 1991).

The perfused liver preparation has also been used extensively to study hepatic

Table I

General Applications of the Isolated Perfused Liver

Application	Representative example	Reference
Hepatic metabolic function		
Hormonal effects	Insulin and glucagon effects	Thomsen and Larsen, 1983
Gluconeogenesis	Rates of gluconeogenesis	Hems et al., 1966
Lipogenesis	Aerobic glycolysis and lipogenesis	Thurman and Scholz, 1973
Ureagenesis	Glutamine and ammonia metabolism	Häussinger, 1983
Ketogenesis	Chylomicron uptake	Sherrill and Dietschy, 1972
Hepatic synthetic function		
Albumin	Plasma proteins	Miller et al., 1951
Lipoproteins	Lipoprotein synthesis	Marsh, 1974
Coagulation factors	Antithrombin III and α_1-antitrypsin	Koj et al., 1978
Glutathione and glutathione disulfide	Intracellular content and biliary efflux	Akerboom et al., 1982
Disease state alterations	Plasma protein synthesis in diabetes	Miller et al., 1990
Biliary excretion		
Bile formation/secretion	Hemodynamic effects	Tavoloni et al., 1978
	α-Adrenergic action and ATP effects	Krell et al., 1985
Choleresis	H_2 antagonists	Bassan et al., 1986
	Dibucaine and procaine	Anwer and Hegner, 1983
Cholestasis	Taurocholate and steroid glucuronides	Durham and Vore, 1986
	Amino acid mixture	Graham et al., 1984
Substrate distribution		
Extraction	Propranolol uptake and metabolism	Shand et al., 1973
Influence of blood flow	Propranolol	Branch et al., 1973; Keiding and Steiness, 1984
	Multiple indicator dilution technique	Pang et al., 1988b
Transport		
Transport interactions	Chloride transport	Scharschmidt et al., 1985
	Cadmium transport; competition by zinc	Kingsley and Frazier, 1979
Diffusional barrier	Acetaminophen glucuronide	Studenberg and Brouwer, 1992
Hepatic processing of formed vs. preformed metabolites	Enalapril and enalaprilat	deLannoy et al., 1993
Influence of binding	Tolbutamide	Schary and Rowland, 1983
	Prazosin and antipyrine	Øie & Fiori, 1985

Physiologic/disease state alterations		
Pregnancy/estrogen coadministration	Estrone and morphine disposition	Brock and Vore, 1982
	Biliary excretion	Auansakul and Vore, 1982
Cirrhosis	Hemodynamic response to vasoactive agents	Ballet et al., 1988
Fatty liver	Ibuprofen disposition	Cox et al., 1985
Hypoxic alterations	Hexobarbital metabolism	Roth and Rubin, 1976b
	Antipyrine metabolism	Brouwer and Vore, 1985
	Harmol conjugation and elimination	Angus et al., 1987
Substrate metabolism		
Phase I	Aminopyrine metabolism	Thurman and Scholz, 1969
Phase II	p-Nitrophenol	Reinke et al., 1981
Limited by cofactor supply	7-Ethoxycoumarin	Belinsky et al., 1983
Inhibition of metabolism	Effects of H_2-receptor antagonists on antipyrine	Mihaly et al., 1982
Nonstationary metabolism	Lidocaine	Tam et al., 1987
Substrate excretion		
Sinusoidal	Dibromosulfophthalein efflux	Meijer et al., 1984
	Harmol sulfate	DeVries et al., 1985
	Glutathione	Ookhtens et al., 1985, 1988
Canalicular	Biliary lipids	Gregory et al., 1978
	Acetaminophen glucuronide	Studenberg and Brouwer, 1992
Lobular heterogeneity		
Extraction	Acinar heterogeneity of taurocholate transport	Groothuis et al., 1982
Drug-metabolizing enzymes	Phenacetin and acetaminophen	Pang and Terrell, 1981
	7-Hydroxycoumarin sulfation and glucuronidation	Conway et al., 1982
	Sublobular compartmentalization	Thurman and Kauffman, 1985
	Gentisamide sulfation and glucuronidation	Morris et al., 1988
Hepatotoxicity		
Drug-induced	Ticrynafen	Zimmerman et al., 1982
	Valproic acid	Olson et al., 1986
Alcohol-induced	Hypoxia as mechanism	Thurman et al., 1984
Allyl alcohol	Biochemical mechanisms underlying zonal toxicity	Badr et al., 1986
Hypoxia	Cell surface changes and enzyme release	Lemasters et al., 1981
Reperfusion injury	Role of purines and xanthine oxidase	Zhong et al., 1989
Mutagenicity testing	Evaluation of carcinogens	Beije et al., 1979

dysfunction in specific regions of the liver lobule and to define biochemical mechanisms underlying the zonal toxicity of chemicals. Miniature oxygen electrodes have allowed assessment of the effects of hepatotoxins on intermediary metabolism in different regions of the liver lobule (Belinsky et al., 1984b). The utility of this technique to probe hepatobiliary function and dysfunction, to examine the hepatic processing of endogenous and exogenous substrates, and to evaluate factors that influence these processes is obvious.

3.2. Specialized Applications

3.2.1. *IN SITU* PERFUSED INTESTINE–LIVER PREPARATION

The sequential processing of xenobiotics and derived metabolites by the gastrointestinal tract and liver, two serially arranged organs primarily responsible for first-pass drug elimination after oral administration, may be evaluated directly with the combined *in situ* perfused rat intestine–liver preparation (Pang et al., 1985; Hirayama et al., 1989; Xu et al., 1989). The intestine is perfused in a single-pass manner with xenobiotic via the superior mesenteric artery; portal venous outflow from the intestine (containing xenobiotic and derived metabolites) as well as hepatic arterial flow (without xenobiotic) provides dual inflow into the liver. This technique allows manipulation of flow rate, perfusate content, substrate concentration, and potential sites of first-pass elimination in the intestine and has been used to quantitate hepatic and intestinal extraction ratios (Pang et al., 1985), determine the contribution of the intestine to first-pass metabolism of substrates (Hirayama et al., 1989; Xu et al., 1989), and investigate intestinal metabolism relative to hepatic metabolism of substrates (Zimmerman et al., 1991).

3.2.2. HEPATIC ARTERY/PORTAL VEIN PERFUSION

Until recently, most studies using the perfused rat liver were performed with only a single inflow, the cannulated portal vein. This differs from the *in vivo* situation, in which the hepatic artery supplies 20–30% of the total hepatic flow with well-oxygenated blood. Different methods of perfusing both the hepatic artery and portal vein have been reported (Conway et al., 1985; Pang et al., 1988a) and reviewed (Huet et al., 1991). This technique is suited particularly for examining the relative zonal enrichment of drug-metabolizing activity in the periportal region and also may be useful in examining the distribution patterns of enzymes in sequential or parallel metabolic pathways or in defining co-substrate requirements in zonal regions of the liver.

3.2.3. PHARMACOKINETIC MODELING

The perfused liver is employed frequently to investigate the hepatic disposition (extraction, binding, metabolism, and excretion) of substrates. The data obtained in such experiments may be incorporated into comprehensive pharmacokinetic models to predict substrate disposition *in vivo* or to extrapolate disposition from experimental animals to humans. For example, measurement of transhepatic extraction in the isolated perfused rat liver allows estimation of hepatic clearance *in vivo* as the product of extraction and hepatic blood flow, assuming that flow is known. Hepatic clearance then can be predicted across mammalian species either by allometric scaling (Boxenbaum, 1980) or through incorporation of extraction into physiologically based pharmacokinetic models (Dedrick, 1974).

Pharmacokinetic modeling of data generated from the perfused liver may also be used to explore mechanisms underlying substrate disposition. For example, data obtained in the isolated perfused rat liver have been used to identify the most appropriate model (parallel tube vs. well-stirred) for the hepatic disposition of a particular substrate (Pang and Rowland, 1977a). Accurate predictions of the influence of hepatic blood flow, protein binding, and intrinsic hepatic clearance on transhepatic extraction and total hepatic clearance rely on selection of an appropriate mathematical model (Pang and Rowland, 1977b). Pharmacokinetic modeling of data from the isolated perfused liver system also has been used to (1) determine rate-limiting steps and (2) identify sites of drug interactions within the hepatobiliary system that are not evident based on conventional mass-balance analysis (Studenberg and Brouwer, 1992; Booth *et al.*, 1996), as well as to (3) assess the influence of albumin on sinusoidal efflux (Proost *et al.*, 1993). The development of pharmacokinetic models based on *in vitro* data capable of describing translocation processes within the hepatobiliary system may improve the ability to predict alterations in the disposition of drugs and derived metabolites in response to *in vivo* perturbations (e.g., interacting drugs or disease states).

4. ADVANTAGES AND DISADVANTAGES OF THE ISOLATED PERFUSED LIVER AS COMPARED TO OTHER MODELS

Essentially, there are five commonly used whole-cell preparations for the study of hepatic metabolism: isolated hepatocytes, hepatocytes in culture, liver slices, perfused livers, and livers *in vivo*. As detailed in Table II, each of these methods has distinct advantages and disadvantages that should be considered in selecting the experimental design most likely to yield information suitable to test the specific hypothesis posed.

Many advantages of isolated hepatocytes, including convenience and the large

Table II
Advantages and Disadvantages of the Isolated Perfused Liver Compared to Other Models[a]

Feature	Isolated	Cultured	Liver slices	Perfused liver	In vivo
	Hepatocytes				
Lobular architecture maintained	−	−	+	+	+
Microcirculation intact	−	−	−	+	+
Neural–hormonal signals intact	−	−	−	−	+
Enzyme systems maintained	+	−	+	+	++
Bile formation	−	−/+[b]	−	+	+
Viability	Hours	Days	Hours	Hours	Days
Efficient for data collection	+++	+++	++	++	−
Flexibility in experimental design	++	++	+	+	−
Reproducibility	+	+	+	+	+
Convenience	+++	+++	++	++	+
Minimal use of experimental animals	+	++	+	−	−
Representative of physiologic state	−	−/+[b]	+	++	+++

[a]+ indicates relative advantages, − indicates relative disadvantages
[b]LeCluyse et al., 1994.

quantity of data generated from a single animal, have been identified since the development of an efficient technique for isolating hepatocytes (Berry and Friend, 1969). However, several disadvantages of the hepatocyte system have become apparent. Lobular architecture is lost with this model, disrupting regional distribution of enzyme systems, and cells in this form evidence diminished activity of many key enzymes. Furthermore, nonparenchymal cells, which play an important and only recently studied role in hepatic function, are absent.

Cultured hepatocytes share some of the advantages of isolated hepatocytes (e.g., convenience, ease of data collection, reproducibility of experiments), as well as some of the disadvantages, particularly regarding enzyme activity. Many enzyme systems revert to fetal states, and cytochrome P450 content declines, limiting the use of cultured cells in toxicity and drug metabolism studies. The loss of lobular architecture prohibits studies assessing zonality of events within the liver lobule. Hepatocytes cultured in a collagen-sandwich configuration (Dunn et al., 1989; LeCluyse et al. 1994) may serve as a more reliable and representative model of hepatic function than conventional hepatocyte culture methods.

In contrast to isolated or cultured cells, liver slices retain lobular architecture while allowing multiple preparations from a single animal. However, cells in this form leak potassium and do not produce bile. Liver slices were abandoned in the 1950s when the perfused liver became a popular technique, but use of this model system has experienced a recent renaissance in toxicity studies (Smith et al., 1985).

Perfused liver systems simulate in vivo conditions more than any of the above techniques. Although studies in intact animals are the most physiologically accurate, the multitude of variables introduced by changes in hormonal, circulatory, and neural systems often complicate data interpretation. Normal hepatic architecture, microcirculation, and bile production are maintained in perfused liver preparations, and studies of the role of different cell types in specific events, impossible with the isolated hepatocyte method, can be undertaken. Biochemical processes may be monitored continuously in the perfused liver, making it an ideal model for the study of intermediary metabolism, biotransformation of xenobiotics, and interactions between these processes. Furthermore, intracellular events may be monitored noninvasively with optical methods in the hemoglobin-free model. The isolated perfused liver preparation is quite sensitive to chemical agents and, in a number of instances, results in biological responses that are very similar to those observed in intact animals. Thus, this model can be a useful laboratory procedure for the study of chemically induced hepatic damage as well as for mechanistic studies that would be difficult or impossible to perform in intact animals. Because hepatic toxicity often involves infiltration of immune cells, hemoglobin-free liver perfusion allows one to distinguish between intrinsic hepatic and extrinsic mechanisms involving neutrophils or other invading cells.

Regardless of the advantages, the potential shortcomings of the perfused liver preparation also must be recognized. This preparation usually is devoid of hepatic innervation. Loss of the neural and hormonal signals present *in vivo*, the absence of nutrients supplied from the diet and from peripheral tissues, and perfusion only via the portal vein may affect hepatic hemodynamics and function. Investigations examining the biotransformation of substrates in the isolated perfused liver require confirmation of relevance, both qualitatively and quantitatively, to the same processes in the intact animal. Moreover, pathological processes requiring days to evolve to completion (e.g., liver regeneration and return to normal function after toxicant insult) cannot be assessed by the organ perfusion technique unless one follows *in vivo* pretreatment by organ perfusion. Finally, the efficiency of the perfused liver preparation in data generation must be considered. While the technique has distinct advantages for the control of experimental conditions, it is relatively slow and inefficient compared to the use of isolated or cultured cells.

Despite these limitations, studies comparing drug metabolism in the perfused liver and *in vivo* indicate that a good correlation exists between the two approaches. In summary, the decision to use the isolated perfused liver preparation depends on the nature of the hypothesis to be addressed. Undoubtedly, extensive use of this preparation will continue, and new applications for this model most assuredly will be developed in the future.

ACKNOWLEDGMENTS

This work was supported in part by grants GM41935 (K.L.R.B.) as well as AA03624, AA09156, DK37034, and ES04325 (RGT) from the National Institutes of Health. The authors thank Dr. Gary M. Pollack and Dr. Arno Nolting for helpful insights in the preparation of this manuscript.

REFERENCES

Akerboom, T. P. M., Bilzer, M., and Sies, H., 1982, The relationships of biliary glutathione disulfide efflux and intracellular glutathione disulfide content in perfused rat liver, *J. Biol. Chem.* **257:**4248–4252.

Angus, P. W., Mihaly, G. W., Morgan, D. J., and Smallwood, R. A., 1987, Hypoxia impairs conjugation and elimination of harmol in the isolated perfused rat liver, *J. Pharmacol. Exp. Ther.* **240:**931–936.

Anundi, I., King, J., Owen, D. A., Schneider, H., Lemasters, J. J., and Thurman, R. G., 1987, Fructose prevents hypoxic cell death in liver, *Am. J. Physiol.* **253:**G390–G396.

Anwer, M. S., and Hegner, D., 1983, Sodium and chloride dependence of dibucaine- and procaine-induced choleresis in isolated perfused rat liver, *J. Pharmacol. Exp. Ther.* **225:**284–290.

Asp, G., 1873, Zur Anatomie und Physiologie der Leber, *Arbeit. Physiol. Anst.* **8:**124–158.

Auansakul, A. C., and Vore, M., 1982, The effect of pregnancy and estradiol-17ß treatment on the biliary transport maximum of dibromosulfophthalein, and the glucuronide conjugates of 5-phenyl-5-*p*-hydroxyphenyl[^{14}C]hydantoin and [^{14}C]morphine in the isolated perfused rat liver, *Drug Metab. Dispos.* **10:**344–349.

Badr, M. Z., Belinsky, S. A., Kauffman, F. C., and Thurman, R. G., 1986, Mechanism of hepatotoxicity to periportal regions of the liver lobule due to allyl alcohol: Role of oxygen and lipid peroxidation, *J. Pharmacol. Exp. Ther.* **238:**1138–1142.

Ballet, F., and Thurman, R. G. (eds.), 1991, *Research in Perfused Liver: Clinical and Basic Applications*, John Libbey & Company Ltd./INSERM, London.

Ballet, F., Chretien, Y., Rey, C., and Poupon, R., 1988, Differential response of normal and cirrhotic liver to vasoactive agents. A study in the isolated perfused rat liver, *J. Pharmacol. Exp. Ther.* **244:**283–289.

Bartosek, I., Guaitani, A., and Garattini, S., 1973, Prolonged perfusion of isolated rat liver, in: *Isolated Liver Perfusion and Its Applications* (I. Bartosek, A. Guaitani, and L. L. Miller, eds.), Raven Press, New York, pp. 63–72.

Bassan, H., Zimmerman, H. J., Jacob, L., Gillespie, J., and Lukacs, L., 1986, Effects of three H$_2$ antagonists on the isolated perfused rat liver. Correlation of bile flow changes with potential for causing hepatic disease in patients, *Biochem. Pharmacol.* **35:**4519–4522.

Beije, B., Jenssen, D., Arrhenius, E., and Zetterqvist, M. A., 1979, Isolated liver perfusion—a tool in mutagenicity testing for the evaluation of carcinogens, *Chem. Biol. Interact.* **27:**41–57.

Belinsky, S. A., Kauffman, F. C., Ji, S., Lemasters, J. J., and Thurman, R. G., 1983, Stimulation of mixed-function oxidation of 7-ethoxycoumarin in periportal and pericentral regions of the perfused rat liver by xylitol, *Eur. J. Biochem.* **137:**1–6.

Belinsky, S. A., Popp, J. A., Kauffman, F. C., and Thurman, R. G., 1984a, Trypan blue uptake as a new method to investigate hepatotoxicity in periportal and pericentral regions of the liver lobule: Studies with allyl alcohol in the perfused liver, *J. Pharmacol. Exp. Ther.* **230:**755–760.

Belinsky, S. A., Matsumura, T., Kauffman, F. C., and Thurman, R. G., 1984b, Rates of allyl alcohol metabolism in periportal and pericentral regions of the liver lobule, *Mol. Pharmacol.* **25:**158–164.

Bergmeyer, H. V., 1988, *Methods of Enzymatic Analysis*, Academic Press, New York.

Bernard, C., 1855, Sur le mécanisme de la formation du sucre dans le foie, *C. R. Acad. Sci.* **41:**461–469.

Berry, M. N., and Friend, D. S., 1969, High-yield preparation of isolated rat liver parenchymal cells. A biochemical and fine structural study, *J. Cell Biol.* **43:**506–520.

Booth, C. L., Pollack, G. M., and Brouwer, K. L. R., 1996, Hepatobiliary disposition of valproic acid and valproate glucuronide: Use of a pharmacokinetic model to examine the rate-limiting steps and potential sites of drug interactions, *Hepatology* **23:**771–780.

Boxenbaum, H., 1980, Interspecies variation in liver weight, hepatic blood flow, and antipyrine intrinsic clearance: Extrapolation of data to benzodiazepines and phenytoin, *J. Pharmacokinet. Biopharm.* **8:**165–176.

Boyer, J. L., and Klatskin, G., 1970, Canalicular bile flow and bile secretory pressure: Evidence for a non-bile salt dependent fraction in the isolated perfused rat liver, *Gastroenterology* **59:**853–859.

Bradford, B. U., Marotto, M., Lemasters, J. J., and Thurman, R. G., 1986, New, simple models to evaluate zone-specific damage due to hypoxia in the perfused rat liver: Time course and effect of nutritional state, *J. Pharmacol. Exp. Ther.* **236:**263–268.

Bradford, B. U., Forman, D. T., and Thurman, R. G., 1993, 4-Methylpyrazole inhibits fatty acyl coenzyme synthetase and diminishes catalase-dependent alcohol metabolism: Has the contribution of alcohol dehydrogenase to alcohol metabolism been previously overestimated?, *Mol. Pharmacol.* **43:**115–119.

Branch, R. A., Nies, A. S., and Shand, D. G., 1973, The disposition of propranolol. VIII. General implications of the effects of liver blood flow on elimination from the perfused rat liver, *Drug Metab. Dispos.* **1:**687–690.

Brauer, R. W., Pessotti, R. L., and Pizzolato, P., 1951, Isolated rat liver preparation. Bile production and other basic properties, *Proc. Soc. Exp. Biol. Med.* **78:**174–181.

Brauer, R. W., Leong, G. F., McElroy, R. F., and Holloway, R. J., 1956, Circulatory pathways in the rat liver as revealed by P^{32}chromic phosphate colloid uptake in the isolated perfused liver preparation, *Am. J. Physiol.* **184:**593–598.

Brauser, B., Bücher, T., Sies, H., and Versmold, H., 1972, Control of mitochondrial activity by metabolites in the hemoglobin-free perfused liver, in: *Molecular Basis of Biological Activity* (K. Gaede, B. L. Itorecker, and W. J. Whelan, eds.), Academic Press, New York, pp. 197–200.

Brock, W. J., and Vore, M., 1982, Hepatic morphine and estrone glucuronyltransferase activity and morphine biliary excretion in the isolated perfused rat liver. Effect of pregnancy and estradiol-17β treatment, *Drug Metab. Dispos.* **10:**336–343.

Brouwer, K. L. R., and Vore, M., 1985, Effect of hypoxia and pregnancy on antipyrine metabolism in isolated perfused rat livers, *J. Pharmacol. Exp. Ther.* **234:**584–589.

Brunengraber, H., Boutry, M., Daikuhara, Y., Kopelovick, L., and Lowenstein, J. M., 1981, Use of the perfused liver for the study of lipogenesis, *Methods Enzymol.* **35:**597–607.

Carey, M. C., 1982, The enterohepatic circulation, in: *The Liver: Biology and Pathobiology* (I. Arias, H. Popper, D. Schacher *et al.*, eds.), Raven Press, New York, pp. 429–466.

Conway, J. G., Kauffman, F. C., Ji, S., and Thurman, R. G., 1982, Rates of sulfation and glucuronidation of 7-hydroxycoumarin in periportal and pericentral regions of the liver lobule, *Mol. Pharmacol.* **22:**509–516.

Conway, J. G., Popp, J. A., and Thurman, R. G., 1985, Microcirculation in periportal and pericentral regions of lobule in perfused rat liver, *Gastrointest. Liver Physiol.* **12:**G449–G456.

Conway, J. G., Kauffman, F. C., Tskuda, T., and Thurman, R. G., 1987, Glucuronidation of 7-hydroxy-coumarin in periportal and pericentral regions of the lobule in livers from untreated and 3-methylchol-anthrene-treated rats, *Mol. Pharmacol.* **33:**111–119.

Cox, J. W., Cox, S. R., VanGiessen, G., and Ruwart, M. J., 1985, Ibuprofen stereoisomer hepatic clearance and distribution in normal and fatty *in situ* perfused rat liver, *J. Pharmacol. Exp. Ther.* **232:**636–642.

Dedrick, R. L., 1974, Animal scale up, in: *Pharmacology and Pharmacokinetics* (T. Teorell, R. L. Dedrick, and P. G. Condliffe, eds.), Plenum Press, New York, pp. 117–145.

deLannoy, I. A. M., Barker, F., and Pang, K. S., 1993, Formed and preformed metabolite excretion clearances in liver, a metabolite formation organ: Studies on enalapril and enalaprilat in the single-pass and recirculating perfused rat liver, *J. Pharmacokinet. Biopharm.* **21:**395–422.

De Vries, M. H., Groothuis, G. M. M., Mulder, G. J., Nguyen, H., and Meijer, D. K. F., 1985, Secretion of the organic anion harmol sulfate from liver into blood. Evidence for a carrier-mediated mechanism, *Biochem. Pharmacol.* **34:**2129–2135.

Dunn, C. Y., Yarmush, M. L., Koebe, H. G., and Tompkins, R. G., 1989, Hepatocyte function and extracellular matrix geometry: Long-term culture in a sandwich configuration, *FASEB J.* **3:**174–177.

Durham, S., and Vore, M., 1986, Taurocholate and steroid glucuronides: Mutual protection against cholestasis in the isolated perfused rat liver, *J. Pharmacol. Exp. Ther.* **237:**490–495.

Fiserova-Bergerova, V., and Hughes, H. C., 1983, Species differences on bioavailability of inhaled vapors and gases, in: *Modeling of Inhalation Exposure to Vapors: Uptake, Distribution and Elimination* (V. Fiserova-Bergerova and H. C. Hughes, eds.), CRC Press, Boca Raton, Florida, pp. 97–106.

Fraser, R., Bowler, L. M., Day, W. A., Dobbs, B., Johnson, H. D., and Lee, D., 1980, High perfusion pressure damages the sieving ability of sinusoidal endothelium in rat livers, *Br. J. Exp. Pathol.* **61:**222–228.

Ganong, W. F., 1983, *Review of Medical Physiology*, 11th ed., Lange Medical Publications, Los Altos, California, pp. 533–535.

Gibaldi, M., and Perrier, D., 1982, *Pharmacokinetics*, 2nd ed., Marcel Dekker, New York.

Goodman, M. N., Parrilla, R., and Toews, C. J., 1973, Influence of fluorocarbon emulsions on hepatic metabolism in perfused rat liver, *Am. J. Physiol.* **225:**1384–1388.

Gores, G. J., Kost, L. J., and LaRusso, N. F., 1986, The isolated perfused rat liver: Conceptual and practical considerations, *Hepatology* **6:**511–517.

Graham, M. F., Tavill, A. S., Halpin, T. C., and Luis, N. L., 1984, Inhibition of bile flow in the isolated perfused rat liver by a synthetic parenteral amino acid mixture: Associated net amino acid fluxes, *Hepatology* **4:**69–73.

Gregory, D. H., Vlahcevic, Z. R., Prugh, M. F., and Swell, L., 1978, Mechanism of secretion of biliary lipids: Role of a microtubular system in hepatocellular transport of biliary lipids in the rat, *Gastroenterology* **74:**93–100.

Groothuis, G. M. M., Hardonk, M. J., Keulemans, K. P. T., Nieunenhuis, P., and Meijer, D. K. F., 1982, Autoradiographic and kinetic demonstration of acinar heterogeneity of taurocholate transport, *Am. J. Physiol.* **243:**G455–G462.

Guarino, A. M., Anderson, J. B., Starkweather, D. K., and Chignell, C. F., 1973, Pharmacologic studies of camptothecin (NSC-100880): Distribution, plasma protein binding, and biliary excretion, *Cancer Chemother. Rep.* **57:**125–140.

Haft, D. E., and Miller, L. L., 1958, Alloxan diabetes and demonstrated direct action of insulin on metabolism of isolated perfused rat liver. *Am. J. Physiol.* **192:**33–42.

Hamilton, R. L., Berry, M. N., Williams, M. C., and Severinghaus, E. M., 1974, A simple and inexpensive membrane "lung" for small organ perfusion, *J. Lipid Res.* **15:**182–186.

Häussinger, D., 1983, Hepatocyte heterogeneity in glutamine and ammonia metabolism and the role of an intercellular glutamine cycle during ureagenesis in perfused rat liver, *Eur. J. Biochem.* **133:**269–275.

Hems, R., Ross, B. D., Berry, M. N., and Krebs, H. A., 1966, Gluconeogenesis in the perfused rat liver, *Biochem. J.* **101:**284–292.

Hirayama, H., Xu, X., and Pang, K. S., 1989, Viability of the vascularly perfused, recirculating rat intestine and intestine–liver preparation, *Am. J. Physiol.* **257:**G249–G258.

Huet, P. M., Kassissia, I., and Semret, M., 1991, Haemodynamics in perfused rat liver, in: *Perfused Liver* (F. Ballet and R. G. Thurman, eds.), John Libbey & Company Ltd., London, pp. 33–42.

Jacobj, C., 1890, Apparat zur Durchblutung isolirter überlebender Organe, *Arch. Exp. Pathol. Pharmakol.* **26:**388–400.

Ji, S., Lemasters, J. J., and Thurman, R. G., 1981, A fluorometric method to measure sublobular rates of mixed-function oxidation in the hemoglobin-free perfused rat liver, *Mol. Pharmacol.* **19:**513–516.

John, D. W., and Miller, L. L., 1969a, Effect of aflatoxin B1 on net synthesis of albumin, fibrinogen, and α_1-acid-glycoprotein by the isolated perfused rat liver, *Biochem. Pharmacol.* **18:**1135–1146.

John, D. W., and Miller, L. L., 1969b, Regulation of net biosynthesis of serum albumin and acute phase plasma proteins. Induction of enhanced net synthesis of fibrinogen, α_1-acid glycoprotein, α_2-(acute phase) globulin, and haptoglobin by amino acids and hormones during perfusion of the isolated normal rat liver, *J. Biol. Chem.* **244:**6134–6142.

Jones, D. B., Mihaly, G. W., Smallwood, R. A., Webster, L. K., Morgan, D. J., and Madsen, N. P., 1984, Differential effects of hypoxia on the disposition of propranolol and sodium taurocholate by the isolated perfused rat liver, *Hepatology* **4:**461–466.

Kari, F. W., Kauffman, F. C., and Thurman, R. G., 1985, Effect of bile salts on rates of formation, accumulation, and export of mutagenic metabolites from benzo(a)pyrene produced by the perfused rat liver, *Cancer Res.* **45:**1621–1627.

Kashiwagi, T., Ji, S., Lemasters, J. J., and Thurman, R. G., 1982, Rates of alcohol dehydrogenase-dependent ethanol metabolism in periportal and pericentral regions of the perfused rat liver, *Mol. Pharmacol.* **21:**438–443.

Kauffman, F. C., and Matschinsky, F. M., 1986, Quantitative histochemical measurements within sublobular zones of the liver lobule, in: *Regulation of Hepatic Metabolism: Intra- and Intercellular Compartmentation* (R. G. Thurman, F. C. Kauffman, and K. Jungermann, eds.), Plenum Press, New York, pp. 119–136.

Keiding, S., and Steiness, E., 1984, Flow dependence of propranolol elimination in perfused rat liver, *J. Pharmacol. Exp. Ther.* **230:**474–477.

Kingsley, B. S., and Frazier, J. M., 1979, Cadmium transport in isolated perfused rat liver: Zinc–cadmium competition, *Am. J. Physiol.* **236:**C139–C143.

Klaassen, C. D., 1971, Does bile acid secretion determine canalicular bile production in rats?, *Am. J. Physiol.* **220:**667–673.

Koj, A., Regoeczi, E., Toews, C. J., Leveille, R., and Jauldi, J., 1978, Synthesis of antithrombin III and alpha-1 antitrypsin by the perfused rat liver, *Biochim. Biophys. Acta* **539:**496–504.

Krebs, H. A., 1966, The regulation of the release of ketone bodies by the liver, *Adv. Enzyme Regul.* **4:** 339–354.

Krebs, H. A., and Henseleit, K., 1932, Untersuchungen über die Harnstoffbildung im Tierkörper, *Hoppe-Seyler's Z. Physiol. Chem.* **210:**33–66.

Krell, H., Jaeschke, H., and Pfaff, E., 1985, Regulation of canalicular bile formation by adrenergic action and by external ATP in the isolated perfused rat liver, *Biochem. Biophys. Res. Commun.* **131:**139–145.

LeCluyse, E. L., Audus, K. L., and Hochman, J. H., 1994, Formation of extensive canalicular networks by rat hepatocytes cultured in collagen-sandwich configuration, *Am. J. Physiol.* **266:**C1764–C1774.

Lemasters, J. J., Ji, S., and Thurman, R. G., 1981, Centrilobular injury following low-flow hypoxia in isolated, perfused rat liver, *Science* **213:**661–663.

Lemasters, J. J., Ji, S., and Thurman, R. G., 1986, New micromethods for studying sublobular structure and function in the isolated, perfused rat liver, in: *Regulation of Hepatic Metabolism: Intra- and Intercellular Compartmentation* (R. G. Thurman, F. C. Kauffman, and K. Jungermann, eds.), Plenum Press, New York, pp. 159–184.

Lloyd, M. H., Iles, R. A., Simpson, B. R., Strunin, J. M., Layton, J. M., and Cohen, R. D., 1973, The effect of stimulated metabolic acidosis on intracellular pH and lactate metabolism in the isolated perfused rat liver, *Clin. Sci. Mol. Med.* **45:**543–549.

Lupton, A. M., 1947, The effect of perfusion through isolated liver on the prothrombin activity of blood from normal and dicumarol treated rats, *J. Pharmacol. Exp. Ther.* **89:**306–312.

Marsh, J. B., 1974, Lipoproteins in a nonrecirculating perfusate of rat liver, *J. Lipid Res.* **15:**544–550.

Matsumura, T., and Thurman, R. G., 1983, Measuring rates of oxygen uptake in periportal and pericentral regions of the liver lobule: Stop-flow experiments with perfused liver, *Am. J. Physiol.* **244:**G656–G659.

Matsumura, T., Kauffman, F. C., Meren, H., and Thurman, R. G., 1986, O_2 uptake in periportal and pericentral regions of liver lobule in perfused liver, *Am. J. Physiol.* **250:**G800–G805.

Meijer, D. K. F., Keulemans, K., and Mulder, G. J., 1981, Isolated perfused rat liver technique, *Methods Enzymol.* **77:**81–94.

Meijer, D. K. F., Blom, A., Weitering, J. G., and Hornsveld, R., 1984, Pharmacokinetics of the hepatic transport of organic anions: Influence of extra- and intracellular binding on hepatic storage of dibromosulfophthalein and interactions with indocyanine green, *J. Pharmacokinet. Biopharm.* **12:**43–65.

Mihaly, G. W., Smallwood, R. A., Anderson, J. D., Jones, D. B., Webster, L. K., and Vajda, F. J., 1982, H_2-receptor antagonists and hepatic drug disposition, *Hepatology* **2:**828–831.

Miller, L. L., 1965, Direct actions of insulin, glucagon, and epinephrine on the isolated perfused rat liver, *Fed. Proc.* **24:**737–754.

Miller, L. L., 1973a, History of isolated liver perfusion and some still unsolved problems, in: *Isolated Liver Perfusion and Its Applications* (I. Bartosek, A. Guaitani, and L. L. Miller, eds.), Raven Press, New York, pp. 1–9.

Miller, L. L., 1973b, Technique of isolated rat liver perfusion, in: *Isolated Liver Perfusion and Its Applications* (I. Bartošek, A. Guaitani, and L. L. Miller, eds.) Raven Press, New York, pp. 11–52.

Miller, L. L., Bly, C. G., Watson, M. L., and Bale, W. F., 1951, The dominant role of the liver in plasma protein synthesis: Direct study of isolated perfused rat liver with aid of lysine-ε-C14, *J. Exp. Med.* **94:**431–453.

Miller, L. L., Hanavan, H. R., Titthasiri, N., and Chowdhury, A., 1964, Dominant role of the liver in biosynthesis of the plasma proteins with special reference to the plasma mucoprotein (seromucoid), ceruloplasmin, and fibrinogen, *Adv. Chem. Ser.* **44:**17–40.

Miller, L. L., Treat, D. E., Fridd, B., and Wemett, D., 1990, Effects of streptozotocin diabetes in the rat on blood levels of ten specific plasma proteins and on their net biosynthesis by the isolated perfused liver, *Hepatology* **11:**636–645.

Mitzkat, H. J., and Meyer, U., 1973, Metabolic state of isolated perfused rat liver and model-induced metabolism modifications, in: *Isolated Liver Perfusion and Its Applications* (I. Bartosek, A. Guaitani, and L. L. Miller, eds.) Raven Press, New York, pp. 79–86.

Morris, M. E., Yuen, V., and Pang, K. S., 1988, Competing pathways in drug metabolism. II. An identical, anterior enzymic distribution for 2- and 5-sulfoconjugation and a posterior localization for 5-glucuronidation of gentisamide in the rat liver, *J. Pharmacokinet. Biopharm.* **16:**633–656.

Ngo, L. Y., Tam, Y. K., and Coutts, R. T., 1995, Lack of residual effects of diethyl ether, methoxyflurane, and sodium pentobarbital on lidocaine metabolism in a single-pass isolated rat liver perfusion system, *Drug Metab. Dispos.* **23:**525–528.

Øie, S., and Fiori, F., 1985, Effects of albumin and alpha-1 acid glycoprotein on elimination of prazosin and antipyrine in the isolated perfused rat liver, *J. Pharmacol. Exp. Ther.* **234:**636–640.

Olson, M. J., Handler, J. A., and Thurman, R. G., 1986, Mechanism of zone-specific hepatic steatosis caused by valproate: Inhibition of ketogenesis in periportal regions of liver lobule, *Mol. Pharmacol.* **30:**520–525.

Ookhtens, M., Hobdy, K., Corvasce, M. C., Aw, T. Y., and Kaplowitz, N., 1985, Sinusoidal efflux of glutathione in the perfused rat liver. Evidence for a carrier-mediated process, *J. Clin. Invest.* **75:** 258–265.

Ookhtens, M., Lyon, I., Fernandez-Checa, J., and Kaplowitz, N., 1988, Inhibition of glutathione efflux in the perfused rat liver and isolated hepatocytes by organic anions and bilirubin. Kinetics, sidedness and molecular forms, *J. Clin. Invest.* **82:**608–616.

Pang, K. S., and Gillette, J. R., 1978, Kinetics of metabolite formation and elimination in the perfused rat liver preparation: Differences between the elimination of preformed acetaminophen and acetaminophen formed from phenacetin, *J. Pharmacol. Exp. Ther.* **207:**178–194.

Pang, K. S., and Rowland, M., 1977a, Hepatic clearance of drugs, I. Theoretical considerations of a "well-stirred" model and a "parallel tube" model. Influence of hepatic blood flow, plasma and blood cell binding, and the hepatocellular enzymatic activity on hepatic drug clearance, *J. Pharmacokinet. Biopharm.* **5:**625–653.

Pang, K. S., and Rowland, M., 1977b, Hepatic clearance of drugs, II. Experimental evidence for acceptance of the "well-stirred" model over the "parallel tube" model using lidocaine in the perfused rat liver *in situ* preparation, *J. Pharmacokinet. Biopharm.* **5:**655–680.

Pang, K. S., and Terrell, J. A., 1981, Retrograde perfusion to probe the heterogeneous distribution of hepatic drug metabolizing enzymes in rats, *J. Pharmcol. Exp. Ther.* **216:**339–346.

Pang, K. S., Cherry, W. F., and Ulm, E. H., 1985, Disposition of enalapril in the perfused rat intestine-liver preparation: Absorption, metabolism and first-pass effect, *J. Pharmacol. Exp. Ther.* **233:**788–795.

Pang, K. S., Cherry, W. F., Accaputo, J., Schwab, A. J., and Goresky, C. A., 1988a, Combined hepatic arterial–portal venous and hepatic arterial–hepatic venous perfusions to probe the abundance of drug metabolizing activities: Perihepatic venous O-deethylation activity for phenacetin and periportal sulfation activity for acetaminophen in the once-through rat liver preparation, *J. Pharmacol. Exp. Ther.* **247:**690–700.

Pang, K. S., Lee, W.-F., Cherry, W. F., Yuen, V., Accaputo, J., Fayz, S., Schwab, A. J., and Goresky, C. A.,

1988b, Effects of perfusate flow rate on measured blood volume, Disse space, intracellular water space and drug extraction in the perfused rat liver preparation: Characterization by the mulitple indicator dilution technique, *J. Pharmacokinet. Biopharm.* **16:**595–632.

Proost, J. H., Nijssen, H. M. J., Strating, C. B., Meijer, D. K. F., and Groothuis, G. M. M., 1993, Pharmacokinetic modeling of the sinusoidal efflux of anionic ligands from the isolated perfused rat liver: The influence of albumin, *J. Pharmacokinet. Biopharm.* **21:**375–394.

Reinke, L. A., Belinsky, S. A., Evans, R. K., Kauffman, F. C., and Thurman, R. G., 1981, Conjugation of *p*-nitrophenol in the perfused rat liver: The effect of substrate concentration and carbohydrate reserves, *J. Pharmacol. Exp. Ther.* **217:**863–870.

Riedel, G. L., Scholle, J. L., Shepherd, A. P., and Ward, W. F., 1983, Effects of hematocrit on oxygenation of the isolated perfused rat liver, *Am. J. Physiol.* **245:**G769–G774.

Rosini, S., Benetti, D., and Kvetina, J., 1976, The functional capacity of the isolated perfused rat liver in relation to the colloidal-osmotic composition of the perfusion medium, *Farmaco. Prat.* **31:**625–629.

Roth, R. A., and Rubin, R. J., 1976a, Role of blood flow in carbon monoxide- and hypoxia-induced alterations in hexobarbital metabolism in rats, *Drug Metab. Dispos.* **4:**460–467.

Roth, R. A., and Rubin, R. J., 1976b, Comparison of the effect of carbon monoxide and of hypoxic hypoxia. II. Hexobarbital metabolism in the isolated, perfused rat liver, *J. Pharmacol. Exp. Ther.* **199:**61–66.

Russel, F. G. M., Weitering, J. G., Oosting, R., Groothuis, G. M. M., Hardonk, M. J., and Meijer, D. K. F., 1983, Influence of taurocholate on hepatic clearance and biliary excretion of asialo intestinal alkaline phosphatase in the rat *in vivo* and in isolated perfused rat liver, *Gastroenterology* **85:**225–234.

Scharschmidt, B. F., Van Dyle, R. W., and Stephens, J. E., 1985, Chloride transport by intact rat liver and cultured rat hepatocytes, *Am. J. Physiol.* **242:**G628–G633.

Schary, W. L., and Rowland, M., 1983, Protein binding and hepatic clearance: Studies with tolbutamide, a drug of low intrinsic clearance, in the isolated perfused rat liver preparation, *J. Pharmacokinet. Biopharm.* **11:**225–243.

Schmucker, D. L., and Curtis, J. C., 1974, A correlated study of the fine structure and physiology of the perfused rat liver, *Lab. Invest.* **30:**201–212.

Schmucker, D. L., Jones, A. L., and Michielsen, C. E., 1975, An improved system for hemoglobin-free perfusion of isolated rat livers, *Lab. Invest.* **33:**168–175.

Scholz, R., and Bücher, T., 1965, Haemoglobin-free perfusion of rat liver, in: *Control of Energy Metabolism* (B. Chance, ed.), Academic Press, New York, pp. 393–414.

Scholz, R., Schwarz, F., and Bücher, T., 1966, Barbiturate und energieliefernder Stoffwechsel in der hämoglobinfrei durchströmten Leber der Ratte, *Z. Klin. Chem.* **4:**179–187.

Scholz, R., Thurman, R. G., Williamson, J. R., Chance, B., and Bücher, T., 1969, Flavin and pyridine nucleotide oxidation–reduction changes in perfused rat liver. Anoxia and subcellular localization of fluorescent flavoproteins, *J. Biol. Chem.* **244:**2317–2324.

Scholz, R., Hansen, W., and Thurman, R. G., 1973, Interaction of mixed function oxidation with biosynthetic processes, I. Inhibition of gluconeogenesis by aminopyrine in perfused rat liver, *Eur. J. Biochem.* **38:**64–72.

Sestoff, L., and Kristensen, L. Ø., 1979, Determination of unidirectional fluxes of phosphate across plasma membrane in isolated perfused rat liver, *Am. J. Physiol.* **236:**C202–C210.

Shand, D. G., Branch, R. A., Evans, G. H., Nies, A. S., and Wilkinson, G. R., 1973, The disposition of propranolol. VII. The effects of saturable hepatic tissue uptake on drug clearance by the perfused rat liver, *Drug Metab. Dispos.* **1:**679–686.

Sherrill, B. C., and Dietschy, J. M., 1972, Characterization of the sinusoidal transport process responsible for uptake of chylomicrons by the liver, *J. Biol. Chem.* **253:**1859–1867.

Sies, H., 1978, The use of perfusion of liver and other organs for the study of microsomal electron-transport and cytochrome P-450 systems, *Methods Enzymol.* **52:**48–59.

Smith, P. F., Gandolfi, A. J., Krumdieck, C. L., Putnam, C. W., Zukoski, C. F., Davis, W. M., and Brendel, K., 1985, Dynamic organ culture of precision liver slices for *in vitro* toxicology, *Life Sci.* **36:**1367–1375.

Studenberg, S. D., and Brouwer, K. L. R., 1992, Impaired biliary excretion of acetaminophen glucuronide in the isolated perfused rat liver after acute phenobarbital treatment and *in vivo* phenobarbital pretreatment, *J. Pharmacol. Exp. Ther.* **261**:1022–1027.

Takei, Y., Kauffman, F. C., Misra, U. K., Yamanaka, H., and Thurman, R. G., 1990, Regulation of urea synthesis in sublobular regions of the liver lobule by oxygen, *Biochim. Biophys. Acta* **1036**:242–244.

Tam, Y. K., Yau, M., Berzins, R., Montgomery, P. R., and Gray, M., 1987, Mechanisms of lidocaine kinetics in the isolated perfused rat liver. I. Effects of continuous infusion, *Drug Metab. Dispos.* **15**:12–16.

Tavoloni, N., Reed, J. S., and Boyer, J. R., 1978, Hemodynamic effects or determinants of bile secretion in isolated rat liver, *Am. J. Physiol.* **234**:E584–E592.

Thomsen, O. O., and Larsen, J. A., 1983, Importance of perfusate hematocrit for insulin- and glucagon-induced choleresis in the perfused rat liver, *Am. J. Physiol.* **245**:G59–G63.

Thurman, R. G., and Kauffman, F. C., 1985, Sublobular compartmentation of pharmacologic events (SCOPE): Metabolic fluxes in periportal and pericentral region of the liver lobule, *Hepatology* **5**:144–151.

Thurman, R. G., and Scholz, R., 1969, Mixed function oxidation in perfused rat liver. The effect of aminopyrine on oxygen uptake, *Eur. J. Biochem.* **10**:459–467.

Thurman, R. G., and Scholz, R., 1973, Interaction of mixed-function oxidation with biosynthetic processes. II. Inhibition of lipogenesis by aminopyrine in perfused rat liver, *Eur. J. Biochem.* **38**:73–78.

Thurman, R. G., Ji, S., Matsumura, T., and Lemasters, J. J., 1984, Is hypoxia involved in the mechanism of alcohol-induced liver injury?, *Fundam. Appl. Toxicol.* **4**:125–133.

Thurman, R. G., Kauffman, F. C., and Jungermann, K., 1986, *Regulation of Hepatic Metabolism: Intra- and Intercellular Compartmentation*, Plenum Press, New York.

Trowell, O. A., 1942, Urea formation in the isolated perfused liver of the rat, *J. Physiol.* **100**:432–458.

Veneziale, C. M., Walter, P., Kneer, M., and Lardy, H. A., 1967, Influence of L-tryptophan and its metabolites on gluconeogenesis in the isolated perfused liver, *Biochemistry* **6**:2129–2138.

von Frey, M., and Gruber, M., 1885, Ein respirationsapparat für isolierter organe, *Arch. Physiol.* **9**:519–532.

Watkins, J. B., Siegers, C.-P., and Klaassen, C. D., 1984, Effect of diethyl ether on the biliary excretion of acetaminophen, *Proc. Soc. Exp. Biol. Med.* **177**:168–175.

Weibel, E. R., 1984, *The Pathway for Oxygen: Structure and Function in the Mammalian Respiratory System*, Harvard University Press, Cambridge, Massachusetts.

Williamson, J. R., Browning, E. T., Thurman, R. G., and Scholz, R., 1969, Inhibition of glucagon effects in perfused liver by (+)-decanoyl-carnitine, *J. Biol. Chem.* **244**:5055–5064.

Xu, X., Hirayama, H., and Pang, K. S., 1989, First-pass metabolism of salicylamide: Studies in the once-through vascularly perfused rat intestine–liver preparation, *Drug Metab. Dispos.* **17**:556–563.

Yoshihara, H., Matsumura, T., Jeffs, R., Kauffman, F. C., Lemasters, J. J., Liang, M., and Thurman, R. G., 1988, Role of calcium in regulation of hepatic O_2 uptake, in: *Integration of Mitochondrial Function* (J. J. Lemasters, C. Hackenbrock, R. G. Thurman, and H. Westerhoff, eds.), Plenum Press, New York, pp. 605–616.

Yu, V. C., DeLamirande, E., Horning, M. G., and Pang, K. S., 1982, Dose-dependent kinetics of quinidine in the perfused rat liver preparation. Kinetics of formation of active metabolites, *Drug Metab. Dispos.* **10**:568–572.

Zhong, Z., Lemasters, J. J., and Thurman, R. G., 1989, Role of purines and xanthine oxidase in reperfusion injury in perfused rat liver, *J. Pharmacol. Exp. Ther.* **250**:470–475.

Zimmerman, H. J., Abernathy, C. O., Lukaco, L., and Ezekiel, M., 1982, Effects of ticrynafen on hepatic excretory function in the isolated perfused rat liver, *Hepatology* **2**:255–257.

Zimmerman, C. L., Ratna, S., Leboeuf, E., and Pang, K. S., 1991, High-performance liquid chromatographic method for the direct determination of 4-methylumbelliferone and its glucuronide and sulfate conjugates. Applications to studies in the single-pass *in situ* perfused rat intestine–liver preparation, *J. Chromatogr.* **563**:83–94.

Chapter 11

Isolated Renal Brush Border and Basolateral Membrane Vesicles and Cultured Renal Cells

Marcelo M. Gutierrez, Claire M. Brett, and Kathleen M. Giacomini

1. INTRODUCTION

The two principal organs of drug elimination are the liver and the kidney. Although the liver is the main organ for biotransformation, the kidney is the primary site for excretion of the chemically unchanged drug as well as its biotransformed products. Understanding the mechanisms of excretion and reabsorption by the kidney is clinically relevant to rational drug therapy, since these mechanisms play an important role in the pharmacology, toxicology, and disposition of many drugs and xenobiotics (Bisel *et al.*, 1970; Grever *et al.*, 1981).

Macromolecules (up to 5 kDa) are easily filtered through the glomerulus; the ability of larger macromolecules to be filtered is a function of their size, shape, and ionic charge. In cases in which the renal clearance of a substance (unbound in plasma) exceeds the glomerular filtration rate (GFR), transport processes in the renal tubules which function in the secretory direction must be responsible in part for the substance's disposition. In contrast, when the renal clearance of a substance is less than the GFR, transport processes in the proximal tubules may be responsible for their net

Marcelo M. Gutierrez • Forest Laboratories Inc., New York, New York 11696. *Claire M. Brett* • Department of Anesthesia, University of California, San Francisco, California 94143. *Kathleen M. Giacomini* • Department of Biopharmaceutical Science, University of California, San Francisco, California 94143.

Models for Assessing Drug Absorption and Metabolism, Ronald T. Borchardt *et al.*, eds., Plenum Press, New York, 1996.

reabsorption. Depending upon their hydrophobicity, compounds may also undergo passive reabsorption in the renal tubules. Metabolism in the kidney may also result in a renal clearance less than the GFR.

Substances are transported into and out of cells by three mechanisms: simple diffusion, facilitated diffusion via carriers or channels, and active transport via carriers or pumps. Small lipophilic substances are able to diffuse through the membrane bilayer with relative ease whereas small hydrophilic substances pass through aqueous pathways between cells. In either case, the transport rate for these diffusional processes depends upon the size of the substance. In cases in which the transport rate does not obey the general principles of simple diffusion, a facilitated mechanism, either active or passive, must be responsible for the movement of the substance across the cellular membrane. Whereas substances transported via passive mechanisms (simple and facilitated diffusion) move down their electrochemical potential/ gradient, active transport mechanisms are able to drive substances across cell membranes against their concentration gradient at the expense of energy. These plasma membrane-associated active transport systems are divided into two major types depending on their energy source: primary- and secondary-active transport systems. Primary-active systems mediate transport across the cell membrane by a process directly coupled to ATP hydrolysis. In secondary-active transport, the movement of a substrate against its electrochemical gradient is coupled to the movement of a second substrate (usually an ion) down its electrochemical gradient. The gradient of the second substrate is maintained in turn by primary-active transport systems (Stein, 1990).

A variety of techniques are available to study the mechanisms of transport across the renal epithelium: *in vivo* clearance techniques (for a review, see Giacomini *et al.*, 1988), isolated cortical slices (Bojesen and Leyssac, 1965), isolated renal tubules (Burg and Knepper, 1986), micropuncture (Lang *et al.*, 1978; Ullrich *et al.*, 1969), isolated brush border and basolateral membrane vesicles (Aronson, 1981; Kinne and Schwartz, 1978; Mürer and Gmaj, 1986; Sachs *et al.*, 1980), and renal cell culture (Handler, 1986; Hull, 1976; Hull *et al.*, 1965; Koyama *et al.*, 1978). In this chapter, we will focus on two methods for studying renal transport: isolated plasma membrane vesicles and renal cell culture. We will discuss the specific advantages of each method.

2. ISOLATED RENAL PLASMA MEMBRANE VESICLES

2.1. Advantages and Disadvantages of Vesicles

The secretion or reabsorption of drugs in the renal tubule is possible because transport systems are asymmetrically distributed between the two surfaces of the epithelial cell. This allows net flux of a substance into the tubular fluid (secretion) or into the plasma (reabsorption). Isolated brush border membrane vesicles (BBMV) and basolateral membrane vesicles (BLMV) provide experimental systems for investigation of transport processes in each membrane separately. In addition, isolated membrane vesicles are devoid of enzymes important for the *in vivo* metabolism of drugs. Thus, vesicles provide a unique system for analyzing transport of drugs in the renal epithelium without the confounding factor of metabolism of the substrate.

Because membrane vesicles are essentially devoid of cytoplasmic components, the ion and solute gradients which exist in intact tissue cannot be maintained. This is the basis of another advantage of membrane vesicles: the ability to experimentally control the composition of the buffers on either side of the membrane. That is, vesicles can be suspended or preloaded in a series of buffers containing various ions. By imposing these various inwardly or outwardly directed chemical gradients, the energetics of membrane transport are experimentally controlled to identify driving forces (Hopfer, 1978).

The advantages of vesicles must be balanced against their limitations. Although methods for preparing membrane vesicles result in enhanced yield of the desired membrane, contamination with other cellular components is inevitable. Although the contamination is generally small, it can result in variability in the transport data. In addition to this heterogeneity of the origin of the membrane obtained, the vesicles obtained are often heterogeneous with respect to the size and orientation (right side out, inside out, or mixed) of the vesicles and the relative proportions of leaky and intact vesicles. The lack of homogeneity of membrane vesicles creates problems in analyzing data for initial rates and kinetics of transport. BBMV are generally more homogeneous than BLMV.

2.2. Materials

2.2.1. ISOLATION OF BRUSH BORDER MEMBRANE VESICLES (BBMV)

Surgical instruments/equipment: Surgical scissors; surgical blades; 23- and 27-gauge needles; 3- and 50-ml syringes; superspeed centrifuge with a fixed-angle rotor to hold 50-ml centrifuge tubes; Sorvall Omni-Mixer.

Chemicals: $MgSO_4$; HK buffer = 10 mM 4-(2 hydroxyethyl)-1-piperazine-ethanesulfonic acid (HEPES) + 150 mM KCl (pH to 7.4 using KOH); HK-EGTA buffer = 10 mM HEPES + 150 mM KCl + 5 mM ethyleneglycol-bis-(β-aminoethyl ether)-N,N'-tetraacetic acid (EGTA).

2.2.2. ISOLATION OF BASOLATERAL MEMBRANE VESICLES (BLMV)

Equipment: Waring blender; Sorvall RC-5B centrifuge and Sorvall SS-34 rotor.

Chemicals: $MgCl_2$; Percoll; homogenizing buffer = 300 mM mannitol + 1 mM EDTA + 0.1 mM phenylmethylsulfonyl fluoride (PMSF) + 18 mM Tris HCl (pH 7.4); washing buffer = 300 mM mannitol + 1 mM EDTA + 2 mM magnesium gluconate + 50 mM HEPES (pH 7.5).

Materials for transport experiments: Scintillation fluid; scintillation vials; test tubes; vacuum filtration apparatus; filters (0.3 μm, PH type); tweezers.

2.3 Procedures

Physical differences among the various cellular membranes are the basis of established procedures to obtain enriched quantities of one membrane versus another. In particular, brush border and basolateral membranes differ in the relative amounts of lipid and protein, surface charge density, hydrophobicity (determined by the degree of glycosylation of membrane proteins), surface properties (i.e., receptor and enzyme composition), and resistance to shearing forces. Such differences among cellular membranes allow their separation by a variety of techniques such as divalent-cation precipitation, differential centrifugation, and Percoll or sucrose gradients. Other biochemical differences are the basis of procedures which are essential to monitor the purity of the isolated membranes (e.g., BBMV or BLMV).

2.3.1. ISOLATION OF BRUSH BORDER MEMBRANE VESICLES (BBMV)

The most frequently used method for the isolation of BBMV is the divalent-cation precipitation method. This method takes advantage of the differences in reactivity of the brush border membrane and the other cellular components with calcium or magnesium (Booth and Kinney, 1974). Epithelial brush border membranes contain abundant negative charges (primarily from sialic acid residues) which are able to neutralize the charges of the divalent cations within the surface of the membrane. Other membrane organelles and the basolateral membrane have a relatively smaller surface density of charge-neutralizing groups and are, therefore, cross-linked by the divalent cations. Thus, divalent-cation precipitation is the initial step to precipitate other cellular membranes away from the brush border membranes. After this, a series of differential centrifugations will produce an enriched suspension of BBMV.

To isolate BBMV:

1. Kidneys are obtained from anesthetized animals (typically 1–2 rabbits or 5–6 rats are used in a single isolation). In rabbits, before excising of the kidney, the renal artery can be isolated and perfused *in situ* with HK buffer. This will reduce contamination from red blood cells and enhance the purity of the BBMV.
2. The kidney is sliced longitudinally, and the capsid (the transparent membrane that envelops the kidney) is removed.
3. The cortex, the lighter colored outer section of the kidney, is separated from the medulla using surgical scissors.
4. The cortex (15–20 g) is coarsely minced with surgical scissors and then placed in 150 ml of cold HK-EGTA buffer.
5. The minced cortex is homogenized using the Sorvall Omni-mixer at the highest speed.
6. $MgSO_4$ or $MgCl_2$ (16 mM) is added to the homogenate, and the solution is stirred on ice for 20 min.

7. The homogenate is centrifuged on a superspeed centrifuge at $7740 \times g$ for 15 min, and the supernatant (S1) is collected. A superspeed centrifuge is used in steps 8–12 below.

8. S1 is then centrifuged at 35,000 $\times$ g for 30 min, and the pellet (P2) is collected and resuspended in 80 ml of HK buffer by passing through a 50-ml syringe fitted with a 23-gauge needle.

9. The resulting P2 suspension is then centrifuged at $7740 \times g$ for 15 min, and the supernatant (S3) is collected.

10. S3 is centrifuged at 48,000 $\times$ g for 25 min.

11. The pellet (P4) is resuspended in 1 ml of HK buffer by passing through a 3-ml syringe fitted with a 27-gauge needle.

12. The P4 suspension is centrifuged at 48,000 $\times$ g for 20 min. The resulting pellet (BBMV) is resuspended in 1 ml of HK buffer by passing through a 3-ml syringe fitted with a 27-gauge needle.

13. The BBMV are stored at 4°C prior to uptake experiments. For best results the vesicles should be used within 24 hr after preparation. To resuspend, the BBMV should be passed through a 27-gauge needle prior to use.

2.3.2. ISOLATION OF BASOLATERAL MEMBRANE VESICLES

Basolateral membrane vesicles have been prepared from renal epithelium using sucrose density gradient centrifugation (Kinsella *et al.*, 1979; Mamelok *et al.*, 1982) or free-flow electrophoresis (Heidrich *et al.*, 1972). More recently, a technique for preparation of BLMV from dog kidney has been described (Hilden *et al.*, 1989) which is simpler, faster, and more efficient than other techniques previously described for BLMV isolation. In this technique, BBMV may also be prepared in conjunction with BLMV isolation.

To isolate BLMV:

1. Kidneys are obtained from anesthesized animals (typically 3–4 rabbits, 10–12 rats, or 1 dog are used in a single isolation). In larger species, before excising of the kidney, the renal artery is isolated and perfused *in situ* with HK buffer.

2. The kidney is sliced longitudinally, and the capsid (the transparent membrane that envelops the kidney) is removed.

3. The cortex, the lighter colored outer section of the kidney, is separated from the medulla using surgical scissors.

4. The cortex (23–45 g) is homogenized in 250 ml of homogenizing buffer (see Section 2.2.2) using a Waring blender. This procedure is carried out in a cold room (4°C) for 1 min.

5. The resulting homogenate is then centrifuged for 10 min at 5000 rpm. For this and subsequent steps, a Sorvall centrifuge (RC-5B) with an SS-34 rotor is used. (Comparable rotors and centrifuges from other manufacturers may also be used.)

6. The supernatant, S1, is separated from the pellet, P1, and the volume of S1 is measured. A volume of 1 M $MgCl_2$ equal to 1% of the total volume is added, and the $S1/MgCl_2$ solution is kept on ice for 20 min.
7. The $S1/MgCl_2$ solution is centrifuged at 4000 rpm for 10 min.
8. The resulting supernatant (S2) may be used to isolate BBMV (see Hilden *et al.*, 1989).
9. The pellet (P2) is resuspended in homogenizing buffer and centrifuged for 20 min at 20,000 rpm.
10. This step is repeated twice, and the resulting pellet (P3) is resuspended in approximately 30 ml of the desired medium (e.g., 300 mM mannitol, 18 mM Tris, 75 mM KCl).
11. The resuspended pellet is combined with Percoll (7.5 g added to 30.5 g of suspension).
12. The Percoll suspension is centrifuged at 20,000 rpm for 30 min.
13. After the centrifugation, two major bands should be apparent. The upper layer is removed and washed with washing buffer three times by centrifugation at 20,000 rpm to remove the Percoll.
14. The BLMV pellet, which is above the clear Percoll pellet, is separated from the Percoll pellet and is resuspended in a volume of the desired medium.

2.3.3. ENZYME MARKERS TO DETERMINE THE ENRICHMENT OF THE PREPARATION

The purity of the vesicle preparation is monitored by determining the activities of enzyme markers in the final suspension and comparing these activities to those obtained in the original homogenate. An enhanced activity of the enzyme markers known to be unique to the membrane of interest is an indication of the purity of the preparation. No enhancement of the activities of enzyme markers that are known to be present in other cellular components provides an additional check on the purity of the vesicular preparation. Enzyme markers commonly assayed for the brush border membrane include γ-glutamyl transpeptidase (Tsao and Curthoy, 1980), alkaline phosphatase (Masuzawa and Sato, 1983), maltase (Dahlqvist, 1964; Sacktor, 1968), and aminopeptidase N (Tsao and Curthoy, 1980). Na^+/K^+-ATPase (Schoner *et al.*, 1967; Mamelok *et al.*, 1982) and adenylate cyclase (Mürer *et al.*, 1977; Hopfer, 1978) are assayed to evaluate for the presence of basolateral membranes, acid phosphatase for lysozomes (Masuzawa and Sato, 1983; Moss, 1984), succinate dehydrogenase for mitochondria, (Gibbs and Reimers, 1965), and glucose 6-phosphatase for the endoplasmic reticulum (Masuzawa and Sato, 1983; Aronson and Touster, 1974). Analytical procedures for these enzyme markers are well described (γ-glutamyl transpeptidase = kit no. 418, Sigma Chemical Co.; Masuzawa and Sato, 1983; Dahlqvist, 1964; Tsao and Curthoy, 1980; Schoner *et al.*, 1967; Mürer *et al.*, 1977; Hopfer, 1978; Kinne and Schwartz, 1978; Gibbs and Reimers, 1965). Enhancement is normalized per milligram of protein in the vesicle suspension and per milligram of protein in the homogenate and calculated as

$$\frac{\text{Activity of enzyme marker in vesicular preparation/mg of protein}}{\text{Activity of enzyme marker in homogenate/mg of protein}}$$

If an experimental method is designed to produce an enriched preparation of renal brush border membranes, the activity of alkaline phosphatase in the final pellet of vesicles should be at least 8- to 10-fold higher than that measured in the initial homogenate of renal cortex. None of the enzyme markers for other cellular membranes should increase. One must exercise caution in interpreting enhancement data if the enzyme is present in other cellular components.

2.3.4. VACUUM FILTRATION TO DETERMINE UPTAKE IN VESICLES

The transport characteristics of many compounds have been determined by measuring uptake into vesicles under a variety of conditions. If the compound of interest is available in the radiolabeled form with a specific activity generally greater than 1 mCi/ mmol, the ease and rapidity of the studies is greatly enhanced. If the compound of interest is not available in the radiolabeled form, one may carry out inhibition experiments in which the compound is used as a putative inhibitor of a radiolabeled substrate (see Section 4.3 on inhibition studies). Uptake of radiolabeled substances is measured using an inhibitor-stop filtration technique (Lee *et al.*, 1988) under vacuum, often termed "rapid vacuum filtration." In these studies, filters (0.3–0.5 μm) are used to retain the vesicles but allow the reaction solutions to pass freely. It is important that the compound not bind extensively to the filter. A variety of filters are available and can be tested for binding. A commonly used filter is Millipore PH Filter, 0.3 μm. In general, hydrophobic compounds tend to bind more extensively to filters. To reduce binding, filters may be treated with various compounds. Alternatively, inclusion of high concentrations of unlabeled substrate in the stop solution may reduce filter binding.

To perform an uptake study:

1. 40-μl aliquot of the appropriate buffer (e.g., H/Na$^+$ buffer, if Na$^+$-driven transport is being tested) containing the radiolabeled compound (i.e., reaction mixture) is added to a 10-μl aliquot of BBMV (or BLMV) suspension (approximately 10–20 mg of protein/ml) and incubated for various times, depending on the experiment. In general, approximately 0.45 μCi of radiolabeled compound is present in 50 μl of reaction mix. The uptake reaction begins when the reaction mixture is added to the vesicle suspension; a vortex mixer is used to facilitate complete mixing of the vesicles and the substrate in the reaction mixture.
2. At the end of each incubation, the uptake is stopped by adding 3 ml of ice-cold buffer.

3. The suspension is filtered using a vacuum filtration apparatus under a 15–20 in. Hg vacuum through a membrane filter.

4. The filter is washed 3 times with ice-cold buffer under vacuum and placed into 5 ml of scintillation fluid. The filter is dissolved in the scintillant overnight.

5. The same process is repeated using a 40-μl sample of each reaction mix without vesicles for determination of filter blanks.

6. The radioactivity associated with the filters is measured by liquid scintillation counting.

In each set of experiments, the radioactivity measured after filtering the transport medium (reaction mixture) in the absence of membrane vesicles (i.e., filter blanks) is subtracted from the radioactivity associated with the uptake of radiolabeled compound into the membrane vesicles to obtain the actual uptake values. Although unlikely, it is possible that a compound may be metabolized or degraded during these procedures. Since total radioactivity is determined, caution should be exercised in interpreting the data until it has been documenteded that no metabolism of the specific compound of interest occurs. Metabolism of the radioligand should be checked using specific analytical procedures such as HPLC or thin-layer chromatography. If metabolism occurs, then the specific analytical procedure should be used in the uptake experiments to measure the unchanged compound.

2.3.5. STUDIES TO DETERMINE BINDING OF A SUBSTRATE TO THE VESICLES

Uptake is defined as the amount of compound associated with the vesicles and is usually expressed as an amount per milligram of protein. Thus, uptake includes both the amount of compound bound to the membrane of the vesicle and the amount present in the intravesicular space. Transport refers to the process of uptake involved in the intravesicular accumulation of the compound and is usually expressed as a rate (i.e., amount per unit time per milligram of protein). Therefore, in order to obtain accurate transport parameters, binding must be distinguished from intravesicular uptake.

Two methods have been generally used to estimate the degree of binding of a compound. The first method involves lysis of the membrane vesicles. Uptake of the compound is determined as described in Section 2.3.4, except that ice-cold distilled water (rather than buffer) is used to stop the reaction. Subsequently, the filters are rinsed with either ice-cold buffer or water. Presumably, the vesicles rupture due to the hypo-osmotic media and the intravesicular contents are spilled. The remaining radioactivity reflects radioligand bound to the vesicles. Binding is expressed as a percentage as follows:

$$\% \text{ Bound} = \frac{\text{Uptake in the lysed vesicles}}{\text{Uptake in the intact vesicles}} \times 100$$

A more commonly used method to measure binding involves determining the uptake of the radioligand at equilibrium in the presence of progressively increasing concentrations of an impermeable solute such as sucrose or mannitol (50–500 mM). A plot of uptake (y-axis) versus the reciprocal of the osmolarity of the reaction mix (x-axis) will generate a line. The y-axis intercept, which reflects the uptake when the intravesicular space is infinitely small (infinite osmolarity), represents binding to the vesicles. By this method, binding to the membrane of the vesicle can be distinguished from uptake of the radioligand into an osmotically reactive intravesicular space. The percent bound at equilibrium can be calculated as follows:

$$\% \text{ Bound} = \frac{\text{Intercept}}{\text{Equilibrium uptake in the absence of sucrose}} \times 100$$

3. CULTURED RENAL EPITHELIAL CELLS

Epithelial cells are ubiquitous cells that line all body cavities and make up over 60% of the cell types in the body (Alberts *et al.*, 1989). While epithelial cells vary in their functional characteristics, a common property is their distinct functional polarity. An epithelial cell is polarized into an apical (brush border) membrane which faces the lumen and a serosal (basolateral) membrane which is exposed to the bloodstream. Epithelial cells are interconnected by tight junctions which form an impermeable barrier between cells. Although the exact role of tight junctions has not been determined, it is reasonable to assume that they play a functional role in the maintenance of polarity. Transport proteins localized on either the brush border or basolateral membrane surface are responsible for the transepithelial transport of solutes. In the kidney, substances that are secreted traverse the epithelial cell in a net direction from the blood to the lumen of the proximal tubules. On the other hand, for solutes that are reabsorbed, there is a net flow across the epithelial cell from the lumen to the bloodstream.

3.1. Advantages and Disadvantages of Studies in Cells

In studying transport processes in cells, it is often important to consider intracellular regulatory events and their direct effects on the transport mechanism. Vesicles provide little information regarding acute or chronic regulation of transport by hormones or substrates. This major limitation of vesicles is circumvented by using intact cells. Renal epithelial cells grow as monolayers in culture with the apical side facing the media and the basal side attached to the solid support. Cultured monolayers can be used to make direct transport measurements at both the brush border and basolateral membrane surfaces and to study transmembrane flux of substances. Cells are well suited for studying intracellular trafficking of the imported drug. On the other hand, transport studies in cells are limited by the extensive metabolism that can occur when the substance enters the cells.

There are a variety of cell lines that have been used to study renal transport (Table

Table I
Most Commonly Used Renal Cell Lines

Cell line	Source	Reference
LLC-PK$_1$	Porcine kidney	Hull, 1976
LLC-RK$_1$	Rabbit kidney	Hull *et al.*, 1965
MDCK	Canine kidney	Madin and Darby, 1958; Gausch *et al.*, 1966
MDBK	Bovine kidney	Madin and Darby, 1958
OK	Opossum kidney	Koyama *et al.*, 1978

I). Cell lines may reflect proximal tubule or distal tubule functions, depending upon their origin. Methods to directly culture renal cells (primary cell lines) have also been developed and have some advantages and disadvantages over continuous cell lines (Gstraunthaler, 1988). In this chapter, we will focus on continuous renal cell lines.

3.2. Materials

Equipment and supplies: T75 or T150 flasks; sterile pipets; centrifuge tubes; hemocytometer; water bath; cell culture plates; detergent (0.5% Triton X-100); scintillation vials; scintillation fluid.

Chemicals: L-Glutamine; phosphate-buffered saline, Ca^{2+}- and Mg^{2+}-free (PBS-CMF); trypsin (0.05%), Versene (0.02%) in saline A (STV); desired growth media; trypan blue; Fungizone (25 µg/ml); penicillin (10 mg/ml), streptomycin (10,000 units/ml) (Pen-Strep).

3.3. Procedures

3.3.1. PROCUREMENT OF CELLS

Cells are obtained from the institutional tissue/cell culture facility or from American Type Culture Collection, Rockville, MD. Cells are maintained at 37°C in a humidified 5% CO_2/95% air atmosphere. The passage number of the cells is important information and should be noted because cells develop different characteristics with age.

3.3.2. Passaging of Cells

The following procedure is employed for passaging cells:

1. The media, PBS-CMF, glutamine and STV, Fungizone, and Pen-Strep are placed in a water bath (37°C) to thaw.
2. The growth medium is supplemented with glutamine, Fungizone, and Pen-Strep (1 ml per 100 ml of growth media).
3. The growth medium in which the cells have been growing is removed by careful suctioning (i.e., do not agitate the cells).
4. The cells are then washed twice with 10 ml of PBS-CMF to remove as much growth medium as possible.
5. STV (5 ml) is added to the cells. The flask containing the cells and the STV is shaken and tapped constantly to detach the cells from the flask. (The cells should not be deprived of media for longer than 5 min.)
6. At the end of 5 min, the trypsin is neutralized with 5 ml of growth media.
7. The resulting cell suspension is transferred into a 50-ml centrifuge tube. The flask is then washed with PBS-CMF (10 ml), and this wash is added to the cell suspension to recover as many cells as possible.
8. The cells are then centrifuged for 5 min at 3000 rpm.
9. The supernatant (S1) is suctioned off, and the pellet (cells) is resuspended with growth media (25 ml), replaced in T75 flasks, and stored in the incubator.

3.3.3.   SEEDING OF CELLS

The procedure for seeding cells is the same as for passaging cells with the following additional steps:

1. After suctioning off S1 (see Section 3.3.2), the cell pellet is resuspended in 10 ml of growth media.
2. For counting cells, 80 µl of cell suspension is placed into a microcentrifuge tube and 80 µl of Trypan blue added.
3. The cells are then counted using a hemocytometer. Multiplying the surface area of a well in each plate by the desired density of the cells per unit well area (approximately 4×10^4 cells/cm^2) and dividing by the number of cells per volume of cell suspension gives the volume of cell suspension to be added to each well. Cells may be grown on a solid support (e.g., Falcon) or on porous filters (e.g., Costar Transwells). Generally, 12-well plates are used, but larger or smaller wells may be used.

3.3.4.   TRANSPORT STUDIES IN CULTURED MONOLAYERS GROWN ON A SOLID SUPPORT

For studies of the transport of radiolabeled substrates, the cell monolayer is washed three times with uptake buffer (e.g., phosphate-buffered saline). The uptake is initiated by adding 500 µl of uptake buffer containing radiolabeled substrate, and the wells are incubated at 24°C (or other suitable temperature) for variable periods of time depending on the experiment. The uptake is stopped by removing the uptake medium by gentle aspiration , and the monolayers are washed immediately with ice-cold uptake buffer three times. The cells are then solubilized in 1 ml of detergent, and an aliquot (500 μl) of the solubilized cells is transferred into scintillation vials for radioactivity measurements. The protein content of the cells is measured with the Bio-Rad™ Protein Assay using the method of Bradford (1976).

3.3.5. TRANSPORT STUDIES IN CULTURED MONOLAYERS GROWN ON MICROPOROUS MEMBRANES

If epithelial cells are grown on microporous membranes, the solutions bathing the apical and serosal surfaces of the epithelium can be manipulated and sampled separately (Fig. 1). Transport studies are conducted in a similar fashion as with cells grown on a solid support. The solution containing the radiolabeled compound is placed on one side of the monolayer, and flux is monitored by taking samples on the other side of the monolayer and measuring the radioactivity by liquid scintillation counting. To count the radioactivity associated with the cells, the membrane filter is first dried by dabbing once with tissue paper on the side not containing the cells. The filter is then excised from the support and immersed in scintillation fluid for counting.

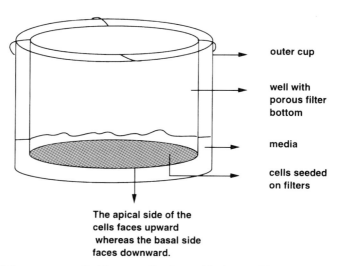

outer cup

well with
porous filter
bottom

media

cells seeded
on filters

The apical side of the
cells faces upward
whereas the basal side
faces downward.

Figure 1.   Cells grown on a well with a porous filter bottom. The inner well hangs on to the outer cup for easy manipulation. The media are first suctioned off, the radiolabeled substance is then placed on one side of the monolayer (the side chosen being dependent on the experiment; e.g., for basolateral uptake, the radiolabeled substance is placed inside the outer cup, with the mixture bathing the bottom of the inner well) and uptake is determined as described in Section 3.3.5.

A marker compound that permeates the monolayer minimally and exhibits similar physicochemical properties as the test compound is used to monitor the integrity of the monolayer.

Electrical measurements can be performed to obtain the resistance of the cell monolayer to electric current. Commercial electrical resistance devices can be used to measure the resistance of the monolayer. Briefly, a pair of matched Ag/AgCl electrodes is used to deliver 5–100 μA of current across the monolayer through salt bridges filled with saturated 3% agar/KCl. The voltage is then measured using a multimeter and Hg/HgCl electrodes which are connected across the cell monolayer with another pair of salt bridges. The resistance is then calculated using Ohm's law. The resistence across a confluent monolayer of renal cells tends to be low (approximately 80–100 Ω·cm²) but is dependent on the cell type.

4. TRANSPORT STUDIES IN MEMBRANE VESICLES AND CELLS

The primary experiments initially performed to determine the mechanisms of transport of a specific compound include studies of saturability, driving forces, and inhibition. We will discuss these types of experiments in detail. Usually, additional studies (which we will not discuss) are performed to further elucidate the characteristics of a transporter: stoichiometry and electrogenicity studies, further inhibition studies, and *in vivo* studies.

4.1. Saturability Studies

Saturability and inhibition studies must be performed at times known to represent "initial rate of transport" to minimize the effects of the substrate leaking back out of the vesicle or cell (substrate backflow) and inhibiting its own uptake (*cis*-inhibition). To determine this initial rate of transport, the uptake of substrate is measured as a function of time. The uptake (*y*-axis) is plotted versus time (*x*-axis); at initial times, uptake is a linear function of time. At times beyond "initial," the uptake versus time plot becomes hyperbolic.

Compounds transported via carrier-mediated mechanisms (facilitated diffusion or active transport) exhibit saturable uptake kinetics. That is, as the substrate concentration increases, the rate of uptake reaches a plateau, and further increases in the rate are not attainable. A plot of initial rate of uptake versus concentration conforms to the Michaelis–Menten equation:

$$\text{Rate} = V_{max} \cdot C/(K_m + C) \tag{1}$$

where V_{max} is the maximal rate of transport of the substrate, and K_m is the concentration of the substrate that produces half the maximal rate. The V_{max} reflects the number of transporters in the vesicular membrane and its turnover number, whereas the K_m is a measure of the affinity of a substrate for the transporter—the higher the affinity, the lower the K_m value. (Sometimes it may be necessary to include a linear component of transport in the equation. This is discussed in Section 4.5.) In these studies the initial rate of transport of substrate over a range of concentrations is defined. The concentrations may be selected based upon pharmacologic relevance or an estimate of the K_m of the compound. (See Sections 2.3.4, 2.3.5, 3.3.4, and 3.3.5 for details of uptake experiments.)

4.2. Driving Force Studies

Determining the driving forces of a transporter is important for understanding its mechanism of action. Knowledge of driving forces can be used to manipulate the pharmacology of drugs known to be substrates of a specific transporter. In addition, understanding mechanisms of transport across specific membranes is vital when attempting to design drugs that must be delivered across an epithelial barrier toward or away from a site of action.

Secondary-active transporters require the presence of a specific ion or an ion gradient to be effective. That is, the energy for transport is dependent on an ion (or substrate) gradient. Vesicles are ideal for identifying ion gradients that are driving forces for secondary-active transport systems. In cells, ion gradients are more difficult to control since the cells are able to self-regulate their concentrations of physiologic ions.

To determine if an ion is a driving force of transport of a compound, the uptake of the substrate is determined in the presence of different ions (e.g., Na^+, K^+, Ca^+, Li^+, and Rb^+) and ion gradients as a function of time. In vesicles, when a transport process is driven by an ion gradient (e.g., Na^+, H^+), an "overshoot" phenomenon is apparent in the presence, but not in the absence, of the gradient (Fig. 2). An "overshoot" phenomenon implies that the uptake of a substance into the vesicles is enhanced above the equilibrium value while the ion gradient exists. For example, in the presence of an inwardly directed Na^+ gradient, the uptake of nucleosides and many amino acids is enhanced, reaches a maximum, and then tapers down to equilibrium. This "overshoot" phenomenon is apparent in vesicles and is indicative of the concentrating capacity of certain transport processes.

For the study of transport systems that are dependent on the hydrolysis of ATP, cells provide a better method than vesicles, since vesicles are devoid of ATP. One method of determining if a transport process is coupled to ATP is to deplete cells of their ATP and determine if the uptake of a compound of interest is inhibited. For example, when cells are preincubated with 2,4-dinitrophenol (250 μM) or other substances that decrease cellular ATP, such as a low-glucose medium, the active transport processes of a compound that is ultimately dependent on ATP will be inhibited. Care must be taken in interpreting these types of data because many

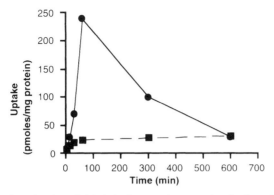

Figure 2. Simulated uptake of a radiolabeled substance, demonstrating the "overshoot" phenomenon. Circles represent uptake in the presence of an ion gradient driving force whereas squares represent uptake in the absence of driving forces.

secondary-active transporters that are driven by ion gradients created by ATPases will also exhibit reduced activity under ATP-depleted conditions. If ATP-regenerating systems are used to supply ATP, vesicles may be used to study ATP-dependent transporters (McKinney and Hosford, 1993).

4.3. Inhibition Studies

   To allow regulated movement of substances across cellular membranes, carrier-mediated transport must be selective. That carrier-mediated transport is both saturable and selective is the basis for perfoming inhibition studies. That is, the uptake of a radiolabeled compound known to be a substrate of a specific transporter is likely to be inhibited in the presence of the same (or a chemically closely related) unlabeled compound. By determining the uptake of known concentrations of radiolabeled substrate in the presence of fixed concentrations of unlabeled inhibitors, the specificity of a transporter is initially characterized (see also Section 4.4 on counterflux studies).
   The nature of inhibition may be investigated further by performing a Michaelis–Menten kinetic experiment in the absence or presence of increasing extravesicular or extracellular inhibitor concentrations. An increase in the apparent K_m of the substrate in the presence of an inhibitor without a change in the V_{max} represents a competitive inhibition whereas a decrease in the V_{max} is consistent with noncompetitive inhibition. Moreover, the IC_{50} (the inhibitor concentration that produces a 50% decrease in the maximal transport) of a compound may be determined. Typically, the initial rate of transport of radiolabeled substrate (at one concentration) is determined over a range of concentrations of unlabeled "inhibitor." Concentrations of inhibitor are selected based upon pharmacologic relevance or an estimate of the IC_{50} of the compound. (See

Sections 2.3.4, 2.3.5, 3.3.4, and 3.3.5 for details of uptake experiments in vesicles or cultured renal cells.)

Thus, if a specific transport process is involved in facilitating the movement of a substance across a membrane, the transport of that substance is inhibited by itself and/or another substance. Inhibition studies determine which substances interact with a transporter and the range of concentrations over which the interaction occurs. Since the inhibitor is not radiolabeled, inhibition studies provide a method to study compounds not available as radioligands.

4.4. Counterflux and *Trans*-stimulation Studies

Inhibition of the transport of a compound by a second compound does not necessarily imply that the two compounds are transported by the same carrier. In fact, a compound may inhibit the transport of a second compound without being translocated. If two compounds are transported by the same carrier, then when compound A is saturated on one side of a membrane, it stimulates the transport of compound B moving in the opposite direction (Stein, 1990). This phenomenon is known as *trans*-stimulation. Vesicles are ideally suited for conducting *trans*-stimulation studies because the intravesicular and extravesicular concentrations can be initially controlled. Such studies may also be performed in cells; however, because of metabolism and difficulty in controlling concentration gradients, caution should be exercised in the interpretation of the data.

In conducting *trans*-stimulation experiments, vesicles (or cells) are "loaded" with compound A by incubation for 1 hr (or longer periods as necessary) with the desired concentration. After this, the initial rate of transport of compound B is determined and compared to its transport rate in "unloaded" vesicles. If the rate is faster in the loaded vesicles, the phenomenon of *trans*-stimulation is presumed. If the uptake of compound B at various times actually exceeds the equilibrium value in the loaded vesicles, then it is presumed that compound A has driven the transport of compound B against a concentration gradient. This phenomenon is termed "counterflux." In vesicles, this phenomenon is temporary, because the concentration gradient of the driving compound (A) will dissipate eventually.

4.5. Calculation of Transport Parameters

Kinetic parameters are obtained by fitting data to the Michaelis–Menten model, including a linear, nonsaturable transport component:

$$\text{Rate} = [(V_{max} \cdot C)/(K_m + C)] + (K_{ns} \cdot C)$$

where V_{max} is the maximal rate of transport, K_m represents the concentration at which the rate of transport is half of V_{max}, K_{ns} is the coefficient for the linear, nonsaturable component, and C is the concentration of substrate in the extravesicular solution.

The IC_{50} is estimated by a sigmoidal inhibition model represented by the following equation:

$$V = \frac{V^o}{1 + (I/IC_{50})^n}$$

where V is the uptake of substrate in the presence of the inhibitor, V^o is the uptake of substrate in the absence of any inhibitor, I is the inhibitor concentration, and n is the slope. Assuming a competitive mechanism of interaction, the inhibition constant, K_I is determined by the following equation:

$$K_I = \frac{IC_{50}}{1 + (C/K_m)}$$

where C represents the concentration of substrate used in the inhibitor studies, and K_m represents the substrate affinity determined in preliminary Michaelis–Menten studies.

ACKNOWLEDGMENTS

We are grateful for support from the National Institutes of Health (GM36780).

REFERENCES

Alberts, B., Bray, D., Lewis, J., Raff, M., Roberts, K., and Watson, J. D., 1989, *Molecular Biology of the Cell*, 2nd ed., Garland Publishing, New York.

Aronson, P., 1981, Identifying secondary active solute transport in epithelia, *Am. J. Physiol.* **240**:F1–F11.

Aronson, N. N., and Touster, O., 1974, Isolation of rat liver plasma membrane fragments in isotonic sucrose, *Methods Enzymol.* **XXXI**, Part A: 90–102.

Bisel, H. F., Ansfield, F. J., Mason, J. H., and Wilson, W. L., 1970, Clinical studies with tubercidin administered by direct intravenous injection, *Cancer Res.* **30**:76–78.

Bojesen, E., and Leyssac, P. P., 1965, The kidney cortex slice technique as a model for sodium transport *in vivo*, *Acta Physiol. Scand.* **65**:20–32.

Booth, A. G., and Kinney, A. J., 1974, A rapid method for the preparation of microvilli from rabbit kidney, *Biochem. J.* **142**:575–581.

Bradford, M. M., 1976, A rapid and sensitive method for the quantitation of μg quantities of protein using the principle of protein dye binding, *Anal. Biochem.* **72**:248–254.

Burg, M. B., and Knepper, M. A., 1986, Single tubule perfusion techniques, *Kidney Int.* **30**:166–170.

Dahlqvist, A., 1964, Method for assay of intestinal disaccharidases, *Anal. Biochem.* **7**:18–25.

Gausch, C. R., Hark, W. L., and Smity, T. F., 1966, Characterization of an established cell line of canine kidney cells (MDCK), *Proc. Soc. Exp. Biol. Med.* **122**:931–935.

Giacomini, K. M., Hsyu, P.-H., and Gisclon, L. G., 1988, Renal transport of drugs: An overview of methodology with application to cimetidine, *Pharm. Res.* **5**:465–471.

Gibbs, G. E., and Reimers, K., 1965, Quantitative microdetermination of enzymes in sweat gland III. Succinic dehydrogenase in cystic fibrosis, *Proc. Soc. Exp. Biol. Med.* **119**:470–478.

Grever, M. R., Siaw, M. F. E., Jacob, W. F., Neidhart, J. A., Miser, J. S., Coleman, M. S., Hutton, J. J., and Balcerzak, S. P., 1981, The biochemical and clinical consequences of 2′ deoxycoformycin in refractory lymphoproliferative malignancy, *Blood* **57**:406–417.

Gstraunthaler, G. J. A., 1988, Epithelial cells in tissue culture, *Renal Physiol. Biochem.* **11**:1–42.

Handler, J. S., 1983, Use of cultured epithelia to study transport and its regulation, *J. Exp. Biol.* **106**:55–69.

Handler, J. S., 1986, Studies of kidney cells in culture, *Kidney Int.* **30**:208–215.

Heidrich, H. G., Kinne, R., Kinne-Saffran, E., and Hannig, K., 1972, The polarity of the proximal tubule cell in rat kidney. Different surface charges for the brush border microvilli and plasma membranes from the basal infoldings, *J. Cell Biol.* **54:**232–245.

Hilden, S. A., Johns, C. A., Guggino, W. B., and Madias, N. E., 1989, Techniques for isolation of brush border and basolateral membrane vesicles from dog kidney cortex, *Biochim. Biophys. Acta* **983:**77–81.

Hopfer, U., 1978, Transport in isolated plasma membranes, *Am. J. Physiol.* **234:**F89–F96.

Hull, R. N., 1976, Origin and characteristics of a pig kidney cell strain, LLC-PK1, *In Vitro* **12:**670–677.

Hull, R. N., Dwyer, A. C., Cherry, W. R., and Tritch, O. J., 1965, Development and characteristics of the Rabbit Kidney Cell Strain, LLC-RK1, *Proc. Soc. Exp. Biol. Med.* **118:**1054.

Kinne, R., and Schwartz, I. L., 1978, Isolated membrane vesicles in the evaluation of the nature, localization, and regulation of renal transport processes, *Kidney Int.* **14:**547–556.

Kinsella, J. L., Holohan, P. D., Pessah, N. I., and Ross, C. R., 1979, Isolation of luminal and antiluminal membranes from dog kidney, *Biochim. Biophys. Acta* **552:**468–477.

Koyama, H., Goodparture, C., Miller, M. M., Teplitz, R. L., and Riggs, A. D., 1978, Establishment and characterization of a cell line from the American opossum, *In Vitro* **14:**239–246.

Lang, F., Greger, R., Lechene, C., and Knox, F.G., 1978, Micropuncture techniques, in: *Methods in Pharmacology* (M. Martinez-Maldonado, ed.), Vol. 4B, Plenum Press, New York, pp. 75–103.

Lee, C. W., Cheeseman, C. I., and Jarvis, S. M., 1988, Na+- and K+-dependent uridine transport in rat renal brush-border membrane vesicles, *Biochim. Biophys. Acta* **942:**139–149.

Madin, S. H., and Darby, N. B., 1958, Established kidney cell lines of normal adult bovine and ovine origin, *Proc. Soc. Exp. Biol. Med.* **98:**574–576.

Mamelok, R. D., Tse, S. S., Newcomb, K., Bildstein, C. L., and Liu, D., 1982, Basal-lateral membranes from rabbit renal cortex prepared on a large scale in a zonal rotor, *Biochim. Biophys. Acta* **692:** 115–125.

Masuzawa, T., and Sato, F., 1983, The enzyme histochemistry of the choroid plexus, *Brain* **106:**55–99.

McKinney, P. D., and Hosford, M. A., 1993, ATP-stimulated tetraethylammonium transport in rabbit renal brush border membrane vesicles, *J. Biol. Chem.* **268:**6886–6895.

Moss, D. W., 1984, Acid phosphatases, in: *Methods in Enzymatic Analysis* (J. Bergmyer and M. Grabl, eds.), 3rd ed., Vol. IV, *Enzymes 2*, Verlag Chemie, Weinheim.

Mürer, H., and Gmaj, P., 1986, Transport studies in plasma membrane vesicles isolated from renal cortex, *Kidney Int.* **30:**171–186.

Mürer, H., Hopfer, U. and Kinne, R., 1977, Adenylate cyclase system in the enterocyte: Cellular localization and possible relation to transepithelial transport, in: *Hormonal Receptors in Digestive Tract Physiology* (F. Rosselin, ed.), North Holland Publishing, Amsterdam, pp. 425–434.

Sachs, G., Jackson, R. J., and Rabon. E. C., 1980, Use of plasma membrane vesicles, *Am. J. Physiol.* **238:**G151–G164.

Sacktor, B., 1968, Trehalase and the transport of glucose in the mammalian kidney and intestine, *Proc. Natl. Acad. Sci. USA* **60:**1007–1014.

Schoner, W., Ilberg, C. V., Kramer, R., and Seubert, W., 1967, On the mechanism of Na+- and K+-stimulated hydrolysis of adenosine triphosphate, *Eur. J. Biochem* **1:**334–343.

Sheikh, I. M., Kragh-Hansen, U., Jorgensen, K. E., and Roigaard-Petersen, H., 1982, Techniques for isolation of brush border and basolateral membrane vesicles from dog kidney cortex, *Biochem. J.* **80:**649–659.

Stein, W. D., 1990, *Channels, Carriers, and Pumps*, Academic Press, San Diego, pp. 174–176.

Tsao, B., and Curthoy, N. P., 1980, The absolute asymmetry of orientation of γ-glutamyl transpeptidase and amino peptidase on the external surface of the rat renal brush border membrane, *J. Biol. Chem.* **255:**7708–7711.

Turner, R. J., 1984, *Membrane Transport Driven by Ion Gradients*, The New York Academy of Sciences, New York, pp. 10–25.

Ullrich, K. J., Frometer, E., and Baumann, K., 1969, *Laboratory Techniques in Membrane Biophysics*, (H. Passow and R. Stampfli, eds.), in: Micropuncture and Microanalysis in Kidney Physiology, Springer-Verlag, Berlin, pp. 106–129.

Chapter 12

Use of an Isolated Perfused Kidney to Assess Renal Clearance of Drugs

Information Obtained in Steady-State and Non-Steady-State Experimental Systems

Noriko Okudaira and Yuichi Sugiyama

1. INTRODUCTION

The kidney plays an important role in eliminating foreign compounds that enter the body as well as in regulating the body pool of endogenous substances. The appearance of drug in the urine is the net result of glomerular filtration, tubular secretion and reabsorption (Fig. 1).

The isolated perfused kidney (IPK) is a useful tool to assess the renal clearance of drugs. The IPK permits the measurement of renal clearance in the absence of nonrenal factors such as hormones and the nervous system.

IPK systems to assess the renal clearance of drugs can be classified into two categories, according to whether data are obtained at steady state or under non-steady-state conditions. In this chapter, we describe the advantages and disadvantages of both these methods.

Noriko Okudaira • Pharmaceutical Research Center, Meiji Seika Kaisha, Ltd., Yokohama 222, Japan.
Yuichi Sugiyama • Faculty of Pharmaceutical Sciences, University of Tokyo, Tokyo 113, Japan.

Models for Assessing Drug Absorption and Metabolism, Ronald T. Borchardt *et al.*, eds., Plenum Press, New York, 1996.

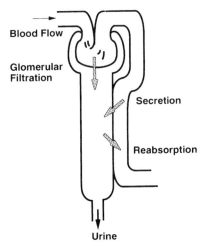

Figure 1.   Schematic of renal clearance in the nephron.

2.   ISOLATED PERFUSED KIDNEY

2.1.   Isolation and Perfusion of Rat Kidney

In our laboratory, we use the method of Nishitsutsuji-Uwo *et al.* (1967) with some modifications. The right kidney of male Wistar rats weighing 300–380 g (10–12 weeks old) is isolated and perfused. Under light anesthesia with ethyl ether, the peritoneal cavity is opened and the right ureter, superior mesenteric artery, right renal artery, and vena cava are dissected out. The right adrenal artery ($\langle A \rangle$ in Fig. 2) is ligated. Loose ligatures are placed as indicated in Fig. 2. The ureter is cannulated with PE-10 polyethylene tubing (0.58 mm i.d., 0.61 mm o.d.). The renal vein is then cannulated with polyethylene tubing (2 mm i.d., 3 mm o.d.). Ligature $\langle C \rangle$ is left loose at this time. A perfusion cannula [an 18-gauge needle connected to silicone tubing (3 mm i.d., 5 mm o.d.)] with a low perfusion flow rate is inserted into the renal artery via the mesenteric artery across the aorta. The perfusion flow rate is set immediately, and site $\langle C \rangle$ is ligated. This procedure prevents the interruption of renal perfusion during cannulation. After a few minutes of preperfusion, the kidney is isolated and placed on the perfusion apparatus (Fig. 3).

The composition of the basic cell-free perfusate used for the filtering kidney (FK) is Krebs–Henseleit buffer (116 mM NaCl, 4 mM KCl, 2 mM $CaCl_2$, 1.5 mM KH_2PO_4, 2.4 mM $MgSO_4$, and 25 mM $NaHCO_3$) containing 5–6% bovine serum albumin (BSA, fraction V). Glucose (1.8 mg/ml) or glucose (1 mg/ml) + a mixture of amino acids (0.5 mM L-methionine, 2 mM L-alanine, 2 mM glycine, 2 mM L-serine,

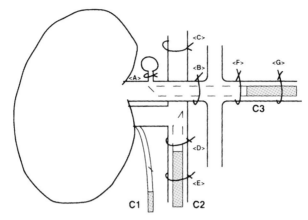

Figure 2. Surgical procedure for isolation and perfusion of rat kidney. Cannulas are inserted into the right ureter (C1), vena cava (C2), and renal artery via the mesenteric artery (C3). ⟨A⟩–⟨G⟩ are sites of ligation (see text).

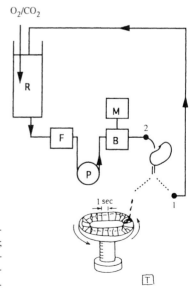

Figure 3. Schematic representation of the rat kidney perfusion system. P, Pump; F, filter; B, bubble trap; M, manometer; R, reservoir; T, turntable. O_2/CO_2 gas in flow into the reservoir. 1, effluent returned to the reservoir in the case of recirculation; 2, injection site for the single-pass MID method.

2 mM L-proline, 1 mM L-isoleucine, and 3 mM L-glutamate) is added to improve stability and viability. Addition of 0.1% mannitol to the perfusate ensures adequate volumes of urine. The perfusion pressure is 100 mm Hg, and the pH of the perfusate is adjusted to 7.4 by gassing with a 95% O_2/5% CO_2 mixture.

To achieve a steady state with test compounds, these are added to the perfusate at designated concentrations.

2.2. Hemodynamic Properties and Viability of the IPK

The hemodynamic and functional properties of the IPK system that we use are shown in Table I (Kim et al., 1992b). The perfusion flow rate in the IPK is higher than the physiological plasma flow rate. This is because when artificial perfusate (red blood cell-free) is used, the oxygen supply is not sufficient at a physiological perfusion flow rate. Also, the glomerular filtration rate (GFR) under the perfusion conditions described above is lower than the GFR in vivo. Hemodynamic properties specific to the IPK have been reviewed in detail by Maack (1980, 1986).

The viability of the IPK is monitored by glucose reabsorption and electrolyte reabsorption involving ions such as sodium and potassium. The stability of the flow rate, pressure, and GFR are also indices of viability. It should be noted that the values of all these parameters are not necessarily coincident with those seen in in vivo studies.

2.3. Single-Pass and Recirculating Perfused Kidney Systems

In the recirculating perfusion system, effluent from the renal vein enters the reservoir, and thus the drug concentration in the reservoir decreases gradually as a

Table I
Overall Functional Properties of the Filtering
and Nonfiltering Isolated Perfused Rat Kidneys[a]

	Filtering kidney	Nonfiltering kidney
Rat body weight (g)	361 ± 15	360 ± 10
Perfusate flow rate (ml $min^{-1}kidney^{-1}$)	17.0 ± 1.0	16.3 ± 0.5
Pressure (mm Hg)	101 ± 2	85 ± 4
GFR (μl $min^{-1}kidney^{-1}$)	413 ± 181	NA[b]
Urine flow (μl $min^{-1}kidney^{-1}$)	25 ± 7	NA
Glucose reabsorption (%)	98.3 ± 1.7	NA
Na^+ reabsorption (%)	96.5 ± 1.9	NA

[a]From Kim et al., 1992b.
[b]NA, Not applicable because no urine was formed.

result of urinary elimination and metabolism, and the metabolites and degradation products formed during the perfusion accumulate in the perfusate. On the other hand, in the single-pass perfusion system, the kidney is always perfused with fresh perfusate without any interaction involving metabolites and other products. The concentrations of substances added to the perfusate are kept constant.

2.4. Assessment of Renal Clearance in the IPK

Renal clearance, CL_R, is defined in terms of loss of drug across the kidney as

$$CL_R = Q \times (1 - C_{out}/C_R) \tag{1}$$

where Q is the perfusion flow rate, and C_{out} and C_R are drug concentrations in the venous effluent and reservoir, respectively. The term in parentheses is the extraction ratio of the drug. In the recirculating perfusion system, the concentration profile in the reservoir is described by the following equation:

$$dC_R/dt = -(CL_R/V_R) \times C_R \tag{2}$$

where V_R is the volume of perfusate. The slope of a logarithmic plot of C_R versus time corresponds to CL_R/V_R. By selecting an appropriate V_R and sampling time, the decrease in C_R is detected with great sensitivity. Renal clearance (CL_R) is also calculated from the urinary excretion data:

$$CL_R = (dXu/dt)/C_R \tag{3}$$

where Xu represents the amount excreted in the urine. Integrating Eq. (3) over the urine collection period, CL_R can be determined as

$$CL_R = Xu/AUC_R \tag{4}$$

where AUC_R is the area under the concentration–time curve.

2.5. Factors that Affect Renal Clearance

CL_R is described by the following general equation representing the contributions of three component processes, glomerular filtration, tubular secretion, and tubular reabsorption:

$$CL_R = (fu \times GFR + CL_{sec}) \times (1 - R) \tag{5}$$

where fu represents the fraction unbound in the perfusate, GFR the glomerular filtration rate, CL_{sec} the tubular secretion clearance, and R the tubular reabsorption fraction. Assuming that only unbound drug is secreted, CL_{sec} is described by Eqs. (6) and (7) based on the "well-stirred" model and the "parallel-tube" model (Pang and Rowland, 1977), respectively:

$$CL_{sec} = Q \times fu \cdot CL_{sec,int}/[Q + fu \cdot CL_{sec,int}] \qquad (6)$$

$$CL_{sec} = Q \times [1 - \exp(-fu \cdot CL_{sec,int}/Q)] \qquad (7)$$

where $CL_{sec,int}$ is the intrinsic clearance of tubular secretion. A CL_R greater than GFR $\times$ fu indicates net secretion, and one lower than GFR $\times$ fu indicates net reabsorption.

2.5.1. GLOMERULAR FILTRATION

Since the mechanism of glomerular filtration is ultrafiltration, drugs bound to macromolecules are not filtered. The GFR is determined by measuring the clearance of compounds such as inulin, creatinine, or sucrose which do not bind to the macromolecules in the perfusate and are eliminated only by glomerular filtration. The balance between the osmotic pressure and oncotic pressure of the perfusate determines the GFR. As discussed above, physiological GFR values cannot be applied to the IPK system. Since the GFR depends on the perfusate composition and perfusion pressure, the GFR of a system must be determined under the conditions used. Also, the fraction unbound of a test compound is altered by the perfusate pH and the concentrations of proteins, the test drug, and some other compounds present in the perfusate.

2.5.2. TUBULAR SECRETION

Several active secretion mechanisms in the proximal tubules have been reported. Among them, organic anion and cation transport systems and peptide transport systems have been extensively studied. Kinetic analysis of the data obatined from various *in vivo* and *in vitro* experiments has elucidated substrate specificity, kinetic parameters (K_m and V_{max}), driving forces, and location of carrier proteins. The properties of organic cation and anion transport systems were recently reviewed by Pritchard and Miller (1993). The contributions of specific transport mechanisms are usually assessed by studying the mutual inhibition of the compound, specific substrates for the transport system, and metabolic inhibitors. In the IPK, the effect of competitive and noncompetitive inhibitors and other chemicals can be studied over wide concentration ranges regardless of their pharmacological effects and systemic toxicity. Figure 4 shows the analysis of the secretion mechanism of triamterene, a potassium-sparing diuretic, and its active metabolite, *p*-hydroxytriamterene sulfate, reported by Muirhead and Somogyi (1991). Triamterene is an organic cation and has been reported to undergo both secretion and reabsorption. In the absence of any inhibitors, the ratio of the unbound clearance to the GFR was found to be greater than 1 for both triamterene and its metabolite, indicating the net secretion of these compounds. H_2 receptor antagonists and probenecid were added to the perfusate as inhibitors of the organic cation and the organic anion transport system, respectively. The ratio of the unbound clearance to the GFR for triamterene was reduced by the H_2

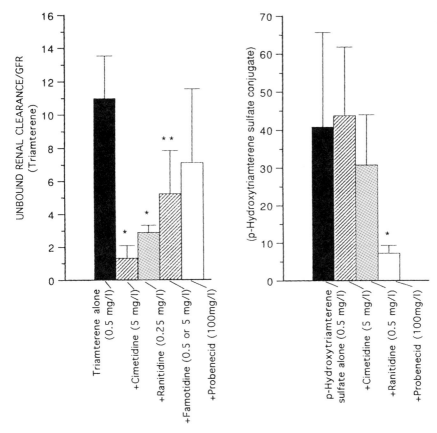

Figure 4. Effect of H_2 antagonists and probenecid on the renal clearance of triamterene and its metabolite, *p*-hydroxytriamterene sulfate. The ratios of renal clearance of triamterene (0.5 mg/l) and *p*-hydroxytriamterene sulfate (0.5 mg/l) to fu·GFR were determined in the recirculating perfusion system in the presence and absence of inhibitors of the organic cation and the organic anion transport system (H_2 receptor antagonists and probenecid, respectively). The data are presented as means ± SD. *$P < 0.05$, **$P < 0.01$ compared with triamterene or *p*-hydroxytriamterene sulfate alone. Modified from Muirhead and Somogyi (1991).

receptor antagonists at clinically observed concentrations, whereas it was not affected by probenecid. For *p*-hydroxytriamterene sulfate, the ratio decreased in the presence of probenecid but was not affected by any H_2 receptor antagonists. These observations indicate that triamterene undergoes tubular secretion by the organic cation transport system, whereas its metabolite, *p*-hydroxytriamterene sulfate, is secreted by the organic anion transport system.

2.5.3. REABSORPTION

There are two mechanisms of reabsorption. An active reabsorption system is reported to exist on the brush border membrane of renal tubules and to transport nutrients and endogenous ions such as glucose, choline, and uric acid (Zins and Weiner, 1968; Acara and Rennick, 1973; Wright et al., 1992). In addition, nonpolar compounds are passively reabsorbed throughout the nephron.

Passive reabsorption is assumed to be specific to unionized drug species. Therefore, urinary pH affects the reabsorption rate by changing the fraction of nonionized molecules in the urine. The fraction of nonionized molecules for weak acids and bases is calculated based on the pH partition theory. For weak acids:

$$C_{mol}/C_{ion} = 10^{(pK_a - pH)} \qquad (8)$$

where C_{mol} and C_{ion} are the concentrations of nonionized and ionized drug, respectively. For weak bases, the term in parentheses becomes pH $-$ pK_a. Table II shows the parameters for the renal excretion of triamterene, an organic cation (pK_a = 6.2), obtained in the IPK system by Kau (1978). He added 1 N HCl or 1 N NaOH to the perfusate to make the urine acidic or alkaline. In the control kidney, the clearance ratio [$(U/F)_{[^3H]-TA} \cdot V$/GFR in Table II] was greater than 1, indicating net secretion. In acidified kidneys the ratio rose by 260%, whereas in alkalinized kidneys the ratio fell

Table II
Influence of Perfusate pH on the Handling of [³H]Triamterene ([³H]-TA)
by the Isolated Perfused Rat Kidney[a,b]

Parameter[c]	Control (n = 5)	Acidified (n = 4)	Alkalinized (n = 4)
Perfusate pH	7.4	6.9–7.1	7.6–7.8
GFR (μl/min)	524 ± 99	498 ± 98	470 ± 23
T_{H_2O} (%)	93.4 ± 2.1	91.4 ± 1.7	96.2 ± 1.0
$(U/P)_{[^3H]-TA}$	7.5 ± 1.6	16.0 ± 3.6[d]	3.2 ± 0.6[d]
$C_{[^3H]-TA}$/GFR	0.39 ± 0.02	1.62 ± 0.59[d]	0.12 ± 0.03[d]
$(U/F)_{[^3H]-TA}$	30.0 ± 6.4	60.6 ± 11.6[d]	13.4 ± 2.1[d]
$(U/F)_{[^3H]-TA}$ V/GFR	1.53 ± 0.21	5.40 ± 1.85[d]	0.50 ± 0.09[d]
FL (μg/min)	0.45 ± 0.10	0.48 ± 0.17	0.59 ± 0.24
Excretion (% of FL)	171 ± 15	583 ± 182[d]	48 ± 9[d]
Reabsorption (Ta) or secretion (Tb) (% of FL)	71 ± 15[e]	474 ± 183[e,d]	52 ± 10[f,d]

[a]From Kau (1978).
[b]Average urine pH at the beginning and at the end of clearance periods was estimated as follows: for control, 6.3–6.8; for acidified perfusate, 5.8–6.4; for alkalinized perfusate, 7.1–7.4.
[c]Abbreviations: GFR, Glomerular filtration rate; T, fractional reabsorption; U/P, urine/perfusate concentration ratio; C, clearance; U/F, urine/ultrafiltrate concentration ratio; $U/F > U/P$; FL, flltered load.
[d]Significantly different ($P < 0.001$) from control kidneys.
[e]Tb = Excretion rate $-$ filtered load = $(U \times V) - (GFR \times F)$.
[f]Ta = Filtered load $-$ excretion rate = $(GFR \times F) - (U \times V)$.

below unity. These data indicate that triamterene is transported bidirectionally (secretion and reabsorption) and that the reabsorption is passive and pH-dependent.

The normal urine flow rate in humans (1.5 l/day) is less than 1% of the renal plasma flow rate (700 ml/min); thus, the concentration of a drug in urine may be 100 times higher than that in plasma. The urine flow rate affects the reabsorption of some drugs through its effects on the concentration gradient and the contact time during which the drug can diffuse out of the urine. According to the simulation by Hall and Rowland (1983), if the renal tubules are impermeable to the drug, then the renal clearance is equivalent to the GFR. If the permeability of the renal tubule to the drug is great, then equilibrium is reached between the drug in the urine and that unbound in the perfusate, and CL_R equals the product of the fraction unbound and the urine flow rate. For a drug with intermediate permeability—digitoxin, for example—a nonlinear relationship between renal clearance and urine flow rate was observed, as expected from the simulation. In the IPK system, the urine flow rate is dependent on the perfusate composition and perfusion conditions. Therefore, for drugs that undergo extensive reabsorption, the appropriate perfusion conditions should be selected and the CL_R obtained should be analyzed carefully.

2.5.4.   PROTEIN BINDING

The IPK is a useful tool for the investigation of the effect of protein binding on renal clearance. By replacing part of the BSA in the perfusate by dextran, the unbound fraction of a compound with a high affinity for BSA can be varied over a wide range (Hall and Rowland, 1983, 1985). As described above, glomerular filtration of a compound is affected by the unbound fraction in the perfusate, since only unbound drug can undergo ultrafiltration at glomeruli. If a drug is extensively secreted (fu × $CL_{sec,int}$ ≫ Q), then Eq. (5) becomes

$$CL_R = [fu \times GFR \times (1 - R)] + Q \times (1 - R) \qquad (9)$$

A plot of CL_R versus fu is predicted to be a straight line with a positive y-intercept. When $CL_{sec,int}$ is low (fu × $CL_{sec,int}$ ≪ Q),

$$CL_R = fu \times (GFR + CL_{sec,int}) \times (1 - R) \qquad (10)$$

If a drug does not undergo tubular secretion,

$$CL_R = fu \times GFR \times (1 - R) \qquad (11)$$

In the latter two cases, a plot of CL_R versus fu is predicted to be linear and to pass through the origin. In fact, for both furosemide, which undergoes tubular secretion but has a low extraction (Fig. 5), and digitoxin, which has a low renal clearance owing to extensive reabsorption, linear relationships were observed between renal clearance and the fraction unbound.

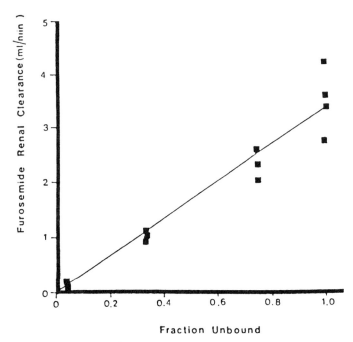

Figure 5. Relationship between the fraction unbound and the renal clearance of furosemide. From Hall and Rowland (1985).

2.6. The Non-Filtering Perfused Kidney System

The nonfiltering perfused kidney (NFK) provides a useful means of evaluating the antiluminal transport/binding of a drug separately from the glomerular filtration and subsequent luminal reabsorption (Kim *et al.*, 1991, 1992a,b; Maack, 1986; Silva, 1990; Sugiyama *et al.*, 1990; Sugiyama, 1991; Johnson and Maack, 1997; Kau and Maack, 1977; Petersen *et al.*, 1982; Suzuki *et al.*, 1987). By increasing the albumin concentration in the perfusate from 5–6% in the FK to 10% in the NFK and decreasing the perfusion pressure by 15% (85 mm Hg), essentially no glomerular filtration takes place, and, thus, luminal reabsorption and catabolism/metabolism after filtration are negligible. The properties of the NFK are compared with those of the FK in Table I. We characterized the biological integrity of the NFK by analyzing the antiluminal uptake of [^{3}H]*p*-aminohippurate ([^{3}H]-PAH), which is known to be a specific substrate for the carrier-mediated transport system on an antiluminal membrane (Kim *et al.*, 1992b). Using the multiple indicator dilution (MID) technique (see Section 3), the distribution volume and extraction ratio of PAH and the extracellular reference, creatinine, and the influx clearance were determined. The distribution volume and extraction ratio of the extracellular reference, creatinine, were comparable in both systems. The influx clearance corrected for the unbound fraction of PAH in the perfusate was almost the same for the NFK and the FK. These observations suggest that the organic anion transport activity through the antiluminal membrane is well preserved in the NFK.

2.7. Application: Analysis of Renal Handling of Epidermal Growth Factor Using the FK and NFK

Our group investigated the renal handling of a polypeptide, epidermal growth factor (EGF), using the FK and NFK (Kim *et al.*, 1991, 1992a,b; Sugiyama *et al.*, 1990; Sugiyama, 1991). In the kidney, EGF exhibits a variety of pharmacological effects such as increasing urine flow and urinary Na^+ and K^+ excretion via receptor binding on the antiluminal membrane (Kim *et al.*, 1991; Scoggins *et al.*, 1984; Fisher *et al.*, 1989). The kidney is the second most important organ in terms of the distribution and elimination of EGF. *In vivo* kinetic analysis indicated that the contribution of the kidney to EGF clearance is 20–30% (Fisher *et al.*, 1989; Kim *et al.*, 1988, 1989; Sugiyama *et al.*, 1990). Two mechanisms can be considered as the renal uptake routes for EGF: (1) reabsorption via the luminal membrane after glomerular filtration, and (2) receptor-mediated endocytosis via the antiluminal membrane. Using acid washing in the FK and NFK, the surface-bound and internalized EGF were separately determined, and the contributions of luminal and antiluminal uptake were estimated.

2.7.1. MATERIALS AND METHODS

The FK and NFK were perfused in the recirculation mode. The perfusate used in this study contained 5% (FK) or 10% (NFK) BSA (fraction V) and amino acids. The tracer [125I]-EGF or [125I]-EGF plus 20 nM unlabeled EGF was added to the reservoir. After the designated sampling times, the perfusate was switched to EGF-free perfusate, and the kidney was washed for 6 min to remove [125I]-EGF remaining in the extracellular space (buffer wash). The 125I activity remaining in the kidney after the buffer wash is the total uptake. Cell-surface-bound and internalized EGF were separated using acid washing. The perfusate was switched to acid buffer (pH 4.0) containing 58 mM NaCl, 4 mM KCl, 2 mM $CaCl_2$, 1.5 mM KH_2PO_4, 2.4 mM $MgSO_4$, 25 mM $NaHCO_3$, and 58 mM CH_3COOH to release cell-surface-bound [125I]-EGF.

2.7.2. RESULTS AND DISCUSSION

In the FK, binding and subsequent internalization take place via both the luminal and antiluminal membranes. The accumulated 125I radioactivity in the renal vein and that in the urinary outflow after acid washing are considered to be the amounts of antiluminal and luminal cell-surface-bound [^{125}I]-EGF, respectively. The ^{125}I radio-activity remaining in the kidney after the acid washing can be regarded as internalized [^{125}I]-EGF.

The NFK was used to investigate the binding on the antiluminal membrane more quantitatively and to evaluate the internalization from the luminal and antiluminal sides separately, since, in the NFK, binding and internalization take place only from the antiluminal side.

The time courses of cell-surface-bound and internalized ^{125}I radioactivity were analyzed based on the compartmental model shown in Fig. 6, assuming that (1) the binding and uptake of [^{125}I]-EGF follow first-order kinetics, (2) the externalization and metabolism of internalized [^{125}I]-EGF can be ignored during the relatively short time period considered, and (3) the single-pass renal extraction ratio of [^{125}I]-EGF in this system is low enough that the [^{125}I]-EGF in the extracelluar space can be approximated to be the same as that in the perfusate. In this experiment the extraction ratio was less than 3% and the latter assumption was validated.

The mass-balance equations for cell-surface-bound [^{125}I]-EGF (LR$_s$) and inter-nalized [^{125}I]-EGF (LR$_i$) are

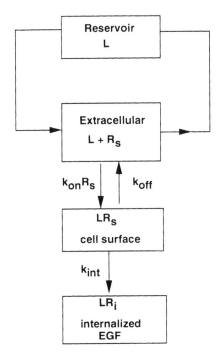

Figure 6. Compartmental model for the renal handling of [^{125}I]-EGF in the NFK. From Kim *et al.* (1991).

$$dLR_s/dt = k_{on} \cdot R_s \cdot L - (k_{off} + k_{int}) \cdot LR_s \qquad (12)$$

$$dLR_i/dt = k_{int} \cdot LR_s \qquad (13)$$

where k_{on} is the association rate constant of EGF with the cell-surface receptor, R_s is the density of the receptors, and k_{off} and k_{int} represent the dissociation rate constant and internalization rate constant, respectively, of the EGF–receptor complex.

The time profiles of LR_s and LR_i were fitted to the above equations using the nonlinear least-squares program Multi (Runge), described by Yamaoka and Nakagawa (1983) and the following parameters were obtained: $k_{on} \cdot R_s = 0.49$ ml min^{-1} (kidney)$^{-1}$, $k_{off} = 0.87$ min^{-1}, and $k_{int} = 0.2$ min^{-1}. We also estimated k_{int} by means of a graphical method using a plot called an "integration plot." By integrating both sides of Eq. (13) from time zero to t, the following equation can be derived:

$$LR_i(t) = k_{int} \int_0^t LR_s \, dt \qquad (14)$$

The plot of LR_i versus $\int_0^t LR_s \, dt$ at various times (Fig. 7) is a straight line passing through the origin, and the slope of the line gives k_{int}. The value of k_{int} obtained by this method was 0.18 min^{-1}, in good agreement with the value obtained from the compartmental analysis.

Finally, internalization via the luminal [LR_i(LM)] and antiluminal [LR_i(ALM)] membrane was calculated by comparing the amount of ^{125}I radioactivity in the NFK and the FK:

$$LR_i(ALM) = LR_i(NFK) \qquad (15)$$

$$LR_i(LM) = LR_i(FK) - LR_i(NFK) \qquad (16)$$

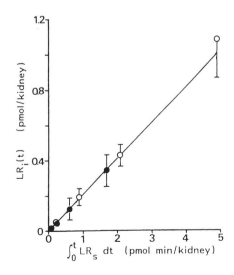

Figure 7. Relationship between internalized EGF and the area under the concentration–time curve (AUC) of cell-surface-bound EGF in the NFK. Internalized EGF at time t (min) is plotted against the AUC of cell-surface-bound EGF from time zero to t (min) according to Eq. (14) (integration plot). Closed and open circles represent results obtained when tracer [^{125}I]-EGF and tracer [^{125}I]-EGF plus 0.5 nM unlabeled EGF, respectively, were perfused. From Kim et al. (1991).

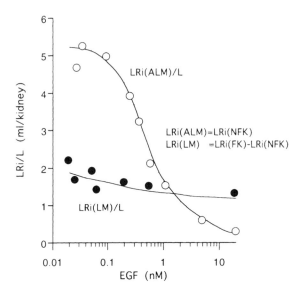

Figure 8. Dependence of the internalization of [^{125}I]-EGF on the concentration of unlabeled EGF in the perfusate. Internalization from the luminal side and from the antiluminal side was calculated from Eqs. (15) and (16), respectively.

Figure 8 shows the luminal and antiluminal internalization at various concentrations of EGF. At low concentrations of EGF, which correspond to the physiological situation, the contribution of the antiluminal uptake was approximately 70%. However, antiluminal internalization decreases dramatically as the concentration of unlabeled EGF increases, and thus nonsaturable luminal internalization may become predominant if EGF concentration increases, for example, in a pathological state.

3. MULTIPLE INDICATOR DILUTION METHOD

We have presented a method for estimating renal clearance using the IPK. However, the parameters obtained under steady-state conditions are hybrids of multiple kinetic parameters. For instance, $CL_{sec,int}$ calculated from Eqs. (6) and (7) is a hybrid of rate constants for the influx from the extracellular space into tubular cells, efflux from the cell to the extracellular space, and sequestration (disappearance by metabolism and/or excretion into urine, etc.).

The multiple indicator dilution (MID) method using the isolated perfused kidney has been a useful tool for investigating capillary permeability, transmembrane transport kinetics, and ligand–receptor kinetics (Chinard *et al.*, 1964, 1965a,b; Crone 1963; Itoh *et al.*, 1986a,b; Silverman *et al.*, 1970a,b, 1981, 1989a,b; Trainor and Silverman, 1982; Whiteside and Silverman, 1983) in the whole kidney, where the organ's structural and spatial architechture are maintained. The basic principle underlying

MID is as follows: (1) A test substance and one or more reference substances are injected simultaneously (in rat kidneys, albumin is used as a plasma reference, and creatinine or sucrose is used as an extracellular reference), (2) the outflow response to the pulse injection of tracers is analyzed at non-steady state; and (3) comparison of the venous or urinary outflow response of a test substance with that of a reference substance yields information on intrarenal events. Lumsden and Silverman (1990) have discussed the hypotheses of MID in detail with regard to techniques, mathematical approaches, and applications.

3.1. Pulse-Injection MID Method Using the Rat IPK

The reference substances for the renal MID are T1824-labeled albumin as a plasma reference (0.7 mg T1824 and 12 mg BSA were added to 0.2 ml of injection solution) and [^{14}C]-creatinine or [^{14}C]-sucrose as the extracelluar reference (0.17 μCi in 0.2 ml of injection solution).

The right kidney of a male Wistar rat is isolated and perfused in a single-pass perfusion mode (see Section 2.1). After 10 min of single-pass preperfusion of unlabeled test compound to achieve steady state, 0.2 ml of the injection solution containing the tracer amount of labeled reference substances and test substance was injected into the silicone tube connecting the arterial cannula and perfusion pump at the site indicated in Fig. 3. Effluent from the venous cannula was collected for 20 sec at 1-sec intervals using a handmade turntable as shown in Fig. 3. T1824 was measured spectrophotometrically (absorbance at 610 nm), and the radioactivity of the radiolabeled compounds was determined using a liquid scintillation spectrometer.

Figure 9 shows the outflow response of T1824-labeled albumin (plasma reference), [^{14}C]-creatinine (extracellular reference), and the test substance, [^{3}H]-cimetidine. Cimetidine is known to undergo active secretion by an organic cation transport system (Lauritsen *et al.*, 1990; Lin *et al.*, 1988). The curves plotted in Fig. 9 are called dilution curves. Note that the values on the abscissa represent the time in seconds. Figure 9 shows that T1824-labeled albumin appeared in the outflow first and then disappeared rapidly compared with the other compounds. The dilution curve for creatinine lies beneath and then crosses over the curve for T1824-labeled albumin. The down slope of the cimetidine curve initially lies under the creatinine curve and later crosses it. These differences arise from the distribution and extraction of the compounds by the renal tubules.

3.2. Analysis of Dilution Curves

Dilution curves are analyzed in model-independent and model-dependent fashions.

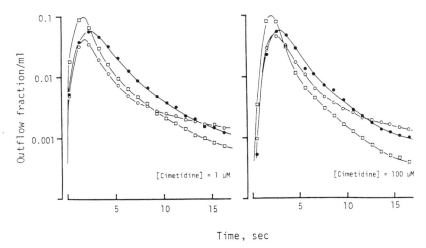

Figure 9. Outflow response of T1824-labeled albumin (plasma reference), [^{14}C]-creatinine (extracellular reference), and [^{3}H]-cimetidine (test compound) in the pulse-injection MID method. Times are corrected for large-vessel transit time. From Itoh *et al.* (1986a).

3.2.1. MODEL-INDEPENDENT PARAMETERS

The mean transit time (MTT) for each material is calculated based on the outflow fraction (C_{out}) during the sampling period:

$$\mathrm{MTT} = \frac{\int_0^T t\, C_{out}(t)\, dt}{\int_0^T C_{out}(t)\, dt} \tag{17}$$

If all the material entering the cells returns to the outflow, the product of the perfusion flow rate (Q) and the mean transit time yields the volume of distribution:

$$V_d = Q \cdot (\mathrm{MTT} - t_o) \tag{18}$$

where t_o is a large-vessel transit time which includes the transit time of the cannula. The renal tubular transport of *p*-aminohippurate (PAH) and tetraethylammomium (TEA) was analyzed by moment analysis of dilution curves (Hori *et al.*, 1988; Kamiya *et al.*, 1990; Saito *et al.*, 1991; Tanigawara *et al.*, 1990). The distribution volumes of eliminated drugs such as PAH and TEA are calculated from the equation

$$V_{d,drug} = (Q \times \mathrm{MTT}_{drug}) + (fu \times \mathrm{CL}_{int} \times \overline{T}_{cell}) \tag{19}$$

where CL_{int} is the apparent tubular secretion intrinsic clearance calculated in Eq. (20), based on the "well-stirred" model [Eq. (6)], from the availability for the tubular transport process [Ftu, Eq. (21)]:

$$fu \times \mathrm{CL}_{int} = Q(1 - Ftu)/Ftu \tag{20}$$

$$F_{tu} = F_{v,drug}/[1 - fu(1 - F_{v,ec})] \qquad (21)$$

where $F_{v,drug}$ and $F_{v,ec}$ are the organ availability for the test compound and the extracellular reference, respectively, which were calculated as the ratio of recovery from venous outflow to total recovery from venous outflow plus urine plus kidney homogenate. $\overline{T}_{cell}$ is the mean residence time in the renal epithelial cell (Fig. 10) and is calculated as follows (Hori *et al.*, 1988):

$$\overline{T}_{cell} = MTT_{u,s} - MTT_{u,g} \qquad (22)$$

where $MTT_{u,s}$ and $MTT_{u,g}$ are the mean transit times for the urinary outflow curve for the secreted and filtered fractions, respectively. Table III shows the effect of probenecid (0–3 mM) on the $\overline{T}_{cell}$ and V_d of PAH. The parameter $\overline{T}_{cell}$ reflects the time required for diffusion in the cytosol and transfer across the luminal membrane

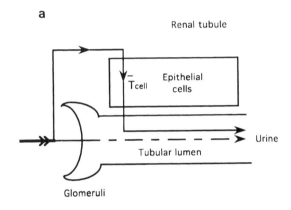

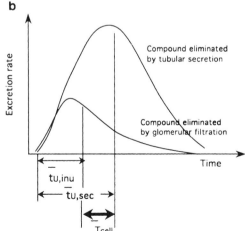

Figure 10. Hypothetical representation of the mean residence time in the renal epithelial cell ($\overline{T}_{cell}$). (a) Renal handling of the secreted and filtered compounds in the single-pass perfusion system. (b) Urinary excretion ratio versus time curve for compounds eliminated by tubular secretion and glomerular filtration. $\overline{t}_{u,inu}$ and $\overline{t}_{u,sec}$ are mean transit times for the urinary outflow curve of the filtered and secreted compounds, respectively. From Tanigawara (1991).

Table III
Effect of Probenecid on the Kinetic Parameters for Tubular Transport
of p-Aminohippurate (PAH): Mean Transit Time for the Renal Vein
Outflow Curve (MTT$_v$), Mean Residence Time in Renal Epithelial
Cells ($\bar{T}_{cell}$), Tubular Secretion Intrinsic Clearance (CL$_{int}$),
and Steady-State Equivalent Volume of Distribution ($V_{d,PAH}$) for PAH
Calculated at the Different Concentrations of Probenecid[a]

Probenecid (mM)	MTT$_v$ (sec)	$\bar{T}_{cell}$ (sec)	CL$_{int}$ (ml/min)	$V_{d,PAH}$ (ml/g)	No. of expts.[b]
0	18.3 ± 0.9[c]	47 ± 7	6.8 ± 0.8	5.8 ± 0.8	6
0.1	14.4 ± 1.4[c]	71 ± 11	3.7 ± 1.0[c]	4.1 ± 0.6	3
1	13.9 ± 1.1[c]	66 ± 14	1.4 ± 0.1[c]	2.5 ± 0.3[c]	3
2	11.0 ± 1.2[c]	90 ± 6	0.4 ± 0.2[c]	1.3 ± 0.3[c]	3
3	8.5 ± 0.7[c]	144 ± 41[c]	0.1 ± 0.0[c]	0.9 ± 0.1[c]	4

[a]From Saito *et al.* (1991).
[b]Number of experiments using different kidney preparations. Each value represents the mean ± SE.
[c]$P < 0.05$ compared with control.

because uptake is a very rapid process (Tanigawara *et al.*, 1990) . On the other hand, the change in antiluminal membrane transport is reflected in $V_{d,drug}$, since the antiluminal transport is a cellular distribution process. Thus, the antiluminal membrane transport is demonstrated as being the rate-limiting step in PAH secretion.

3.2.2. MODEL-DEPENDENT ANALYSIS

The analysis based on mathematical modeling enabled us to estimate separately the kinetic parameters for sets of phenomena underlying renal elimination. Renal tubular secretion consists of three processes: influx from plasma to the tubular cells, efflux from the cells to plasma, and sequestration from the cells. We have applied the MID method to rat kidney (Itoh *et al.*, 1986a,b; Itoh-Okudaira *et al.*, 1987; Sawada *et al.*, 1985), and the rate constants of influx, efflux, and sequestration were separately analyzed based on the mathematical model.

3.3. Mathematical Model

The dilution curves of a test and a reference substance may be compared quantitatively based on the distributed model developed by Goresky and co-workers (Goresky, 1963; Goresky *et al.*, 1970, 1973, 1982, 1983). The kidney is considered to be an assembly of capillaries with the structure shown in Fig. 11. The capillary consists of three compartments: plasma space, extracelluar space, and cellular space. The assumptions made in the development of the model are as follows:

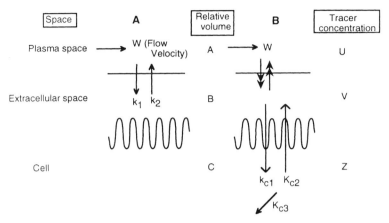

Figure 11. Kinetic models used in the analysis of dilution curves. (A) Model for the estimation of capillary permeability. (B) Model for the estimation of tubular secretion parameters. Arrows show directions of flow and transport of substances. Double arrows show flow-limited distribution. From Itoh *et al.* (1986a).

1. Flow is confined to the vascular compartment A.
2. Diffusion along the length of compartments A and B is zero.
3. Diffusible substances in the plasma space undergo flow-limited distribution into the extracellular space.
4. The equilibration time of the diffusible substance in the lateral direction has a negligible effect on the capillary transit time.
5. The secretory parameters (K_{c1}, K_{c2}, and K_{c3}) are constant throughout the cortex of the kidney.
6. Large-vessel transit time (t_0) is uniform.
7. Renal reabsorption of the test compound is ignored.
8. Metabolism of the test compound is negligible.

In the IPK, the injected materials undergo glomerular filtration before they reach the entrance of the proximal tubule. However, the changes in concentration due to the process of glomerular filtration and the glomerular transit time were calculated to be negligible (Itoh *et al.*, 1986a).

According to the model, the outflow response of the test substance from the whole kidney is described by

$$
\begin{aligned}
C_{\text{drug}}(t') = \exp(K_{C1} \cdot t') \cdot C_{\text{ec}}(t') + \{\exp[-(K_{C2} + K_{C3}) \cdot t'] \\
\times \int_0^{t'} \exp[(-K_{C1} - K_{C2} - K_{C3}) \cdot \tau'] \cdot C_{\text{ec}}(\tau') \cdot \sqrt{\frac{K_{C1} \cdot K_{C2} \cdot \tau'}{t - \tau'}} \\
\times I_1[2\sqrt{K_{C1} \cdot K_{C2} \cdot \tau' \cdot (t - \tau')}] \, d\tau'\}
\end{aligned}
\tag{23}
$$

where

$$K_{Cl} = k_{cl} \cdot \theta/(1 + \gamma)$$

k_{cl} is the rate constant for influx from the extracellular space to the cellular space, K_{c2} and K_{c3} are the rate constants for efflux and sequestration, respectively, from the cellular space to the luminal side, t_o represents the large-vessel transit times, and θ and γ are the ratios of the cellular and the extracellular space, respectively, to the capillary space. Using the distribution volumes of T1824-labeled albumin and [^{14}C]-creatinine, the parameter γ in Eqs. (23) and (24) was calculated to be 0.78 (Itoh *et al.*, 1986a).

3.3.1. SECRETORY PARAMETERS

By fitting the outflow curves of the extracellular reference and the test substance to Eq. (23), the parameters K_{cl}, K_{c2}, and K_{c3} are obtained. A rough estimate of K_{cl} can be obtained from the natural logarithmic plot of the ratio $[C(t')_{ec}/C(t')_{test}]$ versus time, since when t' is small, the second term in Eq. (23) is negligible, and the initial slope of the plot of $\log [C(t')_{ec}/C(t')_{test}]$ versus time equals K_{cl}. This plot is known as the ratio plot.

3.3.2. CLEARANCE

Influx, efflux, and sequestration clearances (expressed as milliliters per minute per gram of kidney) were calculated using Eqs. (25)–(27). A value of 1.56 for Θ (Chinard *et al.*, 1964) was used for the calculation.

$$CL_{int,1} = K_{cl} \times V_{d,creatine} \tag{25}$$

$$CL_{int,2} = K_{c2} \times V_{d,albumin} \times \theta \tag{26}$$

$$CL_{int,3} = K_{c3} \times V_{d,albumin} \times \theta \tag{27}$$

The apparent secretion intrinsic clearance ($CL_{int,app}$) can be calculated as

$$CL_{int,app} = \frac{CL_{int,1} \times CL_{int,3}}{CL_{int,2} + CL_{int,3}} \tag{28}$$

3.4. Estimation of Capillary Permeability

Capillary permeability was estimated by the same approach (Itoh *et al.*, 1986a; Trainor and Silverman, 1982). In this case, the rate constants for influx from plasma into extracellular space and efflux from extracellular space back to plasma were estimated based on the model shown in Fig. 11A.

The permeability clearance of creatinine in the rat IPK was estimated to be five times the perfusion flow rate, whereas that of inulin was comparable to the perfusion flow rate. Therefore, we chose creatinine rather than inulin as the extracellular reference for the kinetic analysis of tubular secretion by the MID method.

3.5. Application: Kinetic Analysis of the Renal Tubular Secretion of Organic Anions and Cations by the MID Method Combined with a Mathematical Model

We have applied the MID method to investigate the renal tubular secretion of cimetidine in isolated perfused rat kidney (Itoh *et al.*, 1986a,b; Itoh-Okudaira *et al.*, 1987; Sawada *et al.*, 1985). Cimetidine, a histamine H_2-receptor antagonist, undergoes tubular secretion by an organic cation transport system; it is also partly eliminated by metabolism (Lauritsen *et al.*, 1990). However, the MID method detects a process whose time frame is on the order of seconds, and thus the metabolism during a single run (usually 20 sec) can be ignored.

3.5.1. MATERIALS AND METHODS

The FK was perfused in the single-pass mode with perfusate containing 6% BSA, 0.2 mg creatinine/ml, and 1–1000 μM unlabeled cimetidine. The IPK was placed on the apparatus, and 0.2 ml of a solution containing 0.7 mg of T1824, 12 mg of BSA, and 0.17 μCi of [^{14}C]-creatinine in 0.2 ml was injected. The effluent was collected at 1-sec intervals for 20 sec. Each kidney received 1–4 injections at different concentrations of unlabeled cimetidine. After each switch to perfusate of a different cimetidine concentration, the kidney was perfused for 10 min to obtain the new steady state.

3.5.2. RESULTS AND DISCUSSION

By computer fitting the data to Eq. (23), the influx, efflux, and sequestration rate constants were obtained. The data indicated saturation of the influx process as the concentration of cimetidine in the perfusate increased.

Using Eqs. (25)–(27), the intrinsic clearance of each process was calculated, and the contribution of each process was evaluated separately. The change in influx rate constant is manifested in the dilution curves and ratio plots as follows. Comparing the two sets of dilution curves shown in Fig. 9, representing input concentrations of cimetidine of 1 μM (left) and 100 μM (right), the curve for cimetidine remained closer to the curve for creatine at the higher concentration (right). The initial slope of the ratio plot decreased as the cimetidine concentration increased (Fig. 12).

The parameters obtained were compared with the secretory parameters obtained

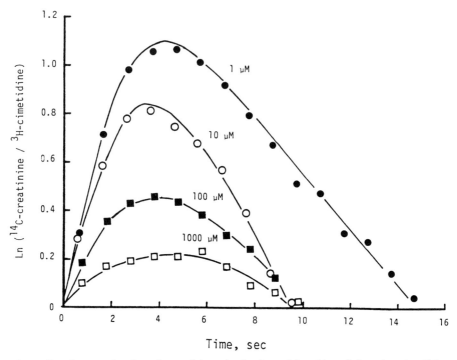

Figure 12. Concentration dependence of the ratio plot (natural logarithm of the ratio extracellular reference/test compound vs. time plot). The concentration of unlabeled cimetidine in the perfusate varied from 1 to 1000 μM. From Itoh *et al.* (1986a).

in vivo. First, assuming that cimetidine does not distribute in erythrocytes, the secretion clearance (CL_{sec}) was calculated to be 3.9 ml/min according to Eq. (29) below. The values of the parameters used in the calculation for a 250-g rat were as follows: $CL_{int,app}$, 10 ml min^{-1} (g kidney)$^{-1}$ [Eq. (28)]; kidney weight, 2.0 g; plasma flow rate (Fp), 5.1 ml/min (Iga *et al.*, 1985); and GFR, 2.0 ml/min (Adolph, 1949). The unbound fraction in rat plasma was assumed to be equal to that in the perfusate (0.826; Itoh *et al.*, 1986).

$$CL_{sec} = Fp \times fu \times CL_{int,app}/[Fp + (fu \times CL_{int,app})] \tag{29}$$

Assuming that reabsorption is negligible, the ratio of CL_R(GFR × fu + CL_{sec}) to GFR was calculated to be 2.8, which is comparable to the value reported by Weiner and Roth (1981), who determined this ratio *in vivo* in rats at low plasma concentrations of cimetidine (2 μg/ml).

Finally, we have attempted to explain the parameters in terms of the transport processes across antiluminal and luminal membranes (ALM and LM, respectively). In the tubular transport model used in the MID analysis, influx and efflux are considered to reflect the transport process across the ALM. The sequestration includes any process resulting in disappearance from the cellular compartment except efflux back to the extracellular space. If a tracer is metabolized or incorporated into an intracellular deep compartment and does not appear in the outflow during a sample collection period, those processes are estimated as sequestration. However, the metabolism of cimetidine is negligible during the 20-sec duration of the experiment, and distribution in an intracellular deep compartment is improbable. Therefore, the sequestration process was considered to be transport across the brush border membrane (BBM) into the lumen. To evaluate the transport kinetics across the membrane, protein binding in the perfusate and the tissue were corrected for, and the rate constants for unbound cimetidine were plotted as a function of unbound drug concentration in the extracellular or intracellular space (Fig. 13; Itoh *et al.*, 1986a). A concentration dependence was noted for the influx and sequestration rate constants. Kinetic analysis (equations are shown in Fig. 13) suggested that the affinity of the saturable portion of transport across the BBM was much higher and the contribution of passive diffusion was greater than for transport across the basolateral membrane. In a study of the transport of cimetidine in the BBM vesicles isolated from rabbit renal cortex, Gisclon *et al.* (1987) observed the existence of a saturable process with high affinity and a nonsaturable process, although their estimate of K_m value was higher than the value that we obtained in the IPK.

4. ADVANTAGES AND DISADVANTAGES OF THE IPK

Compared with the *in vivo* clearance technique, the IPK technique using an artificial perfusate allows investigators to analyze renal elimination in a system free from nonrenal factors. The effects of the nervous system and hormones can be excluded in the IPK. If the kidney is perfused in the single-pass mode, the effect of metabolites formed in the kidney is also eliminated. Furthermore, compounds can be added to the perfusate at chosen concentrations, and the analysis can be performed at steady state, which is advantageous for the kinetic analysis of renal excretion. For the same experiment to be performed *in vivo*, the pharmacokinetic properties of the compounds must be taken into consideration to achieve the desired concentrations, compounds with systemic toxicity must be avoided, and those with pharmacological action make the analysis complicated.

We have illustrated the usefulness of the IPK, not only in determining renal clearance, but also in the investigation of uptake and transport mechanisms. Recently, various new methods have been developed to study renal transport processes (Giacomini *et al.*, 1988). In particular, isolated tubules, isolated membrane vesicles, and cell culture techniques are powerful tools for investigating the kinetics and mechanism of renal uptake mediated by carrier proteins and receptors (see Chapter 11). Isolated membrane vesicles allow the analysis of transport systems on each mem

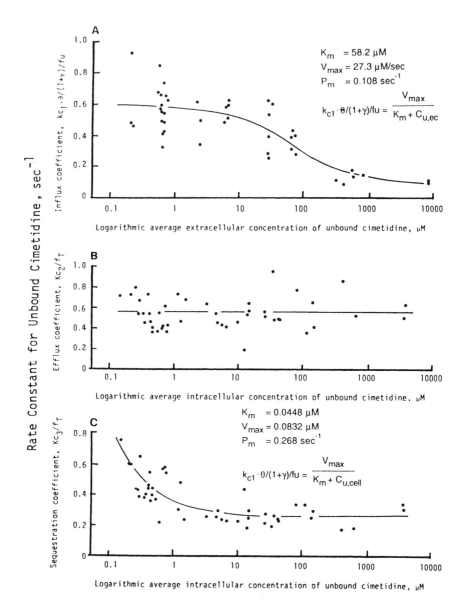

Rate Constant for Unbound Cimetidine, sec^{-1}

A

Influx coefficient, $k_{c1} \cdot \theta/(1+\gamma)/f_u$

$K_m = 58.2 \ \mu M$
$V_{max} = 27.3 \ \mu M/sec$
$P_m = 0.108 \ sec^{-1}$

$$k_{c1} \cdot \theta/(1+\gamma)/f_u = \frac{V_{max}}{K_m + C_{u,ec}}$$

Logarithmic average extracellular concentration of unbound cimetidine, μM

B

Efflux coefficient, k_{c2}/f_T

Logarithmic average intracellular concentration of unbound cimetidine, μM

C

Sequestration coefficient, k_{c3}/f_T

$K_m = 0.0448 \ \mu M$
$V_{max} = 0.0832 \ \mu M$
$P_m = 0.268 \ sec^{-1}$

$$k_{c1} \cdot \theta/(1+\gamma)/f_u = \frac{V_{max}}{K_m + C_{u,cell}}$$

Logarithmic average intracellular concentration of unbound cimetidine, μM

brane separately without the need to take into account the effects of undesired factors, and the composition of the medium inside and outside the vesicles can be modified. These techniques have clarified various mechanisms of membrane transport systems. Monoclonal cell lines provide information about the transport system in a homogeneous population of a single cell type. However, the kidney is an assembly of heterogeneous cells which are highly structured in order to function effectively, and these *in vitro* systems are too simplified to permit the data obtained to be extrapolated quantitatively to *in vivo* situations. The advantage of the IPK over these *in vitro* systems is that the IPK preserves the structural and functional integrity of the organ. As shown in this chapter, by using the IPK, we can quantitatively predict how the transport mechanism observed *in vitro* works *in vivo*.

There are some disadvantages associated with the IPK. First of all, preparation of the IPK is not easy. Although the surgical procedure was designed to prevent interruption of the blood flow into the kidney during preparation, rapid handling is required for better viability. As discussed by Maack (1986), the IPK tends to be in a hypoxic condition, especially when it is perfused with cell-free medium. Thus,the viability must be checked carefully to ensure that the process in question is functioning satisfactorily in the system. Finally, when the IPK is used in pharmacokinetic studies, one must always take into consideration that some hemodynamic parameters, such as GFR and urine flow rate, are easily modified by the conditions of perfusion. To obtain meaningful information, an appropriate perfusion system needs to be selected, and the data obtained must be carefully analyzed.

←——

Figure 13. Relationship between rate constants for unbound cimetidine and the average extracellular or intracellular concentration of unbound cimetidine: (A) influx rate constant; (B) efflux rate constant; and (C) sequestration rate constant. Using the area under the concentration–time curves (AUC) of cimetidine (AUC_{CMD}), albumin (AUC_{alb}), and creatinine (AUC_{cre}), the availability of tubular secretion (Ftu) and the extracellular drug concentrations at the inlet ($C_{ec,in}$) and outlet ($C_{ec,out}$) of the proximal tubules under the steady-state condition are described by the following equations:

$$Ftu = (AUC_{CMD}/AUC_{alb}) \cdot (AUC_{alb}/AUC_{cre})^{fu}$$
$$C_{ec,in} = C_R \times (AUC_{alb}/AUC_{cre})$$
$$C_{ec,out} = C_{ec,in} \times Ftu$$

The concentration in the intracellular space is calculated using the influx, efflux, and sequestration rate constants (see text) as

$$C_{cell} = C_{ec} \cdot k_{c1}/(K_{c2} + K_{c3})$$

The logarithmic average concentrations of unbound cimetidine in the extracellular and intracellular space are described by the following equations:

$$Cu_{ec} = fu \times (C_{ec,in} - C_{ec,out})/[\ln(C_{ec,\,in}/C_{ec,out})]$$
$$Cu_{cell} = f_T \times (C_{cell,in} - C_{cell,out})/[\ln(C_{cell,in}/C_{cell,out})]$$

where f_T is the unbound fraction in the homogenate of renal cortex. From Itoh *et al.* (1986a).

ACKNOWLEDGMENTS

We would like to express our great thanks to Dr. Yasufumi Sawada, Tatsuji Iga, Manabu Hanano, and Dong-Chool Kim for their important roles in establishing the IPK systems in the Department of Biopharmaceutics, Faculty of Pharmaceutical Sciences, University of Tokyo.

REFERENCES

Acara, M., and Rennick, B., 1973, Regulation of plasma choline by the renal tubule: Bidirectional transport of choline, *Am. J. Physiol.* **225:**1123–1128.

Adolph, E. F., 1949, Quantitative relations in the physiological constitutions of mammals, *Science* **109:**579.

Chinard, F. P., Enns, T., and Nolan, M. F., 1964, Arterial hematocrit and separation of cells and plasma in the dog kidney, *Am. J. Physiol.* **207:**128–132.

Chinard, F. P., Enns, T., Goresky, C. A., and Nolan, M. F., 1965a, Renal transit times and distribution volumes of T-1824, creatinine and water, *Am. J. Physiol.* **209:**243–252.

Chinard, F. P., Goresky, C. A., Enns, T., Nolan, M. F., and House, R. W., 1965b, Trapping of urea by red cells in the kidney, *Am. J. Physiol.* **209:**253–263.

Crone, C., 1963, The permeability of capillaries in various organs as determined by use of the indicator diffusion methods, *Acta Physiol. Scand.* **58:**292–305.

Fisher, D., Salido, E., and Barajas, L., 1989, Epidermal growth factor and the kidney, *Annu. Rev. Physiol.* **51:**67–80.

Giacomini, K. M., Hsyu, P. H., and Gisclon, L. G., 1988, Renal transport of drugs: An overview of methodology with application to cimetidine, *Pharm. Res.* **5:**465–471.

Gisclon, L., Wong, F. M., and Giacomini, K. M., 1987, Cimetidine transport in isolated luminal membrane vesicles from rabbit kidney, *Am. J. Physiol.* **253:**F141–F150.

Goresky, C. A., 1963, A linear method for determining liver sinusoidal and extravascular volumes, *Am. J. Physiol.* **204:**626–640.

Goresky, C. A., Ziegler, W. H., and Bach, G. G., 1970, Capillary exchange modeling: Barrier-limited and flow-limited distribution, *Circ. Res.* **27:**739–764.

Goresky, C. A., Bach, G. G., and Nadeau, B. E., 1973, On the uptake of materials by the intact liver: The transport and net removal of galactose, *J. Clin. Invest.* **52:**991–1009.

Goresky, C. A., Huet, P. M., and Villeneuve, J. P., 1982, Blood–tissue exchange and blood flow in the liver, in: *Hepatology: A Textbook of Liver Disease* (D. Zakin and T. Boyer, eds.), W. B. Saunders, Philadelphia, pp. 32–63.

Goresky, C. A., Bach, G. G., and Rose, C. P., 1983, Effects of saturating metabolic uptake on space profiles and tracer kinetics, *Am. J. Physiol.* **244:**G215–G232.

Hall, S., and Rowland, M., 1983, Relationship between renal clearance, protein binding and urine flow for digitoxin, a compound of low clearance in the isolated perfused rat kidney, *J. Pharmacol. Exp. Ther.* **227:**174–179.

Hall, S., and Rowland, M., 1985, Influence of fraction unbound upon the renal clearance of furosemide in the isolated perfused rat kidney, *J. Pharmacol. Exp. Ther.* **232:**263–268.

Hori, R., Tanigawara, Y., Saito, Y., Hayashi, Y., Aiba, T., Okumura, K., and Kamiya, A., 1988, Moment analysis of drug disposition in kidney: Transcellular transport kinetics of *p*-aminohippurate in the isolated perfused rat kidney, *J. Pharm. Sci.* **77:**471–476.

Iga, T., Sawada, Y., and Sugiyama, Y., 1985, Physiological pharmacokinetics, in: *Applied Pharmaco-kinetics—Theory and Experiments* (M. Hanano, K. Umemura, and T. Iga, eds.), Soft Science, Inc., Tokyo, pp. 431–473.

Itoh, N., Sawada, Y., Sugiyama, Y., Iga, T., and Hanano, M., 1986a, Kinetic analysis of rat renal tubular transport based on multiple-indicator dilution method, *Am. J. Physiol.* **251**:F103–F114.

Itoh, N., Sawada, Y., Sugiyama, Y., Iga, T., and Hanano, M., 1986b, Na^+- dependent *p*-aminohippurate transport at the basolateral side of the isolated perfused rat kidney, *Biochim. Biophys. Acta* **860**: 592–599.

Itoh-Okudaira, N., Sawada, Y., Sugiyama, Y., Iga, T., and Hanano, M., 1987, Effect of procainamide on renal transport of cimetidine in the isolated perfused kidney, *Biochim. Biophys. Acta* **981**:1–7.

Johnson, V., and Maack, T., 1977, Renal extraction, filtration, absorption and catabolism of growth hormone, *Am. J. Physiol.* **233**:F185–F196.

Kamiya, A., Tanigawara, Y., Saito, Y., Hayashi, Y., Aiba, T., Inui, K., and Hori, R., 1990, Moment analysis of drug disposition in kidney: II: Urine pH-dependent tubular secretion, *J. Pharm. Sci.* **79**:692–697.

Kau, S. T., 1978, Handling of triamterene by the isolated perfused rat kidney, *J. Pharmacol. Exp. Ther.* **206**:701–709.

Kau, S. T., and Maack, T., 1977, Transport and catabolism of parathyroid hormone in isolated rat kidney, *Am. J. Physiol.* **233**:F445–F454.

Kim, D. C., Sugiyama, Y., Sato, H., Fuwa, T., Iga, T., and Hanano, M., 1988, Kinetic analysis of *in vivo* receptor dependent binding of human epidermal growth factor by rat tissues, *J. Pharm. Sci.* **77**: 200–207.

Kim, D. C., Sugiyama, Y., Fuwa, T., Sakamoto, S., Iga, T., and Hanano, M., 1989, Kinetic analysis of the elimination process of human epidermal growth factor (hEGF) in rats, *Biochem. Pharmacol.* **38**: 241–249.

Kim, D. C., Hanano, M., Sawada, Y., Iga, T., and Sugiyama, Y., 1991, Kinetic analysis of clearance of epidermal growth factor in isolated perfused kidney, *Am. J. Physiol.* **261**:F988–F997.

Kim, D. C., Hanano, M., Yanai, Y., Ohnuma, N., and Sugiyama, Y., 1992a, Localization of binding sites for epidermal growth factor (EGF) in rat kidney: Evidence for the existence of low affinity EGF binding sites on the brush border membrane, *Pharm. Res.* **9**:1394–1401.

Kim, D. C., Sugiyama, Y., Sawada, Y., and Hanano, M., 1992b, Renal tubular handling of *p*-aminohippurate and epidermal growth factor (EGF) in filtering and nonfiltering perfused rat kidneys, *Pharm. Res.* **9**:271–275.

Lauritsen, K., Laursen, L. S., and Rask-Madsen, J., 1990, Clinical pharmacokinetics of drugs used in the treatment of gastrointestinal disease (Part 1), *Clin. Pharmacokinet.* **19**:11–31.

Lin, J. H., Los, L. E., Ulm, E. H., and Duggan, D. E., 1988, Kinetic studies on the competition between famotidine and cimetidine in rats: Evidence of multiple secretory systems for organic cations, *Drug Metab. Dispos.* **16**:52–56.

Lumsden, B. J., and Silverman, M., 1990, Multiple indicator dilution and the kidney: Kinetics, permeation and transport *in vivo, Methods Enzymol.* **191**:34–72.

Maack, T., 1980, Physiological evaluation of the isolated perfused rat kidney, *Am. J. Physiol.* **238**:F71–F78.

Maack, T., 1986, Renal clearance and isolated kidney perfusion techniques, *Kidney Int.* **30**:142–151.

Muirhead, M. R., and Somogyi, A. A., 1991, Effect of H_2 antagonists on the differential secretion of triamterene and its sulfate conjugate metabolite by the isolated perfused rat kidney, *Drug Metab. Dispos.* **19**:312–316.

Nishitsutsuji-Uwo, J. M., Ross, B. D., and Krebs, H. A., 1967, Metabolic activities of the isolated perfused rat kidney, *Biochem. J.* **103**:852–862.

Pang, K. S., and Rowland, M., 1977, Hepatic clearance of drugs: I. Theoretical considerations of a "well-stirred" model and a "parallel-tube" model. Influence of hepatic blood flow, plasma and blood cell binding and the hepatocellular enzymatic activity on hepatic drug clearance, *J. Pharmacokinet. Biopharm.* **5**:625–653.

Petersen, J., Kitaji, J., Duckworth, W. C., and Rabkin, R., 1982, Fate of ^{125}I-insulin from the peritubular circulation of isolated perfused rat kidney, *Am. J. Physiol.* **243**:F126–F132.

Pritchard, J. B., and Miller, D. S., 1993, Mechanisms mediating renal secretion of organic anions and cations, *Physiol. Rev.* **73**:765–796.

Saito, Y., Tanigawara, Y., Okumura, K., Shimizu, H., Kamiya, A., and Hori, R., 1991, Moment analysis of drug disposition in rat kidney: Role of basolateral membrane transport of p-aminohippurate, *J. Pharm. Pharmacol.* **43**:311–316.

Sawada, Y., Itoh, N., Sugiyama, Y., Iga, T. and Hanano, M., 1985, Analysis of multiple indicator dilution curves for estimation of renal tubular transport parameters, *Comput. Prog. Biomed.* **20**:51–61.

Scoggins, B. A., Butkus, A., Coghlan, J. P., Fei, D. T. W., McDougall, J. G., Niall, H. D., Walsh, J. R., and Wang, X., 1984, *In vivo* cardiovascular renal and endocrine effects of epidermal growth factor in sheep, in: *Endocrinology* (F. Labrie and L. Prouix, eds.), Elsevier, New York, pp. 573–575.

Silva, P., 1990, Isolated perfused and nonfiltering kidney, *Methods Enzymol.* **191**:31–34.

Silverman, M., Aganon, M. A., and Chinard, F. P., 1970a, D-Glucose interactions with renal tubule cell surfaces, *Am. J. Physiol.* **218**:735–742.

Silverman, M., Aganon, M. A., and Chinard, F. P., 1970b, Specificity of monosaccharide transport in dog kidney, *Am. J. Physiol.* **218**:743–750.

Silverman, M., Vinary, P., Shinobu, L., Gougoux, A., and Lemieux, G., 1981, Luminal and antiluminal transport of glutamine in dog kidney, *Kidney Int.* **20**:359–365.

Silverman, M., Whiteside, C., and Trainor, C., 1989a, Glomerular and postglomerular transcapillary exchange in dog kidney, *Fed. Proc.* **43**:171–179.

Silverman, M., Whiteside, C., Lumsden, C. J., and Steinhart, H., 1989b, *In vivo* indicator dilution kinetics of PAH transport in dog kidney, *Am. J. Physiol.* **256**:F255–F265.

Sugiyama, Y., 1991, Kinetics of receptor-mediated endocytosis of polypeptide hormones that governs the overall hormone disposition in the body: Analysis of the uptake process of epidermal growth factor by the liver and kidney, *Yakugaku Zasshi* **111**:709–736.

Sugiyama, Y., Kim, D. C., Sato, H., Yanai, S., Satoh, H., Iga, T., and Hanano, M., 1990, Receptor-mediated disposition of polypeptides: Kinetic analysis of the isolated perfused organs and *in vivo* system, *J. Controlled Release* **13**:157–174.

Suzuki, M., Almeida, F. A., Nussenzveig, D. R., Sawyer, D., and Maack, T., 1987, Binding and functional effect of atrial natriuretic factor in isolated rat kidney, *Am. J. Physiol.* **353**:F917–F928.

Tanigawara, Y., 1991, Moment analysis, in: *Modern Biopharmaceutics* (S. Awazu and T. Koizumi, eds.), Nanko-do, Tokyo, pp. 257–282.

Tanigawara, Y., Saito, Y., Aiba, T., Ohoka, K., Kamiya, A., and Hori, R., 1990, Moment analysis of drug disposition in kidney. III: Transport of p-aminohippurate and tetraethylammonium in the perfused kidney isolated from uranyl nitrate-induced acute renal failure rats, *J. Pharm. Sci.* **79**:249–256.

Trainor, C., and Silverman, M., 1982, Transcapillary exchange of molecular weight markers in the postglomerular circulation: Application of a barrier-limited model, *Am. J. Physiol.* **242**:F436–F446.

Weiner, I. M., and Roth, L., 1981, Renal excretion of cimetidine, *J. Pharmacol. Exp. Ther.* **216**:516–520.

Whiteside, C., and Silverman, M., 1983, Determination of glomerular permselectivity to neutral dextrans in the dog, *Am. J. Physiol.* **245**:F485–F495.

Wright, S. H., Wunz, T. M., and Wunz, T. P., 1992, A choline transporter in renal brush-border membrane vesicles: Energetics and structural specificity, *J. Membr. Biol.* **126**:51–65.

Yamaoka, K., and Nakagawa, T., 1983, A nonlinear least squares program based on differential equations, Multi (Runge), for microcomputers, *J. Pharmacobio.-Dyn.* **6**:595–606.

Zins, G. R., and Weiner, I. M., 1968, Bidirectional urate transport limited to the proximal tubule in dogs, *Am. J. Physiol.* **215**:411–422.

Chapter 13

Brain Microvessel Endothelial
Cell Culture Systems

*Kenneth L. Audus, Lawrence Ng, Wen Wang,
and Ronald T. Borchardt*

1. INTRODUCTION

The cellular basis of the blood–brain barrier (BBB) was defined as the endothelial lining of the brain microvessels in the late 1960s (Reese and Karnovsky, 1967; Brightman and Reese, 1969). This unique endothelial lining was recognized as the sole restrictive permeability barrier to the passage of nutrients, drugs, and metabolic waste products between the blood and the central nervous system. Consequently, investigations on the BBB have focused on developing an understanding of the transport and functional properties of this specialized endothelium (Bradbury, 1993).

The first cell culture system representing brain microvessel endothelium was described in 1978 (Panula *et al.*, 1978). Since that time, a variety of primary and passaged cell culture systems have been described in the literature (Joo, 1992). This chapter describes the establishment of a primary culture system that has been employed in one configuration or another by a number of research groups to study BBB transport and metabolic functions. The isolation and seeding methods for this system are based on the original protocol of Bowman *et al.* (1983) and have also been described in less detail in other formats (Audus and Borchardt, 1986, 1987; Miller *et al.*, 1992). Included in this chapter are summaries of potential pharmaceutical

Kenneth L. Audus, Lawrence Ng, Wen Wang, and Ronald T. Borchardt • Department of Pharmaceutical Chemistry, The University of Kansas, Lawrence, Kansas 66045.

Models for Assessing Drug Absorption and Metabolism, Ronald T. Borchardt *et al.*, eds., Plenum Press, New York, 1996.

applications and some of the advantages and disadvantages of the primary and related brain microvessel endothelial cell (BMEC) monolayer culture systems.

2. METHODS

2.1. Materials

Minimum essential medium (MEM) and Ham's F-12 medium were purchased from either Fisher or JR Scientific, dispase and collagenase/dispase were obtained from Boehringer Mannheim, and endothelial cell growth supplement (ECGS, from bovine neural tissue) and rat tail collagen were from Collaborative Biomedical Products; other chemicals and reagents were obtained from Sigma. All preparations are made up in either glass distilled or Milli-Q filtered water.

2.2. Solutions and Reagents

All of the solutions are made in advance, sterile filtered, and stored under refrigeration unless specifically indicated in the text.

MEM, pH 7.4: 9.5 mg MEM/ml, 11.92 mg HEPES/ml, 50 μg gentamicin/ml, 50 μg polymixin B/ml, 2.5 μg amphotericin B/ml.

MEM 3X, pH 7.4: MEM, pH 7.4, containing penicillin G (300 μg/ml) and streptomycin (300 μg/ml).

MEM, pH 9.4: 9.5 mg MEM/ml, 11.92 mg HEPES/ml, 50 μg gentamicin/ml, 50 μg polymixin B/ml, 2.5 μg amphotericin B/ml.

10X MEM: 95 mg MEM/ml. Autoclave the solution and store in the refrigerator.

1 M HEPES, pH 7.6.

12.5% dispase: Add 2.5 g of dispase to 20 ml of MEM, pH 7.4, in a 50-ml disposable centrifuge tube, and incubate the tube for 30 min in a 37°C water bath with constant shaking. Centrifuge the solution for 30 min in a DYNAC centrifuge (Becton Dickinson and Co., Parsippany, NJ) at maximum speed (setting of 100). Sterile filter the supernatant, and store the filtrate in the freezer. Thaw the dispase solution immediately prior use.

4-mg/ml collagenase/dispase: Add 20 mg of collagenase/dispase to 5 ml of MEM, pH 7.4, in a 15-ml disposable centrifuge tube, and incubate the mixture for 30 min in a 37°C water bath with constant shaking. Sterile filter the solution, and store the filtrate in the freezer. Thaw it immediately before use.

13% dextran: Dissolve 65 g of dextran (average molecular weight 71,000) in 422 ml of water; then autoclave the solution. After the dextran solution is cool, add 50 ml of 10X MEM and 25 ml of 1M HEPES, pH 7.6, and add polymixin B, gentamicin, and amphotericin B to final concentrations of 50, 40, and 2.5 μg/ml, respectively.

50% Percoll: Mix 75 ml of Percoll with 52 ml of sterile water, 15 ml of 10X MEM, and 7.5 ml of 1 M HEPES, pH 7.6, and add polymixin B, gentamicin, and amphotericin B to final concentrations of 50, 40, and 2.5 µg/ml, respectively. MEM-F12, pH 7.4: 4.75 mg MEM/ml, 5.3 mg F-12/ml, 2.58 mg HEPES/ml, 1.09 mg sodium bicarbonate/ml, 50 µg gentamicin/ml.

Freezing medium: MEM-F12 medium containing 20% platelet-poor horse serum and 10% dimethyl sulfoxide (DMSO).

BMEC culture medium: MEM-F12 medium containing 10% platelet-poor horse serum, 125 µg heparin/ml, and 25 µg ECGS/ml. Addition of the endothelial cell growth supplement is optional, and researchers are advised to characterize the effects of the supplement on the cells.

Collagen coating solution: A commercially purchased 1-mg/ml solution of rat tail collagen in 60% ethanol may be used. Alternatively, collagen strands may be removed from 3–4 rat tails, sterilized under UV light for 24 hr, suspended in 0.1% aqueous acetic acid at a concentration of 3 mg/ml, and stirred at 4°C for 48 hr. The resulting suspension is centrifuged at $100 \times g$ for 10 min, and then the supernatant is decanted and stored in a refrigerator.

Fibronectin coating solution: 0.04-mg/ml solution of either bovine or human fibronectin in MEM-F12.

2.3. Brain Microvessel Isolation

The method described here for the isolation of brain microvessels is essentially based on the procedures developed by Bowman *et al.* (1983) and, subsequently, Audus and Borchardt (1986, 1987), with minor modifications. The key modifications to the original Bowman method include changes in times of incubation for cells with enzymes and quantitatively defining the amount of the enzyme (collagenase/dispase) required for enzymatic digestion of microvessels to help ensure the successful and consistent isolation of a pure population of healthy BMECs. Figure 1 outlines the general protocol for the isolation of the BMECs, which includes collection of brain gray matter, enzymatic treatment of the gray matter and differential centrifugation to separate microvessels from neural tissues, removal of the basement membrane and pericytes, and separation of contaminated cells and cell debris from the microvessels. Although this protocol was originally designed for isolating brain microvessels from a bovine brain, it can be applied to isolate brain microvessels from other species (Shi and Audus, 1994). The detailed procedure for the isolation of microvessels from bovine brain is as follows:

(a) Obtain two or three fresh bovine brains from a local slaughterhouse, place them in ice-cold MEM 3X, pH 7.4, immediately, and transport to the laboratory on wet ice. All the subsequent procedures for collecting brain gray matter are then performed preferably on ice in a laminar flow hood and under aseptic conditions.

(b) Transfer the brains to a sterile beaker containing cold MEM 3X. Cut away

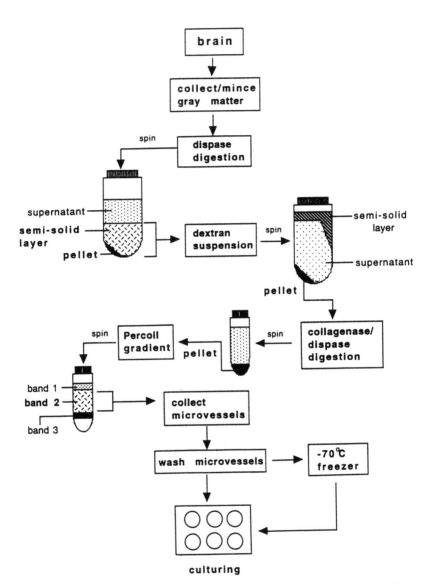

Figure 1.   General scheme for isolating and culturing brain microvessel endothelial cells.

the brain stems and the cerebellums. Remove brain surface vessels and outer membrane (meninges) with hands or a pair of forceps. Transfer the cleaned brains to another beaker containing cold MEM, pH 7.4.

(c) Scrape the gray matter from the brain using a sterile surgical blade or a sterile razor blade. Collect the gray matter in a sterile beaker containing approximately 50 ml of ice-cold MEM, pH 7.4.

(d) Mince the gray matter into 1- to 2-mm cubes with a sterile multirazor blade (5 razor blades glued together). Collect the minced gray matter into a 500-ml preweighed sterile Nalgene bottle. Remove the excess MEM from the bottle and weigh the gray matter. We usually can get approximately 250–300 g of wet gray matter from two brains. The procedure was optimized for 250 g of wet tissue.

(e) Add 12.5% dispase to the minced gray matter at a ratio of 4 ml of dispase per 50 g of gray matter, and incubate for 30 min in a 37°C shaker water bath at about 100 oscillations/min. The enzyme treatment results in a dispersal of the tissue, releasing low-pH cell materials and reducing the pH of the incubation medium within the first 30 min. After 30 min, remove the bottle from the water bath, and add to it a volume of MEM, pH 9.4, equal to the weight of the gray matter to give a final dispase concentration of 0.5%. This restores the pH of the medium to the neutral range, where dispase is active, and cell damage in the presence of prolonged low-pH conditions will be minimized. Incubate in the 37°C water bath for an additional 2 hr with shaking.

(f) Remove the bottle from the water bath after no more than a 2.5-hr dispase digestion, distribute the content equally into four preweighed 250-ml sterile centrifuge bottles, and centrifuge the suspension for 10 min at $2000 \times g$ (4000 rpm in a Beckman JA-14 rotor) at room temperature. At the end of centrifugation, there are three distinct layers formed in the bottles: a red pellet and a large pink-colored semisolid layer, both of which contain microvessels, and a brown-colored liquid supernatant containing enzyme solution. Remove and discard only the liquid supernatant, being careful not to disturb the soft pellet.

(g) Resuspend the soft pellet with the 12.5% dextran solution, and divide the resuspended material equally among four 250-ml centrifuge tubes. Further dilute the suspensions with the remaining 12.5% dextran solution. Centrifuge the suspension for 10 min at $9000 \times g$ (7700 rpm in a Beckman JA-14 rotor) at room temperature. After centrifugation, there is a large red pellet containing microvessels and erythrocytes, a clear supernatant, and a semisolid brown-colored layer on the top of the supernatant and on the side of the bottle. Pour off all of the liquid supernatant and semisolid layer, and wipe out the remaining supernatant and semisolid material on the side of the bottles with a sterile cotton ball wrapped with cheesecloth. This step isolates a crude population of microvessels which are further purified in the remaining steps.

(h) The purpose of this step is to enzymatically remove the basement membrane, pericytes, and any remaining adherent cell types from microvessels using a collagenase/dispase preparation. In previously published procedures, there was no quantitative information about the amount of enzyme required based on the amount of microvessels present. As a consequence, application of previous procedures often resulted in inconsistent microvessel isolations, harmed endothelial cells, or a high percentage of contamination from other cell types. Therefore, we have been working on quantitating and optimizing the amount of collagenase/dispase needed for microvessel treatment to achieve consistent and successful isolation. We have found a ratio of collagenase/dispase to microvessels of 2.5 mg of collagenase/dispase per gram of microvessels and a final collagenase/dispase concentration of 0.5 mg/ml to be the optimal conditions for producing consistent microvessel isolations of healthy endothelial cells.

(i) To determine the amount of the collagenase/dispase needed, the weight of the isolated microvessels must first be obtained. To do that, reweigh the bottles now containing the microvessel pellet from step g, and then obtain the weight of the microvessels by subtracting the weight of the preweighed bottles (without microvessels) from the total weight. Second, dilute 4-mg/ml collagenase/dispase stock to 0.5 mg/ml. Then calculate the amount and volume of the enzyme needed according the formula below:

$$\text{Amount of 0.5-mg/ml collagenase/dispase (ml)}$$
$$= \frac{\text{Weight of microvessels (g)} \times 2.5 \text{ mg}}{0.5 \text{ mg/ml}}$$

Therefore, for each gram of microvessels, one would require 5 ml of 0.5-mg/ml collagenase/dispase for the digestion, which gives the optimal ratio of enzyme to microvessels (2.5 mg of enzyme per gram of microvessels).

(j) Resuspend the microvessel pellets in the volume of collagenase/dispase solution calculated from step i. Collect the cell suspension into a sterile 50-ml disposable centrifuge tube. Incubate the cell suspension for approximately 4 hr in a 37°C shaker water bath at 100 oscillations/min.

(k) To prepare the Percoll gradient, add 35 ml of well-mixed 50% Percoll solution to each of four 40-ml centrifuge tubes, and centrifuge them for 1 hr at 39,200 × *g* (18,000 rpm in a Beckman JA-20 rotor) at 4°C. At end of spin, remove the tubes containing Percoll gradients carefully and store at 4°C.

(l) After a 4-hr collagenase/dispase incubation, dilute the microvessel suspension with MEM, pH 7.4, to 50 ml and centrifuge for 10 min in the DYNAC centrifuge at a setting of 100 at room temperature to terminate enzymatic digestion and sediment the microvessels.

(m) Remove and discard the supernatant from the tube. Resuspend the microvessel pellet in 10 ml of MEM, pH 7.4. Some of the microvessel pellet may not be resuspendable due to the formation of large fibrous aggregates. Therefore, to release the microvessels trapped in the aggregates, transfer the large fibrous aggregates to another tube and wash them in 30 ml of MEM, pH 7.4. Remove and discard the washed fibrous aggregates. Combine the 30-ml microvessel resuspension with the 10-ml original microvessel resuspension in one 50-ml centrifuge tube. Centrifuge it for 10 min in the DYNAC centrifuge at a setting of 100.

(n) Resuspend the microvessel pellet in 8 ml of MEM, pH 7.4. This microvessel resuspension contains microvessels, endothelial cells, and other components including red blood cells, small amounts of other cell types including pericytes, and cell debris. To separate the microvessels and endothelial cells from those components, apply 2 ml of the suspension onto the top of each of the four preformed Percoll gradients (see step k), and spin for 10 min at $1700 \times g$ (3700 rpm in a Beckman JA-20 rotor). At the end of the centrifugation, there are three layers of bands formed: band 1, top white layer containing cell debris and contaminating cell types; band 2, under band 1, a diffuse layer with red clumps containing microvessel fragments and some endothelial cells; and band 3, a red band near the bottom containing red blood cells.

(o) Collect band 2 from the four Percoll gradients into four 50-ml centrifuge tubes using a 5-ml syringe with an 18-gauge needle attached. Dilute the cell suspension in each tube with MEM-F12 to 50 ml, and centrifuge for 10 min in the DYNAC centrifuge at a setting of 100 at room temperature to remove Percoll.

(p) The microvessel fragments and endothelial cells are now ready for culturing or for freezing for long-term storage. For freezing, resuspend the microvessel endothelial cell pellet in the freezing medium, aliquot 1.5 ml into a cryovial, and store at $-70°C$. These cells can be stored for future use for up to 2 months. Isolates may be stored for longer periods of time under liquid nitrogen.

The cells isolated by this procedure are generally 85–90% viable by trypan blue exclusion. The yield of microvessel endothelial cells from the gray matter of about two bovine brains is 30–200 million cells, depending on the efficiency of the isolation procedure and, more often, the age and condition of the starting tissues. One further note—it has been the purpose of this procedure to isolate microvessel fragments. Isolates of single cells have very poor plating efficiency and generally will not proliferate to form confluent monolayers (Bowman *et al.*, 1983).

2.4. Preparation of Growth Surfaces for Brain Microvessels

The primary brain microvessel fragments can be seeded onto and grown successfully on a substrate-treated solid plastic surface (tissue culture plate), a filter membrane (polycarbonate membrane), or on a filter membrane insert (Transwell®). Seeding of cells onto uncoated growing surfaces generally leads to low plating efficiency. Here, we describe the protocol for culturing the BMECs onto Transwell™ (Costar) inserts with a 0.4-μm-pore polycarbonate filter. Culturing the BMECs on a 3-μ-pore Transwell membrane is unsatisfactory, since the BMECs can migrate through these pores and form cell monolayers on both sides of the Transwell membrane (Raub *et al.*, 1992). However, BMECs will not migrate through a 3-μm-pore filter placed in a plastic dish such that the abluminal face of the filter is placed against the plastic dish bottom. The following procedure is employed:

(a) Coat the filter membrane of the Transwell insert with collagen. Apply the collagen coating solution (e.g., 1 mg/ml in 60% ethanol) to the Transwell insert chamber side at a volume of 0.1 ml/cm^2, and let it dry for 3 hr in a laminar flow hood with exposure to UV light. Alternatively, the membrane can be coated with a crude cross-linked collagen as follows. First, add collagen solution (e.g., 3 mg/ml in 0.1% acetic acid) to the Transwell inserts in a volume of 0.1 ml/cm^2, and coat for 5 min. Remove the excess collagen solution from the Transwell inserts. Expose the inserts to ammonia fumes for 30 min to promote cross-linking of the collagen. Then, let the coated surface dry for 3 hr in a laminar flow hood with exposure to UV light. The coating process is similar for plastic surfaces or for filters placed on plastic surfaces of 100-mm culture dishes.

(b) Treat the collagen-coated surface with fibronectin. Add fibronectin coating solution to the collagen-coated Transwell inserts at a volume of 0.2 ml/cm^2 and incubate for 1 hr. Then, remove the excess fibronectin solution from the inserts. Wash the treated growth surface once with MEM-F12. The growth surface is now ready for plating of the BMECs.

2.5. Seeding of Brain Microvessels onto Growth Surfaces

(a) Thaw the frozen BMEC vials rapidly under tap water and wash three times in BMEC culture medium without ECGS by centrifuging the cell suspension for 10 min in a DYNAC centrifuge at maximum speed (setting of 100).

(b) Resuspend the final pellet in an appropriate volume of the BMEC culture medium. In this resuspension, there are still some small fibrous aggregates. Small visible aggregates will not interfere with the BMECs attaching to the growing surface. To remove larger aggregates, filter the suspension through a 75-μm sterilized mesh nylon or polypropylene filter. Collect the filtrate which contains the BMECs. Take a small sample from the suspension, stain the nuclei with crystal violet, and estimate the total cell number using a hemocytometer.

(c) Seed the BMECs on the collagen/fibronectin-coated surfaces at a density of approximately 50,000 cells/cm^2. Add 2.6 ml of culture medium to the receiver chamber and a final volume of 1.5 ml in the donor chamber of the Transwell™ system or a final volume of 10 ml in 100-mm culture dishes. Place the cells under standard culture conditions of 37°C, 5% CO_2, and 95% humidity.

(d) Leave the seeded cells unperturbed for 3 days before changing the culture medium on the third day after plating. Continue changing the medium every other day thereafter.

Using the procedure described above, we found that the BMECs reach confluence on day 7 or 8 and form a tight monolayer on approximately day 9 or 10 as shown in Fig. 2. Subsequent experiments, such as transport or uptake experiments, can be conducted from day 9 to 12. The cells will begin to undergo noticeable morphological and functional changes after about day 16 (Raub *et al.*, 1992).

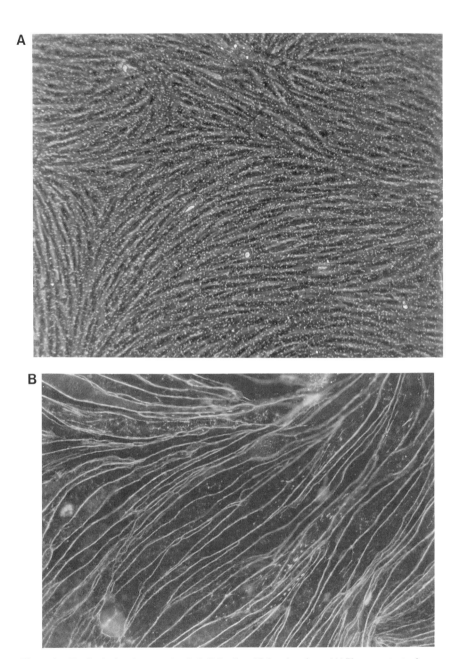

Figure 2. Bovine brain microvessel endothelial cells at 10 days in culture. (A) Phase-contrast microscopy of BMECs. BMECs were grown on a clear Transwell® membrane and observed with a phase-contrast microscope using a 10× objective lens. (B) Actin staining of the BMECs, showing the actin bundles formed on the peripheral region of the BMECs which outline the cell boundary. BMECs were stained with rhodamine-pholloidin to reveal the actin distribution and observed with a fluorescence microscope using a 50× objective lens.

3. EXPERIMENTAL PROTOCOLS FOR UPTAKE AND TRANSPORT STUDIES

3.1. Uptake Studies

For uptake studies, BMECs are seeded into collagen-coated and fibronectin-treated 24-well tissue culture dishes or Costar Transwell™ inserts (12 mm or 24 mm) at a concentration of 50,000 cells/cm². Typically, cells will reach confluence and be ready for uptake studies in about 9–12 days. Upon confirming establishment of confluence (usually by light or fluorescence microscopy), the BMEC monolayers are washed 2 to 3 times with 37°C buffer containing 122 mM NaCl, 25 mM NaHCO₃, 10 mM D-glucose, 3 mM KCl, 2.5 mM MgSO₄, 0.4 mM K₂HPO₄, 1.4 mM CaCl₂, and 10 mM HEPES (hereinafter referred to as Buffer). Alternatively, Hanks' balanced salt solution (HBSS) containing 10 mM HEPES buffer, pH 7.4, can be used. After washing, uptake is initiated by incubating the BMEC monolayers with a suitable volume of 37°C Buffer (1 ml for 24-well tissue culture dish, 0.5 ml for 12-mm Transwell®, and 1.5 ml for 24-mm Transwell®) containing an appropriate concentration of the tested substrate (frequently radiolabeled). If, however, the tested substrate is believed to be taken up into the cells via an active process (carrier- or receptor-mediated), uptake studies can be carried out in the presence of various concentrations of unlabeled substrate or potential competitors. Alternatively, uptake studies can also be carried out at cold temperature (4°C) or in the presence of metabolic inhibitors. Uptake is usually measured for 30 sec–1 min at 37°C while gently shaking the 24-well tissue culture dish or 6-well or 12-well cluster tray containing the Transwell inserts to avoid creating undesirable unstirred aqueous layers. Incubations can, however, be performed for any reasonable time intervals. The uptake is stopped by removing the Buffer, followed by immediate rinsing with ice-cold Buffer, pH 7.4. A volume (0.5 ml for 24-well tissue culture dish and 12-mm Transwell and 1 ml for 24-mm Transwell) of 0.25% aqueous trypsin–EDTA mixture is then added to the monolayers and incubated at 37°C overnight on an orbital shaker at low speed in order to solubilize the BMECs. Cell-associated radioactivity is assayed by liquid scintillation spectrometry following addition of the solubilized material to 4 ml of scintillation cocktail.

3.2. Transport Studies

While the uptake and absorption of the tested substrate can be examined using cells cultured on a solid support, actual transport studies require culturing of the cells onto permeable filter or filter supports. Our laboratory has had success with two procedures, and detailed descriptions of these procedures are given below.

The first procedure involves growing BMECs onto a collagen-coated and fibronectin-treated polycarbonate membrane (13-mm diameter and 3-μm pore size) placed in a 100-mm culture dish. Upon reaching confluence, the polycarbonate membranes containing BMEC monolayers are carefully removed and placed between side-by-side diffusion cells (Crown Glass Co., Somerset, NJ). A 3-ml aliquot of Buffer at 37°C is added to both sides (apical side and basolateral side) of the diffusion cell. The cells and the Buffer are then allowed to equilibrate at 37°C for 15–30 min by running thermostated water into the water jacket surrounding the donor chamber (apical side) and the receiver chamber (basolateral side). A transport study is started by addition of a small aliquot (10–100 μl) of the tested substrate at an appropriate concentration to the donor chamber and an equivalent amount of the tested substrate's solution to the receiver chamber. Stirring in each side of the diffusion cell is maintained by a magnetic stir bar (rotating at 600 rpm). Samples (10–200 μl) are taken from the receiver chamber at designated times and replaced with fresh Buffer.

The second procedure that is frequently applied in our laboratory to study transendothelial transport employs the 24-mm Transwell® culture-insert system (0.4-μm pore size). In general, this system allows independent access to both the apical and basolateral plasma domains and is very easy to use. BMECs grown on collagen-coated and fibronectin-treated Transwell polycarbonate membrane are pre-incubated at 37°C in pH 7.4 Buffer for 15–30 min. Prior to the transendothelial transport studies, the Buffer in both the apical and basolateral sides is removed. Fresh Buffer (2.6 ml) is then added to the basolateral side. To start the transport experiment, 1.5 ml of Buffer containing an appropriate concentration of the tested substrate is added to the apical side. To avoid the effect of an unstirred aqueous layer, the cluster tray containing the Transwell inserts is gently shaken during the course of the transport experiment. If the unstirred aqueous layer becomes a significant transport barrier, one can resort to a newly designed side-by-side diffusion apparatus as reported recently by our laboratory (Ng *et al.*, 1993). Samples (50 μl) are taken from the basolateral side at designated time points and replaced with an equivalent volume of fresh Buffer.

As with the uptake studies, if transport of the tested substrate is via an active pathway, one can systematically study the transport process by varying the unlabeled substrate concentrations or by addition of various competitors or metabolic inhibitors. Alternatively, the transport study can be performed at low temperature (4°C) to block cell-mediated mechanisms. Detection of substrate transported is usually accomplished by radiolabel detection as described for the uptake studies. Depending on the nature of the tested substrate, passage across the monolayers may be assayed by HPLC with UV or fluorescence detection, or conventional spectroscopy.

3.3. Protein Estimation

When uptake and transport of substrates are mediated by active processes, uptake and transport data are usually normalized by dividing the amount (moles) of substrate taken up or transported per unit time (minute or second) by the total protein content (milligrams or micrograms) of the cells. This is because active uptake or transport processes are mainly mediated by proteins that are embedded in the cellular plasma membrane, and the amount of protein per cell is considered consistent. To determine the total protein content in BMECs after the uptake or transport studies, BMEC monolayers are first washed twice with Buffer. A volume (0.5 ml for the side-by-side setup and 2 ml for 24-mm Transwell) of 0.2 N NaOH containing 0.2% Triton X-100 is then added to the apical side of the monolayer for overnight incubation at room temperature. At the end of the incubation, 100 μl of the cell lysis in NaOH is taken and diluted 10-fold with water. The total protein content of 100 μl of the diluted cell lysis is then measured with a Bio-Rad Protein Assay Kit using bovine serum albumin as the standard.

4. CALCULATIONS OF DATA

4.1. Permeability Coefficients

Since different compounds have different abilities to passively diffuse across the same biological membrane, it is essential to express this ability in terms of a parameter that allows meaningful comparison between the permeability of compounds to be made. One such physical parameter is the apparent permeability coefficient (P), which is defined by the following equation:

$$P = \text{flux}_{\text{monolayer}} \times 1/A \times 1/C$$

where C (pmol/ml) is the initial concentration of the tested substrate on the apical side (or the basolateral side if basolateral-to-apical transport is being studied) of the monolayer, A (cm^2) is the surface area of the monolayer available for transport (0.636 cm^2 for the side-by-side setup and 4.7 cm^2 for 24-mm Transwell), and flux$_{\text{monolayer}}$ (pmol/sec) is the steady-state rate of appearance of apically or basolaterally applied tested substrate on the basolateral side or apical side, respectively, of the monolayers and is calculated as the linearly regressed slope through linear transport data. Permeability data must be carefully generated to allow determination of the contributions of transcellular and paracellular pathways to the total permeability (Adson *et al.*, 1994). A recent review published by Ho *et al.* (1996) is a good source of information for those who are interested in a more extensive mathematical treatment and interpretation of transcellular and paracellular permeability data.

4.2. Kinetic Parameters for Active Processes

To determine the kinetic parameters (K_m and V_{max}) for active uptake and transport processes, the apical-to-basolateral (or basolateral-to-apical) uptake or transport rates (expressed as picomoles per minute per milligram of protein) as a function of substrate concentration on the apical side (or basolateral side) of the monolayers are first determined. These rates are then plotted against the substrate concentration on the apical side (or basolateral side) of the monolayers. The kinetic parameters K_m and V_{max} of such processes are then determined by fitting the rate versus concentration data with the use of a nonlinear estimation program (e.g., PCNONLIN, SCI Software).

5. PHARMACEUTICAL APPLICATIONS

5.1. Uptake and Transport

The major application of BMEC cultures in the field of pharmaceutics is in the investigation of the relative permeability of the BBB to conventional drugs and therapeutic peptides, proteins, and other biotechnology products. BMEC monolayers grown in primary culture have been used to investigate a variety of carrier systems, endocytotic and transcytotic mechanisms, and latentiation and have the potential for examining experimental chimeric nutrient and peptide delivery systems. It is beyond the scope of this review to list all of the uptake and permeability studies conducted with BMEC monolayers to date. Arbitrarily selected examples of the recent use of BMEC monolayers to study BBB permeability properties include characterization of the transcellular passage of glucose (Takakura et al., 1991b), biotin (Shi et al., 1993a), cholesterol synthesis inhibitors (Guillot et al., 1993; Saheki et al., 1994), imaging agents (Pirro et al., 1994), quinolone antibacterials (Jaehde et al., 1993), dextromethorphan and dextrorphan (Shi et al., 1993b), zidovudine (AZT; Masereeuw et al., 1994), peptides (Weber et al., 1993; Chikhale et al., 1994), and viral vectors (Hurwitz et al., 1994) and the endocytosis and/or transcytosis of peptides and proteins such as modified albumins (Smith and Borchardt, 1989; Vorbrodt and Trowbridge, 1991b), transferrin (Raub and Newton, 1991), and ricin (Raub and Audus, 1990). The role of P-glycoprotein overexpression (Tsuji et al., 1992) and the development of chimeric carrier systems (Fukuta et al., 1994) have also been investigated with BMECs in primary culture. The use of BMEC cultures to characterize low-molecular-weight and macromolecule permeability properties has been more extensively considered in several recent reviews (Audus and Borchardt, 1991; Takakura et al., 1991a; Miller et al., 1992; Audus et al., 1992; Audus and Raub, 1993). While generally basic in nature, all of these studies are intended to contribute to the development of a better understanding of the role of specific cell processes in regulating the transfer of substances across the BBB.

5.2. Metabolism

The delivery of blood-borne agents to the central nervous system can be limited by inactivation or activation by metabolism at the BBB. By comparison with permeability processes, metabolism related to drug transport has received less attention. However, enzyme pathways relevant to degradative or synthetic modifications of therapeutic agents are retained in primary cultures of BMECs. Selected examples of enzyme pathways that have been investigated with primary cultures of BMECs include synthetic and degradative pathways for catecholamines (Baranczyk-Kuzma *et al.*, 1989a; Scriba and Borchardt, 1989a, 1989b), peptidases (Baranczyk-Kuzma and Audus, 1987; Thompson and Audus, 1994a), and hydrolases (Baranczyk-Kuzma *et al.*, 1989b). Recent reviews by Joo (1992, 1993) summarize a broad range of investigations on more general cellular metabolism and biochemical properties of BMECs.

5.3. Permeability Regulation

Potential approaches to improving the transfer of therapeutic substances across the BBB include alteration of the interface by chemical or biological factors (Audus *et al.*, 1992). Primary cultures of BMECs offer a useful system for the examination of the mechanistic aspects of these treatments, their reversibility, and possible toxicological/pathological consequences prior to or in conjunction with studies in animal models. The permeability-regulating effects and mechanisms for vasoactive peptides (Guillot and Audus, 1991; Reardon and Audus, 1993), leucine enkephalin (Thompson and Audus, 1994b; Thompson *et al.*, 1994), α- and β-adrenergic agents (Borges *et al.*, 1994), and bacterial factors (Tunkel *et al.*, 1991) have all been recently investigated with primary cultures of BMECs.

6. ADVANTAGES AND DISADVANTAGES OF BMEC CULTURE SYSTEMS

6.1. Advantages Over Other *in Vitro* Systems

The significant advantage in using cultures of BMEC monolayers is the ability to grow the cells on a permeable support, allowing the study of transcellular transport and access to both luminal and abluminal surfaces (Audus and Borchardt, 1991). This allows investigation of polarized transport, receptor, and enzyme systems and other surface or asymmetrical properties that may define the nature of the BBB.

The alternative *in vitro* system, isolated brain capillaries in suspension, has and will continue to contribute important information on the BBB (Joo, 1985, 1992, 1993). This system is convenient and easy to use. However, the capillary suspension does not allow one to assess or examine transcellular transport processes. Additionally, unless other than mechanical methods of isolation are employed and steps are taken to modify the suspension medium, metabolic deficiencies are often introduced in the isolation procedures (Williams *et al.*, 1980; Lasbennes and Gayet, 1984; Sussman *et al.*, 1988; McCall *et al.*, 1988).

6.2.   Appropriate Roles and Relationship to the BBB *in Vivo*

Many of the morphological and biochemical features of BMECs *in vitro* are, to varying degrees, consistent with the BBB *in vivo* (Joo, 1985, 1992, 1993). Recent literature supporting this observation relates to the potential use of cultures of BMEC monolayers as a *qualitative* indicator system for BBB permeability to various experimental and therapeutic agents. This growing list of reports confirms a qualitative correlation between the permeability characteristics of cultures of BMECs (with and without astroglial factors or cAMP stimulators present) and the permeability characteristics of *in situ/in vivo* BBB models for a variety of low-molecular-weight substances (Dehouck *et al.*, 1992; Guillot *et al.*, 1993; Masereeuw *et al.*, 1994; Pirro *et al.*, 1994; Saheki *et al.*, 1994) and peptides or proteins (Pardridge *et al.*, 1990; Weber *et al.*, 1993; Chikhale *et al.*, 1994). A similar relationship is observed for a lengthy list of metabolic and biochemical properties of BMECs *in vivo* and *in vitro* (Joo, 1985, 1992, 1993). Because of the significant differences between the simple nature of the *in vitro* models and the complex *in vivo* situation, researchers cannot and should not try to establish direct quantitative correlations between the systems.

6.3.   Current Limitations

Primary cultures of BMECs form confluent monolayers that retain many morphological and biochemical properties (Audus and Borchardt, 1986, 1987; Miller *et al.*, 1992) and are functionally polarized (Raub and Audus, 1990; Guillot and Audus, 1991; Tsjui *et al.*, 1992; Borges *et al.*, 1994) like their *in vivo* counterparts. However, the obvious limitation of the primary BMEC cultures has been the higher than desirable paracellular permeability, attributed to alterations in the development of tight intercellular junctions. The often-cited transendothelial electrical resistance (TEER) for primary cultures of BMECs, for example, is maximally around 160 $\Omega\cdot cm^2$. Although higher than the TEER values obtained for cultures of either passaged BMECs or bovine adrenal endothelial cells (<9 $\Omega\cdot cm^2$; Raub *et al.*, 1992), the TEER measured for primary BMEC monolayers is still well below the *in vivo* estimates of 400–2000 $\Omega\cdot cm^2$ (i.e., a range dependent upon several factors including the complexity of experimental techniques used, vessel type, and size) (Oleson and Crone, 1986). In general, the relationship between TEER measures and monolayer permeability to molecules other than ions does not hold. A better characterization of the "tightness" of BMEC monolayers should be drawn from studies in which the permeability to a series of markers varying in molecular size is determined (Milton and Knutson, 1990; Adson *et al.*, 1994). From the earlier discussions, it is clear that while the permeability of BMECs in culture is less restrictive, qualitative relationships with the *in vivo* situation can be developed.

Primary cultures of BMECs do not incorporate all of the factors necessary to create an *in vitro* system that precisely reflects the BBB *in vivo*. This system was developed as a simple tool with which one can begin to study both the permeability-regulating and metabolic properties of the BBB. Factors absent in the artificial *in vitro* environment include neuronal and astroglial input, the cylindrical geometry of the capillary, blood pressure and flow, blood-borne factors, and blood cells that can and may influence BMEC function and differentiation (Joo, 1985, 1992; Reardon and Audus, 1993). The ideal of developing an *in vitro* system that is equivalent to the *in vivo* situation may be unattainable for some time to come, owing mainly to our incomplete understanding of the role of each of the factors listed. On the other hand, the study of astroglial:endothelial cell co-culture systems by a number of research groups over the past 15 years has contributed to an understanding of how glial interactions may influence BBB endothelial cell structure and metabolism (Joo, 1992, 1993). Therefore, the ongoing research projects considering the importance of incorporation of such induction factors into the tissue culture medium should result in the evolution of *in vitro* systems that more closely approximate the *in vivo* BBB in structure, metabolism, and permeability. In addition, such studies also advance our knowledge of the fundamental basis of the BBB (Joo, 1992, 1993).

6.4. Status of Cell Line Development

Efforts have been made to establish continuous cell lines representative of BBB endothelium. These efforts include generating conventional subcultured or passaged brain microvessel endothelial cell systems from mouse (DeBault and Cancilla, 1980; DeBault, 1981; DeBault *et al.*, 1981), porcine (Tontsch and Bauer, 1991), ovine (Vorbrodt and Trowbridge, 1991a,b), and bovine (Dehouck *et al.*, 1992; Durieu-Trautmann *et al.*, 1991; Minikawa *et al.*, 1991; Raub *et al.*, 1992) brain tissues. In general, passaged cells appear to more accurately present morphological and biochemical markers for the BBB only when combinations of astrocyte, neuronal, and pericyte influences are restored by either establishing co-cultures or adding conditioned medium to the tissue culture environment (Debault, 1981; Dehouck *et al.*, 1990; Minikawa *et al.*, 1991; Tontsch and Bauer, 1991; Raub *et al.*, 1992).

A few reports have appeared on transformed cell systems. However, these cell systems have not been characterized to the same extent as either the primary or passaged cell culture systems. Examples include a transformed microvascular endothelial cell line from rat brain which exhibited anchorage-independent growth and elevated levels of γ-glutamyl transpeptidase (Diglio *et al.*, 1983; Caspers and Diglio,

1984) and a similar system derived from mouse brain that found applications in the study of mechanisms related to cerebrovascular endothelial cell growth functions and control (Robinson *et al.*, 1986).

7. CONCLUSIONS AND FUTURE PERSPECTIVES

The extensive reviews of Joo (1985, 1992, 1993) summarize the expanding knowledge base with respect to the many investigations on BMEC cultures over the past few decades. There continues to be an optimistic view that the *in vitro* approach has been and will remain an important tool in understanding the biochemical basis of the BBB. Although not perfect, the primary BMEC culture system described here has been rather successfully employed by a number of investigators to study transport, metabolic, and permeability-regulating properties of the BBB. The future contributions of such *in vitro* systems and progress in our understanding of the BBB will likely depend on researchers continuing to explore, manipulate, and exploit a variety of similar models. In particular, advances in the development of cell lines may eventually lead to the establishment of more convenient *in vitro* systems for study of the BBB.

Acknowledgments

Research summarized in this chapter has been supported by the American Heart Association—Kansas Affiliate, Hoffmann-LaRoche, INTERx Research Corporation, a subsidiary of Merck & Co., Lawrence, Kansas, and The Upjohn Company, Kalamazoo, Michigan.

REFERENCES

Adson, A., Raub, T. J., Burton, P. S., Barshun, C. L., Hilgers, A. R., Audus, K. L., and Ho, N. F. H., 1994, Quantitative approaches to delineate paracellular diffusion in cultured epithelial monolayers, *J. Pharm. Sci.* **83**:1529–1536.

Audus, K. L., and Borchardt, R. T., 1986, Characterization of an *in vitro* blood–brain barrier model system for studying drug transport and metabolism, *Pharm. Res.* **3**:81–87.

Audus, K. L., and Borchardt, R. T., 1987, Bovine brain microvessel endothelial cell monolayers as a model system for the blood–brain barrier, *Ann. N. Y. Acad. Sci.* **507**:9–18.

Audus, K. L., and Borchardt, R. T., 1991, Transport of macromolecules across the capillary endothelium, *Handb. Exp. Pharmacol.* **100**:43–70.

Audus, K. L., and Raub, T. J., 1993, Lysosomes of brain and other vascular endothelia, in: *The Blood–Brain Barrier* (W. M. Pardridge, ed.) Raven Press, New York, pp. 201–227.

Audus, K. L., Chikhale, P. J., Miller, D. W., Thompson, S. E., and Borchardt, R. T., 1992, Brain uptake of drugs: The influence of chemical and biological factors, *Adv. Drug Res.* **23**:1–64.

Baranczyk-Kuzma, A., and Audus, K. L., 1987, Characteristics of aminopeptidase activity from bovine brain microvessel endothelium, *J. Cereb. Blood Flow Metab.* **7**:801–805.

Baranczyk-Kuzma, A., Audus, K. L., and Borchardt, R. T., 1989a, Substrate specificity of phenol sulfotransferase from primary cultures of bovine brain microvessel endothelium, *J. Neurochem.* **46:**1956–1960.

Baranczyk-Kuzma, A., Raub, T. J., and Audus, K. L., 1989b, Demonstration of acid hydrolase activity in primary cultures of bovine brain microvessel endothelium, *Neurochem. Res.* **14:**689–691.

Borges, N., Shi, F., Azevedo, I., and Audus, K. L., 1994, Changes in brain microvessel endothelial cell monolayer permeability induced by adrenergic drugs, *Eur. J. Pharmacol.* **269:**243–248.

Bowman, P. D., Ennis, S. R., Rarey, K. E., Betz, A. L., and Goldstein, G. W., 1983, Brain microvessel endothelial cells in tissue culture: A model for study of blood–brain barrier permeability, *Ann. Neurol.* **14:**396–402.

Bradbury, M. W. B., 1993, The blood–brain barrier, *Exp. Physiol.* **78:**453–472.

Brightman, M. W., and Reese, T. S., 1969, Junctions between intimately opposed cell membranes in the vertebrate brain, *J. Cell Biol.* **40:**648–677.

Caspers, M. L., and Diglio, C. A., 1984, Expression of gamma-glutamyl transpeptidase in a transformed rat cerebral endothelial cell line, *Biochim. Biophys. Acta* **803:**1–6.

Chikhale, E. G., Ng, K.-Y., Burton, P. S., and Borchardt, R. T., 1994, Hydrogen bonding potential as a determinant of the *in vitro* and *in situ* blood–brain barrier permeability of peptides, *Pharm. Res.* **11:**412–419.

DeBault, L. E., 1981, γ-glutamyltranspeptidase induction mediated by glial foot process-to-endothelium contact in co-culture, *Brain Res.* **220:**432–435.

DeBault, L. E., and Cancilla, P. A., 1980, Gamma-glutamyl transpeptidase in isolated brain endothelial cell: Induction by glial cells *in vitro, Science* **207:**653–655.

DeBault, L. E., Henriquez, E., Hart, M. N., and Cancilla, P. A., 1981, Cerebral microvessels and derived cells in tissue culture: Establishment, identification, and preliminary characterization of an endothelial cell line, *In Vitro* **15:**480–494.

Dehouck, M.-P., Jolliet-Riant, P., Bree, F., Fruchart, J.-C., Cecchelli, R., and Tillement, J.-P., 1992, Drug transfer across the blood–brain barrier: Correlation between *in vitro* and *in vivo* models, *J. Neurochem.* **58:**1790–1797.

Diglio, C. A., Wolfe, D. E., and Meyers, P., 1983, Transformation of rat cerebral endothelial cells by Rous sarcoma virus, *J. Cell Biol.* **97:**15–21.

Durieu-Trautmann, O., Foignant, N., Strosberg, A. D., and Couraud, P. O., 1991, Coexpression of 1- and 2-adrenergic receptors on bovine brain capillary endothelial cells in culture, *J. Neurochem.* **56:** 775–781.

Fukuta, M., Okada, H., Iinuma, S., Yanai, S., and Toguchi, H., 1994, Insulin fragments as a carrier for peptide delivery across the blood–brain barrier, *Pharm. Res.* **11:**1681–1688.

Guillot, F. L., and Audus, K. L., 1991, Angiotensin peptide regulation of bovine brain microvessel endothelial cell monolayer permeability, *J. Cardiovasc. Pharmacol.* **18:**212–218.

Guillot, F. L., Misslin, P., and Lemaire, M., 1993, Comparison of fluvastatin and lovastatin blood–brain barrier transfer using *in vitro* and *in vivo* methods, *J. Cardiovasc. Pharmacol.* **21:**339–346.

Ho, N. F., Raub, T. J., Burton, P., Barsuhn, C. L., Adson, A., Audus, K. L., and Borchardt, R. T., 1996, Quantitative approaches to delineate passive transport mechanisms in cell culture monolayers, in: *Transport Processes in Pharmaceutical Systems* (K. J. Himmelstein, G. L. Amidon, and P. I. Lee, eds.), Marcel Dekker, New York, in press.

Hurwitz, A. A., Berman, J. W., and Lyman, W. D., 1994, The role of the blood–brain barrier in HIV infection of the central nervous system, *Adv. Neuroimmunol.* **4:**249–256.

Jaehde, U., Goto, T., de Boer, A. G., and Breimer, D. D., 1993, Blood–brain barrier transport rate of quinolone antibacterials evaluated in cerebrovascular endothelial cell cultures, *Eur. J. Pharm. Sci.* **1:**49–55.

Joo, F., 1985, The blood–brain barrier *in vitro:* Ten years of research on microvessels isolated from the brain, *Neurochem. Int.* **7:**1–25.

Joo, F., 1992, The cerebral microvessels in culture, an update, *J. Neurochem.* **58:**1–17.

Joo, F., 1993, The blood–brain barrier *in vitro*: The second decade, *Neurochem. Int.* **23**:499–521.

Lasbennes, F., and Gayet, J., 1984, Capacity for energy metabolism in microvessels isolated from rat brain, *Neurochem. Res.* **9**:1–10.

Masereeuw, R., Jaehde, U., Langemeijer, M. W. E., de Boer, A. G., and Breimer, D. D., 1994, *In vitro* and *in vivo* transport of zidovudine (AZT) across the blood–brain barrier and the effect of transport inhibitors, *Pharm. Res.* **11**:324–330.

McCall, A. L., Valente, J., Cordero, R., Ruderman, N. B., and Tornheim, K., 1988, Metabolic characterization of isolated cerebral microvessels: ATP and ADP concentrations, *Microvasc. Res.* **35**:325–333.

Miller, D. W., Audus, K. L., and Borchardt, R. T., 1992, Application of cultured endothelial cells of the brain microvasculature in the study of the blood–brain barrier, *J. Tissue Cult. Methods* **14**:217–224.

Milton, S. G., and Knutson, V. P., 1990, Comparison of the function of the tight junctions of endothelial cells and epithelial cells in regulating the movement of electrolytes and macromolecules across the cell monolayer, *J. Cell. Physiol.* **144**:498–504.

Minikawa, T., Bready, J., Berliner, J., Fisher, M., and Cancilla, P. A., 1991, *In vitro* interaction of astrocytes and pericytes with capillary-like structures of brain microvessel endothelium, *Lab. Invest.* **65**:32–40.

Ng, K., Grass, G., Lane, H., and Borchardt, R. T., 1993, Characterization of the unstirred water layer in cultured brain microvessel endothelial cells, *In Vitro Cell. Dev. Biol.* **29A**:627–629.

Oleson, S. P., and Crone, C., 1986, Substances that rapidly augment ionic conductance of endothelium in cerebral venules, *Acta Physiol. Scand.* **127**:233–241.

Panula, P., Joo, F., and Rechardt, L., 1978, Evidence for the presence of viable endothelial cells in cultures derived from dissociated rat brain, *Experientia* **34**:95–97.

Pardridge, W. M., Triguero, D., Yang, J., and Cancilla, P. A., 1990, Comparison of *in vitro* and *in vivo* models of drug transcytosis through the blood–brain barrier, *J. Pharm. Exp. Ther.* **253**:884–891.

Pirro, J. P., Di Rocco, R. J., Narra, R. K., and Nunn, A. D., 1994, The relationship between *in vitro* transendothelial permeability and *in vivo* single-pass brain extraction of several SPECT imaging agents, *J. Nucl. Med.* **35**:1514–1519.

Raub, T. J., and Audus, K. L., 1990, Adsorptive endocytosis and membrane recycling by cultured primary bovine brain microvessel endothelial cell monolayers, *J. Cell Sci.* **97**:127–138.

Raub, T. J., and Newton, C. R., 1991, Recycling kinetics and transcytosis of transferrin in primary cultures of bovine brain microvessel endothelial cells, *J. Cell. Physiol.* **149**:141–151.

Raub, T. J., Kuentzel, S. L., and Sawada, G. A., 1992, Permeability of bovine brain microvessel endothelial cells *in vitro*: Barrier tightening by a factor released from astroglioma cells, *Exp. Cell Res.* **199**: 330–340.

Reardon, P. M., and Audus, K. L., 1993, Applications of primary cultures of brain microvessel endothelial cell monolayers in the study of vasoactive peptide interaction with the blood–brain barrier, *S.T.P. Pharm. Sci.* **3**:63–68.

Reese, T. S., and Karnovsky, M. J., 1967, Structural localization of a blood–brain barrier to exogenous peroxidase, *J. Cell Biol.* **34**:207–217.

Robinson, R. A., TenEyck, C. J., and Hart, M. N., 1986, Establishment and preliminary growth characteristics of a transformed mouse cerebral microvessel endothelial cell line, *Lab. Invest.* **54**:579–588.

Saheki, A., Terasaki, T., Tamai, I., and Tsuji, A., 1994, *In vivo* and *in vitro* blood–brain barrier transport of 3-hydroxy-3-methylglutaryl coenzyme A (HMG-CoA) reductase inhibitors, *Pharm. Res.* **11**:305–311.

Scriba, G. K., and Borchardt, R. T., 1989a, Metabolism of catecholamine esters by cultured bovine brain microvascular endothelium, *J. Neurochem.* **53**:610–615.

Scriba, G. K., and Borchardt, R. T., 1989b, Metabolism of 1-methyl-4-phenyl-1,2,3,6-tetrahyropyridine (MPTP) by bovine brain microvessel endothelial cells, *Brain Res.* **501**:175–178.

Shi, F., and Audus, K. L., 1994, Biochemical characteristics of primary and passaged cultures of primate brain microvessel endothelial cells, *Neurochem. Res.* **19**:427–433.

Shi, F., Bailey, C., Malick, A. W., and Audus, K. L., 1993a, Biotin uptake and transport across bovine brain microvessel endothelial cell monolayers, *Pharm. Res.* **10**:282–288.

Shi, F., Cavitt, J. L., Bailey, C., Malick, A. W., and Audus, K. L., 1993b, Characterization of dextromethorphan and dextrorphan uptake by a putative glutamic acid carrier and passive diffusion across brain microvessel endothelium, *Drug Deliv.* **1**:113–118.

Smith, K. R., and Borchardt, R. T., 1989, Permeability and mechanism of albumin, cationized albumin, and glycosylated albumin transcellular transport across monolayers of cultured bovine brain capillary endothelial cells, *Pharm. Res.* **6**:466–473.

Sussman, I., Carson, M. P., McCall, A. L., Shulz, V., Ruderman, N. B., and Tornheim, K., 1988, Energy state of bovine cerebral microvessels: Comparison of isolation methods, *Microvasc. Res.* **35**:167–178.

Takakura, Y., Audus, K. L., and Borchardt, R. T., 1991a, Blood–brain barrier: Transport studies in isolated brain capillaries and in cultured brain endothelial cells, *Adv. Pharmacol.* **22**:137–165.

Takakura, Y., Trammel, A. M., Kuentzel, S. L., Raub, T. J., Davies, A., Baldwin, S. A., and Borchardt, R. T., 1991b, Hexose uptake in primary cultures of bovine brain microvessel endothelial cells. I. Basic characteristics and effects of D-glucose and insulin, *Biochim. Biophys. Acta* **1070**:1–10.

Thompson, S. E., and Audus, K. L., 1994a, Leucine enkephalin metabolism by bovine brain microvessel endothelial cells, *Peptides* **15**:109–116.

Thompson, S. E., and Audus, K. L., 1994b, Leucine enkephalin effects on brain microvessel endothelial cell monolayer permeability, *Pharm. Res.* **11**:1367–1370.

Thompson, S. E., Cavitt, J., and Audus, K. L., 1994, Leucine enkephalin effects on endocytosis, membrane structure, tight junction integrity and passive permeability in brain microvessel endothelial cells, *J. Cardiovasc. Pharmacol.* **24**:818–825.

Tontsch, U., and Bauer, H. C., 1991, Glial cells and neurons induce blood/brain barrier related enzymes in cultured cerebral endothelial cells, *Brain Res.* **539**:247–253.

Tsuji, A., Terasaki, T., Takabatake, Y., Tenda, Y., Tamai, I., Yamashima, T., Moritani, S., Tsuruo, T., and Yamashita, J., 1992, P-Glycoprotein as the drug efflux pump in primary cultured bovine brain capillary endothelial cells, *Life Sci.* **51**:1427–1437.

Tunkel, A. R., Rosser, S. W., Hansen, E. J., and Scheld, W. M., 1991, Blood–brain barrier alterations in bacterial meningitis: Development of an *in vitro* model and observations on the effects of lipopolysaccharide, *In Vitro Cell. Dev. Biol.* **27A**:113–120.

Vorbrodt, A. W., and Trowbridge, R. S., 1991a, Ultracytochemical characteristics of cultured sheep brain microvascular endothelial cells, *J. Histochem. Cytochem.* **39**:1555–1563.

Vorbrodt, A. W., and Trowbridge, R. S., 1991b, Ultrastructural study of transcellular transport of native and cationized albumin in cultured sheep brain microvascular endothelium, *J. Neurocytol.* **20**:998–1006.

Weber, S. J., Abbruscato, T. J., Brownson, E. A., Lipkowski, A. W., Polt, R., Misicka, A., Haaseth, R. C., Bartosz, H., Hruby, V. J., and Davis, T. P., 1993, Assessment of an *in vitro* blood–brain barrier model using several [Met^5]enkephalin opioid analogs, *J. Pharmacol. Exp. Ther.* **266**:1649–1655.

Williams, S. K., Gillis, J. F., Matthews, M. A., Wagner, R. C., and Bitensky, M. W., 1980, Isolation and characterization of brain endothelial cells: Morphology and enzyme activity, *J. Neurochem.* **35**:374–381.

Chapter 14

Methods to Study Drug Transport in Isolated Choroid Plexus Tissue and Cultured Cells

Carla B. Washington, Kathleen M. Giacomini, and Claire M. Brett

1. INTRODUCTION

1.1. Role and Function of the Choroid Plexus

The choroid plexuses, which comprise the blood–cerebrospinal fluid (CSF) barrier, are situated within the third, fourth, and lateral cerebral ventricles (Fig. 1). The choroid plexus functions in the secretion and reabsorption of a variety of compounds and is similar in morphology to other epithelia that are involved in such transport processes (i.e., kidney and intestine) (Spector and Johanson, 1989). The choroid plexus villi are composed of a single layer of simple columnar or cuboidal epithelial cells that rest on a basement membrane. Similar to other epithelia, the choroid plexus cell is polar, having distinct brush border (faces the CSF) and basolateral (faces the blood) surfaces. Each polar membrane has distinct characteristics, and, in particular,

Carla B. Washington • Department of Pharmacy, University of California, San Francisco, California 94143. *Kathleen M. Giacomini* • Departments of Biopharmaceutical Sciences, University of California, San Francisco, California 94143. *Claire M. Brett* • Department of Anesthesia, University of California, San Francisco, California 94143.

Models for Assessing Drug Absorption and Metabolism, Ronald T. Borchardt *et al.*, eds., Plenum Press, New York, 1996.

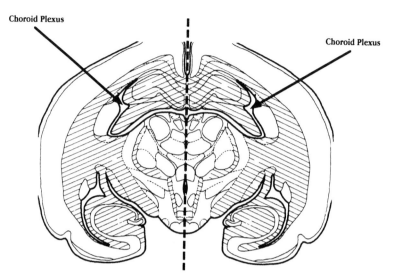

Figure 1.   Lateral view of the rabbit brain. The choroid plexuses within the lateral ventricles are outlined.

transporters are uniquely distributed between the two surfaces. This polar arrangement allows for the net secretion of solutes and water from the blood to the CSF as well as the net reabsorption of other compounds in the opposite direction, from CSF to blood. In addition, the epithelial cells of the choroid plexus are laterally joined to each other by a continuous band of tight junctions (zonulae occludens) located near the brush border surface. This prevents significant paracellular movement of solutes into and out of the CSF via the choroid plexus.

The choroid plexus has two major functions: CSF production and transport of water and solutes. This epithelium produces up to 70% of the CSF, depending on the species (Pollay, 1975). Of more significance for this discussion, the choroid plexus plays an important role in maintaining biochemical homeostasis within the CSF via multiple transport systems distributed on the brush border and basolateral membranes. Together with the blood–brain barrier, the choroid plexus (blood–CSF barrier) maintains the protected microenvironment of the brain by regulating the transmembrane movement of various solutes. That is, the blood–brain barrier and the choroid plexus are the only two routes by which many biologically active substances enter and leave the brain. Over the last decade, the mechanisms of transport across this epithelium have received increasing attention, since several transport systems have been identified in the choroid plexus that are absent in the blood–brain barrier (Spector and Eells, 1984).

1.2. Importance of the Choroid Plexus in Drug Delivery and Targeting to the Brain

Disabilities caused by disorders of the brain affect more than 50 million people in the United States (Pardridge *et al.*, 1992). Over the last decade there has been an explosion of information about the cellular and molecular basis of many of these neurological and psychiatric disorders. As a result, new classes of drugs have been designed based on the three-dimensional structures of the receptors thought to be involved in mediating such diseases. However, these structure–function approaches are ineffective if these compounds are then unable to gain access to a site of action within the brain. Thus, a specific understanding of drug delivery across the barriers of the brain is crucial to the future design of compounds targeted for sites within the brain.

Recent studies suggest that the choroid plexus may play an important role in the selective delivery of water-soluble compounds from the blood into the CSF (Neuwelt, 1989) and eventually the brain, since the CSF is in free communication with the extracellular fluid of the brain. By taking advantage of the unique structural and functional characteristics of the blood–CSF barrier (i.e., permeability, kinetics, carrier specificity, etc.), it is possible to target certain compounds toward the extracellular fluid of the brain via the choroid plexus. Of particular interest is targeting of certain antiviral compounds, such as the $2',3'$-dideoxynucleosides, including azidothymidine (AZT) and dideoxyinosine (DDI), to the brain via the choroid plexus. These agents are currently used to inhibit the human immunodeficiency virus (HIV) to treat AIDS-related dementia complex. Previous studies suggest that the mode of entry of these compounds may be at the level of the choroid plexus (Anderson *et al.*, 1990).

1.3. Importance of the Choroid Plexus in Pharmacokinetics and Pharmacodynamics

A clear understanding of pharmacologic principles is needed when administering drugs to treat disabilities affecting the central nervous system. In addition to the challenge of targeting drugs across the selective barriers of the brain, once a compound gains access to its site of action, a mechanism for elimination is often necessary to avoid long-term exposure which might produce neurotoxicity. Other drugs may cause neurotoxicity as a side effect of therapy when their chemical structure allows free entry into the central nervous system. Thus, an understanding of the mechanisms of transport of various classes of compounds across the barriers of the brain provides a basis for the rational targeting of drugs away from (as well as into) the brain.

Determining the sidedness (basolateral membrane vs. brush border membrane) of various transporters can be an important issue, since their location often determines net direction of movement of a compound across a barrier. For example, a transport system in the basolateral membrane of the choroid plexus for a specific compound may exhibit high-affinity, low-capacity kinetics for entry from the blood into the CSF; another system for the same compound in the brush border membrane may exhibit low-affinity, high-capacity kinetics for elimination of the same compound from the CSF into the blood. This difference in kinetics between the two membranes would allow for the net influx of the compound into the CSF when plasma concentrations are low and net efflux at high plasma concentrations.

1.4. Techniques for the Study of Drug Transport in the Choroid Plexus

The mechanisms of drug transport may be elucidated in the intact animal using a variety of *in vivo* and *in situ* techniques. Ventriculocisternal perfusion and intracerebral injection techniques can be used to study mechanisms for elimination of substances from the CSF (i.e., absorption) via the choroid plexus. Recently, choroidal artery perfusion methods have advanced our knowledge of the role of the choroid plexus in mediating the entry of substances into the CSF. These *in vivo* techniques may be coupled with microdialysis methods to gain further information on the relative contribution of the blood–brain and the blood–CSF barriers to the mechanism of a particular compound's entry into and elimination from the brain.

Isolated choroid plexus tissue slices comprise an uncomplicated *in vitro* system that provides an ideal initial approach for uptake studies to characterize mechanisms of transport in this epithelium. Isolated brush border and basolateral membrane vesicles can be prepared from the choroid plexus; such vesicles allow the study of each membrane separately and, thereby, provide a technique to identify the location of a transporter. Finally, cultured choroid plexus cells, which form polarized monolayers, provide another important *in vitro* system to further define drug transport and are particularly useful for the study of kinetics of flux across the epithelium and for the investigation of mechanisms of regulation of transporters.

In this chapter, we will focus on two methods for studying the transport of drugs in the choroid plexus: isolated choroid plexus tissue slices and primary cell culture. The advantages of each method are discussed in detail.

2. TRANSPORT STUDIES IN ISOLATED CHOROID PLEXUS TISSUE SLICES

The transport of many drugs and other molecules occurs by simple or facilitated diffusion. These processes are "passive," requiring no energy, because molecules are moving down their concentration or electrochemical gradients. A number of other drugs and molecules interact with active transport systems in order to bypass epithelial barriers. Active transport implies the movement of a substrate against its concentration (or electrochemical) gradient and therefore is energy-dependent. There are two major types of active transport: primary-active and secondary-active. Primary-active transport occurs when the energy to move against a gradient is directly coupled to the breakdown of ATP (or, less frequently, light energy) (Wainer, 1993). The Na^+/K^+-ATPase pump is an example of primary-active transport. Secondary-active transport involves the coupling of a substrate moving up its concentration gradient to an ion (or another substrate) moving down its concentration gradient (Stein, 1990). The Na^+-glucose transporter is secondary-active (Semenza, 1982).

There are two methods by which isolated choroid plexus tissue may be used to study mechanisms of transport across the blood–CSF barrier: the use of whole tissue slices and of ATP-depleted slices. Whole isolated choroid plexus tissue slices are necessary to study ATP-dependent transporters and have been used to examine the disposition of a number of compounds (Spector and Boose, 1979; Spector, 1982; Kim and Pritchard, 1993; Spector, 1987). In addition, intact tissue slices are important to initially determine if the transport of a particular compound is "energy-dependent." After this question is answered, ATP-depleted choroid plexus slices offer a number of advantages over whole choroid plexuses. The experiments are simpler and less expensive. In addition, ATP-depleted choroid plexus tissue slices are reminiscent of vesicles, and, because no ATP is available to drive the pumps which maintain the normal distribution of ions and solutes, intracellular and extracellular concentrations of ions and substrates can be experimentally controlled. That is, ion gradients may be imposed to determine driving forces, stoichiometry, and other mechanisms of transport. ATP-depleted choroid plexus slices have been used by this laboratory to characterize nucleoside and amino acid transport (Wu et al., 1992, 1994; Chung et al., 1994).

The techniques for performing studies in whole versus ATP-depleted tissue are similar. In the following sections, to avoid repetition, we have concentrated on materials and methods for studies in ATP-depleted tissue slices. However, we will emphasize several important differences in preparation and handling of the two types of tissue preparations.

2.1. Materials

Equipment and supplies: Pieces of aluminum foil (1 cm × 1 cm); shaking water bath (37°C); 24-well cell culture plates; glass vials; Petri dishes; tweezers; scissors; scalpel and blades; rongeur; dissecting instrument; vortexer; infrared (RI) lamp; microcentrifuge tubes; scintillation counter; scintillation vials.

Chemicals: 2,4-Dinitrophenol (250 µM) in ethanol; NaCl-HEPES buffer; KCl-

HEPES buffer; ^{3}H-labeled compounds; [^{14}C]mannitol; reaction mixture; 3 N HCl; 3 N KOH.

Additional materials for whole tissue slices: Artificial CSF; metabolic shaker (temperature controlled).

2.2. Procedures

2.2.1. ISOLATION OF CHOROID PLEXUS

New Zealand white rabbits are anesthetized with ketamine (40 mg/kg). When an adequate depth of anesthesia is achieved, the rabbit is decapitated using a guillotine. A midline scalp incision is then made, and the soft tissues overlying the parieto-occipital region are removed. A rongeur is used to remove bone over the parietal lobes bilaterally, extending from the torcular posteriorly to bregma anteriorly. The remainder of the dissection can be performed with the brain *in situ*, or the brain can be removed by severing the optic nerves and the brain stem at the level of the pons or medulla. In either case, the dura is opened using a knife with an 11 blade, exposing the interhemispheric fissure. The fissure is split with a dissecting instrument to reveal the splenium and the body of the corpus callosum. The callosal fibers are separated longitudinally just to the right and left of midline until the ependymal lining of the lateral ventricles is exposed. The ependyma is opened using the dissecting instrument to expose the floor of the lateral ventricles. The choroid plexus is then visible as a pink band of friable tissue lying on the floor of the lateral ventricles between the thalamus and caudate nucleus. Using fine forceps, the choroid plexus is elevated and removed. The tissue is placed into KCl-HEPES buffer (see Section 2.2.2) which has been incubated at 37°C.

2.2.2. PREPARATION OF ATP-DEPLETED CHOROID PLEXUS SLICES

The preparation of whole and ATP-depleted choroid plexus slices is similar; we have chosen to describe in detail the procedures for ATP-depleted slices. These methods can be easily adapted to intact tissue slices. We have divided this section into three parts: setup prior to harvesting choroid plexus, experimental procedures after harvesting the choroid plexus, and procedures in preparation for scintillation counting.

2.2.2a.   Setup Prior to Harvesting Choroid Plexus Tissue

1.   Prepare 100 ml of KCl-HEPES buffer (120 mM KCl, 40 mM mannitol, 25 mM HEPES, pH 7.4 with 1 M Tris) and NaCl-HEPES buffer (120 mM NaCl, 40 mM mannitol, 25 mM HEPES, pH 7.4 with 1 M Tris). For whole choroid plexus slices, prepare artificial CSF (Merlis, 1940).

2. Cut pieces of aluminum foil ($1 \text{ cm} \times 1 \text{ cm}$), one for each choroid plexus slice. Weigh, record weight, and place each piece of aluminum foil into the well of a cell culture plate; number each well. Aluminum foil is used because it is inexpensive and allows one to easily handle the choroid plexus slices.

3. Number microcentrifuge tubes to correspond to the numbers of the wells in the cell culture plate. One microcentrifuge tube will be used per choroid plexus slice.

4. Prepare a 10-ml solution of 2,4-dinitrophenol (DNP; 250 μM) in KCl-HEPES buffer from a stock solution (50 mM). Maintain at 37°C (we use a shaking water bath).

5. Pipet equivalent dpm quantities of the ^{3}H-labeled compound of interest and [^{14}C] mannitol (i.e., 200,000–300,000 dpm per 50 μl of reaction mix) into 1.5-ml polycarbonate microcentrifuge tubes. Add DNP (250 μM final concentration). Evaporate the solution under a stream of nitrogen. Add buffer (KCl-HEPES or NaCl-HEPES). Prepare enough reaction mixture so that there is at least 140 μl for each choroid plexus slice and so that each time/data point may be performed in triplicate. Place 140 μl of reaction mixture into each labeled microcentrifuge tube, and incubate at 37°C in a shaking water bath. The [^{14}C]mannitol serves as an extracellular marker.

6. Incubate 10 ml solution of KCl-HEPES buffer at 37°C.

2.2.2b. Experimental Procedures after Harvesting the Choroid Plexus

1. Initially place choroid plexuses in the 10-ml solution of KCl-HEPES buffer which has been previously incubated at 37°C. [For studies in intact choroid plexus slices which are not ATP-depleted, the tissue is placed into a modified artificial CSF (Merlis, 1940) and is maintained in a 95% O_2/5% CO_2 environment. The pH should be carefully monitored. A metabolic shaker is necessary to keep the gases mixing uniformly throughout the tissue, and the temperature should be maintained at 37°C.]

2. Transfer choroid plexuses into a Petri dish to cut into 2- to 3-mm pieces. To perform experiments on intact choroid plexus, investigators often do not cut the tissue into smaller pieces.

3. To deplete the tissue of ATP, the 2- to 3-mm choroid plexus slices are placed into DNP (250 μM, 10 ml, 37°C) in KCl-HEPES buffer for 20 min. Previous studies have shown that, under these conditions, ATP levels are reduced to approximately 9% of control (Carter and Kimmich, 1979; Wu et al., 1994). Following the 20-min incubation period, the tissue slices should remain in the DNP solution but are stored on ice until used during the experiment.

4. To determine the uptake of a radiolabeled compound, use tweezers to carefully remove individual choroid plexus slices from iced-DNP–KCl buffer, blot on laboratory tissue, and then place into the microcentrifuge tube containing 140 μl of reaction mixture (37°C).

5. At the end of the incubation period, remove the tissue from the reaction mixture with tweezers, blot on laboratory tissue, and place on the corresponding numbered, preweighed piece of aluminum foil in the cell culture plate. Do not discard the 140-μl reaction mixture.
6. Dry the tissue slices at room temperature overnight or under an infrared lamp for 1 hr.

2.2.2c. Procedures in Preparation for Scintillation Counting

1. Place 50 μl of each reaction mixture in separate, numbered scintillation vials with 5 ml of scintillant, and vortex.
2. When dry, the choroid plexus tissue slices should be weighed and removed from the aluminum foil and placed in individually numbered scintillation vials. Do not discard the aluminum foil.
3. After the tissue is dried, add 100 μl of 3N KOH to dissolve the tissue; this takes approximately 3 hr or the tissue may be dissolved overnight.
4. Add 100 μl of 3N HCl to neutralize the KOH. Add 5 ml of scintillation fluid.
5. Place each individual piece of aluminum foil into the corresponding scintillation vial and vortex.
6. The radioactive content from each choroid plexus tissue slice is expressed as a volume of distribution (V_d) (Whittico *et al.*, 1990; Wu *et al.*, 1992; see Section 2.5).

2.2.3. CRITERIA FOR IDENTIFICATION OF FUNCTIONAL ATP-DEPLETED CHOROID PLEXUS TISSUE SLICES

A transporter for the neutral amino acid L-proline is present in the brush border membrane of the choroid plexus (Ross and Wright, 1984). Control experiments measuring the Na^+-stimulated uptake of this amino acid should be performed to obtain supportive evidence that the tissue obtained is the choroid plexus. The methods for procuring and ATP-depleting the choroid plexus to perform a Na^+-proline uptake experiment are the same as described in Section 2.2.2.

To perform a control study documenting the presence of Na^+-driven L-proline transport, a time-dependent study should be conducted in the presence and absence of an initial inwardly directed Na^+ gradient (see Section 2.3.1). If an "overshoot phenomenon" is observed, this is supportive evidence that the tissue has been ATP-depleted (i.e., a Na^+ gradient was present transiently).

2.3. Mechanisms of Transport

At least three types of studies are performed to initially characterize the mechanism of transport for a particular compound: time-dependent studies, concentration-dependent (saturation or Michaelis–Menten) kinetic experiments, and inhibition studies. These are described in detail below.

2.3.1. TIME-DEPENDENT STUDIES

Studies of time dependency establish the time course of uptake of a substrate and the times at which an "initial rate" of uptake can be determined, as well as the time at which equilibrium is achieved. In addition, time-dependent studies may also be performed at different temperatures to establish the temperature dependency of an uptake process. In general, a high degree of temperature dependency is indicative of an active or facilitated transport process.

In these experiments, choroid plexus slices (whole or ATP-depleted) are prepared and incubated in the reaction mixture (37°C) for a range of times (e.g., 5, 15, 30 sec; 1, 5, 15, 30, 60 min). Uptake of a radiolabeled compound is then plotted as a function of time. Uptake is expressed as either tissue-to-media ratio (whole choroid plexus slices) or volume of distribution (ATP-depleted choroid plexus slices) (see Section 2.5).

To perform a time-dependent study:

1. Prepare reaction mixtures (see Section 2.2.2). Prepare enough reaction mixture so that each time/data point may be obtained in triplicate. Choosing the concentration of substrate (radiolabeled plus cold) used in this study is important. Typically, the concentration used should be well below the K_m. Unfortunately, in most cases the K_m is not known. Therefore, a concentration is estimated based on clinically relevant concentrations or on data available for structurally related compounds. Typically, for active transport systems, an appropriate concentration is in the micromolar range.
2. Harvest tissue (see Section 2.2.1).
3. A typical range of time points to measure uptake (37°C) includes: 5, 15, and 30 sec and 1, 5, 15, 30, and 60 min.
4. After incubation, blot choroid plexus on laboratory tissue, and place on the preweighed piece of aluminum foil in an individual well of a 24-well cell culture plate to dry.
5. See Section 2.2.2 for further details on preparation of tissue, reaction mixtures, and foil for scintillation counting.

2.3.2. CONCENTRATION-DEPENDENT (MICHAELIS–MENTEN) STUDIES

In these experiments, the uptake of a compound is studied as a function of change in its concentration. A linear relationship between uptake and concentration is characteristic of passive diffusion, whereas saturability is characteristic of carrier-mediated transport.

A time-dependent study must be performed before the Michaelis–Menten study to determine the range of time over which the uptake of the solute is linear. In a

Michaelis–Menten study, uptake should be measured during this linear phase to ensure that efflux of the radiolabeled compound is negligible. Michaelis–Menten parameters for a radiolabeled compound are calculated by determining initial rates of transport in the presence of increasing concentrations of the unlabeled compound. Facilitated diffusion as well as high- and low-affinity saturable transport processes may be identified by fitting the data to the following equation:

$$\text{Rate of uptake} = V_{\max} \cdot C/(K_m + C)$$

where $V_{\max}$ is the maximal rate of transport, K_m is the concentration of the compound of interest when the initial rate is at one-half of maximum, and C is the concentration of the compound of interest in the reaction mixture. Rate of uptake is expressed as nanomoles per gram of tissue per second.

To perform a Michaelis–Menten study:

1. Solutions containing the radiolabeled compound (reaction mixture; see Section 2.2.2) should contain twice the final desired concentrations (i.e., instead of 250 μM DNP, prepare 500 μM; instead of 15 μl of radiolabeled compound, use 30 μl).

2. A series of solutions containing various concentrations (e.g., 0, 2, 5, 10, 25, 50, 75, 100, 150, 200, 300, and 400 μM) of the unlabeled compound should be prepared. These concentrations should be twice the final desired concentrations (i.e., if the final concentration should be 10 μM, prepare a 20 μM solution). If studying a Na^+-dependent transporter, prepare the solution in NaCl-HEPES buffer.

3. To make the final reaction mixture, add 70 μl of solution containing the radiolabeled substrate and 70 μl of the mixture containing the unlabeled compound, for each corresponding concentration, to an appropriately labeled microcentrifuge tube or glass vial. This technique ensures that each reaction mixture contains the same amount of radiolabel. These solutions should be incubated at 37°C.

4. After harvesting (see Section 2.2.1) and ATP-depleting the choroid plexus (see Section 2.2.2), incubate individual tissue slices in the reaction mixture for a time period known to represent an "initial time" point.

5. After incubation, blot choroid plexus on laboratory tissue and place on the preweighed piece of aluminum foil in an individual well of a 24-well cell culture plate to dry.

6. See Section 2.2.2 for further details on preparation of tissue, reaction mixtures, and foil for scintillation counting.

2.3.3. INHIBITION STUDIES

A transporter is generally selective for substrates that are closely related structurally. The purpose of inhibition studies is to define this structural specificity of a particular transporter. Compounds to be screened as potential inhibitors are added to the reaction mixture containing a radiolabeled compound known to be a substrate of a particular transport system. Because transport via a carrier-mediated system is saturable, the uptake of a radiolabeled substrate will be inhibited in the presence of an unlabeled compound that is transported by or interacts with the same protein. That is, the unlabeled compound is an "inhibitor."

To perform an inhibition study, uptake of the radiolabeled substrate is measured in the absence (control) and presence of a series of potential "inhibitors." As in the Michaelis–Menten studies, an initial time should be selected to measure uptake. If the uptake of the radiolabeled substrate is significantly decreased from that measured with the control, this suggests that the inhibitor interacts with the same transporter. If a compound is found to be an inhibitor, other mechanistic studies (e.g., Michaelis–Menten, IC_{50}, counterflux) may then be performed to determine if the inhibition is competitive, uncompetitive, or noncompetitive (Stein, 1990).

To perform an inhibition study:

1. Solutions containing the radiolabeled compound should be twice the final desired concentrations (i.e., instead of 250 μM DNP, prepare 500 μM; instead of 15 μl of radiolabeled compound, use 30 μl).
2. Solutions of inhibitors should contain twice the desired concentration (i.e., if the final concentration should be 100 μM, prepare a 200 μM solution). If studying a Na^+-dependent transporter, prepare the solution in NaCl-HEPES buffer.
3. To make the final reaction mixture, add 70 μl of solution containing the radiolabeled substrate and 70 μl of the inhibitor solution, for each corresponding concentration, to an appropriately labeled microcentrifuge tube or glass vial. This technique ensures that each reaction mixture contains the same amount of radiolabel. These solutions should then be incubated at 37°C.
4. Incubate an individual choroid plexus slice in each reaction mixture for a time period known to represent an "initial time" point.
5. After incubation, blot choroid plexus on laboratory tissue and place on the preweighed piece of aluminum foil in an individual well of a 24-well cell culture plate to dry.
6. See Section 2.2.2 for further details on preparation of tissue, reaction mixtures, and foil for scintillation counting.

2.3.4. IDENTIFICATION OF DRIVING FORCES

The uphill transport of a number of compounds across epithelial barriers has been demonstrated to be coupled to an ion moving down its concentration gradient (Le Hir and Dubach, 1985b). In general, an inwardly directed Na^+ or proton gradient has been identified as a major driving force in a number of secondary-active transporters (e.g., glucose, nucleosides, and many amino acids; Semenza, 1982; Wu *et al.*, 1992; Kragh *et al.*, 1984). After being ATP-depleted, choroid plexus slices cannot maintain the normal transmembrane ion gradients, since these gradients require ATP-dependent, membrane-bound pumps. Thus, studies to identify the driving forces of a particular transport system can be accomplished in ATP-depleted choroid plexus slices, since various gradients can be experimentally controlled.

To determine what ions are essential to a particular transporter, a time-dependent study is performed in the presence of a particular substrate and a gradient of various cations (e.g., H^+ or Na^+) or anions (e.g., Cl^-, SCN^-, SO_4^{2-}, etc.). If the transport of a substrate is enhanced in the presence of a particular ion gradient, an "overshoot phenomenon" occurs. An "overshoot phenomenon" is seen when uptake is plotted versus time; the intracellular concentration of substrate transiently exceeds the equilibrium concentration (Le Hir and Dubach, 1985a). This phenomenon suggests that uphill transport of a substrate (i.e., against a concentration gradient) is coupled to the movement of an ion down its concentration gradient.

To identify driving forces (e.g., Na^+-dependency):

1. At least two reaction mixes are prepared (i.e., one with and one without the ion in question). For example, to determine if a transporter is dependent on an inwardly directed Na^+ gradient, one reaction mix should be prepared in KCl-HEPES buffer and the other in NaCl-HEPES buffer. A 140-μl aliquot of each should be placed in individually labeled microcentrifuge tubes and incubated at 37°C.
2. After harvesting (see Section 2.2.1) and ATP-depleting the choroid plexus (see Section 2.2.2), incubate individual tissue slices for various times (e.g., 5, 15, 30 sec; 1, 5, 15, 30, 60 min) in the reaction mixtures.
3. Blot choroid plexus on laboratory tissue and place on the preweighed piece of aluminum foil in an individual well of a 24-well cell culture plate to dry.
4. See Section 2.2.2 for further details on preparation of tissue, reaction mixtures, and foil for scintillation counting.

After these initial studies of driving forces, stoichiometry studies may be performed to determine the specific mechanism of interaction of an ion with a transporter (Wu *et al.*, 1992).

2.3.5. COUNTERFLUX STUDIES

Many compounds can inhibit a transporter without being translocated but by simply binding to the protein. To determine whether two compounds share a common transporter, counterflux or countertransport studies may be conducted. The counterflux phenomenon usually depends on competition between structurally similar molecules for the same transporter (Hofer and Hogget, 1980). Counterflux implies that a compound on the *trans* side of the membrane can drive the uphill transport of a radiolabeled compound added to the opposite side of the membrane. These studies are usually performed in ATP-depleted choroid plexus slices that have been "preloaded" with a compound to be tested (i.e., concentration equilibrated across membranes of the tissue) for counterfluxing the radiolabeled substrate contained in the reaction mixture. The energy necessary for this transport is provided by the outwardly directed concentration gradient of the unlabeled compound. If an "overshoot phenomenon" is observed in the preloaded choroid plexus tissue slices (and not observed in nonloaded tissue), then the phenomenon of counterflux has been demonstrated.

To perform a counterflux study:

1. To make the reaction mixtures, pipet equivalent dpm quantities of ^{3}H-labeled compound and [^{14}C]mannitol (i.e., 200,000–300,000 dpm per 50 μl of reaction mixture). Add DNP (250 μM). Evaporate the solution under a stream of nitrogen.

2. After harvesting (see Section 2.2.1) and ATP-depleting the choroid plexus (see Section 2.2.2), preincubate (preload) tissue slices in a buffer containing the potential counterfluxing compound, DNP (250 μM), and NaCl-HEPES buffer (120 mM, pH 7.4) for 30 min. Then quickly wash in ice-cold NaCl-HEPES buffer and blot on laboratory tissue. Incubate individual choroid plexus slices at a series of time points (e.g., 5, 15, 30 sec; 1, 5, 15, 30, 60 min) in the reaction mixture.

3. Blot choroid plexus on laboratory tissue and place on the preweighed piece of aluminum foil in an individual well of a 24-well cell culture plate to dry.

4. See Section 2.2.2 for further details on preparation of tissue, reaction mixtures, and foil for scintillation counting.

2.4. Potential Problems

A major problem encountered when handling whole choroid plexus slices that have not been ATP-depleted is tissue death due to inadequate oxygenation. Tissue must be immediately placed in oxygenated buffer following isolation. Even with adequate oxygenation, intact tissue is probably viable for only 1–2 hr.

Because transporters may be sensitive to pH changes, the pH of buffers and reaction mixtures must be checked carefully. In particular, adding compounds to buffers to perform inhibitor studies may change the pH significantly; adjust the pH to 7.4 before performing experiments.

To study driving forces in ATP-depleted tissue, the choroid plexus tissue must be incubated in the DNP at 37°C for 20 min. If ATP depletion is incomplete, ion and substrate gradients cannot be accurately controlled experimentally.

Isolated choroid plexus tissue contains a mixture of cell types: epithelium, endothelial cells, fibroblasts, etc. Many transporters in the epithelia of the choroid plexus are not likely to be found in these other cell types, but it is important to recognize the possibility that they may be. In addition, it is impossible to determine if a transporter is located on the brush border or basolateral membrane or both by means of the above-described whole-tissue techniques. Performing studies in isolated membrane vesicles (Whittico *et al.*, 1991) or in pure cell cultures (see Section 3) is essential to identify the specific location and to determine characteristics and function of the transporter. For example, if a monolayer of choroid plexus epithelium and a monolayer of fibroblasts are obtained, time-dependent uptake studies of a particular substrate in the two cell types can be easily compared to identify if and where a transporter is present. Isolated membrane vesicles will also allow separate access to the brush border and basolateral transporters.

2.5.　Calculation of Transport Parameters

The tissue-to-media ratio (T/M) is calculated as

$$T/M = \frac{\text{dpm } ^{3}\text{H-labelled compound/g of choroid plexus}}{\text{dpm } ^{3}\text{H-labelled compound/ml of media}}$$

where the weight of choroid plexus is wet weight. The volume of distribution (V_d) is calculated as

$$V_d = \frac{\text{dpm } ^{3}\text{H-labelled compound/g of choroid plexus}}{\text{dpm } ^{3}\text{H-labelled compound/ml of media}}$$
$$- \frac{\text{dpm } [^{14}\text{C}]\text{mannitol/g of choroid plexus}}{\text{dpm } [^{14}\text{C}]\text{mannitol/ml of media}}$$

where the weight of choroid plexus is dry weight.

To calculate kinetic parameters, uptake is expressed as a rate (e.g., nanomoles per milligram of dry tissue weight per second). Data are plotted as initial rate of uptake versus concentration, and kinetic parameters are obtained by fitting the data to a Michaelis–Menten equation which may include several saturable transport components as well as a linear nonsaturable transport component, e.g.,

$$\text{Rate} = [(V_{\max} \cdot C/K_m + C)] + (K_{ns} \cdot C)$$

where $V_{\max}$ is the maximal rate of transport, K_m is the concentration at which the rate of transport is half of $V_{\max}$, K_{ns} is the coefficient for the linear, nonsaturable component, and C is the concentration of substrate in the reaction mixture. In the determination of inhibition potency, an IC_{50} is usually estimated by a sigmoidal inhibition model:

$$V = \frac{V^o}{1 + (I/IC_{50})^n}$$

where V is the uptake of substrate in the presence of the inhibitor, V^o is the uptake of substrate in the absence of any inhibitor, I is the inhibitor concentration, and n is the slope. If the interaction is competitive, n will be 1.0. For a competitive interaction, the K_I is determined from the following equation:

$$K_I = \frac{IC_{50}}{1 + C/K_m}$$

where C represents the concentration of substrate used in the inhibitor studies, and K_m represents the substrate affinity determined in Michaelis–Menten studies.

3. CULTURED CHOROID PLEXUS EPITHELIAL CELLS

Cell culture has been demonstrated to be a powerful tool in identifying mechanisms of transport in various epithelia. When cells are cultured as a monolayer, external physical and chemical environments can be manipulated easily (Taub, 1985). In addition, after the orientation of the monolayer is recognized, the location ("sidedness") of a transporter can be determined (brush border vs. basolateral membrane) by growing cells on filters or inserts in wells (Transwell®), a system that allows separate access to the brush border and the basolateral membranes (Fig. 2). The results of such experimental techniques often provide insight into the physiologic function of a transporter. Does this transporter function in secretion or absorption? Are there different proteins on the two surfaces with different kinetic characteristics transporting the same substrates? In particular, identifying the mechanisms of transport of substrates on each membrane of the choroid plexus can have an important impact on drug targeting into or out of the CSF. Although membrane vesicles may also be used to determine sidedness, the technique requires large amounts of tissue to obtain enriched quantities of particular membranes, especially when it is used to study the choroid plexus epithelium.

Cell culture is an important *in vitro* technique to evaluate the absorption and delivery of new classes of drugs (Wilson, 1990). To be relevant, however, a cell culture system must display morphological and functional characteristics of an *in vivo* cell system. Many continuous cell lines have been developed (e.g., renal and intestinal epithelial cells, brain endothelial cells) which express a variety of *in vivo* transport systems. Because of this, multiple transporters in the kidney and intestine have been extensively studied in various cell culture models. However, this has not been accomplished in the choroid plexus because, currently, a continuous cell line of choroid plexus epithelia is not available. Recently, techniques to culture choroid plexus cells as a primary culture have been developed. It is envisioned that these techniques will be increasingly used to study drug transport across the blood–CSF barrier (Crook *et al.*, 1981; Mayer and Sanders, 1993; Southwell *et al.*, 1993).

At times, primary cell cultures are more representative of the cell types from which they were derived. However, the method is often cumbersome, and meticulous

Brush Border Membrane Chamber

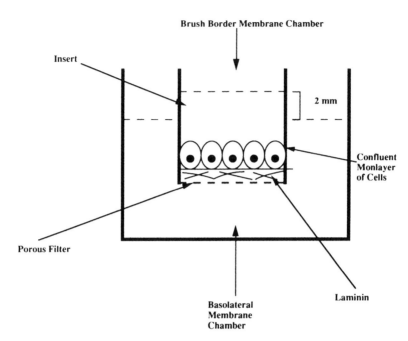

Figure 2. Schematic of a two-chamber cell culture system. A monolayer of epithelial choroid plexus cells is plated on the laminin-coated Transwell® membranes. Cell culture media is added to the upper and lower chambers. Fluid in the upper chamber bathes the apical (brush border) membrane. Fluid in the lower chamber is in contact with the basolateral membrane.

technique is necessary to avoid infection, to prevent overgrowth of fibroblasts, and to obtain sufficient yield to produce a confluent monolayer (Freshney, 1986).

3.1. Materials

Equipment and supplies: Laminar flow hood; inverted microscope; tissue culture CO_2 incubator; culture dishes (2×100 and 1×25 mm); scissors; scalpel and blades; rongeur; dissecting instrument; forceps; cellulose TLC plates; culture plates (24-well); sterile tubes (15 ml and 50 ml) containing Ham's buffer, placed on ice.

Chemicals and media: Hams' F-12; Dulbecco's modified Eagle's (DME) medium; phosphate-buffered saline; penicillin (50 U/ml); gentamicin sulfate (10 μg/ml); streptomycin (50 μg/ml); sodium selenite (5 ng/ml); epidermal growth factor (10 ng/ml); fetal calf serum (10%); glutamine (2 mM); transferrin (5 μg/ml); DNase (20 mg); HEPES (10 mM); pronase (5 mg); prostaglandin E_a (26 μg/ml); insulin (5 μg/ml); laminin (0.006 mg/insert).

Dissecting medium A (complete culture medium): DME/Ham's with penicillin/ streptomycin, HEPES, glutamine, and fetal calf serum. Prewarm 100 ml to 37°C. Check pH after warming; cells will not tolerate alkali media.

Dissecting medium B: Ham's F-12 and DME medium (1:1) with penicillin, streptomycin, HEPES, glutamine, insulin, transferrin, sodium selenite, epidermal growth factor, and prostaglandin E_a.

3.2. Procedures

3.2.1. ISOLATION OF CELLS AND ESTABLISHING A MONOLAYER

The following method is based on that described by Southwell *et al.* (1993). Therefore, the experimental animal is a rat, but the technique can probably be adapted to other species.

1. All dissections are done wearing sterile gloves. Instruments are washed frequently in 70% ethanol.
2. Fifteen to twenty Buffalo rats (20-day-old, male) are anesthetized with ether and then decapitated. (In this laboratory, we have found that Sprague-Dawley rats of the same age may also be used. Initial studies also suggest that adult New Zealand white rabbits may be used.)
3. The brain and spinal cord are removed and placed into a dish of culture medium containing medium B. Keep medium in a warming bath until immediately before use.
4. The plexus is then removed with the brain submerged in medium B. (See Section 2.2.1 for details of obtaining choroid plexus.) Attention to sterile technique is important when obtaining choroid plexus for primary cell culture, as compared to obtaining the tissue for whole or ATP-depleted slices. Cell isolation should be performed in a laminar flow hood.
5. Place choroid plexuses into a culture dish containing medium B. Maintain medium B at 37°C until all plexuses have been removed. Sacrifice the next animal only after the previous plexus has been placed in medium B.
6. After all the choroid plexuses have been isolated, transfer the clean tissue into a second small dish with medium B. Observe cells using an inverted microscope (100× magnification); epithelial cells should be round and plump.
7. Cut choroid plexuses into smaller (¼ size) pieces.
8. Transfer plexuses into a small flask (10 ml) with a 1000-μl pipet, remove the media, and replace with prewarmed trypsin (1.2%)/EDTA (0.1%) solution.
9. Gently swirl cells for 15 min and allow plexuses to settle to the bottom. [Plexuses are gently shaken on an orbital shaker platform for 15 min at 37°C in the trypsin (1.2%)/EDTA (0.1%) solution.]

10. Transfer trypsin solution containing released cells to a sterile plastic centrifuge tube containing 1 ml of fetal calf serum. Maintain at 37°C.

11. Add fresh trypsin to the flask containing the choroid plexuses to further dissociate epithelial cells from the tissue. Maintain at 37°C.

12. Repeat steps 9–11 at least 6 times.

13. Spin (<1000 rpm) the centrifuge tubes containing the trypsin solution (from step 10) for 1–2 min to pellet cells. Discard the trypsin supernatant, resuspend the cells in 1 ml of complete culture medium (dissecting medium A), place into a well of a 24-well plate, and put into the CO_2 incubator for 2 hr. The cells obtained from each 15-min treatment with trypsin are placed into separate wells.

14. Most of the cells obtained in the first 1–2 trypsin treatments are red blood cells and broken epithelial cells. Most of the epithelial cells are obtained in the third and later treatments. It takes about 1.5 hr to disperse the cells from the intact tissue.

15. Examine the 24-well plate under an inverted microscope to confirm which fractions contain the epithelial cells. Cells should be in small sheets or should appear as individual cells. Epithelial cells will be round in complete medium.

16. Collect the fractions containing only epithelial cells into centrifuge tubes, and centrifuge gently (<1000 rpm for 1–2 min) to remove medium. If the epithelial cells are in large clumps, repeat trypsin treatment. Cells should be washed with dissecting medium B to remove any fetal calf serum before trypsinization.

17. Pipet cells gently, and spin to remove trypsin.

18. Add 1 ml of complete culture medium, resuspend, and count cells.

19. A dilute solution of trypan blue may be added to the cells to be counted for viability measurement. However, cells should be counted *immediately*, since choroid plexus epithelial cells tend to be phagocytic and readily take up trypan blue. That is, within 1 min, approximately half of the viable epithelial cells may be lightly stained.

20. Adjust the cell concentration to 5×10^5 cells/ml in complete culture medium.

21. Before seeding cells, precoat Costar transparent collagen-treated membrane (Costar Transwell-COL, 6.5 mm) wells with laminin (0.006 mg/insert). Southwell *et al.* (1993) recommend natural mouse laminin (Gibco/BRL 23017-015). Laminin contains a high density of negative charges which allows cells to attach by cross linkage directly to Ca^{2+} or Mg^{2+}.

22. The unattached epithelial cells should be collected and cultured at a density of 1×10^5 to 3×10^5 cells per well (1.3-cm diameter) in culture medium.

23. Do not disturb the cells for the first couple of days. The culture medium should be carefully changed after two days and, after that, every two days.

It takes approximately 5–7 days for the cells to establish a barrier. Be gentle in changing the media to avoid detaching cells from the culture well.

3.2.2. CRITERIA FOR IDENTIFICATION OF CULTURED CELLS

When initially establishing a primary choroid plexus cell culture system, one must determine that the cells cultured are the desired choroid plexus epithelium. The following procedures attempt to ensure that choroid plexus epithelium has been obtained:

1. By using phase-contrast microscopy, cells possessing a flat, polygonal morphology should be observed, a feature common to epithelial cells in primary culture, and one reported by Crook *et al.* (1981) to be present in the cultured choroid plexus cells.
2. Treat cells with *cis*-hydroxyproline at concentrations of up to 250 µg/ml. These concentrations are lethal to fibroblasts but presumably not to epithelial cells, including the choroid plexus epithelial cells.
3. Measure the levels of γ-glutamyl transpeptidase and alkaline phosphatase. The activity of γ-glutamyl transpeptidase is high in the epithelial cells relative to that in fibroblasts and the activity of alkaline phosphatase is low.
4. Electron microscopy may be used to determine the presence of a microvillous membrane as well as junctional complexes and to ascertain that the cells have grown as monolayers (Fig. 3). Previously, Southwell *et al.* (1993) found that epithelial cells cultured from choroid plexus of the rat formed monolayers with distinct microvilli and junctional complexes.
5. Trypan blue may also be used to determine if cells are viable (see Section 3.2.1, step 19).
6. Transepithelial electrical resistances (TEER values, with a resistance meter) and mannitol fluxes should be measured. Previously, Southwell *et al.* (1993) found that TEER values in cultured choroid plexus epithelial cell monolayers 5 days after seeding were about 100 $\Omega \cdot cm^2$.

3.2.3. TRANSPORT STUDIES IN CULTURED MONOLAYERS

In culture, epithelial cells are oriented with the brush border (apical) surface facing the media and the basolateral surface attached to the solid support or filter. Although epithelial cell monolayers can be grown on a solid support, it is generally preferable to grow such monolayers on filters. Epithelial cells grown on filters polarize and often exhibit more highly differentiated characteristics in comparison to cells grown on a solid support. Moreover, if cells are grown on filters in a Transwell® system, uptake experiments across either the brush border or basolateral membrane can be performed. However, uptake across the brush border surface can also be

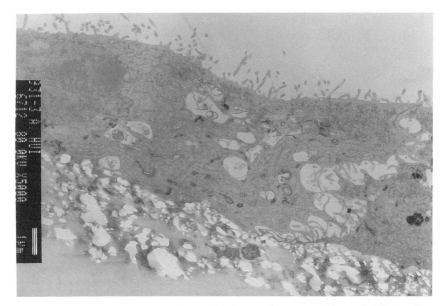

Figure 3. Electron micrograph of rabbit choroid plexus cells grown on Transwell-COL®, collagen-coated permeable membrane filters (5000× magnification). The epithelial cells separate the CSF from the blood. The cells rest upon a thin basement membrane and are joined together at the brush border membrane by desmosomes (tight junctions). The apical (brush border) membrane is composed of numerous micro-villi, visible at the top of the micrograph, which serve to increase the surface area.

determined in cells grown on a solid support, since the cells grow with the brush border facing the media and the basolateral surface attached to the support.

To perform experiments of uptake across the brush border membrane (Transwell® system):

1. Prior to initiating uptake, aspirate media from above each monolayer, and gently rinse three times with phosphate-buffered saline (PBS) at room temperature. Do not flush the cells directly with the media because they are still easily detached from the well. Set aside a few wells in order to perform a protein assay.

2. To initiate uptake, add 500 μl of uptake buffer containing radiolabeled substrate at 24°C to the filter cup (Transwell insert). Uptake is usually performed for a range of times (e.g., 1, 5, 15, 30, 60, 90, 120, 150 min). For the initial experiments, the reaction mixture is made such that there is approximately 500,000 dpm/ml of reaction mix. In subsequent studies, the dpm's can be adjusted, depending on the results of scintillation counting. It is important to minimize the accumulation of substrate in the basolateral compartment. This can be done by placing a large volume of media in the

basolateral compartment or by frequently changing the media in the basolateral compartment.

3. To stop uptake, remove the reaction mixture with gentle aspiration. Remove the filter cup and dip it into ice-cold PBS three times. (For cells grown on a solid support, wash monolayers three times with 500 μl of ice-cold PBS.)

4. Blot the bottom of filter cup on laboratory tissue and flip cup over to drain.

5. Cut out filters, and place them into scintillation vials containing scintillant and allow to sit overnight. Vortex and count. [If the experiment is performed on cells grown on a solid support without filters, the cells are solubilized in 1 ml of Triton X-100 for 1 hr. After this, an aliquot (500 μl) of the solubilized cells is transferred into scintillation vials, and 5 ml of scintillant is added.]

6. To perform a protein assay, aspirate media, and rinse three times with PBS at room temperature. Add 500 μl of 1 N NaOH, and allow to sit for 1 hr. After dissolution of cells, add 500 μl of 1 N HCl to neutralize.

7. Protein concentration may be determined using the Bio-Rad Protein Assay Kit as outlined by Bradford (1976). Bovine serum albumin (BSA; 1 μg/μl) is used as a standard.

8. Dilute Bio-Rad solution 1:5 with water and filter using a Buchner funnel.

9. Dilute the protein (cells) 1:20 and 1:40 with water and vortex. Place 20 μl of 1:20 dilution and 40 μl of 1:40 dilution into test tubes (two samples), and add a sufficient quantity of water to make 100 μl.

10. A standard curve should then be prepared using BSA. Aliquot 0 to 25 μl, in 5-μl increments, of BSA into test tubes. Add a sufficient quantity of water to make 100 μl.

11. Add 5 ml of diluted Bio-Rad solution, and vortex.

12. Let samples stand for 5 min.

13. Analyze samples with a spectrophotometer within 1 hr at 595 nm (visible range).

To perform experiments of uptake across the basolateral (bottom) membrane:

1. Prior to initiating uptake, aspirate media and gently rinse each filter cup which contains the monolayer three times with PBS at room temperature. Do not flush the cells directly with the media because they are still easily detached from the well. Set aside a few wells in order to perform a protein assay.

2. Drain the filter of PBS by inverting.

3. Add 400 μl of mineral oil to cover the surface of the cells (brush border side). Mineral oil is used to prevent cells from dehydrating.

4. To initiate uptake, add 1 ml of reaction mixture containing radiolabeled substrate at 24°C to the basolateral side. Uptake is usually measured over a range of times (e.g., 1, 5, 15, 30, 60, 90, 120, 150 min). For the initial

experiments, the reaction mixture is made such that there is approximately 500,000 dpm/ml of reaction mixture.

5. To stop uptake, remove the filter cup and dip it into ice-cold PBS three times.
6. See above description of experiments across the brush border membrane for subsequent steps of this method.

3.2.4. TRANSEPITHELIAL FLUX STUDIES IN MONOLAYERS GROWN ON PERMEABLE FILTERS

If cells are grown on permeable filters (Fig. 2), in addition to studying transport via the brush border and basolateral surfaces separately, net directional flux can also be measured. (Generally, to perform flux studies, a substrate is added at one surface, and the concentration of the same substrate is measured from the other surface.) However, it is critical to have a totally confluent monolayer. Otherwise, flux measurements will reflect leaks in the monolayer. By including radiolabeled mannitol in the reaction mix, correction for paracellular flux (or flux through filters not covered with cells) can be ascertained. TEER values should be measured across each monolayer to ascertain that the monolayer is confluent. Low TEER ($\ll 100$ $\Omega \cdot cm^2$) suggests that the monolayer is leaky. For flux studies, it is important to select filters that do not rate-limit flux. Ideally, the flux of mannitol across the filter (without cells) should be rapid in comparison to its flux across filters with monolayers.

To perform flux studies:

1. Prior to initiating uptake, aspirate media and gently rinse each filter cup which contains the monolayer three times with PBS at room temperature. Do not flush the cells directly with the media because they are still easily detached from the well. Set up wells containing approximately 1 ml of PBS (smaller wells may require less fluid). Wells should be labeled with the various sampling times (e.g., 1, 5, 10, 30 min; 1, 2 hr).
2. Invert filter to drain PBS.
3. To initiate uptake, add 1 ml of reaction mixture containing radiolabeled substrate (and radiolabeled mannitol) at 24°C to the bottom or the basolateral side (basolateral to brush border flux). Wells used in flux studies are sampled at different time points (e.g., 1, 5, 10, 30 min; 1, 2 hr). The filter cup should be placed in the first well for the allotted time (e.g., 1 min). Then place filter cup into the next well until the next allotted time (e.g., 5 min) is reached. This is repeated until the endpoint time is reached.
4. Remove fluid from each well and place in scintillation vials containing scintillant. Vortex and count.
5. These experiments can be performed to monitor brush border-to-basolateral flux by placing the initial reaction mixture in the brush border compartment and sampling from the basolateral compartment.

3.3. Calculation of Transport Parameters and Flux

Transport parameter calculations (i.e., Michaelis–Menten) are similar to those described in Section 2.3. Cultured choroid plexus cells may be used to determine time dependence, temperature dependence, and Michaelis–Menten kinetic parameters and to perform inhibition studies. In general, uptake in cultured choroid plexus cells is expressed as picomoles per milligram of protein:

$$\text{Uptake} = \frac{\text{Intracellular dpm/Specific activity}}{\text{mg protein}}$$

The apparent permeability coefficient (P_{app}) is determined as follows (Artursson and Magnusson, 1990):

$$\text{Flux or } P_{app} = \frac{\Delta v Q}{\Delta t \times 60 \times A \times C_0}$$

where $\Delta Q/\Delta t$ is the permeability rate (μg/min), C_0 is the initial concentration in the donor chamber (μg/ml), and A is the surface area of the membrane (cm^2).

3.4. Potential Problems

A primary cell culture of choroid plexus cells is difficult to establish. The cells require careful monitoring of pH of the media because they do not survive in alkali media. Fibroblast overgrowth can occur, especially in media containing fetal calf serum. Finally, a high seeding density is essential to obtain a confluent monolayer of cells, which is necessary to perform flux studies. Cells grown in culture may lose some of the properties of the intact cells *in vivo*. Therefore, care must be taken in interpreting data obtained from cultured monolayers. Importantly, transport function may deteriorate (or appear) with time. Therefore, initial studies should be performed to determine the optimum time after seeding to perform transport studies. Because cells are intact, metabolic processes are active. Thus, many drugs may be metabolized in the cells. For drug studies, the transport of the parent compound should be determined specifically.

4. SUMMARY

In order to understand the pharmacokinetics and pharmacodynamics of drugs and molecules in the central nervous system, it is important to have an in-depth knowledge of the transport processes which determine their absorption, distribution, and elimination. The techniques described in this chapter have been successfully used to study transport across the blood–CSF barrier (choroid plexus). There are advantages and disadvantages for each technique. In general, a combination of these techniques as well as others which we have referenced are necessary to identify and characterize a particular transporter.

ACKNOWLEDGMENTS

The authors wish to thank Drs. Bridget Southwell and Gerhard Schreiber for the choroid plexus primary cell culture technique. Work in the authors' laboratories is supported by grants from the National Institutes of Health (GM26691, GM36780, GM42230).

REFERENCES

Anderson, B. D., Hoesterey, B. L., Baker, D. C., and Galinsky, R. E., 1990, Uptake kinetics of 2′,3′-dideoxyinosine into brain and cerebrospinal fluid of rats: Intravenous infusion studies, *J. Pharmacol. Exp. Ther.* **253:**113–118.
Artursson, P., and Magnusson, C., 1990, Epithelial transport of drugs in cell culture. II: Effect of extracellular calcium concentration on the paracellular transport of drugs of different lipophilicities across monolayers of intestinal epithelial (Caco-2) cells, *J. Pharm. Sci.* **79:**595–600.
Bradford, M. M., 1976, A rapid and sensitive method for the quantitation of microgram quantities of protein utilizing the principle of protein–dye binding, *Anal. Biochem.* **72:**248–254.
Carter, S. C., and Kimmich, G. A., 1979, Membrane potentials and sugar transport by ATP-depleted intestinal cells: Effect of anion gradients, *Am. J. Physiol.* **237:**C67–C74.
Chung, S.-J., Ramanathan, V., Giacomini, K., and Brett, C., 1994, Characterization of a sodium-dependent taurine transporter in rabbit choroid plexus, *Biochim. Biophys. Acta* **1193:**10–16.
Crook, R. B., Kasagami, H., and Prusiner, S. B., 1981, Culture and characterization of epithelial cells from bovine choroid plexus, *J. Neurochem.* **37:**845–854.
Freshney, R. I. (ed.), 1986, *Animal Cell Culture: A Practical Approach*, IRL Press, Oxford.
Hofer, M., and Hogget, J. G., 1980, *Transport across Biological Membranes*, Pitman Advanced Publishing Program, Boston.
Kim, C. S., and Pritchard, J. B., 1993, Transport of 2,4,5-trichlorophenoxyacetic acid across the blood–cerebrospinal fluid barrier of the rabbit, *J. Pharmacol. Exp. Ther.* **267:**751–757.
Kragh, H. U., Roigaard, P. H., Jacobsen, C., and Sheikh, M. I., 1984, Renal transport of neutral amino acids. Tubular localization of Na⁺-dependent phenylalanine- and glucose-transport systems, *Biochem. J.* **220:**15–24.
Le Hir, M., and Dubach, U. C., 1985a, Concentrative transport of purine nucleosides in brush border vesicles of the rat kidney, *Eur. J. Clin. Invest.* **15:**121–127.
Le Hir, M., and Dubach, U. C., 1985b, Uphill transport of pyrimidine nucleosides in renal brush border vesicles, *Pflügers Arch.* **404:**238–243.
Mayer, S. E., and Sanders, B. E., 1993, Sodium-dependent antiporters in choroid plexus epithelial cultures from rabbit, *J. Neurochem.* **60:**1308–1316.
Merlis, J. K., 1940, The effect of changes in the calcium content of the cerebrospinal fluid on spinal reflex activity in the dog, *Am. J. Physiol.* **131:**67–72.
Neuwelt, E. A. (ed.), 1989, *Implications of the Blood Brain Barrier and Its Manipulation*, Plenum Medical Book Co., New York.

Pardridge, W. M., Boado, R. J., Black, K. L., and Cancilla, P. A., 1992, Blood–brain barrier and new approaches to brain drug delivery [see comments], *West. J. Med.* **156:**281–286.

Pollay, M., 1975, Formation of cerebrospinal fluid. Relation of studies of isolated choroid plexus to the standing gradient hypothesis, *J. Neurosurg.* **42:**665–673.

Ross, H. J., and Wright, E. M., 1984, Neutral amino acid transport by plasma membrane vesicles of the rabbit choroid plexus, *Brain Res.* **295:**155–160.

Semenza, G., 1982, The Na^+/D-glucose co-transporter of the small-intestinal brush-border membrane, *Biochem. Soc. Trans.* **10:**7 (Abstract).

Southwell, B. R., Duan, W., Alcorn, D., Brack, C., Richardson, S. J., Kohrle, J., and Schreiber, G., 1993, Thyroxine transport to the brain: Role of protein synthesis by the choroid plexus, *Endocrinology* **133:**2116–2126.

Spector, R., 1982, Nucleoside transport in choroid plexus: Mechanism and specificity, *Arch. Biochem. Biophys.* **216:**693–703.

Spector, R., 1987, Hypoxanthine transport through the blood–brain barrier, *Neurochem. Res.* **12:**791–796.

Spector, R., and Boose, B., 1979, Active transport of riboflavin by the isolated choroid plexus *in vitro*, *J. Biol. Chem.* **254:**10286–10289.

Spector, R., and Eells, J., 1984, Deoxynucleoside and vitamin transport into the central nervous system, *Fed. Proc.* **43:**196–200.

Spector, R., and Johanson, C. E., 1989, The mammalian choroid plexus, *Sci. Am.* **261:**68–74.

Stein, W. D. (ed.), 1990, *Channels, Carriers, and Pumps*, Academic Press, San Diego.

Taub, M., 1985, *Tissue Culture of Epithelial Cells*, Plenum Press, New York.

Wainer, I. W. (ed.), 1993, *Drug Stereochemistry: Analytical Methods and Pharmacology*, Marcel Dekker, New York.

Whittico, M. T., Gang, Y. A., and Giacomini, K. M., 1990, Cimetidine transport in isolated brush border membrane vesicles from bovine choroid plexus, *J. Pharmacol. Exp. Ther.* **255:**615–623.

Whittico, M. T., Hui, A. C., and Giacomini, K. M., 1991, Preparation of brush border membrane vesicles from bovine choroid plexus, *J. Pharmacol. Methods* **25:**215–227.

Wilson, G., 1990, Cell culture techniques for the study of drug transport, *Eur. J. Drug Metab. Pharmacokinet.* **15:**159–163.

Wu, X., Yuan, G., Brett, C. M., Hui, A. C., and Giacomini, K. M., 1992, Sodium-dependent nucleoside transport in choroid plexus from rabbit. Evidence for a single transporter for purine and pyrimidine nucleosides, *J. Biol. Chem.* **267:**8813–8818.

Wu, X., Gutierrez, M. M., and Giacomini, K. M., 1994, Further characterization of the sodium-dependent nucleoside transporter (N3) in choroid plexus from rabbit, *Biochim. Biophys. Acta* **1191:**190–196.

Chapter 15

Brain Perfusion Systems for Studies of Drug Uptake and Metabolism in the Central Nervous System

Quentin R. Smith

1. INTRODUCTION

Recent advances in biotechnology and the pharmaceutical sciences have greatly expanded the number of drugs that are being developed for the treatment of central nervous system (CNS) diseases. These drugs include a wide array of antibody, protein, peptide, and recombinant DNA agents as well as novel small agents (e.g., amino acids, nucleic acid precursors, and receptor agonists or blockers) for the treatment of brain tumors, strokes, infections, and neurodegenerative diseases. Though such agents often show excellent activity *in vitro*, many exhibit only restricted activity *in vivo* because of poor brain uptake and penetration. This problem has stimulated new work on factors that control drug uptake into brain and on methods to enhance CNS drug delivery.

One factor that critically limits drug access to brain is the blood–brain barrier (Bradbury, 1992). The barrier is composed of a system of tissue sites, including the brain capillary endothelium, choroid plexus epithelium, and arachnoid membrane, which together restrict and regulate the flux of hydrophilic ions, proteins, and nonelectrolytes from plasma to brain extracellular fluid and cerebrospinal fluid (Fig. 1). The barrier at each site is formed by a single layer of cells that are joined by multiple bands of continuous tight junctions (Bundgaard, 1986; Brightman, 1989). These tight junctions, which have at least three associated proteins—ZO-1, ZO-2, and

Quentin R. Smith • Neurochemistry and Brain Transport Section, National Institute on Aging, National Institutes of Health, Bethesda, Maryland 20892.

Models for Assessing Drug Absorption and Metabolism, Ronald T. Borchardt *et al.*, eds., Plenum Press, New York, 1996.

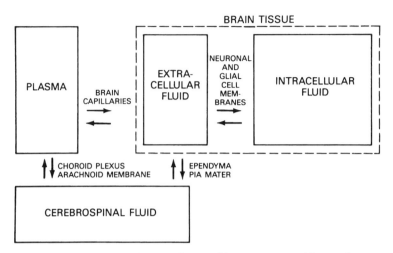

Figure 1. Model for solute exchange between plasma and the compartments of the central nervous system illustrating the components of the blood–brain barrier.

cingulin (Citi *et al.*, 1988; Watson *et al.*, 1991; Dermietzel and Krause, 1991; Petrov *et al.*, 1994)—virtually fuse adjacent barrier cell membranes, thereby blocking intercellular diffusion. This, together with the fact that barrier cells contain few aqueous pores and exhibit only limited vesicular transport activity, bestows upon the barrier many of the properties of a continuous cell membrane (Rapoport *et al.*, 1979). Therefore, most solutes can cross the barrier only by either dissolving in and diffusing across barrier cell membranes, based on solute lipid solubility, hydrogen-bonding, conformation, and size (Ohno *et al.*, 1978; Rapoport *et al.*, 1979; Levin, 1980; Smith and Takasato, 1986; Greig *et al.*, 1990; Chikhale *et al.*, 1994), or being transported across by specific carrier-or receptor-mediated mechanisms (Smith, 1995). Uptake is also limited at the barrier through the presence of various degradative enzymes (Hardebo *et al.*, 1980; Djuričić and Mrsulja, 1988; Minn *et al.*, 1991; Brownson *et al.*, 1994) and active efflux pumps (Cordon-Cardo *et al.*, 1989; Tatsuta *et al.*, 1992; Dykstra *et al.*, 1993) that attack solutes before they have a chance to cross into brain. Genetic or competitive blockage of these enzymatic or active transport systems markedly enhances brain uptake for selected agents (e.g., AZT, MPTP, vinblastine, and peptides; Kalaria *et al.*, 1987; Wong *et al.*, 1992; Schinkel *et al.*, 1994; Chikhale *et al.*, 1995). Once within brain, drug access to critical active sites can be restricted further by intracerebral sequestration, binding, or metabolism. These latter limitations are especially important for agents that act at membrane receptors based on their local brain extracellular concentration.

Due to the multiplicity of factors that influence drug uptake into brain, it has been difficult to develop simple *in vitro* systems that fully model all aspects of the *in vivo* situation. On the other hand, standard *in vivo* preparations are frequently too difficult and time-consuming for use as simple drug screening tools.

A compromise approach that we have pursued in our laboratory is to study drug penetration into brain using an *in situ* perfusion system that combines many of the best aspects of *in vitro* and *in vivo* systems (Smith, 1992). With the brain perfusion approach, the circulation to the brain is taken over briefly by infusion of artificial blood or physiologic saline into the heart or carotid artery. Perfusion allows the drug to be delivered directly to the brain at a constant, defined concentration that is set readily by the investigator in the perfusion fluid (Takasato *et al.*, 1984; Smith, 1992). Similarly, perfusion allows absolute control of vascular concentrations of plasma proteins, ions, and competing substrates for studies of transport mechanism or the effects of plasma protein binding (Levitan *et al.*, 1984; Smith *et al.*, 1992; Takada *et al.*, 1992; Rabin *et al.*, 1993). With nonrecirculating systems, the drug has no access to peripheral metabolizing enzymes prior to cerebral exposure, and thus uptake of metabolites is not a complicating factor (Levitan *et al.*, 1984; Fukui *et al.*, 1991; Samii *et al.*, 1994). If metabolites are detected in brain, they arise most likely from intracerebral metabolism, either at the barrier or within the brain parenchyma by neuronal or glial enzymes. As a consequence, the method provides a powerful tool for studying both drug uptake and metabolism in brain.

The simplicity and utility of the perfusion approach have generated considerable interest in the method as a brain research tool. This chapter will review work over the past 10 years on *in situ* perfusion models for brain uptake and metabolism. Details will be given on the procedure followed in a typical experiment and the calculation and interpretation of the data. Further, the advantages and disadvantages of the method in comparison to other approaches will be summarized.

2.   *IN SITU* BRAIN PERFUSION METHOD

2.1.   General Considerations

The primary objective of a brain perfusion approach is to take over the circulation of the brain for a short period of time via intracarotid infusion of artificial blood or saline. This allows the brain to be exposed for a defined interval to a known, constant concentration of drug under controlled conditions. At varying times the perfusion is stopped and the amount of drug in brain is determined. From these measurements, the kinetics of brain uptake can be analyzed, and appropriate transport or permeability constants calculated (Smith, 1989).

The perfusion approach is not new. In fact, it has been used on and off in neurochemical research for over 50 years (for reviews, see Woods and Youdim, 1978; Gilboe, 1982). However, early methods focused primarily on long-term (30 min–4 hr) perfusion of the isolated brain and required extensive surgical preparation. Transport measurements were based on single-pass uptake or steady-state arteriovenous difference methods that were of limited sensitivity for poorly penetrating solutes (Smith, 1989). Brain uptake and metabolism of several drugs have been examined with the isolated brain method (Horst and Jester, 1971; Gilboe, 1982). However, owing to the effort involved, the method did not receive wide attention as a drug screening tool.

The problems associated with the perfusion approach were overcome in the early 1980s with the development of the *in situ* rat brain perfusion technique. The *in situ* method provided a simple means for perfusion of the adult CNS for short-term studies (5 sec–30 min) of brain uptake and metabolism. Surgery was reduced by perfusion of the intact brain without complete isolation of the head or cranium. Transport measurements were based on single- or multiple-time-point, continuous uptake methods, which allow excellent control and sensitivity (Smith, 1989). The first of these methods was developed by Takasato *et al.* in 1982 and 1984. Since then, several variants have been published that modify and extend the original method (Hervonen and Steinwall, 1984; Greenwood *et al.*, 1985; Zlokovic *et al.*, 1986; Fishman *et al.*, 1987; Luthert *et al.*, 1987; Smith *et al.*, 1990; Deane and Bradbury, 1990; Triguero *et al.*, 1990; Takada *et al.*, 1991; Smith et al, 1992; Rabin *et al.*, 1993; Ennis *et al.*, 1994; Skarlatos *et al.*, 1995).

This chapter will focus primarily on the Takasato method, for which the largest literature exists. However, comparisons will be made with other methods where appropriate. Considerable flexibility exists with the brain perfusion approach, and it is expected that novel advances will continue to appear.

2.2. Surgical Preparation

In the Takasato method, rats are the experimental animal. However, other species (e.g., mouse, guinea pig, or rabbit) may be used with appropriate modifications (Zlokovic *et al.*, 1986; Deane and Bradbury, 1988; Richerson and Getting, 1990). The primary consideration is that the animal be large enough for arterial catheterization.

Anesthesia is induced with sodium pentobarbital [40–50 mg/kg, intraperitoneal (i.p.)] or other suitable medium- or long-acting anesthetic agent. Deep anesthesia is required for surgery on the carotid circulation. Care should be taken to maintain anesthesia throughout the experiment, which may require addition of anesthetic to the perfusion fluid if the perfusion time is longer than 1 min. With short perfusions (<1 min), loss of pentobarbital from brain is trivial, based on washout of [^{14}C]pentobarbital (Q. Smith, unpublished observations). The level of anesthesia can be monitored during perfusion by EEG (Woods and Youdim, 1978; Gilboe, 1982; Richerson and Getting, 1990). The animal should not be allowed to regain consciousness during the experiment.

Two approaches are used for placement of perfusion catheters. In the original Takasato method, the perfusion catheter [usually polyethylene (PE-50) or silicone tubing containing 100 IU sodium heparin/ml in 0.9% NaCl] is placed in the external carotid artery just distal to the bifurcation of the common carotid artery (Fig. 2). In addition, the ipsilateral pterygopalatine, superior thyroid, and occipital arteries are ligated and cut. This latter action allows the carotid circulation of one side of the body to be completely isolated without collaterals to other organs. Perfusion fluid is infused retrograde down the external carotid artery and up the internal carotid artery toward the brain. The common carotid artery is ligated just before perfusion is initiated to prevent mixing of perfusion fluid with systemic blood at the carotid bifurcation (Fig. 2). Once the fluid has passed through the cerebral capillaries, it exits into the venous circulation. The infusion rate is set so that the perfusion pressure in the carotid artery slightly exceeds that of the systemic circulation so that the perfusate is not contaminated with systemic blood at the circle of Willis (Fig. 2; Takasato *et al.*, 1984). During perfusion, systemic blood volume can be held constant, if desired, by simultaneous withdrawal of blood from the femoral artery or vein at a rate equivalent to the infusion rate (Takasato *et al.*, 1984).

The Takasato method provides complete perfusion of one cerebral hemisphere, with partial perfusion of the contralateral cerebral hemisphere, cerebellum, and brain stem. The flow rate is fixed by the fact that there must be sufficient perfusion pressure

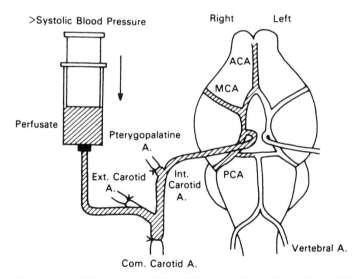

Figure 2. Diagram of the Takasato *et al.* (1982, 1984) method for *in situ* perfusion of the rat brain hemisphere. The perfusion catheter is placed in the external carotid artery, and the pterygopalatine artery is closed. Just before the perfusion is begun, the common carotid artery is ligated just proximal to the bifurcation with the external carotid artery to prevent fluid mixing with systemic blood. In the Takasato *et al.* (1982, 1984) method the heart is maintained intact during the perfusion, and only one cerebral hemisphere is completely perfused. ACA, Anterior cerebral artery; MCA, middle cerebral artery; PCA, posterior cerebral artery. Modified from Smith (1989).

in the internal carotid artery to prevent flow contributions from the animal's own blood at the circle of Willis (Fig. 2; Takasato *et al.*, 1984). As a consequence, the flow rate cannot be reduced without producing significant mixing.

The surgical and catheterization procedures required for the Takasato method are not simple and require practice and training. We have found that successful surgery requires the use of appropriate microdissecting forceps, scissors, and clamps (Roboz, Rockville, MD), as well as a good dissecting microscope (4–20×; Storz, St. Louis, MO). For ligation of small blood vessels, 6-0 surgical silk works well, whereas 4-0 silk is good for catheterization of the external carotid artery. Small blood vessels can also be cauterized using a Malis Bipolar coagulator (Codman, Randolph, MA). With practice, an investigator can complete surgery on a single animal in <30 min and do six or more perfusions per day.

Although the original Takasato method works well for perfusion of a single cerebral hemisphere at a constant rate, more recently we have developed and tested several modifications that require less effort and allow greater control of flow rate and perfusion pressure (Smith *et al.*, 1990; Takada *et al.*, 1991, 1992; Rabin *et al.*, 1993). The new procedures are illustrated in Fig. 3.

With the new methods, surgery is simplified by placement of the perfusion catheter (PE-50-80) in the common carotid artery, followed by ligation of the external carotid artery. The pterygopalatine artery can either be ligated or left open, depending upon the choice of the investigator (Fig. 3). For short perfusions (5–60 sec), it is often

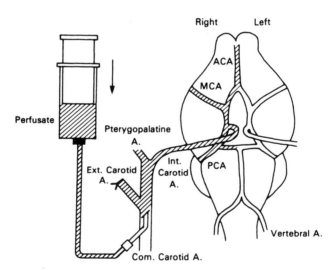

Figure 3.   Diagram of modified Takasato method with catheter placement in the common carotid artery and ligation of the external carotid artery. The pterygopalatine artery can be either ligated or left open. The heart is stopped just prior to the start of perfusion to minimize mixing and to allow perfusion of both cerebral hemispheres. ACA, Anterior cerebral artery; MCA, middle cerebral artery; PCA, posterior cerebral artery.

easier to keep the pterygopalatine artery open. Following catheter placement in the common carotid artery, blood flow to the ipsilateral cerebral hemisphere is maintained by crossover at the circle of Willis from the contralateral circulation (Salford and Siesjö, 1974). Cannulation of the common carotid artery is simple to perform and can be completed by most scientists in ~15 min. The procedures are no more rigorous than those required for other blood–brain barrier transport methods, such as the brain uptake index (Oldendorf, 1970; Pardridge, 1983) or the arterial injection (Ohno *et al.*, 1978; Rapoport *et al.*, 1979) methods.

With this alternative approach, the thoracic cavity is opened at the beginning of perfusion, and the cardiac ventricles are severed to stop blood flow from the systemic circulation. Then, perfusion fluid is infused up the common carotid artery at a rate sufficient to perfuse both cerebral hemispheres as well as the brain stem at a reasonable pressure. Because only one carotid artery is perfused, flow in the ipsilateral cerebral hemisphere exceeds that in the contralateral cerebral hemisphere by 3- to 10-fold. Because the heart is stopped, there is no contribution to flow from the systemic circulation, and the brain flow rate can be set at will for studies of the flow-dependent transport or metabolism (Smith *et al.*, 1990; Takada *et al.*, 1991; Rabin *et al.*, 1993).

Other groups have found that it is also possible to simplify the preparation by placing the infusion catheter in the left cardiac ventricle or in the aorta (Thompson *et al.*, 1968; Greenwood *et al.*, 1985; Luthert *et al.*, 1987). Such systems provide equal perfusion to both hemispheres of the brain but require higher infusion rates.

The physiologic status of the animal should be monitored both during and after surgery. Body temperature should be maintained at 37°C with a heating pad or lamp attached to a feedback device, such as the YSI Indicating Controller (YSI Instruments, Yellow Springs, OH). Additional anesthetic should be given as needed to maintain anesthesia throughout the experiment.

2.3. Perfusion Fluid

A number of perfusion fluids have been developed for use with the *in situ* brain perfusion technique. The most common fluids are rat whole blood, artificial blood, and buffered Ringer or Krebs–Henseleit physiologic saline (Takasato *et al.*, 1984; Momma *et al.*, 1987). The optimum fluid depends upon the experimental goals. In most experiments, the primary objective is to keep the perfusate simple and yet to supply sufficient nutrients and salts to maintain the metabolic and structural integrity of the brain. Each fluid is a compromise. Several well-characterized perfusates are presented below.

One of the simplest fluids is a buffered Ringer or Krebs–Henseleit physiologic saline that contains 128 mM NaCl, 24 mM $NaHCO_3$, 4.2 mM KCl, 2.4 mM NaH_2PO_4, 1.5 mM $CaCl_2$, and 0.9 mM $MgSO_4$ (Momma *et al.*, 1987). The solution is bubbled with humidified 95% O_2/5% CO_2 to pH 7.4. D-Glucose (5–10 mM) is usually added to maintain cerebral glucose metabolism and ATP production. Other substrates (e.g., amino acids, fatty acids, vitamins, and metals) may also be added but are not required for short perfusions (<60 sec). We have found that the barrier will accept considerable variation in perfusate composition for short intervals (<5 min) as long as the pH (7.0–7.5) and osmolarity (260–330 mOsm/kg) are maintained within normal limits. Isotonic sucrose has been used with good retention of barrier integrity (Momma et al., 1987). Exchange or substitution of specific ions, such as sodium and potassium, is also well tolerated (Deane and Bradbury, 1990; Smith et al., 1992; Ennis et al., 1994). Bicarbonate can be replaced or supplemented with HEPES to obtain a more stable buffering system.

Serum proteins are not required in the perfusate for oncotic pressure, as the brain capillaries have a low permeability to both large and small solutes. However, serum proteins often serve critical roles with regard to drug binding and transport and may be added for that purpose. Albumin, the primary plasma protein, is found in serum normally in concentrations of 2.5–4.0%. Transferrin, γ-globulin, α_1-acid glycoprotein, and α_2-macroglobulin also have critical binding roles and are found in plasma at lower concentrations. High-molecular-weight, nonprotein polymers, including dextran, hydroxyethyl starch, and polyvinylpyrrolidone, are available as nonbinding controls. Studies of choroid plexus transport should include a high-molecular-weight, oncotic agent as choroid plexus capillaries, unlike brain capillaries, are leaky to small solutes.

For long perfusions, a fluid with adequate oxygen-carrying capacity is required to sustain normal cerebral metabolic and electrical activity (Gilboe, 1982; Richerson and Getting, 1990). Most investigators achieve this by supplementing their physiologic saline or artificial plasma with washed erythrocytes to a hematocrit of 20–40% (Gilboe, 1982; Takasato et al., 1984; Zlokovic et al., 1986; Ennis et al., 1994). Erythrocytes from rats, dogs, cattle, and sheep have all been shown to work well for this purpose. With good oxygenation, cerebral oxygen metabolism and EEG can be maintained for over 1 hr (Kintner et al., 1986a). However, with long perfusions, greater care must be taken to supply a balanced mix of critical nutrients, hormones, and cofactors in the perfusate to sustain metabolism. With the perfused dog brain, Kintner et al. (1986a) noted changes in the CMR-O_2 and EEG after only 20 min of perfusion with a simple artificial blood perfusate, but maintained much better viability with a more complete blood perfusate. They attributed the changes to the absence of an essential nutrient, possibly fatty acids.

An alternative means to enhance oxygen delivery to brain is to use whole blood from donor animals. Whole blood contains all the appropriate nutrients, metals and proteins at physiologic concentrations. However, whole blood can have problems with clotting and aggregation. To minimize this, an appropriate anticoagulant (e.g., heparin) must be added to the blood, and the fluid must be carefully filtered prior to perfusion. Whole blood may also contain vasoconstricting substances from platelets and white cells, which may increase vascular resistance during perfusion (Kintner *et al.*, 1986b). Such problems can be overcome through the use of artificial oxygen carriers, such as fluorocarbons (Dirks *et al.*, 1980; Lowe, 1987) and cross-linked hemoglobins (Chang, 1993). However, the erythrocyte is the normal oxygen-delivering device, and it is recommended on that basis. Kintner *et al.* (1986a) avoided some of the problems of whole blood by using washed red cells combined with buffy-coat-poor plasma to a hematocrit of 30%.

Once the perfusion fluid is prepared, it must be warmed to 37°C, filtered, and stored in a sterile container. Drugs can be added directly to the perfusate prior to perfusion or can be introduced to the perfusion line once the perfusion is started via a mixing port (Zlokovic *et al.*, 1986). This latter approach is valuable for compounds with limited stability that may be metabolized by blood enzymes if added too early before the perfusion is begun (Zlokovic *et al.*, 1989, 1990). Care should also be taken to maintain clean, aseptic conditions to minimize contamination from fungi or bacteria.

2.4. Perfusion Apparatus

With the Takasato method, perfusion fluid is infused into the carotid circulation with either a peristaltic or a constant-rate pump. Pulsatile flow is believed generally to be better than nonpulsatile flow for most organs (Deane and Bradbury, 1988). However, for short perfusions (<1–2 min), the effect appears to be minor. We have found that with the use of a Harvard model 944 constant-rate infusion pump (Harvard Apparatus, South Natick, MA) that cerebral perfusion flow remains stable for at least 60 sec (Momma *et al.*, 1987) and that barrier integrity is maintained for at least 4 min (Takasato *et al.*, 1984; Smith and Takasato, 1986). For the Harvard constant-rate infusion pump, we generally use 5- to 50-ml glass LEUR-LOK syringes (Becton Dickinson, Franklin Lakes, NJ).

In-line filters are valuable for removal of particulate matter and clots (Takasato *et al.*, 1984; Luthert *et al.*, 1987; Ennis *et al.*, 1994). Perfusion pressure can be measured using a strain gauge transducer connected to a chart recorder (Gould, Cleveland, OH), as described by Takasato *et al.* (1984). The transducer can be joined to the perfusion line via a T connector. Finally, the temperature of the experimental animal and the perfusate must be maintained carefully at 37°C. We use either a heating pad (Casco, New York, NY) or light connected to a feedback device (YSI Indicating Controller, YSI Instruments, Yellow Springs, OH) for regulation of the animal's body temperature and heat the perfusate and syringe using a water bath system (Haake D8, Haake, Berlin, Germany). An alternative means is to put the entire perfusion apparatus in a heated box that is maintained at 37°C. However, for short perfusions, adequate temperature control can be obtained with the simpler system.

   Other components of the perfusion apparatus have been described in previous sections. For short saline perfusions, all that is required is an infusion pump and a mechanism to maintain temperature at 37°C.

   In some experiments, it is desirable to include a brief wash with drug-free fluid either at the start of perfusion to preequilibrate the capillaries to the fluid or at the end of perfusion to remove drug from the brain intravascular space. The former is valuable for perfusion experiments in which the fluid differs markedly from *in vivo*, whereas the latter is valuable for agents that bind significantly to the luminal surfaces of barrier membranes. Vascularly bound agents can be rapidly removed by brain perfusion with drug-free saline or albumin solution for 5–20 sec. In such experiments, we use a dual-syringe Harvard infusion pump and a four-way valve (Fig. 4) that allows simultaneous switching of the infusion lines in a fraction of a second (Momma *et al.*, 1987; Rabin *et al.*, 1993). Similar experiments can also be performed with a simpler three-way valve, but at the cost of a significant interruption in fluid flow.

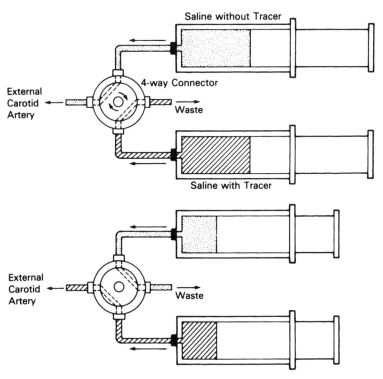

Figure 4.   Diagram of four-way valve for perfusion of brain with tracer- or drug-free saline at the start or end of the perfusion experiment. The valve allows rapid switching of the infusion lines so that the infusion rate is not interrupted.

2.5. Perfusion Experiment

To start the perfusion, the carotid catheter is connected to the perfusion syringe, and the common carotid artery, if open, is ligated. With the modified perfusion procedure, the heart is stopped by severing the right and left ventricles. Then, perfusion fluid is infused into the carotid artery at a rate that maintains physiologic perfusion pressure.

Recommended infusion rates for the original and modified Takasato methods are summarized in Table I. In general, saline has a lower viscosity than blood and requires a higher infusion rate to obtain the same pressure. Ideally, the infusion rate should be the minimum necessary to obtain complete perfusion of the cerebral hemisphere with minimal contributions from systemic blood. Pressures in excess of 200 mm Hg should be avoided as they may damage the blood–brain barrier. With the original Takasato method, an infusion rate of 6.7×10^{-2}–8.3×10^{-2} ml/sec (4–5 ml/min) was required to obtain complete perfusion with physiologic saline (Fig. 5; Takasato *et al.*, 1984). Infusion rates with rat whole or artificial blood were correspondingly lower (3.0×10^{-2}–4.2×10^{-2} ml/sec or 1.8–2.5 ml/min). With the heart-cut modification, the infusion rate should be doubled to maintain the same cerebral perfusion fluid flow (Takada *et al.*, 1991). Similarly, if the pterygopalatine artery is left open, an additional factor of 2 must be incorporated to adjust for fluid loss to the extracerebral circulation. Thus, an infusion rate of 20 ml of normal physiologic saline per minute would be required with the heart-cut and open-pterygopalatine modifications to obtain the same perfusion fluid flow rate in the brain as with the original Takasato method. However,

Table I

Carotid Infusion Rates for *in Situ* Brain Perfusion of the Adult Rat[a]

Perfusion preparation	Perfusion fluid	Carotid infusion rate (ml/min)	Cerebral perfusion fluid flow (ml $sec^{-1}g^{-1}$)
Takasato *et al.* (1984) (ligated pterygopalatine artery with intact heart)	Whole blood	1.8	3.8×10^{-2}
	Artificial blood	2.5	3.1×10^{-2}
	Physiologic saline	5	12.8×10^{-2}
Modified Takasato (ligated pterygopalatine artery with heart cut)	Physiologic saline	1.2	1.1×10^{-2}
		5	5.4×10^{-2}
		10	12.1×10^{-2}
		15	16.2×10^{-2}
Modified Takasato (open pterygopalatine artery with heart cut)	Physiologic saline	20	12×10^{-2}

[a]Values represent means for $n = 3$–12 animals for the parietal cerebral cortex (Takasato *et al.*, 1984; Takada *et al.*, 1991). Infusion rates are valid for animals with body weights from 240 to 450 g.

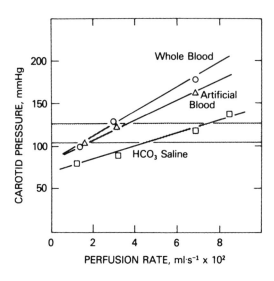

Figure 5. Relation of carotid pressure to perfusion rate of whole blood, artificial blood and physiologic saline with the *in situ* brain perfusion method of Takasato *et al.* (1984). From Takasato *et al.* (1984).

with the hear-cut method, lower infusion rates can be used without sacrificing the completeness of perfusion (Smith *et al.*, 1990).

At the end of perfusion, the animal is decapitated and the pump is turned off. The brain is removed from the skull and dissected on ice to obtain samples from appropriate regions (Takasato *et al.*, 1984). The total concentration of drug or radiotracer in brain is then determined by scintillation counting, GC-MS, HPLC, or other suitable analytical means. When metabolism is a factor, it is often necessary to perform chromatography to separate and independently quantitate the various metabolites. Drug passage across the barrier can be demonstrated either by separating the cerebral microvessels from the brain parenchyma by physical means, such as the capillary depletion technique of Triguero *et al.* (1990), or by analyzing drug distribution in brain by thaw-mount autoradiography (Duffy and Pardridge, 1987; Skarlatos *et al.*, 1995). If the former method is used, great care must be taken to prevent drug loss from capillaries during the isolation procedure. The method may be adequate for proteins and large peptides, but problems may be encountered with small solutes as they will more readily leak out from cerebral microvessels during the brain homogenization procedure.

2.6. Calculations

Data from the brain perfusion technique can be analyzed by both compartmental and noncompartmental methods (Smith, 1989).

The simplest approach is to examine the initial, "unidirectional" uptake of solute into brain at early times during perfusion before backflux and metabolism become important. When backflux and metabolism are negligible, the rate of drug uptake into brain (J_{in}) is given by

$$J_{in} = dC_{br}/dt = K_{in}C_{pf} \tag{1}$$

where C_{br} is the amount of drug that has crossed the blood–brain barrier into brain (in units of mass drug/g brain), C_{pf} is the concentration of drug in the perfusion fluid (mass drug/volume fluid), K_{in} is the blood-to-brain transfer coefficient for drug, and t is the perfusion time. K_{in} is a proportionality constant that gives a measure of the ability of the drug to cross into brain from the perfusion fluid. It is determined by the barrier permeability (P) to the drug, the cerebral perfusion fluid flow rate (F), the surface area of the barrier for exchange (A), and the fraction of drug in the perfusate in the unionized and unbound form (f) (Smith, 1989, 1992). With the Crone Renkin model of capillary transport, K_{in} is defined as $F[1 - \exp(-PA/F)]$. If the drug binds minimally to plasma proteins ($f \approx 1.0$) and the transfer constant (K_{in}) is small relative to the flow rate F (i.e., $K_{in} < 0.2F$), then K_{in} reduces to a PA product which is essentially flow independent (Smith, 1989). On the other hand, if K_{in} is significant relative to flow ($K_{in} \geq 0.3F$), then uptake will depend on both flow and permeability.

Equation (1) can be rearranged and integrated from the start of the perfusion ($t = 0$) to the end (T), to give

$$C_{br} = K_{in}C_{pf}T \tag{2}$$

At the end of perfusion, the total amount of drug in brain (C_{tot}) is the sum of that which has left the perfusate and crossed into brain (C_{br}) and that which remains in perfusate in the brain blood vessels (C_{vas}),

$$C_{tot} = C_{br} + C_{vas} \tag{3}$$

Equations (2) and (3) can be combined and divided by C_{pf} to give the Patlak equation (Patlak et al., 1983) which is in the form of a straight line:

$$C_{tot}/C_{pf} = K_{in}T + (C_{vas}/C_{pf}) \tag{4}$$

To measure K_{in}, C_{tot}/C_{pf} is determined at several different perfusion times and the data are plotted as C_{tot}/C_{pf} versus T. K_{in} is then obtained as the slope of the initial linear portion of the uptake curve by least-squares regression. The accuracy and sensitivity of the method can be improved if C_{vas}/C_{pf} is determined directly in each animal with a vascular volume marker, such as [^{3}H] or [^{14}C]inulin, which does not measurably cross the blood–brain barrier during short perfusions (Takasato et al., 1984; Smith et al., 1988). With a vascular volume marker, C_{br}/C_{pf} can be calculated directly as $C_{tot}/C_{pf} - C_{vas}/C_{pf}$, where C_{vas}/C_{pf} is obtained from the brain distribution of the vascular marker at the end of the perfusion. However, care should be taken to ensure that the vascular volume of the marker tracer matches that of the test compound (Smith et al., 1988).

Some drugs bind or accumulate in the vascular endothelium so that C_{vas}/C_{pf} exceeds that measured with an inert vascular marker.

An example of this analysis method is shown in Fig. 6 for L-[^{14}C]-phenylalanine, which is taken up into brain by the large neutral amino acid transport system of the blood–brain barrier. Rats were perfused with physiologic saline containing 0.0005 mM L-[^{14}C]phenylalanine, with or without 0.10 mM unlabeled L-phenylalanine. [^{3}H]inulin was included in the perfusate for vascular volume determination. Brain uptake of L-[^{14}C]phenylalanine tracer was linear for 40 sec with both fluids. However, the magnitude of uptake was far greater in the absence of unlabeled L-phenylalanine because of reduced competition for the transport system. Determination of K_{in} over a wide range of perfusate L-phenylalanine concentrations (0–10 mM) allowed calculation of the maximal transport capacity ($V_{max} = 41$ nmol min^{-1}g^{-1}) and half-saturation constant ($K_m = 0.011$ mM) for the transporter (Momma et al., 1987). The K_m was 10-fold lower than previous in vivo estimates (Pardridge, 1983) owing to reduced mixing of perfusate with blood and efflux of unlabeled amino acid from brain (Smith et al., 1985; Momma et al., 1987; Smith et al., 1987).

Once the linear portion of the uptake curve is known, it is often more efficient to determine K_{in} in individual animals using the single-time-point method. For this, a single perfusion time is chosen over which uptake is unidirectional, and that time is used in all experiments. At the end of perfusion, vascular drug (C_{vas}) is either removed from the brain by a short washout (5–15 sec) with drug-free fluid (Deane and

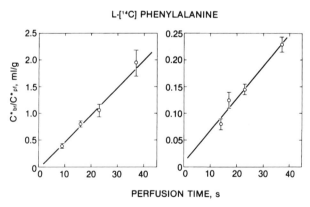

L-[^{14}C] PHENYLALANINE

PERFUSION TIME, s

Figure 6.   Time course of L-[^{14}C]phenylalanine uptake into brain during perfusion with physiologic saline containing 0.0005 mM L-[^{14}C]phenylalanine, with (right) or without (left) 0.1 mM unlabeled L-phenylalanine. Values were corrected for intravascular tracer using [^{3}H]inulin. Best-fit K_{in} values equaled 5.12 ± 0.42 × 10^{-2} ml sec^{-1} g^{-1} at 0.0005 mM and 6.0 ± 0.7 × 10^{-3} ml sec^{-1} g^{-1} at 0.10 mM L-phenylalanine. Data were obtained with the perfusion technique of Takasato et al. (1984). Data points are means ± SEM for $n = 3$–6 animals. Modified from Momma et al. (1987).

Bradbury, 1990; Rabin *et al.*, 1993) or is measured indirectly using a vascular marker. K_{in} is then calculated as,

$$K_{in} = (C_{tot} - V_v C_{pf})/C_{pf}T \tag{5}$$

where V_v = brain vascular volume, defined as the ratio of the vascular marker concentration in brain to that in perfusion fluid, and C_{vas} is determined as $V_v C_{pf}$ for drug. If brain washout is performed, $C_{vas} \approx 0$. The only critical requirements of a vascular marker are that it does not cross the blood–brain barrier and that it gives a brain vascular distribution space similar to that of the drug of interest (Takasato *et al.*, 1984; Smith *et al.*, 1988). Other vascular markers that have been used include radioactive mannitol, sucrose, raffiniose, dextran, and albumin (Smith, 1989).

Ideally, investigators should conduct all perfusion experiments so that over half of the drug in brain has crossed the blood–brain barrier ($C_{tot}/C_{pf} \geqslant 2 \times C_{vas}/C_{pf}$). Otherwise, small errors in intravascular drug distribution can appreciably affect the brain permeability calculations. In addition, investigators should ensure that they are on the linear portion of the uptake curve and that the brain uptake space extrapolates to zero (at $T = 0$) after vascular correction (Smith, 1989). Finally, it may be appropriate in some instances to confirm that the drug does not modify blood–brain barrier permeability. Such modifications have been shown to occur for some vasoactive peptides and drugs.

Finally, to convert K_{in} to a blood–brain barrier *PA* product, the cerebral perfusion fluid flow rate must be known. *F* can be measured in brain perfusion experiments with radioactive diazepam, iodoantipyrine, or microspheres (Takasato *et al.*, 1984). In most experiments, we use [^{3}H]diazepam because it is completely extracted during a single pass through brain (Takasato *et al.*, 1984) and because its uptake is linear with time for at least 30 sec. At high flow rates, dissociation of diazepam from albumin can become limiting. However, this is not usually seen until *F* reaches values of >3 ml min^{-1}/g^{-1} (Q. R. Smith, unpublished observation).

3. APPLICATIONS

In the 10 years since publication of the Takasato *et al.* (1984) method, the perfusion technique has been widely used to study blood–brain barrier transport. Because of the control of perfusate concentration and composition that the method allows, it has become a standard in studies of carrier- or receptor-mediated transport at the blood-brain barrier for nutrients (Smith *et al.*, 1985, 1987; Stoll *et al.*, 1993; Pardridge *et al.*, 1994), vitamins (Greenwood *et al.*, 1986; Spector *et al.*, 1986), metals (Fishman *et al.*, 1987; Deane and Bradbury, 1990; Rabin *et al.*, 1993; Buxani-Rice *et al.*, 1994; Skarlatos *et al.*, 1995), peptides (Zlokovic *et al.*, 1989, 1990; Begley *et al.*, 1990; Chikhale *et al.*, 1995), and drugs (Takada *et al.*, 1991, 1992; Smith, 1995). The method has proved particularly valuable in studies of poorly penetrating solutes

(Triguero *et al.*, 1990; Begley *et al.*, 1990; Smith *et al.*, 1992; Skarlatos *et al.*,1995), for which the extra sensitivity of the perfusion method is critical, and in studies of unstable or highly metabolizable solutes (Fukui *et al.*, 1991; Takada *et al.*, 1992; Samii *et al.*, 1994), for which brain perfusion allows determination of uptake in the absence of complicating metabolites. The ability also to examine uptake in the presence and absence of plasma proteins has allowed valuable insights into the role of plasma protein binding on brain transport (Levitan *et al.*, 1984; Greig *et al.*, 1990; Smith *et al.*, 1990, 1991; Rabin *et al.*, 1993).

Greenwood and collaborators developed an interesting variant of the brain perfusion method in which brain energy metabolism is blocked by addition of dinitrophenol, an uncoupler of oxidative metabolism, to the perfusate (Greenwood *et al.*, 1985; Luthert *et al.*, 1987). This modification allows evaluation of brain uptake and barrier function in the absence of ATP and other energy-yielding substrates (Greenwood *et al.*, 1986, 1989, 1991).

The perfusion approach has also been used to probe other brain functions, such as metabolism and active transport. For example, Pardridge *et al.* (1994) used brain perfusion to demonstrate the rapid conversion of adenosine in brain to various metabolites as part of the "enzymatic" blood–brain barrier. Similarly, Washizaki *et al.* (1991) used the brain perfusion method to study the rapid cerebral incorporation of fatty acids. Finally, Chikhale *et al.* (1995) recently used the perfusion method to study the effect of verapamil, a blocker of the P-glycoprotein transport system, on peptide uptake into brain. Verapamil significantly and selectively increased peptide uptake into brain, suggesting that the P-glycoprotein may have a significant role in protecting the brain from circulating neuroactive peptides.

In the future, it may be possible to use the perfusion method to study cerebral blood flow and regulation. We have found that cerebral perfusion fluid flow remains stable for up to 60 sec using saline fluid (Fig. 7) and longer (up to 5 min) using blood perfusion (Takasato *et al.*, 1984; Momma *et al.*, 1987; Smith *et al.*, 1990). With the heart-cut method, F can be varied over a 50-fold range, with flow directly proportional to infusion rate (Smith *et al.*, 1990; Takada *et al.*, 1991).

The perfusion method has been used to survey blood–brain barrier permeability to drugs in relation to lipid solubility (Fig. 8; Takasato *et al.*, 1984; Smith and Takasato, 1986; Pardridge *et al.*, 1990; Greig *et al.*, 1990; Chikhale *et al.*, 1994,95). Comparisons were made in at least two studies (Pardridge *et al.*, 1990; Chikhale *et al.*, 1994) with the results obtained with *in vitro* models of the blood–brain barrier. The authors found that permeability values obtained with the two methods correlated, but values with the *in vitro* system were, on average, 100 times greater than corresponding values with the *in situ* system. The authors attributed the difference to the greater leakiness of the *in vitro* blood–brain barrier systems. Thus, the *in situ* perfusion method provides a valuable approach to quickly screen and analyze the *in vivo* brain uptake of a wide variety of new compounds. It complements similar *in vitro* methods and provides a highly accurate view of *in vivo* brain penetration that will be of use for pharmacologic studies.

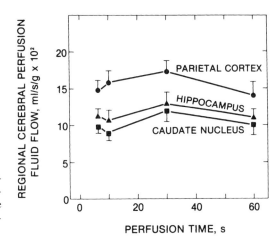

Figure 7. Time course of cerebral perfusion fluid flow rate during brain perfusion with physiologic saline. Data are means ± SEM (bars) for n = 3–5 animals. From Momma *et al.* (1987).

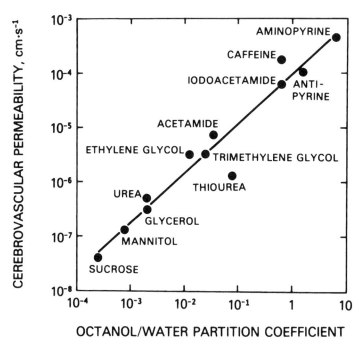

Figure 8. Relation of blood–brain barrier permeability and solute octanol/water partition coefficient for 12 nonelectrolytes as measured with the *in situ* brain perfusion technique. Each point represents the mean for n = 3–5 animals. The line is the least-squares fit to the data.

4. ADVANTAGES AND DISADVANTAGES

The principal advantages of the perfusion method over other *in vivo* methods include the accuracy and sensitivity of the technique, as well as the control of perfusate composition (Takasato *et al.*, 1984; Smith, 1989). Brain perfusion can be used to determine permeability coefficients for both rapidly and slowly penetrating compounds, as well as readily metabolizable substrates. *PA* values for reference compounds obtained with the perfusion method (Fig. 9) agree with values obtained in control animals using the intravenous (i.v.) injection method (Takasato *et al.*, 1984; Smith and Takasato, 1986). As the i.v. injection method is generally considered the

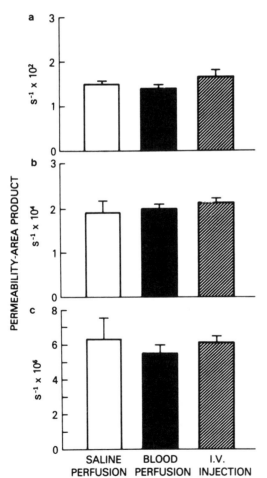

Figure 9. Blood–brain barrier permeability–area products for three reference solutes—(a) antipyrine, (b) thiourea, and (c) sucrose—as measured by the brain perfusion and i.v. injection methods in rats. Values are means ± SEM for $n = 3$–5 animals. Modified from Smith and Takasato (1986).

"gold" standard (Smith, 1989), this agreement suggests that brain perfusion does not grossly alter barrier integrity or function. The lower limit of PA that can be measured with the perfusion method (1×10^{-6}–5×10^{-6} ml sec^{-1} g^{-1}) is one to two orders of magnitude lower than that for single-pass extraction methods, such as the indicator dilution and brain uptake index techniques (Smith, 1989). The perfusion method offers far greater flexibility and simplicity than comparable i.v. injection methods, especially for studies of transport mechanism, and is superior to similar *in vitro* methods because uptake is measured in the intact brain with its full complement of enzymes, proteins, and transport systems. The perfusion method has been used to reinforce the critical importance of solute lipid solubility on drug uptake and blood–brain barrier penetration (Smith and Takasato, 1986).

The principal disadvantages of the brain perfusion technique, relative to *in vitro* barrier systems, are the lack of control of brain extracellular fluid concentration for studies of drug efflux from brain and the greater complexity that the brain matrix provides in assays of brain drug concentration. *In situ* perfusion generally requires use of an anesthetic agent, which can modify results and, in some instances, lead to erroneous interpretations. In addition, as with all model systems, work is required to validate the perfusion system and to demonstrate the functional integrity of the preparation. Brain perfusion systems likely produce some disruption in brain metabolism, as it is extremely difficult to provide all the nutrients and cofactors that are required for long-term brain preservation. However, often the functional consequences of such imbalances are negligible, as shown by the excellent agreement that has been obtained between the perfusion method and the i.v. injection method for nutrients, ions, and small nonelectrolytes (Takasato *et al.*, 1984; Smith *et al.*, 1985, 1987; Ennis *et al.*, 1994).

REFERENCES

Begley, D. J., Squires, L. K., Zloković, B. V., Mitrović, D. M., Hughes, C. C. W., Revest, P. A., and Greenwood, J., 1990, Permeability of the blood–brain barrier to the immunosuppressive cyclic peptide cyclosporin A, *J. Neurochem.* **55**:1222–1230.

Bradbury, M. W. B., 1992, *Physiology and Pharmacology of the Blood–Brain Barrier*, Springer-Verlag, Berlin.

Brightman, M. W., 1989, The anatomic basis of the blood–brain barrier, in: *Implications of the Blood–Brain Barrier and Its Manipulation*, Vol. 1 (E. A. Neuwelt, ed.), Plenum Press, New York, pp. 53–83.

Brownson, E. A., Abbruscato, T. J., Gillespie, T. J., Hruby, V. J., and Davis, T. P., 1994, Effect of peptidases at the blood–brain barrier on the permeability of enkephalin, *J. Pharmacol. Exp. Ther.* **270**:675–680.

Bundgaard, M., 1986, Pathways across the vertebrate blood–brain barrier: Morphological viewpoints, *Ann. N.Y. Acad. Sci.* **481**:7–18.

Buxani-Rice, S., Ueda, F., and Bradbury, M. W. B., 1994, Transport of zinc-65 at the blood–brain barrier during short cerebrovascular perfusion in the rat: Its enhancement by histidine, *J. Neurochem.* **62**:665–672.

Chang, T. M. S., 1993, *Blood Substitutes and Oxygen Carriers*, Marcel Dekker, New York.

Chikhale, E. G., Ng, K. Y., Burton, P. S., and Borchardt, R. T., 1994, Hydrogen bonding potential as a determinant of the *in vitro* and *in situ* blood–brain barrier permeability of peptides, *Pharm. Res.* **11**:412–419.

Chikhale, E. G., Burton, P. S., and Borchardt, R. T., 1995, The effect of verapamil on the transport of peptides across the blood–brain barrier in rats: Kinetic evidence for an apically polarized efflux mechanism, *J. Pharmacol. Exp. Ther.* **273**:298–303.

Citi, S., Sabanay, H., Jakes, R., Geiger, B., and Kendrick-Jones, J., 1988, Cingulin: A new peripheral component of tight junctions, *Nature* **333**:272–276.

Cordon-Cardo, C., O'Brien, J. P., Casals, D., Rittman-Grauer, L., Biedler, J. L., Melamed, M. R., and Bertino, J. R., 1989, Multidrug resistance gene (P-glycoprotein) is expressed by endothelial cells at the blood–brain barrier, *Proc. Natl. Acad. Sci. USA.* **86**:695–698.

Deane, R., and Bradbury, M. W. B., 1988, Is pulsation important for the brain, in: *Peptide and Amino Acid Transport Mechanisms in the Central Nervous System* (L. Rakić, D. J. Begley, H. Davson, and B. V. Zloković, eds.), Stockton Press, New York, pp. 305–316.

Deane, R., and Bradbury, M. W. B., 1990, Transport of lead-203 at the blood–brain barrier during short cerebrovascular perfusion with saline in the rat, *J. Neurochem.* **54**:905–914.

Dermietzel, R., and Krause, D., 1991, Molecular anatomy of the blood–brain barrier as defined by immunocytochemistry, *Int. Rev. Cytol.* **127**:57–109.

Dirks, B., Krieglstein, J., Lind, H. H., Rieger, H., and Schutz, H., 1980, Fluorocarbon perfusion medium applied to the isolated rat brain, *J. Pharmacol. Methods* **4**:95–108.

Duffy, K. R., and Pardridge, W. M., 1987, Blood–brain barrier transcytosis of insulin in developing rabbits, *Brain Res.* **420**:32–38.

Djuričić, B. M., and Mršulja, B. B., 1988, Transport and barrier systems of the cerebral microvasculature: Enzymatic aspects, in: *Peptide and Amino Acid Transport Mechanisms in the Central Nervous System* (L. Rakić, D. J. Begley, H. Davson, and B. K. Zlokovic, eds.), Stockton Press, New York, pp. 269–278.

Dykstra, K. H., Arya, A., Arriola, D. M., Bungay, P. M., Morrison, P. F., and Dedrick, R. L., 1993, Microdialysis study of zidovudine (AZT) transport in rat brain, *J. Pharmacol. Exp. Ther.* **267**:1227–1236.

Ennis, S. R., Xiao-dan, R., and Betz, A. L., 1994, Transport of α-aminoisobutyric acid across the blood–brain barrier with *in situ* perfusion of rat brain, *Brain Res.* **643**:100–107.

Fishman, J. B., Rubin, J. B., Handrahan, J. V., Connor, J. R., and Fine, R. E., 1987, Receptor-mediated transfer of transferrin across the blood–brain barrier, *J. Neurosci. Res.* **18**:299–304.

Fukui, S., Schwarcz, R., Rapoport, S. I., Takada, Y., and Smith, Q. R., 1991, Blood–brain barrier transport of kynurenines: Implications for brain synthesis and metabolism, *J. Neurochem.* **56**:2007–2017.

Gilboe, D. D., 1982, Perfusion of the isolated brain, in: *Handbook of Neurochemistry*, Vol. 2 (A. Lajtha, ed.), Plenum Press, New York, pp. 301–330.

Greenwood, J., Luthert, P. J., Pratt, O. E., and Lantos, P. L., 1985, Maintenance of the integrity of the blood–brain barrier in the rat during an *in situ* saline-based perfusion, *Neurosci. Lett.* **56**:223–227.

Greenwood, J., Luthert, P. J., Pratt, O. E., and Lantos, P. L., 1986, Transport of thiamin across the blood–brain barrier of the rat in the absence of aerobic metabolism, *Brain Res.* **399**:148–151.

Greenwood, J., Hazell, A. S., and Pratt, O. E., 1989, The transport of leucine and aminoacyclopentanecarboxylate across the intact, energy-depleted rat blood–brain barrier, *J. Cereb. Blood Flow Metab.* **9**:226–233.

Greenwood, J., Adu, J., Davey, A. J., Abbott, N. J., and Bradbury, M. W. B., 1991, The effect of bile salts on the permeability and ultrastructure of the perfused, energy-depleted, rat blood–brain barrier, *J. Cereb. Blood Flow Metab.* **11**:644–654.

Greig, N. H., Soncrant, T. T., Shetty, H. U., Momma, S., Smith, Q. R., and Rapoport, S. I., 1990, Brain uptake and anticancer activity of vincristine and vinblastine are restricted by their low cerebrovascular permeability and binding to plasma constituents in rat, *Cancer Chemother. Pharmacol.* **26**:263–268.

Hardebo, J. E., Emson, P. C., Falck, B., Owman, C., and Rosengren, E., 1980, Enzymes related to monoamine metabolism in brain microvessels, *J. Neurochem.* **35:**1388–1393.

Hervonen, H., and Steinwall, O., 1984, Endothelial surface sulfhydryl-groups in blood–brain barrier transport of nutrients, *Acta Physiol. Scand.* **121:**343–351.

Horst, W. D., and Jester, J., 1971, The use of isolated brain perfused rat brains in a study of ^{14}C-L-DOPA metabolism, *Life Sci.* **10:**685–689.

Kalaria, R. N., Mitchell, M. J., and Harik, S. I., 1987, Correlation of 1-methyl-4-phenyl-1,2,3,6-tetrahydropyridine neurotoxicity with blood–brain barrier monoamine oxidase activity, *Proc. Natl. Acad. Sci. USA* **84:**3521–3525.

Kintner, D. B., Kao, J. L., Woodson, R. D., and Gilboe, D. D., 1986a, Evaluation of artificial plasma for maintaining the isolated canine brain, *J. Cereb. Blood Flow Metab.* **6:**455–462.

Kintner, D. B., Kranner, P. W., and Gilboe, D. D., 1986b, Cerebral vascular resistance following platelet and leukocyte removal from perfusate, *J. Cereb. Blood Flow Metab.* **6:**52–58.

Levin, V., 1980, Relationship of octanol/water partition coefficient and molecular weight to rat brain capillary permeability, *J. Med. Chem.* **23:**682–684.

Levitan, H., Ziylan, Z., Smith, Q. R., Takasato, Y., and Rapoport, S. I., 1984, Brain uptake of a food dye, erythrosin B, prevented by plasma protein binding, *Brain Res.* **322:**131–134.

Lowe, K. C., 1987, Perfluorocarbons as oxygen-transport fluids, *Comp. Biochem. Physiol.* **87A:**825–838.

Luthert, P. J., Greenwood, J., Pratt, O. E., and Lantos, P. L., 1987, The effect of metabolic inhibitor upon the properties of the cerebral vasculature during whole-head saline perfusion of the rat, *Quart. J. Exp. Physiol.* **72:**129–141.

Minn, A., Ghersi-Egea, J. F., Perrin, R., Leininger, B., and Siest, G., 1991, Drug metabolizing enzymes in the brain and cerebral microvessels, *Brain Res. Rev.* **16:**65–82.

Momma, S., Aoyagi, M., Rapoport, S. I., and Smith, Q. R., 1987, Phenylalanine transport across the blood–brain barrier as studied with the *in situ* brain perfusion technique, *J. Neurochem.* **48:**1291–1300.

Ohno, K., Pettigrew, K. D., and Rapoport, S. I., 1978, Lower limits of cerebrovascular permeability to nonelectrolytes in the conscious rat, *Am. J. Physiol.* **235:**H299–H307.

Oldendorf, W. H., 1970, Measurement of brain uptake of radiolabeled substances using a tritiated water internal standard, *Brain Res.* **24:**372–376.

Pardridge, W. M., 1983, Brain metabolism: A perspective from the blood–brain barrier, *Physiol. Rev.* **63:**1481–1535.

Pardridge, W. M., Triguero, D., Yang, J., and Cancilla, P. A., 1990, Comparison of *in vitro* and *in vivo* models of drug transcytosis through the blood–brain barrier, *J. Pharmacol. Exp. Ther.* **253:**884–891.

Pardridge, W. M., Yoshikawa, T., Kang, Y. S., and Miller, L. P., 1994, Blood–brain barrier transport and metabolism of adenosine and adenosine analogs, *J. Pharmacol. Exp. Ther.* **268:**14–18.

Patlak, C. S., Blasberg, R. G., and Fenstermacher, J. D., 1983, Graphical evaluation of blood-to-brain transfer constants from multiple-time uptake data, *J. Cereb. Blood Flow Metab.* **3:**1–7.

Petrov, T., Howarth, A. G., Krukoff, T. L., and Stevenson, B. R., 1994, Distribution of tight junction-associated protein ZO-1 in circumventricular organs of the CNS, *Mol. Brain Res.* **21:**235–246.

Rabin, O., Hegedus, L., Bourre, J. M., and Smith, Q. R., 1993, Rapid brain uptake of manganese(II) across the blood–brain barrier, *J. Neurochem.* **61:**509–517.

Rapoport, S. I., Ohno, K., and Pettigrew, K. D., 1979, Drug entry into the brain, *Brain Res.* **172:**354–359.

Richerson, G. B., and Getting, P. A., 1990, Preservation of integrative function in a perfused guinea pig brain, *Brain Res.* **517:**7–18.

Salford, L. G., and Seisjo, B. K., 1974, The influence of arterial hypoxia and unilateral carotid artery occlusion upon regional blood flow and metabolism in the rat brain, *Acta Physiol. Scand.* **92:**130–141.

Samii, A., Bickel, U., Stroth, U., and Pardridge, W. M., 1994, Blood–brain barrier transport of neuropeptides: Analysis with a metabolically stable dermorphin analogue, *Am. J. Physiol.* **267:**E124–E131.

Schinkel, A. H., Smit, J. J. M., van Tellingen, O., Beijnen, J. H., Wagenaar, E., van Deetmer, L., Moi, C. A. A. M., van der Valk, M. A., Robanus-Maandag, E. C., te Riele, H. P. J., Berns, A. J. M., and Borst, P.,

1994, Disruption of the mouse mdr1a P-glycoprotein gene leads to deficiency in the blood–brain barrier and to increased sensitivity to drugs, *Cell* **77**:491–502.

Skarlatos, S., Yoshikawa, T., and Pardridge, W. M., 1995, Transport of [^{125}I]transferrin through the rat blood–brain barrier, *Brain Res.* **683**:164–171.

Smith, Q. R., 1989, Quantitation of blood–brain barrier permeability, in: *Implications of the Blood–Brain Barrier and Its Manipulation*, Vol. 1 (E. A. Neuwelt, ed.), Plenum Press, New York, pp. 85–118.

Smith, Q. R., 1992, Methods of study, *Hand. Exp. Pharmacol.* **103**:23–52.

Smith, Q. R., 1995, Carrier-mediated drug transport at the blood–brain barrier and the potential for drug targeting to the brain, in: *New Concepts of a Blood–Brain Barrier* (J. Greenwood, D. Begley, and M. Segal, eds.), Plenum Press, New York, pp. 265–276.

Smith, Q. R., and Takasato, Y., 1986, Kinetics of amino acid transport at the blood–brain barrier studied using an *in situ* brain perfusion technique, *Ann. N.Y. Acad. Sci.* **481**:186–201.

Smith, Q. R., Takasato, Y., Sweeney, D. J., and Rapoport, S. I., 1985, Regional cerebrovascular transport of leucine as measured by the *in situ* brain perfusion technique, *J. Cereb. Blood Flow Metab.* **5**:300–311.

Smith, Q. R., Momma, S., Aoyagi, M., and Rapoport, S. I., 1987, Kinetics of neutral amino acid transport across the blood–brain barrier, *J. Neurochem.* **49**:1651.

Smith, Q. R., Ziylan, Y., and Rapoport, S. I., 1988, Kinetics and distribution volumes for tracers of different sizes in the brain plasma space, *Brain Res.* **462**:1–9.

Smith, Q. R., Fukui, S., Robinson, P., Rapoport, S. I., 1990, Influence of cerebral blood flow of tryptophan uptake into brain, in: *Amino Acids: Chemistry, Biology and Medicine* (G. Lubec and G. A. Rosenthal eds.), ESCOM Science Publishers, Leiden, pp. 364–369.

Smith, Q. R., Nagura, H., Washizaki, K., DeGeorge, J., Robinson, P., and Rapoport, S. I., 1991, Kinetics of fatty acid dissociation from albumin and transport into brain, *Soc. Neuroscience Abstr.* **17**:239.

Smith, Q. R., Nagura, H., Takada, Y., and Duncan, M. W., 1992, Facilitated transport of a neurotoxin, β-*N*-methylamino-L-alanine, across the blood–brain barrier, *J. Neurochem.* **58**:1330–1337.

Spector, R., Sivesind, C., and Kinzenbaw, D., 1986, Pantothenic acid transport through the blood–brain barrier, *J. Neurochem.* **47**:966–971.

Stoll, J., Wadhwani, K. C., and Smith, Q. R., 1993, Identification of the cationic amino acid transporter (System y+) of the rat blood–brain barrier, *J. Neurochem.* **60**:1956–1959.

Takada, Y., Greig, N. H., Vistica, D. T., Rapoport, S. I., and Smith, Q. R., 1991, Affinity of antineoplastic amino acid drugs for the large neutral amino acid transporter of the blood–brain barrier, *Cancer Chemother. Pharmacol.* **29**:89–94.

Takada, Y., Vistica, D. T., Greig, N. H., Purdon, D., Rapoport, S. I., and Smith, Q. R., 1992, Rapid high-affinity transport of a chemotherapeutic amino acid across the blood–brain barrier, *Cancer Res.* **52**:2191–2196.

Takasato, Y., Rapoport, S. I., Smith, Q. R., 1982, A new method to determine cerebrovascular permeability in the anesthetized rat, *Soc. Neurosci. Abstr.* **8**:850.

Takasato Y., Rapoport, S. I., and Smith, Q. R., 1984, An *in situ* brain perfusion technique to study cerebrovascular transport in the rat, *Am. J. Physiol.* **247**:H484–H493.

Tatsuta, T., Naito, M., Oh-hara, T., Sugawara, I., and Tsuruo, T., 1992, Functional involvement of P-glycoprotein in blood–brain barrier, *J. Biol. Chem.* **267**:20383–20391.

Thompson, A. M., Robertson, R. C., and Bauer, T. A., 1968, A rat head-perfusion technique developed for the study of brain uptake of materials, *J. Appl. Physiol.* **24**:407–411.

Triguero, D., Buciak, J., and Pardridge, W. M., 1990, Capillary depletion method for quantification of blood–brain barrier transport of circulating peptides and plasma proteins, *J. Neurochem.* **54**:1882–1888.

Washizaki, K., Purdon, D., DeGeorge, J., Robinson, P., Rapoport, S. I. and Smith, Q. R., 1991, Fatty acid uptake and esterification by the *in situ* perfused rat brain, *Soc. Neuroscience Abstr.* **17**:864.

Watson, P. M., Anderson, J. M., Vanltaille, C. M., and Doctorow, S. R., 1991, The tight junction-specific protein ZO-1 is a component of the human and rat blood–brain barriers, *Neurosci. Lett.* **129**:6–10.

Wong, S. L., van Belle, K., and Sawchuk, R. L., 1993, Distributional transport kinetics of zidovudine between plasma and brain extracellular fluid/cerebrospinal fluid in the rabbit: Investigation of the inhibitory effect of probenecid utilizing microdialysis, *J. Pharmacol. Exp. Ther.* **264:**899–909.

Woods, H. F., and Youdim, M. B. H., 1978, The isolated perfused rat brain preparation—a critical assessment, *Essays Neurochem. Neuropharmacol.* **3:**49–69.

Zlokovic, B. V., Begley, D. J., Djuričić, B. M., and Mitrovic, D. M., 1986, Measurement of solute transport across the blood–brain barrier in the perfused guinea pig brain: Method and application to *N*-methyl-aminoisobutyric acid, *J. Neurochem.* **46:**1441–1451.

Zlokovic, B. V., Mackic, J. B., Djuričić, B., and Davson, H., 1989, Kinetic analysis of leucine-enkephalin cellular uptake at the luminal side of the blood–brain barrier of an *in situ* perfused guinea pig brain, *J. Neurochem.* **53:**1333–1340.

Zlokovic, B. V., Hyman, S., McComb, J. G., Lipovac, M. N., Tang, G., and Davson, H., 1990, Kinetics of arginine-vasopressin uptake at the blood–brain barrier, *Biochim. Biophys. Acta* **1025:**191–198.

Chapter 16

In Vitro Nasal Models

Patricia M. Reardon

1. INTRODUCTION

Pharmaceutical companies are investing time and money in the development of alternatives to injectable formulations for the systemic delivery of therapeutics. Alternative delivery systems offer enormous market potential and increased patient compliance. The nasal route has proved effective and acceptable for several therapeutics. In fact, several biotechnology nasal products are currently in the U.S. market, including DDAVP (desmopressin acetate, Rhone-Poulenc Rorer), Synarel (narelin acetate, Syntex), Diapid (lypressin, Sandoz), and Syntocinon (oxytocin, Sandoz). Intranasal administration of therapeutics offers many advantages over other routes of administration. Therapeutics administered nasally avoid gastrointestinal degradation and first-pass metabolism associated with oral administration. In addition, the high vascularity of the nasal mucosa allows rapid absorption of some compounds. However, bioavailability of nasally administered therapeutics is normally low, making this route acceptable for only a few potent therapeutics.

The low bioavailability of nasally administered therapeutics is believed to result from both epithelial and protease barriers. An understanding of transport and metabolic properties of these barriers will provide information necessary to facilitate the development of successful nasal formulations for new therapeutic entities as well as for existing therapeutics currently delivered by alternative routes of administration. Several *in vitro* nasal models are currently being employed to study the transport and metabolic properties of the nasal mucosa.

The aim of this chapter is to provide methods to establish *in vitro* nasal models essential for investigating transport and metabolic properties of the nasal mucosa.

Patricia M. Reardon • Amgen, Inc., Thousand Oaks, California 91320.

Models for Assessing Drug Absorption and Metabolism, Ronald T. Borchardt *et al.*, eds., Plenum Press, New York, 1996.

Models discussed include the excised nasal tissue model, isolated airway epithelial membranes, and nasal homogenates. Each model has its own benefits in studying transport and metabolism of potential therapeutics directed at the nasal mucosa as outlined in this chapter.

2. METHODS

2.1. Materials

Common reagents used for *in vitro* nasal model systems are as follows.

Bicarbonate-buffered Ringer solution (BBRS): 112 mM NaCl, 5.0 mM KCl, 1.2 mM $CaCl_2 \cdot 2H_2O$, 1.2 mM $MgCl_2 \cdot 6H_2O$, 1.6 mM $NaHPO_4$, and 25 mM $NaHCO_4$. The BBRS is often oxygenated with 95% O_2/5% CO_2 and incubated at 37°C to maintain a pH of 7.4 (Wheatley *et al.*, 1988).

Isotonic physiological buffer: A number of buffers are appropriate, such as phosphate-buffered saline (PBS), 0.1 M phosphate buffer, 0.9% NaCl solution, or KCl solution.

Mucosal bathing solution: BBRS containing 10 mM mannitol.

Serosal bathing solution: BBRS containing 10 mM glucose.

Membrane incubation buffer: 250 mM sucrose, 5 mM HEPES-Tris, 2 mM EDTA, and 1 mM dithiothreitol, pH 7.8.

Membrane homogenization buffer: 50 mM mannitol, 5 mM HEPES-Tris, 0.25 mM $MgCl_2$, and 1 mM dithiothreitol, pH 7.4.

Membrane isolation medium: 10 mM $MgCl_2$, 100 mM mannitol, and 5 mM HEPES-Tris, pH 7.4.

Alkaline phosphatase assay substrate (Sigma 104 phosphate substrate, Sigma Chemical Co., St. Louis, MO).

Alkaline phosphatase assay medium: 0.1 M Tris (pH 9.0), 2.5 mM $MgCl_2$, and 1% Triton X-100.

Glycine buffer: 133 mM glycine, 83 mM sodium carbonate, and 67 mM sodium chloride.

2.2. Excised Nasal Tissue Model

The utilization of excised nasal tissue mounted in Ussing chambers or modified Ussing chambers provides a rapid method to evaluate the permeability and the mechanisms of permeation of therapeutics across the nasal mucosa. In addition, the model provides a method to quantitate peptidase activity at the mucosal surface as well as to investigate the degradation of therapeutics directed at the nasal mucosa.

2.2.1 TISSUE PREPARATION AND EQUILIBRATION

Fresh nasal mucosal tissue obtained from either rabbit (Corbo *et al.*, 1990; Cremaschi *et al.*, 1990, 1991a,b; Hersey and Jackson, 1987), canine (Hersey and Jackson, 1987), or ovine (Reardon *et al.*, 1993; Wheatley *et al.*, 1988) is dissected to remove the ventral nasal conchae. The nasal mucosa is carefully removed from the underlying cartilage and placed in ice-cold, oxygenated (95% O_2/5% CO_2) BBRS. Tissue is then mounted between leucite half-chambers and joined to glass reservoirs to form the complete Ussing chamber system. Mucosal and serosal bathing solutions are added simultaneously to the mucosal and serosal reservoirs, respectively. The total volume in each reservoir is usually 10–12 ml. The glass reservoirs are water-jacketed and connected to a circulating water bath to maintain the tissue at a constant temperature of 37°C. In addition, the reservoirs are equipped with a gas lift system to provide oxygenation and circulation of the added buffered solutions with 95% O_2/5% CO_2.

The tissue viability and integrity are continuously monitored by measuring the short-circuit current (I_{sc}) and transepithelial conductance (G_t) using a high conductance membrane voltage clamp. The I_{sc}, the current required to nullify the spontaneous potential difference, provides a measure of net active ion transport, an indirect measure of tissue viability. The I_{sc} arises from the active transport of Na^+ across the apical membrane via an amiloride-sensitive conductive pathway and exit across the basolateral membrane via a Na^+/K^+-ATPase. The G_t across the epithelia provides a measure of ionic permeability, from which one can evaluate tissue integrity. The tissue is continuously short-circuited via electrodes at the distal ends of each half-chamber for brief intervals (<10 sec) during which time the transepithelial potential difference (P_D) is measured with reference to the mucosal bathing solution. The transepithelial I_{sc} value, corrected for chamber area, is calculated by dividing I_{sc} in microamperes (μA) by Faraday's constant (26.88 μA·hr/μequiv) to convert it to microequivalents per hour. Subsequently, I_{sc} in microequivalents per hour is divided by the chamber area to convert I_{sc} to units of microequivalents per hour per square centimeter. The G_t (mS/cm^2) is calculated by dividing I_{sc} (μA) by P_D (mV) and by the chamber area in square centimeters (Koefoed-Johnson *et al.*, 1952). At electrical steady state, I_{sc} and G_t values measured in ovine nasal mucosa are approximately 3.5 μEq/cm^2·hr and 8.3 mS/cm^2, respectively (Reardon *et al.*, 1993).

2.2.2. TRANSEPITHELIAL FLUX AND PERMEABILITY MEASUREMENTS

After equilibration has been achieved, chambers and reservoirs are drained and refilled with 10–12 ml of serosal or mucosal bathing solution in the serosal and mucosal reservoirs, respectively. Initially, a 1-hr passive permeability marker flux may be performed to assess tissue permeability under control conditions. In such studies, a radiolabeled passive permeability marker is added either to the serosal reservoir for serosal (s)-to-mucosal (m) flux determination or to the mucosal reservoir for m-to-s flux determination. Samples are taken from the receiver reservoir at 0, 15, 30, and 60 min and from the donor reservoir at 0 and 60 min. After each sample, the volume removed from the receiver reservoir is replaced with the appropriate buffer to maintain a constant volume. Radiolabeled mannitol has been used previously in ovine nasal mucosa studies (Reardon et al., 1993), since it is a known passive permeability marker (Laker et al., 1982). In such studies, 5 μCi of [^{14}C]mannitol was added to the donor reservoir, and 1-ml samples were taken from the receiver reservoir and 100-μl samples were taken from the donor reservoir at the times indicated above. Mannitol m-to-s and s-to-m fluxes were identical at 0.1 $\pm$ 0.01%/(hr·cm^2).

Subsequently, 3-hr flux study in the same tissue is conducted in the absence of a concentration gradient using radiolabeled compounds. Chambers and reservoirs are drained and refilled as before, followed by the addition of unlabeled compound of interest in equimolar quantities to both the serosal and the mucosal chamber. The radiolabeled form of the compound is then added to either the serosal reservoir for s-to-m fluxes or the mucosal reservoir for m-to-s fluxes. Sample aliquots are taken from the receiver reservoirs at 30-min intervals for up to 3 hr. Again, the volume removed from the receiver reservoir is replaced with the appropriate buffer to maintain a constant volume. At 0-, 60-, and 180-min intervals, samples are taken from the donor reservoirs, but these volumes are not replaced. Beta-emitter samples, such as those in which the radiolabel is ^{3}H and ^{14}C, are mixed with 2 to 10 ml of scintillation cocktail and counted in a liquid scintillation counter. Gamma-emitter samples, such as those in which the radiolabel is ^{125}I, are counted in a gamma-counter. The permeability of several compounds have been investigated using radiolabeled compounds and nasal tissue mounted in Ussing chambers or modified Ussing chambers, including inulin and propranolol (Wheatley et al., 1988); growth hormone-releasing peptide (Reardon et al., 1993); insulin, PEG 4000, and sucrose (Carstens et al., 1993); and calcitonin and adrenocorticotropic hormone (Cremaschi et al., 1991).

In addition, the flux of fluorescent compounds may be determined, but a concentration gradient cannot be eliminated. The flux of lucifer yellow, a passive permeability marker (Artigas et al., 1987), was previously determined in ovine nasal mucosa by adding 1 mg of lucifer yellow to the donor reservoir. Samples were then taken at the volumes and times indicated above. The fluorescence of lucifer yellow was measured at an excitation wavelength of 428 nm and an emission wavelength of 540 nm. The flux of lucifer yellow in the m-to-s direction was 0.09 $\pm$ 0.01 %/(hr·cm^2) (Reardon et al., 1993), similar to that of mannitol.

The tissue integrity and viability is measured throughout the experiment by measuring the P_D and I_{sc} as indicated above. At the end of the experiment, 10^{-4} M amiloride, an inhibitor of active Na$^+$ transport, may be added to the mucosal bathing solution, and tissue electrical properties determined as a final measurement of tissue viability.

Results may be presented as either the percentage of the administrated dose over time or concentration of the compound over time. The percentage of the administered dose is determined from the rate of appearance of the compound of interest in the receiver reservoir. Alternatively, the flux of the compound of interest, J, is determined by plotting millimoles measured in the receiver reservoir per square centimeter versus minutes. All calculations should take into account the dilution effect of the replacement buffer. The apparent permeability coefficient, P_C, in centimeters per minute, is calculated from the flux value using Fick's law of diffusion:

$$J = P_C(C_D - C_R)$$

where C_D (mmol/cm^3) is the initial donor concentration and C_R (mmol/cm^3) is the final receiver concentration.

2.2.3. MEASUREMENT OF PROTEASE ACTIVITY

Protease activities at the mucosal surface of nasal tissue can be measured by simple fluorescence or chromogenic assays. Studies are performed by incubating nasal tissue equilibrated in Ussing chambers or modified Ussing chambers with the substrate of the enzyme of interest. Samples are then taken from the mucosal reservoir and analyzed for enzyme activity using a preexisting enzyme assay. Both aminopeptidase and chymotrypsin activity have been quantitated at ovine nasal mucosal surface employing Ussing chambers and standard chromogenic enzyme assays (Reardon, 1992).

Leucine aminopeptidase (LAP) activity was determined by using L-Leucyl-β-naphthylamide as the LAP substrate. L-Leucyl-β-naphthylamide at a concentration of 0.16 mg/ml was added to the mucosal reservoir of an Ussing chamber mounted with equilibrated ovine nasal mucosa. The tissue was incubated for 1.5 hr at 37°C. At the end of the incubation period, 1-ml samples were taken from the mucosal reservoir. LAP activity was determined by using the LAP Diagnostic Kit (Sigma) and quantitated by measuring the absorption of the product at 580 nm (Martinek *et al.*, 1964). LAP activity was detected at significant levels, 27.4 ± 2.3 μg/cm^2, in ovine nasal mucosa (Reardon, 1992).

Chymotrypsin activity was quantitated by using succinylphenylalanin 4-nitroanilide (Suphepa) as the substrate. Suphepa at a concentration of 2.1 mg/ml was added to the mucosal reservoir of an Ussing chamber mounted with equilibrated ovine nasal mucosa. The tissue was incubated for 2 hr at 37°C, and then a 2-ml sample was taken from the mucosal reservoir. A 5-μl aliquot of a 2-mg/ml aprotinin solution was added to the sample to terminate any further reaction. Chymotrypsin activity was quantitated by measuring the absorbance of 4-nitroaniline, the product of the reaction of Suphepa reacting with chymotrypsin, at 405 nm. Chymotrypsin activity was detected at low levels, 4.8 ± 0.7 μg/cm^2, in ovine nasal mucosa (Reardon, 1992).

2.2.4. METABOLISM STUDIES

The metabolism of therapeutic compounds directed at the nasal mucosa can be investigated by analytical techniques. Studies are performed by incubating the compound of interest with nasal tissue mounted in Ussing chambers or diffusion chambers modified for tissues. Samples are taken from both the mucosal and serosal reservoirs and analyzed for the parent compound and metabolites. The methodology of analysis of the compound either has to be developed or may often be adapted from an existing assay. In addition, if the compound of interest is radiolabeled, fractions may be collected during analysis and the radioactivity quantitated to generate an elution profile for radioactivity. The radioactivity profile is then compared with the UV absorbance profile to determine the identities of the radioactive fractions.

The degradation of growth hormone-releasing peptide (GHRP) was investigated by mounting ovine nasal mucosa in diffusion chambers modified for tissues (Reardon *et al.*, 1993). The tissues were equilibrated for 60–120 min in 5 ml of serosal bathing solution in the serosal chamber and 5 ml of mucosal bathing solution in the mucosal chamber. After equilibration, the chambers were drained and refilled with fresh bathing solutions. GHRP (100 μM) and 15 μCi of [^{3}H] GHRP were added to the mucosal chambers and allowed to incubate for up to 3 hr. Samples (1 ml) were taken from both the mucosal and serosal chambers at 0, 60, and 180 min. These samples were not replaced. Acetonitrile was added to each sample to obtain a 20% acetonitrile concentration to terminate any further degradation of GHRP. Mucosal samples were then analyzed for GHRP degradation by HPLC analysis. In addition, 1-min fractions were collected throughout each HPLC run. The fractions were then counted in a liquid scintillation counter to determine the elution profile of radioactivity. The radioactivity elution profiles were then compared with the UV absorbance profiles obtained from the HPLC run to determine the identities of the radioactive fractions.

2.3.   Isolated Airway Epithelial Membranes

Bovine trachea apical membranes have been employed to elucidate potential mechanisms by which therapeutics permeate across epithelial membranes by measuring the membrane structural integrity. The membrane integrity can be monitored by steady-state fluorescence anisotropy techniques.

2.3.1.   BOVINE TRACHEA APICAL MEMBRANE PREPARATION AND CHARACTERIZATION

Bovine trachea apical membrane preparation is performed by a modification of the previously described procedures (Langridge-Smith *et al.*, 1983; Fong *et al.*, 1988). Bovine trachea is obtained from a local slaughterhouse, where it is removed 10–15 min after the animal has been killed and immediately put on ice for transportation. Each trachea is divided into two or three segments, opened anteriorly, and washed in ice-cold BBRS containing 1 mM dithiothreitol to remove debris and mucus from the lumen. The strips of mucosa with underlying connective tissue and cartilage are incubated for 15 min in ice-cold membrane incubation buffer and bubbled vigorously with 95% O_2/5% CO_2. The luminal surface is then firmly scraped with a glass microscope slide to harvest the trachea mucosa. The mucosal scrapings (5 g) are collected in 30 ml of ice-cold membrane homogenization buffer. All subsequent steps are performed at 4°C. The mucosal suspension is then homogenized with 12 strokes in a glass homogenizer with a motor-driven teflon pestle. The resulting homogenate is centrifuged at 300 × g for 8 min. The supernatant is saved, and the pellet is resuspended in 20 ml of membrane homogenization buffer. The resuspended pellet is added to the supernatant and homogenized as before. The combined supernatant and pellet is centrifuged at 2000 × g for 8 min to remove the nuclei and large cellular debris. The resulting supernatant is centrifuged at 9500 × g for 10 min, and a dense pellet with a loose lighter halo results. The lighter halo is gently sloughed off the pellet and collected with the supernatant using a Pasteur pipet. The supernatant suspension is centrifuged for 40 min at 35,000 × g. The resulting pellet contains the mixed plasma fraction enriched in both apical and basolateral membranes. The pellet is resuspended in 20 ml of membrane isolation medium. The suspension is incubated on ice for approximately 1.5 hr with occasional stirring. Following the incubation period, the suspension is centrifuged at 1500 × g for 12 min. The pellet contains basolateral membranes, and the supernatant contains apical membranes. Apical membranes are diluted in the membrane isolation medium containing 1 mM EDTA to remove excess Mg^{2+}, and centrifuged at 100,000 × g for 25 min. The pellet, which contains the apical membranes, is saved, and the supernatant is discarded. Protein concentration of the apical membrane pellet is measured by a standard protein assay kit using bovine serum albumin as the standard. The pellets are then diluted in BBRS to achieve an approximate protein concentration of 5–7 mg/ml. Membranes may be stored at −80°C until use.

To monitor the consistency between apical membrane preparations, alkaline phosphatase activity in micromoles per hour per unit protein concentration is measured. Alkaline phosphatase activity, an apical membrane marker, is measured by a modified procedure previously described (Weiser, 1973). Briefly, a 200-μl aliquot of apical membrane suspension and 50 μl of 1.32-mg/ml of alkaline phosphatase assay substrate solution is diluted to a final volume of 850 μl with alkaline phosphatase assay medium. The reaction is incubated for 15 min at 37°C. The reaction is terminated upon addition of 2.25 μl of ice-cold glycine buffer. A standard curve is prepared using *p*-nitrophenol to calculate alkaline phosphatase activity (μmol/hr). The absorbances of samples and standards are recorded at 410 nm.

2.3.2. FLUORESCENCE LABELING OF MEMBRANES

Fluorophore probes often utilized to label membranes include 1,6-diphenyl-1,3,5-hexatriene (DPH) and [4-(trimethlyammonio)phenyl]-6-phenyl-1,3,5-hexatriene (TMA-DPH) purchased from Molecular Probes (Eugene, OR) (Audus *et al.*, 1991; Reardon and Audus, 1993). DPH localizes at the hydrophobic core of membrane lipid bilayers, whereas TMA-DPH, a cationized probe, localizes at the membrane lipid–water interface. DPH (1 mM) and TMA-DPH (5×10^{-4} M) stock solutions are prepared on the day of the experiment in tetrahydrofuran and dimethylformamide, respectively. Bovine membranes at a final concentration of 200 μg/ml and compounds of interest are added to a quartz cuvette to achieve a final volume of 2.5 ml. The membrane suspensions are labeled with DPH by adding DPH stock solution to the membrane suspension to obtain a final concentration of 2 μM. The probe is equilibrated with the membranes in the dark at room temperature for 30 min. The membrane suspensions are labeled with TMA-DPH by adding TMA-DPH stock solution to the membrane suspension to obtain a final concentration of 1 μM. The probe only requires a few minutes to become equilibrated with the membranes (Bronner *et al.*, 1986).

2.3.3. STEADY-STATE FLUORESCENCE ANISOTROPY AND LIFETIME MEASUREMENTS

Steady-state fluorescence anisotropy of DPH- and TMA-DPH-labeled bovine trachea membranes is measured with a fluorometer equipped with polarization capabilities. Photomultiplier tubes are placed to the right and left of the sample cell with polarizers inserted in emission and excitation beams. The labeled membranes, placed in quartz cuvettes, are gently stirred with a magnetic stirrer and maintained at an appropriate temperature in a dual-chamber sample cell by an external water bath. Steady-state fluorescence anisotropy, r_s, is determined by exciting the sample at an emission wavelength of 360 nm, first with a horizontally polarized beam and then with a vertically polarized beam. Fluorescence intensities are measured at an emission wavelength of 430 nm with a 389-nm-cutoff filter.

The corrected fluorescence anisotropy data are calculated from the relationships:

$$P = \left(\frac{A}{B} - 1\right)\left(\frac{A}{B} + 1\right)$$

$$r_s = (2 \times P)/(3 - P)$$

where P is the fluorescence polarization, A is the ratio of fluorescence intensities parallel and perpendicular to the plane of vertically polarized excitation light, B is the ratio of fluorescence intensities parallel and perpendicular to the plane of horizontally polarized excitation light, and r_s is the polarized anisotropy. The lipid order parameter, S, is calculated for DPH and TMA-DPH from the following relationship (LeCluyse *et al.*, 1991):

$$s^2 = (\tfrac{4}{3}r_s - 0.1)/r_0$$

where r_0 is the maximal fluorescence anisotropy value in the absence of any rotational motion. A value of 0.4 for r_0 has been used in previous studies (Reardon and Audus, 1993). The lipid order parameter of DPH-labeled biomembranes represents the average molecular packing of the hydrophobic core of the lipid bilayer, and the lipid order parameter of TMA-DPH-labeled biomembranes represents the average molecular packing near the lipid–water interface of the lipid bilayer. A decrease in the lipid order parameter signifies an increase in the fluorophore probe's cone rotational angle either within the deeper hydrophobic domains for DPH or at the lipid–water interface for TMA-DPH. A decrease in membrane lipid order consequently signifies an increase in membrane fluidity.

Lifetime measurements are required to evaluate direct interactions between the compound of interest and the fluorophore in the membranes. The excited-state lifetimes (τ) are calculated from phase and modulation measurements as described previously (Lackowicz, 1983; Audus *et al.*, 1991). Briefly, the fluorophore probe's lifetimes are analyzed under control conditions and under test conditions at both 18- and 30-MHz modulation frequencies, utilizing dimethyl-POPOP, which has a lifetime of approximately 1.45 nsec, as the reference probe. The phase angle (Φ) and modulation of each sample are measured alternately five times, with approximately 10-sec intervals between each measurement, and the phase (τ_{Φ}) and modulation (τ_m) lifetimes are calculated using the following relationships:

$$\tau_{\Phi} = 1/\overline{\omega} \tan \Theta$$

$$\tau_m = 1/\overline{\omega}[(1/M^3) - 1]^{1/2}$$

where τ_{Φ} is the phase lifetime in nanoseconds, Θ is the phase shift in degrees caused by a sinusoidally modulated emission from a fluorophore of lifetime τ, $\overline{\omega}$ is the angular frequency of excitation, which is 2π times the modulated frequency (18 or 30 MHz), τ_m is the modulation lifetime, and M is the demodulation factor of sinusoidally modulated emission from a fluorophore of lifetime τ. M is the ratio of M_s/M_r, where M_s is the relative modulation of the fluorescence solution, and M_r is the relative modulation of a scattered (reference) solution. For a decrease in the fluorescence lifetime measurements to significantly affect the anisotropy of DPH and TMA-DPH, and hence, the lipid-packing order measurements, at least 50% reduction in the lifetime would have to occur (Sklar, 1984).

2.4. Nasal Homogenate Systems

Nasal homogenates have been employed to study nasal peptidase activity as well as the degradation of therapeutics by nasal proteases. A number of species have been utilized to obtain nasal homogenates, including human (Aceto *et al.*, 1989; Gervasi *et al.*, 1991), sheep (Holbrook *et al.*, 1991), rabbit (Kashi and Lee, 1986; Stratford and Lee, 1986; Jonsson *et al.*, 1992), and rat (Morimoto *et al.*, 1991). Human and rabbit are the most widely used, so this section will focus on the isolation of human and rabbit nasal homogenates.

2.4.1. PREPARATION OF NASAL HOMOGENATES

Human nasal homogenates are prepared by removing nasal tissue from human patients afflicted by hypertrophy of the inferior turbinates. Tissues are washed thoroughly in ice-cold isotonic physiologic buffer and are then immediately frozen in liquid nitrogen and stored at $-80°C$ until use. A histopathological examination is performed to determine that there are no signs of leukocyte infiltration within the tissues. Tissues are then minced and homogenized. To separate cytosolic and microsomal fractions, tissue homogenates are centrifuged at $100,000 \times g$ for 60 min. The supernatant contains the cytosolic fraction, and the pellet contains the microsomal fraction. The protein concentrations of the cytosolic and microsomal fractions are measured by a standard protein assay kit using bovine serum albumin as the standard.

Rabbit nasal homogenates are prepared similarly as indicated above. Briefly, rabbits weighing 2 to 3 kg are fasted overnight and are then terminated by lethal injection of pentobarbital solution into the marginal ear vein. The nasal mucosa is immediately removed and rinsed with an isotonic physiologic buffer. The tissue is either stored at $-80°C$ for future use or immediately homogenized as indicated below. Frozen tissue is thawed at room temperature for approximately 10 min. Thawed or fresh tissue is rinsed twice with 0.05 M maleate buffer, pH 7.4, and homogenized in 4–6 ml of maleate buffer at 4°C. The homogenate is centrifuged at $3000–5000 \times g$ for 10 min at 4°C. The supernatant, containing the cytosol and relevant plasma and intracellular fractions, is saved, and the pellet, containing the cellular and nuclear debris, is discarded. The protein concentration of the supernatant is measured by a standard protein assay kit using bovine serum albumin as the standard. The supernatant is then diluted with physiological buffer to obtain a final protein concentration of 5 mg/ml.

2.4.2. HOMOGENATE PROTEASE ACTIVITY MEASUREMENTS

Protease activity in nasal homogenates can be measured by simple fluorescence or chromogenic enzyme assays. Experiments are performed by incubating nasal homogenates with the substrate of the enzyme of interest. Protease activity is then determined by a preexisting enzyme assay. The protease activity for a number of proteases has been previously measured in nasal homogenates, including aminopeptidases (Stratford and Lee, 1986) and glutathione transferase (Aceto et al., 1989), as well as oxidative and nonoxidative enzymes (Gervasi et al., 1991).

Aminopeptidase activity was measured in rabbit homogenates by a continuous fluorescence assay which monitors the formation of a fluorescent leaving group from one of four nonfluorescent aminopeptidase substrates (Stratford and Lee, 1986). Briefly, 100 μl of the 5-mg/ml nasal homogenate was incubated in 2.8 ml of maleate buffer for 15 min in a fluorescence cuvette at 37°C. The reaction was initiated by adding 100 μl of a 30 mM solution of one of the four aminopeptidases substrates, namely, 4-methoxy-2-naphthylamine of L-leucine, L-alanine, L-glutamic acid, or L-arginine. The increase in fluorescence intensity was monitored at an excitation wavelength of 342 nm and an emission wavelength of 426 nm for 5 min. Fluorescence intensities were plotted against time to express aminopeptidase activity in terms of nanomoles of substrate hydrolyzed per minute per milligram of protein. The aminopeptidase activities measured were approximately $2-18$ nmol/min^{-1}/(mg protein)$^{-1}$.

2.4.3. HOMOGENATE METABOLISM STUDIES

The metabolism of therapeutic compounds by nasal homogenates can be investigated by analytical techniques. Studies are performed by incubating the compound of interest with nasal homogenates. Samples are taken from the homogenate suspension and analyzed for the parent compound and metabolites. As indicated in the section on the excised tissue model, the methodology of analysis of the compound either has to be developed or may often be adapted from an existing assay. Nasal homogenates have been utilized to determine the enzymatic degradation of therapeutics such as enkephalins (Kashi and Lee, 1986) and desamino[1], D-arginine[8]-vasopressin (Jonsson *et al.*, 1992) as well as small peptides and amino acids (Holbrook *et al.*, 1991).

The degradation of desamino[1], D-arginine[8]-vasopressin (DDAVP) by rabbit nasal homogenates was investigated by incubating nasal homogenates at a protein concentration of 1 g/l with DDAVP at 37°C. The final DDAVP concentration in the homogenate suspension was 3.2 mM. Samples were removed at 5, 20, 30, 45, 60, 90, and 120 min. Acetonitrile was added to each sample to obtain a 34% final concentration to terminate further degradation. Samples were centrifuged at $13,000 \times g$ at 4°C for 15 min to remove precipitated proteins. The supernatants were then analyzed for DDAVP degradation by reversed-phase (RP)-HPLC.

The degradation of enkephalins was investigated in a similar manner. Briefly, 10 μl of the 5-mg/ml homogenate was incubated with 40 μl of a 2.5 mM enkephalin solution, prepared in an isotonic phosphate buffer, at 37°C for up to 180 min. At preset times, 75 μl of acetonitrile was added to the sample to terminate any further degradation. Ten microliters of a 0.25-mg/ml trytophan solution was added to each sample as an internal standard. Samples were centrifuged for 15 min to remove precipitated proteins. The acetonitrile was evaporated under nitrogen, and 10 μl of each sample was analyzed for degradation by HPLC analysis.

3. ABSORPTION AND METABOLISM APPLICATIONS

Excised nasal tissue mounted in Ussing chambers or modified Ussing chambers has been employed to study transepithelial transport properties and determine metabolic capabilities of the nasal mucosa as well as to assess tissue integrity and viability. The mechanisms of permeation across the nasal mucosa have been studied for a number compounds, including inulin and propranolol (Wheatley *et al.*, 1988), growth-hormone releasing peptide and lucifer yellow (Reardon *et al.*, 1993a), adrenocorticotropic hormone and elcatonin (Cremaschi *et al.*, 1991), and insulin and PEG 4000 (Carstens *et al.*, 1993). Limited research has been focused on determining the metabolic capabilities of the nasal mucosa using Ussing chambers (Reardon 1992; Reardon *et al.*, 1993). However, Ussing chambers have been employed to provide information on the metabolic capability of the gastrointestinal mucosal tissue (Matuszewska *et al.*, 1988; Smith *et al.*, 1988). In addition, the effects of absorption promoters on nasal permeation and integrity have been studied for a number of absorption enhancers, including deoxycholate (Wheatley *et al.*, 1988), ammonium glycyrrhizinate (Reardon *et al.*, 1993), and didecanoyl-L-α-phosphatidylcholine (Carstens *et al.*, 1993).

Isolated epithelial membranes are often used to correlate therapeutic absorption and perturbation of membrane integrity. This is especially true when absorption promoters are added to a formulation. In fact, several investigators have demonstrated a correlation between promoting effects of absorption promoters and perturbation of the structural integrity of membranes through the use of steady-state anisotropy techniques (Kajii *et al.*, 1985, 1986; Higaki *et al.*, 1988; Iseki *et al.*, 1988; LeCluyse *et al.*, 1991; Reardon and Audus, 1993). Thus, steady-state anisotropy studies utilizing bovine trachea apical epithelial membranes can provide mechanistic information regarding permeation of therapeutics across nasal membranes.

Nasal homogenate systems have been used to define protease activity in the nasal mucosa as well as to determine the enzymatic degradation of potential therapeutics. Stratford and Lee (1986) determined the type and activity of aminopeptidases in nasal homogenates by using a simple, continuous fluorescence assay that monitors the formation of a fluorescent leaving group from nonfluorescent aminopeptidase substrates. Oxidative and nonoxidative nasal enzyme activities have been investigated in human nasal homogenates (Gervasi *et al.*, 1991). Glutathione transferase activity in nasal homogenates has been investigated in human nasal homogenates (Aceto *et al.*, 1989). The degradation of enkephalins (Kashi and Lee, 1986) and desamino[1],D-arginine[8]-vasopressin (Jonsson *et al.*, 1992) has been investigated utilizing nasal homogenates.

4. ADVANTAGES AND DISADVANTAGES OF *IN VITRO* NASAL MODELS

In vitro nasal models allow the study of mechanistic approaches that are not possible in whole animal models. However, *in vitro* nasal models cannot be employed to study the effects of other factors, such as residence time at the nasal mucosa and site of deposition within the nasal cavity, on nasal absorption. In addition, whole animal models are required to evaluate the therapeutic response and behavior of nasally delivered therapeutics. The main limitation of *in vitro* nasal models involves the availability of nasal tissues. Investigators may find it difficult to obtain a reliable source of required tissue, especially if human tissue is preferred. Also, interspecies variations should be anticipated when animal tissue is used to model human physiology.

The excised nasal tissue model is advantageous as compared to the other *in vitro* nasal models because it most closely represents intact nasal mucosa observed *in vivo*. The excised nasal tissue model is also a versatile model since it can be utilized to study transport across the nasal mucosa and metabolic capabilities of the nasal mucosa, as well as the effects of therapeutics on the nasal mucosa integrity and morphology. Isolated membranes provide a good model for the study of membrane transport events in the absence of cytosolic contents. In addition, apical and basolateral membrane properties can be studied separately. However, protease activities in nasal homogenates must be viewed with some scrutiny, since the protease organization within the mucosa membrane, cytosol, and inner organelle membranes is disrupted during homogenization. As a result, protease activity of homogenates may not represent the true protease activity encountered during absorption across intact nasal mucosa. In addition, variations in protease activity among homogenate samples may result from tissue and species heterogeneity. All in all, *in vitro* nasal models are beneficial in determining the mechanisms by which compounds permeate across the nasal mucosa, but one must be aware of the limitations of the model used.

REFERENCES

Aceto, A., Di Ilio, C., Angelucci, S., Longo, V., Gervasi, P. G., and Federici, G., 1989, Glutathione transferase in human nasal mucosa, *Arch. Toxicol.* **63**:427–431.

Artigas, J., Aruffo, C., Sampaolo, S., Cruz-Sanchez, F., Ferszt, R., and Cervos-Navarro, J., 1987, Lucifer yellow as a morphofunctional tracer of the blood-brain barrier, in: *Stroke and Microcirculation* (J. Cervos-Navarro and R. Ferszt, eds.), Raven Press, New York, pp. 238–243.

Audus, K. L., Guillot, F. L., and Braughler, J. M., 1991, Evidence for 21-aminosteroid association with the hydrophobic domains of brain microvessel endothelial cells, *Free Radical Biol. Med.* **11**:361–371.

Bronner, C., Landry, Y., Fonteneau, P., and Kuhry, J., 1986, A fluorescent hydrophobic probe used for monitoring the kinetics of exocytosis phenomena, *Biochemistry* **25**:2149–2154.

Carstens, S., Danielsen, G., Guldhammer, B., and Frederiksen, O., 1993, Transport of insulin across rabbit nasal mucosa *in vitro* induced by didecanoyl-L-α-phosphatidylcholine, *Diabetes* **42**:1032–1040.

Corbo, D. C., Huang, Y. C., and Chien, Y. W., 1990, Characterization of the barrier properties of mucosal membranes, *J. Pharm. Sci.* **79**:202–206.

Cremaschi, D., Rossetti, C., Draghetti, M. T., Manzoni, C., and Aliverti, V., 1990, Active transport of polypeptides in rabbit respiratory nasal mucosa, *J. Controlled Release* **13**:319–320.

Cremaschi, D., Rossetti, C., Draghetti, M. T., Manzoni, C., and Aliverti, V., 1991, Active transport of polypeptides in rabbit nasal mucosa: Possible role in the sampling of potential antigens, *Pflügers Arch.* **419**:425–432.

Fong, P., Illsely, N. P., Widdicombe, J. H., and Verkman, A. S., 1988, Chloride transport in apical membrane vesicles from bovine tracheal epithelium: Characterization using fluorescent indicator, *J. Membrane Biol.* **104:**233–239.

Gervasi, P. G., Longo, V., Naldi, F., Panattoni, G., and Ursino, F., 1991, Xenobiotic-metabolizing enzymes in human respiratory nasal mucosa, *Biochem. Pharmacol.* **41**(2):177–184.

Gray, T. E., Thomassen, D. G., Mass, M. J., Barrett, J. C., 1983, Quantitation of cell proliferation, colony formation, and carcinogen induced cytotoxicity of rat tracheal epithelial cells grown in culture on 3T3 feeder layers, *In Vitro* **19:**559–570.

Hersey, S. J., and Jackson, R. T., 1987, Effect of bile salts on nasal permeability *in vitro*, *J. Pharm. Sci.* **76:**876–879.

Higaki, K., Kato, M., Hashida, M., and Sezaki, H., 1988, Enhanced membrane permeability to phenol red by medium-chain glycerides: Studies on the membrane permeability and microviscosity, *Pharm. Res.* **5:**309–312.

Holbrook, P. A., Irwin, W. J., Livingstone, C. R., and Dey, M., 1991, A study of the proteolytic activity in sheep nasal mucosa, *Proc. Int. Symp. Controlled Release Bioact. Mater.* **18:**285–286.

Iseki, K., Sugawara, M., Saitoh, H., Miyazaki, K., and Arita, T., 1988, Effect of chlorpromazine on the permeability of β-lactam antibiotics across rat intestinal brush border membrane vesicles, *J. Pharm. Pharmacol.* **40:**701–705.

Jonsson, K., Alfredsson, K., Soderberg-Ahlm, C., Critchley, H., Broeders, A., and Ohlin, M., 1992, Evaluation of the degradation of desamino^1,D-arginine^8-vasopressin by nasal mucosa, *Acta Endocrinol.* **127:**27–32.

Kajii, H., Horie, T., Hayashi, M., and Awazu, S., 1985, Fluorescence study on the interaction of salicylate with rat small intestinal epithelial cells: Possible mechanism for the promoting effects of salicylate on drug absorption *in vivo*, *Life Sci.* **37:**523–530.

Kajii, H., Horie, T., Hayashi, M., and Awazu, S., 1986, Effects of salicylate acid on the permeability of the plasma membrane of the small intestine of the rat: A fluorescence spectroscopic approach to elucidate the mechanism of promoted drug absorption, *J. Pharm. Sci.* **75:**475–478.

Kashi, S. D., and Lee, V. H. L., 1986, Enkephalin hydrolysis in homogenates of various absorptive mucosa of the albino rabbit: Similarities in rates and involvement of aminopeptidases, *Life Sci.* **38:**2019–2028.

Koefoed-Johnsen, V., Levi, H., and Ussing, H. H., 1952, The modes of passage of chloride ions through the isolated frog skin, *Acta Physiol. Scand.* **25:**150–163.

Lackowicz, J. R., 1983, *Principles of Fluorescence Spectroscopy*, Plenum Press, New York.

Laker, M. F., Bull, H. J., and Menzies, I. S., 1982, Evaluation of mannitol for use as a probe marker of gastrointestinal permeability in man, *Eur. J. Clin. Invest.* **12:**485–491.

Langridge-Smith, J. E., Field, M., and Dubinsky, W. P., 1983, Isolation of transporting plasma membrane vesicles from bovine tracheal epithelium, *Biochim. Biophys. Acta* **731:**318–328.

LeCluyse, E. L., Appel, L. E., and Sutton, S. C., 1991, Relationship between drug absorption enhancing activity and membrane perturbing effects of acylcarnitine, *Pharm. Res.* **8:**84–87.

Lee, T. C., Wu, R., Brody, A. R., Barrett, J. C., and Nettesheim, P., 1984, Growth and differentiation of hamster tracheal epithelial cells in culture, *Exp. Lung Res.* **6:**27–45.

Martinek, G. J., Berger, L., and Brioda, D., 1964, Simplified estimation of leucine aminopeptidase [LAP] activity, *Clin. Chem.* **10:**1087.

Matuszewska, B., Liversidge, G. G., Ryan, F., Dent, J., and Smith, P. L., 1988, *In vitro* study of intestinal absorption and metabolism of 8-L-arginine vasopressin and its analogues, *Int. J. Pharm.* **46:**1110–1120.

Morimoto, K., Yamaguchi, H., Iwakura, Y., Miyazaki, M., Nakatani, E., Iwamoto, T., Ohashi, Y., and Nakai, Y., 1991, Effects of proteolytic enzyme inhibitors on the nasal absorption of vasopressin and an analogue, *Pharm. Res.* **8:**1175–1179.

Reardon, P. R., 1992, *In Vitro* Intranasal Study: Effects of Ammonium Glycyrrhizinate on Nasal Mucosal Properties, dissertation, University of Kansas, Pharmaceutical Chemistry Dept.

Reardon, P. R., and Audus, K. L., 1993, Ammonium glycyrrhizinate (AMGZ) effects on membrane integrity, *Int. J. Pharm.* **94:**161–170.

Reardon, P. R., Gochoco, C. H., Audus, K. L., Wilson, G., and Smith, P. L, 1993, *In vitro* nasal transport across ovine mucosa: Effects of ammonium glycyrrhizinate on electrical properties and permeability of growth hormone releasing peptide, mannitol, and lucifer yellow, *Pharm. Res.* **10:**553–561.

Sklar, L. A., 1984, Fluorescence polarization studies of membrane fluidity: Where do we go from here?, in: *Biomembranes* (K. Morris and L. A. Manson, eds.), Plenum Press, New York, pp. 99–127.

Smith, P. L., Mirabelli, C., Fondacaro, J., Ryan, F., and Dent, J., 1988, Intestinal 5-fluorouracil absorption: Use of Ussing chambers to assess transport and metabolism, *Pharm. Res.* **5:**598–603.

Stratford, R. E., and Lee, V. H. L., 1986, Aminopeptidase activity in homogenates of various absorptive mucosae in the albino rabbit: Implications in peptide delivery, *Int. J. Pharm.* **30:**73–82.

Weiser, M. M., 1973, Intestinal epithelial cell surface membrane glycoprotein synthesis, *J. Biol. Chem.* **248:**2536–2541.

Wheatley, M. A., Dent, J., Wheeldon, E. B., and Smith, P. L., 1988, Nasal drug delivery: An *in vitro* characterization of transepithelial electrical properties and fluxes in the presence or absence of enhancers, *J. Controlled Release* **8:**167–177.

Chapter 17

Models for Investigation of Peptide and Protein Transport across Cultured Mammalian Respiratory Epithelial Barriers

Kwang-Jin Kim and Edward D. Crandall

1. INTRODUCTION

In this chapter, we describe *in vitro* methods that can be used for the investigation of peptide and protein transport across respiratory epithelial barriers. We begin with the approaches for culture of alveolar epithelial and tracheo(bronchial) epithelial cells, followed by experimental methods to investigate transport and metabolism utilizing the cultured cells. Where appropriate, advantages and disadvantages of the approaches utilized are discussed.

The airspaces of the lung are continuously lined with epithelial cells. There are some 25 bifurcating generations starting from the upper tracheal region down to the terminal air saccules of the alveolar region. The total surface area offered by these epithelial cells is >100 m² in humans, with the alveolar epithelial surface area occupying greater than 90% of the total area (Scothorne, 1987). The respiratory epithelial barrier is thought to restrict the leak of water and solutes into the airspaces from the surrounding sea of fluid in the interstitial and vascular spaces (Taylor and Gaar, 1970; Crandall and Kim, 1991). This understanding is primarily based on data

Kwang-Jin Kim • Departments of Medicine, Physiology and Biophysics, and Biomedical Engineering, Schools of Medicine and Engineering, University of Southern California, Los Angeles, California 90033. *Edward D. Crandall* • Departments of Medicine and Pathology, School of Medicine, University of Southern California, Los Angeles, California 90033.

Models for Assessing Drug Absorption and Metabolism, Ronald T. Borchardt *et al.*, eds., Plenum Press, New York, 1996.

from experiments on whole lungs *in situ* or isolated perfused lungs. For example, intratracheal instillation of test solutes followed by sampling from the vascular space (e.g., perfusate or blood) has been used extensively to assess permeability properties of the respiratory epithelial tract. Equivalent pore characteristics of the respiratory epithelial barrier as a whole indicate heteroporous properties, with a majority of smaller pores (radius about 0.5 nm) and a few larger pores (4–8 nm) having been reported by a number of investigators (Taylor and Gaar, 1970; Theodore *et al.*, 1975; Berg *et al.*, 1989; McLaughlin *et al.*, 1993).

Unfortunately, information specific to each respiratory epithelial barrier (i.e., alveolar and airway epithelium) is difficult to obtain using the whole lung approach. This has led to the need for models of alveolar or airway epithelium, such as the utilization of purified epithelial cells (Brown *et al.*, 1985), the development of cultured confluent monolayers of specific epithelial cell types present in the lungs (Mason *et al.*, 1982; Coleman *et al.*, 1984; Van Scott *et al.*, 1986, 1987, 1988, 1990; Adler *et al.*, 1987, 1990a,b; Boucher *et al.*, 1987; Cott *et al.*, 1987; Boucher and Larsen, 1988; Whitcutt *et al.*, 1988; Cheek *et al.*, 1989a,b; Gruenert *et al.*, 1990; Jefferson *et al.*, 1990; Kawada *et al.*, 1990; Tournier *et al.*, 1990; Kondo *et al.*, 1991, 1993; Beckmann *et al.*, 1992; Van Scott and Paradiso, 1992; Robison *et al.*, 1993), and the use of isolated tissue [e.g., excised tracheal epithelium (Olver *et al.*, 1975; Knowles *et al.*, 1982, 1991; Boucher and Gatzy, 1983; Cotton *et al.*, 1983; Jarnigan *et al.*, 1983; Nathanson *et al.*, 1983; Vulliemin *et al.*, 1983; Langridge-Smith *et al.*, 1984; Corrales *et al.*, 1986; Langridge-Smith, 1986; Olver and Robinson, 1986; Yankaskas *et al.*, 1987; Croxton, 1993; Smith and Welsh, 1993; Croxton *et al.*, 1994; Smith *et al.*, 1994; Steel *et al.*, 1994) and bronchial epithelium (Boucher *et al.*, 1987; Ballard and Gatzy, 1991a,b; Ballard *et al.*, 1992; Ballard and Taylor, 1994)] or isolated amphibian lungs (Crandall and Kim, 1981; Kim and Crandall, 1983, 1985, 1988; Kim, 1990). Recently, primary cultures of tracheobronchial epithelial cells and alveolar epithelial cells have been successfully developed and used for the acquisition of information pertinent to transport, metabolism, and other cellular functions (e.g., gene regulation) (Olsen *et al.*, 1992). A review on primary culture techniques for obtaining mammalian type II pneumocytes and the approaches for utilization of alveolar epithelial cells in primary culture has appeared elsewhere (Dobbs, 1990). The advantages of utilizing cultured epithelial cell monolayers as opposed to using entire organs or tissues are numerous. Of these, the most important advantage may be the ability to investigate in isolation epithelial barrier properties arising from a specific cell type (e.g., alveolar epithelial cell monolayers).

2. METHODS AND MATERIALS

Animal surgery and lavage are performed on a clean work bench, and all cell isolation procedures are conducted in a laminar flow hood at room temperature, unless indicated otherwise. All solutions are sterilized by filtration through 0.22-μm filters in the hood.

2.1. Primary Culture of Alveolar Epithelial Cells

2.1.1. BACKGROUND

There are about 40 different cell types in the mammalian lung, with alveolar epithelial cells representing about 20% of total lung cells (Scothorne, 1987). Alveolar epithelium is lined by type I and type II cells. Type I pneumocytes cover >95% of the surface area of alveolar airspaces, although the number of type I cells is half that of type II cells in adult mammalian lung (Weibel *et al.*, 1976; Scothorne, 1987; Haies *et al.*, 1981; Crapo *et al.*, 1982).

The morphology of type I cells exhibits protuberant nuclei with very thine (~0.2 μm) cytoplasmic extensions (Weibel *et al.*, 1976), which may serve as a short diffusion path for efficient gas exchange. Type II pneumocytes are located at the corners of alveolar airspaces, are cuboidal in shape, have numerous microvilli on their apical aspect, and possess lamellar bodies (which are thought to be the storage sites for pulmonary surfactant). The cell volume and surface area of type II cells are about 40% and 1.7% of the corresponding values (1800 μm^3 and 5100 μm^2 for human) for type I cells (Crapo *et al.*, 1982; Haies *et al.*, 1981). Compared to type II cells, type I pneumocytes have fewer mitochondria, smaller Golgi complexes, and more numerous pinocytotic vesicles (Gil *et al.*, 1971). Finally, type II pneumocytes are widely believed to be progenitor cells for type I cells following injury to the adult alveolar epithelium (Adamson and Bowden, 1975; Evans *et al.*, 1975; Evans and Shami, 1989; Schneeberger and Lynch, 1994).

2.1.2. SOLUTIONS

Phosphate-buffered saline (PBS) is made by adding 0.385 g of Na_2HPO_4 (monohydrate), 9.65 g of NaH_2PO_4 (pentahydrate), and 8.5 g NaCl to 1 l of MilliQ (Millipore, Boston, MA) water and titrating to pH 7.2. Tris-buffered solution (50 mM TBS) is made by adding 6.079 g of Trizma base to 100 ml of MilliQ water and titrating to pH 9.5. Solution-A (SOL-A, pH 7.4 at 25°C) consists of NaCl (136 mM), KCl (5.3 mM), Na_2HPO_4 (7.2 mM) *N*-2-hydroxyethylpiperazine-*N'*-2-ethanesulfonic acid (HEPES; 10 mM), and glucose (5.6 mM). SOL-B is the same as SOL-A, except for the presence of $CaCl_2$ (1.9 mM) and $MgSO_4$ (1.3 mM). Sterilized SOL-A and -B are stored at 4°C for up to 2 weeks. Immediately before use, 10 mg of gentamicin is added to SOL-A and -B (500 ml each). SOL-C is made fresh by adding 120 U of porcine pancreatic elastase (Worthington, Freehold, NJ) to 60 ml of SOL-B (37°C). SOL-D is made by dissolving 0.1 g of bovine serum albumin, 10 mg of soybean trypsin inhibitor, and 5.84 mg of EDTA in 10 ml of SOL-A. SOL-E contains 10 mg of DNase (Sigma, St. Louis, MO) in 10 ml of SOL-A.

Earle's minimum essential medium (EMEM, Sigma, St. Louis, MO) is further supplemented to yield S-EMEM by adding 1 ml of 200 mM L-glutamine, 1 ml of 10,000 U sodium penicillin G, 1 ml of 10-mg/ml streptomycin, and 1 ml of 1 M HEPES to 100 ml of EMEM. A completely defined, serum-free culture medium (MDSF) consists of 500 ml of DME-F12 (1:1 mixture, Sigma, St. Louis, MO) supplemented with 0.625 g of bovine serum albumin (Collaborative Research, Bedford, MA), 5 ml of 1 M HEPES, 0.5 ml of 100 mM nonessential amino acids (Sigma, St. Louis, MO), 5 ml of 200 mM L-glutamine, 5 ml of 10,000 U sodium penicillin G, and 5 ml of 10-mg/ml streptomycin.

2.1.3. PREPARATION OF IgG PLATES

Rat IgG (Sigma, St. Louis, MO) is dissolved in TBS at 0.5 mg/ml and added to plastic petri dishes (100-mm bacteriologic plates, Becton Dickinson Labware, Franklin Lakes, NJ) at 5 ml/dish. IgG solution is allowed to coat the dish for 3 hr at room temperature, followed by storage at 4°C for up to 4 weeks until use. Prior to use, the IgG plates are washed gently with PBS five times and with S-EMEM once.

2.1.4. ANIMAL SURGERY

For alveolar epithelial cell culture, lungs of small rodents [e.g., mouse (Massey *et al.*, 1987), guinea pig (Sikpi *et al.*, 1986), hamster (Pfleger, 1977), rabbit (Finkelstein and Shapiro, 1982; Lazo *et al.*, 1984)], large animals [e.g., cow (Augustin-Voss *et al.*, 1989)], and resected human lung lobes (Robinson *et al.*, 1984) have been utilized. However, the majority of work on alveolar epithelial cell culture by us and other investigators has utilized rat lungs. Rats (male, specific pathogen-free, weighing about 125–150 g) are anesthetized with 25–50 mg of sodium pentobarbital administered intraperitoneally and weighed. The anesthetized animal is placed on a small animal surgery board, and 300 U of heparin sodium is injected intraperitoneally. A midline incision is made to open the abdominal and chest cavities of the animal. The thymus is removed and the trachea cannulated with a blunted 18-gauge needle, followed by ventilation of the lungs with a tidal volume of 7 ml at a rate of 40 strokes/min. The lungs are perfused with SOL-B at a pressure of 20 cm H_2O) via a polyethylene (PE-90) cannula in the pulmonary artery. After the lungs blanch, ventilation is stopped, and the lungs lavaged with 10 ml of SOL-A 10 times through the tracheal cannula. Lavaged lungs with their tracheal cannula closed by a stopcock are removed from the chest cavity and placed into a beaker containing SOL-A (prewarmed to 37°C). From this point on, the cell isolation procedures are carried out in a laminar flow hood.

2.1.5. ISOLATION OF PNEUMOCYTES

The isolation of pneumocytes has been described in detail by Dobbs (1990) and Cheek et al. (1989a,b). Isolated rat lungs are inflated to near total lung capacity (~10 ml) with SOL-A and drained by gravity. This procedure of filling/draining is repeated 6 times to remove as many macrophages as possible. The lavaged lungs are then filled with 10 ml of SOL-C, placed into a beaker containing SOL-B (~150 ml), and incubated in a shaking water bath for 20 min. Because of leaking of SOL-C, an additional 5–10 ml of SOL-C is intratracheally delivered to the lungs during the 20-min incubation. After elastase treatment, each lung is put into a 50-ml conical centrifuge tube, cut into three pieces [large airways (e.g., trachea and main-stem bronchi) discarded], and incubated with 5 ml of SOL-D to inhibit elastase. The pieces of lung are then minced on a McIlwain tissue chopper (Brinkmann, Westbury, NY) to attain smaller pieces (<1 mm^3). These small blocks of tissue are collected into a plastic flask containing 2 ml of SOL-D and 5 ml of SOL-E, triturated three times using a 10-ml plastic pipet to further dissociate the tissue blocks into isolated cells, and finally agitated rapidly in a shaking water bath at 37°C for 2 min.

2.1.6. PURIFICATION OF TYPE II PNEUMOCYTES

The procedures for purification of type II pneumocytes have been described by Dobbs et al. (1986) and Kim et al. (1992). The crude cell mixtures are passed through a series of filters [100-, 70-, and 35-μm Nitex (Tetko, Elmsford, NY) meshes, pre-sterilized by autoclaving]. The filtered cells are centrifuged at $100 \times g$ for 10 min at room temperature, and the cell pellet is resuspended in S-EMEM. An aliquot is counted using a hemacytometer to obtain cell viability (by trypan blue exclusion) and total cell yield at this stage. The crude cell suspension is adjusted to yield about 2×10^6 cells/ml and poured onto the IgG plates at 10 ml/plate. Macrophages in the crude cell mixture are allowed to bind to IgG at 37°C for 60 min in a 5% CO_2 incubator. The incubated cell mixtures are gently panned with back-and-forth movement 3 times, followed by removal of the unattached cells with a plastic pipet. These partially purified cells are centrifuged at $100 \times g$ for 10 min at room temperature. The cell pellet is resuspended in MDSF, and an aliquot counted. The final cell concentration is adjusted to 2×10^6 cells/ml. At this stage, >90% of isolated cells represent type II pneumocytes with a viability greater than 95%.

2.1.7. CULTURE OF ALVEOLAR EPITHELIAL CELL MONOLAYERS

The procedures for the primary culture of alveolar epithelial cell monolayers have been reported elsewhere (Mason et al., 1985; Cheek et al., 1989a,b; Kim et al., 1990, 1992; Borok et al., 1994). We routinely culture rat alveolar epithelial cell monolayers on tissue culture-treated polycarbonate filter membranes (6-, 12-, and 24-mm Transwells, CoStar-Corning, Cambridge, MA) at 0.5×10^6 to 1.5×10^6 cells/cm^2. The day of plating cells is designated as day 0 (d0). The volumes for the top and bottom sides of the filter are adjusted to yield slightly positive ($\sim$ 2 mm H$_2$O) hydrostatic pressure on the top side of the Transwell filter membrane during the first 2–3 days in culture to help cells attach to the membrane. Typically, cultured mono-layers are fed on d3 with fresh culture medium (e.g., MDSF). For long-term cultures, these monolayers are fed every other day. Bioelectric properties (see Section 4.1) of the monolayers are monitored (before feeding) daily.

Cell plating efficiency as a function of time is determined using Hoechst 33528 fluorochrome for DNA assay (Cesarone *et al.*, 1979). Freshly isolated cells are centrifuged at $100 \times g$ for 10 min, and the resultant cell pellet is stored at $-20°C$. On a predesignated culture day (e.g., d0, d1, d2, d5, d8, and d11), cells are washed once with PBS and stored frozen at $-20°C$. Before assay, cell lysate is obtained by the freeze-thawing method (West *et al.*, 1985), where cells are thawed in MilliQ water, followed by freezing at $-80°C$, and thawed again. A fluorochrome stock solution is made by adding Hoechst 33258 (2 μg/ml or 1.5 μM) to SSC [0.154 M NaCl and 15 mM sodium citrate (pH 7.0, room temperature)]. To measure cell DNA, 200 μl of cell lysate is mixed with 1.8 ml of SSC and 1 ml of fluorochrome stock solution by inversion, followed by monitoring of the fluorescence of the sample (3 ml in a disposable plastic cuvette) at excitation and emission wavelengths of 350 and 455 nm, respectively. Quantitation of DNA contents of cell lysate samples is based on a standard curve similarly generated using 0–10 μg of calf thymus or salmon sperm DNA.

2.2. Primary Culture of Airway Epithelial Cells

2.2.1. BACKGROUND

Airway epithelium, which actively transports ions vectorially between the air-spaces and the albuminal spaces, is lined continuously with epithelial cells, including surface epithelial cells, goblet cells, and basal cells (St. George *et al.*, 1988). Excised trachea from mammalian lungs, especially the membranous posterior portion of the upper trachea, has been widely used for studies of ion (e.g., Na$^+$, Cl$^-$, and K$^+$) and solute (e.g., mannitol, albumin) transport properties (Olver *et al.*, 1975; Welsh *et al.*, 1982; Bhalla and Crocker, 1986; Johnson *et al.*, 1989; Webber and Widdicombe, 1989; Deffebach *et al.*, 1990; Webber *et al.*, 1991; Egan *et al.*, 1992; Kitano *et al.*, 1992; Price *et al.*, 1990, 1993). For example, excised canine upper trachea under short-circuit conditions has been shown to primarily secrete Cl$^-$ actively with water following passively (Olver *et al.*, 1975), while tracheas of other species have been reported to actively absorb Na$^+$ (with a lesser degree of Cl$^-$ secretion). Recently, culture models for mixed cell populations and for surface epithelial cells and goblet cells separately have been developed (Wu and Smith, 1982; Welsh, 1985, 1986; Widdicombe, 1986, 1990; Widdicombe *et al.*, 1985, 1987; Zeitlin *et al.*, 1989a,b; Culp *et al.*, 1992; Yamaya *et al.*, 1991a,b, 1992, 1993; Cozens *et al.*, 1991, 1992, 1994; Yankaskas and Boucher, 1990; Yankaskas *et al.*, 1993; Smith *et al.*, 1994). We will describe the airway cell culture procedures for mixed (i.e., surface, goblet, and basal epithelial) cell populations, which may be a better model for determining drug delivery properties of the airway epithelial barrier.

Airway epithelial cell cultures described herein have been reported to contain three populations of cell types normally present in the upper airway *in vivo* in approximately the same proportions. Those who are interested in characterization of mucin secretion in particular should consult other reports (Adler *et al.*, 1990a,b; Yamaya *et al.*, 1991a,b, 1992, 1993; Zeitlin *et al.*, 1989a,b) dealing with primary cultures of submucosal glandular cells. For the purpose of characterizing systemic drug delivery via upper airways, the tracheobronchial airway epithelial cell monolayer is satisfactory, in that the model provides a unique opportunity to dissect information pertinent to the upper airway epithelial tract alone.

2.2.2. SOLUTIONS

Ca^{2+}- and Mg^{2+}-free Hanks' balanced salt solution (HBSS) is obtained from Gibco BRL (Grand Island, NY). Protease solution (PRON) is made by adding 0.2 g of type XIV pronase (Sigma, St. Louis, MO) to 100 ml of Ca^{2+}-free MEM (S-MEM, Sigma, St. Louis, MO). To stop the pronase reaction and to prevent cell clumping, DNS solution is used, which contains 10 ml of fetal bovine serum (FBS) and 0.1 g of DNase I (type IV, Sigma, St. Louis, MO) in 100 ml of S-MEM. Separately, 10 ml of FBS is added to 90 ml of S-MEM and designated as FS-MEM. Complete culture medium (CCM) is made by adding 1 ml of 200 mM L-glutamine, 1 ml of 10,000 U/ml penicillin G, 1 ml of 10-mg/ml streptomycin, and 1 ml of 5-mg/ml gentamicin to 100 ml of serum-free, defined medium (PC-1, Hycor Biomedical, Portland, OR). CCM is further supplemented (1:100) with attachment factor solution supplied by the manufacturer with the PC-1 solution.

2.2.3. ANIMAL SURGERY

For tracheobronchial cell culture, airways of a number of species have been utilized, including small rodents [e.g., mouse (Massey *et al.*, 1987), rabbit (Wu and Smith, 1982; Van Scott *et al.*, 1987, 1990; Van Scott and Paradiso, 1992; Zeitlin *et al.*, 1989a), guinea pig (Adler *et al.*, 1987; Robison *et al.*, 1993)], cat (Culp *et al.*, 1992), dog (Widdicombe *et al.*, 1981; Widdicombe, 1990; Coleman *et al.*, 1984; Welsh, 1985, 1986; Widdicombe *et al.*, 1987; Boucher and Larsen, 1988; Kondo *et al.*, 1991;

Mochizuki *et al.*, 1994), cow (Beckmann *et al.*, 1992; Kondo *et al.*, 1993), and human (Widdicombe *et al.*, 1985; Boucher *et al.*, 1987; Tournier *et al.*, 1990; Yamaya *et al.*, 1991a,b, 1992, 1993). In this subsection, we describe the approach to obtaining airway cells of rabbits and guinea pigs. Either male New Zealand white rabbits (2.5 to 3 kg, Irish Farms, Los Angeles, CA) or male, specific pathogen-free Hartley guinea pigs [Crl:(HA)BR, 250 to 300 g, Charles River, Wilmington, MA] are euthanized with Eutha-6 (0.5 mg/kg) via the marginal ear vein or with sodium pentobarbital (0.3 g/kg) intraperitoneally, respectively. After opening of the thorax via a midline incision, the airways between the larynx and lobar bronchi are excised under sterile conditions. Surrounding connective tissue is carefully removed by blunt dissection. This tracheo-bronchial segment is cut open longitudinally, transferred to a petri dish containing ice-cold HBSS, and washed once with fresh, ice-cold HBSS.

2.2.4. ISOLATION OF TRACHEOCYTES

Wu and Smith (1982), Kondo *et al.* (1991, 1993), and Robison *et al.* (1993) have described various approaches to the isolation of tracheocytes. Washed airway tissue is cut into smaller pieces and treated with 10 ml PRON at 37°C in a 5% CO_2 incubator for 90 min. The epithelial layer is then gently scraped off with a sterile scalpel blade (size 10 to 15), and the isolated cells are immediately transferred to 10 ml of DNS which has been preequilibrated with 5% CO_2 at 37°C. The cell suspension in DNS is triturated 15 times using a sterile, 5-ml plastic pipet and centrifuged at room tempera-ture for 5 min at $250 \times g$. The cell pellet is resuspended in 10 ml of preequilibrated (37°C, 5% CO_2) FS-MEM and centrifuged again at the same setting. The cell pellet is again resuspended in FS-MEM, filtered through a cell strainer (40 µm, Becton Dickinson Labware, Franklin Lakes, NJ), collected into a 50-ml centrifuge tube, and pelleted a third time at the same setting. This final cell pellet is resuspended in CCM and an aliquot counted using a hemacytometer for assessment of cell number and viability (e.g., by trypan blue dye exclusion). The concentration of these isolated cells is adjusted to 2.9×10^6 cells/ml for plating onto filter membranes.

2.2.5. MONOLAYER CULTURE OF ISOLATED TRACHEOBRONCHIAL
EPITHELIAL CELLS

The confluent monolayer culture of isolated tracheobronchial epithelial cells has been recently described (Robison *et al.*, 1993; Robison and Kim, 1994, 1995). Isolated tracheocytes are plated at $\sim 10^6$ cells/cm^2 onto collagen-treated Transwell filters (Costar-Corning). After 24 hr, the bathing fluids of the cultured airway epithelial cells are replenished with fresh, preequilibrated CCM. The order of removing culture fluids from the filter is first from the basolateral compartment, followed by the apical compartment. Addition of fresh fluid is in the reverse order (i.e., apical first, followed by basolateral compartment). By this feeding procedure, the cells on filters are not facing hydrostatic pressure from the basolateral side. From d1 on, cells on filters are fed every other day using the same procedure. Tracheocytes cultured in this fashion develop confluency by d3 in primary culture.

3. AIR-INTERFACE CULTURE

It has been recently reported that culturing of tracheocytes in an air-interface on their apical aspect led to polarized differentiation of groups of cells with formation of pseudostratified ciliated columnar epithelium that is similar in structure and function to those observed *in vivo* (Adler *et al.*, 1987; Whitcutt *et al.*, 1988; Adler *et al.*, 1990a,b; Robison *et al.*, 1993). For example, tracheocytes cultured in an air interface were reported to contain approximately the same proportion of ciliated surface epithelial cells, basal cells, and goblet cells, whereas those cultured under liquid-covered conditions showed more surface epithelial cells. Apparently, airway epithelial cells cultured in an air-interface may consume more oxygen than those cultured under liquid-covered conditions (Adler *et al.*, 1990a,b), which may play an important role in the development of a well-differentiated airway epithelial barrier in primary culture. For culture in an air interface, conventional liquid-covered culture of tracheocytes is performed as described above. On d1, the bottom and top fluids are removed, and only the bottom compartment is filled with enough fresh CCM to wet the filter bottom (i.e., no hydrostatic pressure across the cell monolayer).

For air-interface culture of alveolar epithelial cells, a similar schedule of removing the bathing fluids can be employed. Our preliminary studies indicate that serum (10%, newborn bovine) helps maintain air-interface cultures of alveolar epithelial cell monolayers. We were able to obtain functional (i.e., exhibiting substantial potential difference and monolayer resistance) cell monolayers or rat pneumocytes cultured in both conventional liquid-covered and air-interface conditions for up to 60 days (Kim and Crandall, unpublished data).

4. APPLICATIONS TO ABSORPTION/METABOLISM

4.1. Bioelectric Measurements

4.1.1. SCREENING OF MONOLAYER ELECTRICAL PARAMETERS (E.G., PD AND R)

From d1 on, cultured cells on filters can be screened for their electrical resistance and potential difference using a MilliCell ERS (Millipore, Bedford, MA) or EVOM device (WPI, Sarasota, FL). Potential difference (PD) across the cell monolayer is measured in millivolts (with the apical bath as reference), and transmonolayer resistance (R) in kilohm-square centimeters. PD reflects the magnitude of active ion transport (see below, I_{eq}) occurring through the epithelial cells, and R reflects the tightness (i.e., resistance to diffusional flow of ions primarily through paracellular pathways) of the epithelial cell monolayer. Possible modulation of PD and R by a drug of interest can be monitored during the entire period of transport studies by this procedure.

Typically, rat alveolar epithelial cell monolayers (cultured with MDSF) exhibit about 6 mV and 1.3 kΩ·cm^2 by d5 (Borok *et al.*, 1994). When cultured in the presence of 10% newborn bovine serum (NBS) in MDSF or EMEM, rat alveolar epithelial cell monolayers develop PD and R up to about 20 mV and 3.5 kΩ·cm^2 by d3–d4 in culture. When alveolar epithelial cells are grown in an air interface, R and PD are maintained at ~60% of the corresponding parameters found with the monolayers cultured under liquid-covered conditions (Kim and Crandall, unpublished results).

Confluent tracheocyte monolayers develop resistance in excess of 1 kΩ·cm^2 by d3 in primary culture. PD and R reach a maximum by d3–d4. Resistance of guinea pig tracheocyte monolayers cultured in an air interface is lower (1.2 kΩ·cm^2) than that of liquid-covered monolayers (1.6 kΩ·cm^2) on d3 in culture. PD, on the other hand, is higher in air-interface cultures than that found for liquid-covered monolayers (Robison *et al.*, 1993). Mochizuki *et al.* (1994) reported PD of 10 mV and R of about 0.5 kΩ·cm^2 for canine tracheal epithelial cells in an air interface under serum-free conditions. In the presence of 5–15% serum, tracheobronchial epithelial cells (of human and other species) grown under liquid-covered conditions were reported to exhibit PD and R of about 10–30 mV and 0.2–0.8 kΩ·cm^2 at d3–d4 in culture (Zeitlin *et al.*, 1989a,b; Widdicombe *et al.*, 1987; Widdicombe, 1990; Kondo *et al.*, 1991, 1993; Yamaya *et al.*, 1992; Boucher, 1994a,b).

4.1.2. ESTIMATION OF ACTIVE ION TRANSPORT (I_{eq})

One of the important aspects of pulmonary epithelial barriers is their ability to actively transport salts into/out of airspaces. For example, rat alveolar epithelial cell monolayers have been confirmed to have an active ion transport (mostly Na$^+$ absorption) rate of about 4–6 μA/cm^2 in studies utilizing Ussing chamber techniques. By contrast, excised tracheal epithelium of a number of species demonstrate I_{eq} values in the range from 20 to 50 μA/cm^2 (Durand *et al.*, 1986; Graham *et al.*, 1992, 1993; Croxton, 1993; McBride *et al.*, 1993; Boucher, 1994a,b; Croxton *et al.*, 1994; Steel *et al.*, 1994), and cultured monolayers of tracheocytes and bronchial epithelial cells show I_{eq} ranging from 10 to 60 μA/cm^2 (Widdicombe *et al.*, 1981, 1985; Widdicombe, 1986; Widdicombe *et al.*, 1987; Yamaya *et al.*, 1992; Boucher, 1994a,b). Since I_{eq} reflects the functionality (e.g., absorption/secretion of salts from/into the lumen) of an epithelial barrier, the change in I_{eq} following instillation of test drug (for transport studies) serves as a useful monitor/index. For example, decreased I_{eq} may suggest interference by the drug with the active ion transport machinery of the epithelium, which may lead to altered fluid transport across the epithelial barrier(s) lining the airspaces.

4.2. Flux Measurements of Peptides and Proteins

Successful systemic delivery of drugs (especially for peptides and proteins) via the respiratory tract appears feasible (Debs *et al.*, 1988; Hubbard *et al.*, 1989; Smith *et al.*, 1989; Adjei and Garren, 1990; Niven *et al.*, 1990; Patton *et al.*, 1990; Colthorpe *et al.*, 1992; Folkesson *et al.*, 1992; Hoover *et al.*, 1992; Okumura *et al.*, 1992; Sakr, 1992), although the exact sites of passage, mechanisms of transport, and possible cellular metabolism of proteins/peptides are not well understood. Reviews on pulmonary drug delivery have recently been published (Lee, 1991; Patton and Platz, 1992). In this and the next subsection, we describe the approach to study the flux and metabolism of peptides and protein drugs by utilizing airway and alveolar epithelial cell monolayers.

Estimation of unidirectional solute (e.g., peptide and protein drugs) fluxes occurring across cultured epithelial cell monolayers can be performed in two different ways. One of these involves using the cells on filters in the culture plate as a mini-Ussing chamber system and studying solute flux under open-circuit conditions (Morimoto *et al.*, 1993, 1994; Yamahara *et al.*, 1994a,b). The other, more flexible (but time-consuming) approach entails using filters mounted in Ussing type flux chambers (Kim *et al.*, 1985; Cheek *et al.*, 1989a,b; Kim *et al.*, 1992). The advantage of this latter approach is the capability of imposing known (e.g., zero) electrical gradients across the monolayer (i.e., short-circuiting) for transport studies of charged solutes (which include most peptide/protein drugs).

For screening of drug absorption via airway/alveolar epithelial cell monolayers, a drug of interest is instilled into the apical fluid. The drug can be used without labeling or appropriately labeled with radioactivity (^{125}I, ^{35}S, ^{3}H, or ^{14}C) or fluorochrome [e.g., fluorescein isothiocyanate (FITC)]. High-performance liquid chromatography (HPLC) or standard radiotrace/fluorescent measurement techniques are employed to estimate the cumulative appearance (Q, mol) of drug in the receiver compartment. Flux (J, $mol \cdot sec^{-1} \cdot cm^{-2}$) is estimated from the drug appearance rate (dQ/dt, mol/sec) in downstream (i.e., receiver) fluid, which occurs through the nominal surface area (S, cm^2) of the monolayer. In mathematical terms, $J = (dQ/dt)/S$, where dQ/dt can be estimated from the steady-state appearance rate of the solute in the receiver fluid. If one knows the specific activity (i.e., the concentration expressed in moles per milliliter, S_{pa}) of the drug in the donor (i.e., upstream) compartment at time $t = 0$ (i.e., the onset of the flux measurement), the apparent permeability coefficient (P_{app}, cm/sec) of the drug can be estimated from the relation $J = P_{app} S_{pa}$ (Kim and Crandall, 1983). Estimation and interpretation of P_{app} for peptide and protein drugs can be complex, since these drugs may be subject to cellular metabolism as they transit the epithelial cells (Morimoto *et al.*, 1993, 1994; Yamahara *et al.*, 1994a,b).

4.3. Metabolism of Peptides and Proteins

The presence of metabolites (i.e., fragmented peptides/amino acids) of the parent peptide/protein in the bathing fluids of the cell monolayers used in flux measurements can be taken to indicate that cells are metabolizing the protein/peptide. The use of relatively pure radiolabeled proteins/peptides is essential to quantify cell metabolism of solutes (Morimoto *et al.*, 1994; Yamahara *et al.*, 1994a,b). HPLC of the bathing fluids and the cell lysates may be used for this purpose. As for HPLC cell lysates, interference from the detergent [e.g., sodium dodecyl sulfate (SDS), Triton X-100] may be minimized by pretreatment of cell lysate samples with detergent-removing agents (e.g., Extracti-Gel, Pierce, Rockford, IL). Utilizing similar approaches for analyses of metabolites in bathing fluids, Yamahara *et al.* (1994a) recently investigated the contribution of peptidase activity to arginine vasopressin (AVP) metabolism during transit across rat alveolar epithelial cell monolayers. These authors reported that the apical presence of aminopeptidase inhibitor (e.g., FOY305) resulted in an increase in the fraction of intact AVP translocated across the rat alveolar epithelial cell monolayer in the apical-to-basolateral direction.

Once the involvement of certain species of peptidases/proteases is suspected, biochemical measurements of the rate of peptide/protein metabolism of a known substrate for these enzymes can be performed. For this purpose, a known substrate for the suspected peptidase/protease is put into either bathing fluid of the cell monolayers, and the activity of the peptidase/proteinase enzyme is measured. One caution would be the use of a substrate large enough so that the substrate itself is not transported across the cell monolayer or transported into the cell. One possible approach to render the substrate large enough would be conjugating the substrate to an inert substance (e.g., bead). If, however, the information on the polarized locale of the enzyme is not critical, the substrate can be added at equal concentrations to both bathing fluids, followed by determination of enzymatic activity.

4.4. Further Considerations

Information specific to each respiratory epithelial barrier (e.g., alveolar versus airway epithelium) is difficult to obtain using the whole lung approach. This problem can be alleviated by using primary cultures of tracheobronchial epithelial cells and alveolar epithelial cells for the acquisition of specific information pertinent to transport, metabolism, and other cellular functions (e.g., gene regulation). The advantages of utilizing cultured epithelial cell monolayers (as opposed to the use of whole organs or intact tissues) are numerous. Of these, the most important may be the ability to investigate in isolation epithelial barrier properties arising from a specific cell type, enabling characterization of transport properties of various (e.g., upper airway, bronchial, bronchiolar, and alveolar epithelial) regions of the respiratory epithelial tract in relation to overall systemic drug delivery via the pulmonary route. Furthermore, the composition (e.g., concentration of drugs and other constituents) and colligative properties (e.g., osmolarity, pH) of fluid compartments can be easily controlled in these experiments as opposed to *in vivo/in situ* and other *ex vivo* experiments performed with whole lungs. As a corollary to this, with cells cultured in defined, serum-free medium, one can assess the effects of a humoral factor or a combination of such factors by simply adding the factor(s) of choice to the culture medium either from the onset of primary culture or acutely at a predesignated time. One such example is an investigation of the effect of epidermal growth factor (EGF) on alveolar epithelial cell monolayer barrier properties (Borok *et al.*, 1994), where EGF was seen to increase PD and R by about 50% (with a half-time of about 16 hr). As compared to isolated tissues (e.g., excised tracheal strip or tubular preparation of upper airways), cultured tracheocyte monolayers offer the epithelial barrier free of interference from underlying lymphoid tissue, nerve cells, and vasculature. Lastly, edge effects inevitably encountered in mounting isolated tissues in Ussing type flux chambers can be reduced or eliminated with cells cultured in filter cups, since no direct mechanical pressure is exerted on the cells themselves.

Cells (e.g., macrophages) resident in the airspaces of the lung or those (e.g., fibroblasts) that are a constituent of lung interstitium have been implicated in regulating a wide range of epithelial cell properties, which may include attachment, spreading, differentiation, and perhaps transport properties (Shannon *et al.*, 1987; Rannels and Rannels, 1989; Kawada *et al.*, 1990; Sannes, 1991; Tanswell *et al.*, 1991). The influence of cytoactive materials (e.g., cytokines) secreted and/or absorbed by the macrophages or fibroblasts on respiratory epithelial cells can be studied with a co-culture system. For example, macrophages can be added to the apical side of the cell monolayer, and the epithelial PD and R can be monitored to elucidate the effect of macrophage-elaborated factors and/or cell–cell interactions (e.g., adhesion of macrophages to the alveolar epithelial cells) on alveolar epithelial barrier properties. This particular arrangement may be useful to assess the contribution of macrophage uptake of drugs to the transport of drugs into normal and stimulated macrophages across the epithelial barrier. The effect of agents that are thought to inhibit/stimulate the uptake of drugs by macrophages on overall drug delivery across the epithelial barrier can also be tested using this approach. Another useful model is co-culture of respiratory epithelial cells with fibroblasts in the basolateral compartment (Mangum *et al.*, 1990; Liu *et al.*, 1993). This can be accomplished, for example, by growing fibroblasts on the bottom side of the filter. Direct addition of fibroblasts into the apical compartment, where the respiratory epithelial cells are located, is not recommended, because the fibroblasts will take over growth/spreading of the epithelial cells there. Using a co-culture system of epithelial cells in the top compartment and fibroblasts in the bottom compartment, epithelial–fibroblast interactions may be dissected.

Although methods for isolating type I cells from rat lungs have been reported (Weller and Karnovsky, 1986), the purity of cells is low (50–70%) and specific identification of type I pneumocytes is not yet definitive. More importantly, the viability and growth of type I cells in primary cell culture have not been demonstrated. Strategies for successful isolation of viable type I cells remain to be developed. On the other hand, alveolar type II epithelial cells (when cultured on tissue culture-treated substrate) exhibit cell morphology with protuberant nuclei and thin cytoplasmic extensions starting about d3 in culture. Morphometric analysis of cultured cells (e.g., mean arithmetic thickness, mean cell surface area, cell volume) as a function of cell culture age indicate that the cells cultured for >3 days on tissue culture-treated polycarbonate filters exhibit the morphological characteristics of type I cells *in vivo* (Cheek *et al.*, 1989a,b). We have recently reported that these tight monolayers of rat pneumocytes react with rat type I cell-specific monoclonal antibody from d3–d4 onward (Danto *et al.*, 1992). This reactivity is maintained throughout a prolonged experimental period (up to 60 days, unpublished data), suggesting that type II cells cultured on tissue culture-treated polycarbonate filters may be on the continuum of cells differentiating toward a type I cell phenotype. Other data available to date, including lectin binding properties (Dobbs *et al.*, 1985) and reactivity with other type I cell-specific markers (Danto *et al.*, 1992; Dobbs *et al.*, 1988; Christensen *et al.*, 1993; Albanese *et al.*, 1993), are consistent with the likelihood that type II cells may differentiate toward type I-like cells in primary culture. However, further delineation of cell phenotypic properties in primary culture requires development of additional cell-type-specific probes and/or a viable type I cell monolayer preparation.

Direct correlation of data obtained in the *in vitro* setting with those found in *in situ/in vivo* lungs is difficult due to the complex anatomy of the mammalian lungs. Data available to date indicate that the distal respiratory tract of various mammalian species (including human) possesses transport processes for actively removing Na^+ (and thus water by osmosis), confirming results obtained utilizing the tight monolayer model of rat alveolar epithelial cells (Goodman *et al.*, 1987; Berg *et al.*, 1989; McLaughlin *et al.*, 1993). Importantly, active Na^+ transport across the alveolar epithelium is regulable by several agents (e.g., beta-agonists) (Berg *et al.*, 1989; Kim *et al.*, 1992), findings evident in both intact whole lung and monolayer experiments. Investigations of transport of peptide and protein drugs via the respiratory tract are still at a relatively early stage, and correlations between *in vitro* and intact models remain to be determined. As for the upper airway epithelial tract, active Cl^- secretion and Na^+ absorption have been shown in a number of airway culture models and intact tissue under short-circuit conditions (Steel *et al.*, 1994; Olver *et al.*, 1975; Boucher, 1994a,b). Similar observations were reported earlier for excised tracheal preparations of sheep lungs (Olver *et al.*, 1975). Paradoxically, however, under open-circuit conditions, net Na^+ absorption (but not appreciable Cl^- secretion) is evident in excised airway epithelium of almost all species.

ACKNOWLEDGMENTS

This work was supported in part by research grants (HL38578, HL38621, and HL38658) from the National Institutes of Health and a grant-in-aid (92-604) from the American Heart Association. The authors thank Drs. Vincent H. L. Lee, Claus-Michael Lehr, Yasuhisa Matsukawa, Kazuhiro Morimoto, Timothy W. Robison, and Hiroshi Yamahara for insights and contributions to the ongoing research in the authors' laboratories. Dr. Crandall is Hastings Professor of Medicine.

REFERENCES

Adamson, I. Y. R., and Bowden, D. H., 1975, Derivation of type I epithelium from type 2 cells in the developing rat lung, *Lab. Invest.* **32:**736–746.

Adjei, A., and Garren, J., 1990, Pulmonary delivery of peptide drugs: Effect of particle size on bioavailability of leuprolide acetate in healthy male volunteers, *Pharm. Res.* **7:**565–569.

Adler, K. B., Shwartz, J. E., Whitcutt, M. J., and Wu, R., 1987, A new chamber system for maintaining differentiated guinea pig respiratory epithelial cells between air and liquid phases, *BioTechniques* **5:**462–465.

Adler, K. B., Cheng, P. W., and Kim, K. C., 1990a, Characterization of guinea pig tracheal epithelial cells maintained in biphasic organotypic culture: Cellular composition and biochemical analysis of released glycoconjugates, *Am. J. Respir. Cell Mol. Biol.* **2:**145–154.

Adler, K. B., Holden-Stauffer, W. J., and Repine, J. E., 1990b, Oxygen metabolites stimulate release of high-molecular weight glycoconjugates by cell and organ cultures of rodent-respiratory epithelium via an arachidonic acid-dependent mechanism, *J. Clin. Invest.* **85:**75–85.

Albanese, S., Rishi, A. K., Williams, M. C., and Brody, J. S., 1993, Regulation of T1alpha, a novel rat lung type I alveolar cell gene (abstract), *Am. Rev. Respir. Dis.* **147:**A466.

Augustin-Voss, H. G., Schoon, H. A., Stockhoefe, N., and Ueberschar, S., 1989, Isolation of bovine type II pneumocytes in high yield and purity, *Lung* **167:**1–10.

Ballard, S. T., and Gatzy, J. T., 1991a, Alveolar transepithelial potential difference and ion transport in adult rat lung, *J. Appl. Physiol.* **70:**63–69.

Ballard, S. T., and Gatzy, J. T., 1991b, Volume flow across the alveolar epithelium of adult rat lung, *J. Appl. Physiol.* **70:**1665–1676.

Ballard, S. T., and Taylor, A. E., 1994, Bioelectric properties of proximal bronchiolar epithelium, *Am. J. Physiol.* **267:**L79–L84.

Ballard, S. T., Schepens, S. M., Falcone, J. C., Meininger, G. A., and Taylor, A. E., 1992, Regional bioelectric properties of porcine airway epithelium, *J. Appl. Physiol.* **73:**2021–2027.

Beckmann, J. D., Takizawa, H., Romberger, D., Illig, M., Claassen, L., Rickard, K., and Rennard, S., 1992, Serum-free culture of fractionated bovine bronchial epithelial cells, *In Vitro Cell. Dev. Biol.* **28A:** 39–46.

Berg, M. M., Kim, K. J., Lubman, R. L., and Crandall, E. D., 1989, Hydrophilic solute transport across rat alveolar epithelium, *J. Appl. Physiol.* **66:**2320–2327.

Bhalla, D. K., and Crocker, T. T., 1986, Tracheal permeability in rats exposed to ozone. An electron microscopic and autoradiographic analysis of the transport pathway, *Am. Rev. Respir. Dis.* **134:** 572–579.

Borok, Z., Danto, S. I., Zabski, S. M., and Crandall, E. D., 1994, Defined medium for primary culture *de novo* of adult rat alveolar epithelial cells, *In Vitro Cell. Dev. Biol.* **30A:**99–104.

Boucher, R. C., 1994a, Human airway ion transport. Part one, *Am. Rev. Respir. Cell Mol. Biol.* **150:**271–281.

Boucher, R. C., 1994b, Human airway ion transport. Part two, *Am. Rev. Respir. Cell Mol. Biol.* **150:** 581–593.

Boucher, R. C., and Gatzy, J. T., 1983, Characteristics of sodium transport by excised rabbit trachea, *J. Appl. Physiol.* **55:**1877–1883.

Boucher, R. C., and Larsen, E. H., 1988, Comparison of ion transport by cultured secretory and absorptive canine airway epithelia, *Am. J. Physiol.* **254:**C535–C547.

Boucher, R. C., Stutts, M. J., and Gatzy, J. T., 1981, Regional differences in bioelectric properties and ion flow in excised canine airways, *J. Appl. Physiol.* **51:**706–714.

Boucher, R. C., Yankaskas, J. R., Cotton, C. U., Knowles, M. R., and Stutts, M. J., 1987, Cell culture approaches to the investigation of human airway ion transport, *Eur. J. Respir. Dis.* **153:**59–67.

Brown, S. E. S., Kim, K. J., Goodman, B. E., Wells, J. R., and Crandall, E. D., 1985, Sodium–amino acid cotransport by type II alveolar epithelial cells, *J. Appl. Physiol.* **59:**1616–1622.

Cesarone, C. F., Bolognesi, C., and Santi, L., 1979, Improved microfluorometric DNA determination in biological material using 33258 Hoechst, *Anal. Biochem.* **100:**188–197.

Cheek, J. M., Evans, M. J., and Crandall, E. D., 1989a, Type I cell-like morphology in tight alveolar epithelial monolayers, *Exp. Cell Res.* **184:**375–387.

Cheek, J. M., Kim, K. J., and Crandall, E. D., 1989b, Tight monolayers of rat alveolar epithelial cells: Bioelectric properties and active sodium transport, *Am. J. Physiol.* **256:**C688–C693.

Christensen, P. J., Kim, S., Simon, R. H., Toews, G. B., and Paine, R., 1993, Differentiation-related expression of ICAM-1 by rat alveolar epithelial cells, *Am. J. Respir. Cell Mol. Biol.* **8:**9–15.

Coleman, D. L., Tuet, I. K., and Widdicombe, J. H., 1984, Electrical properties of dog tracheal epithelial cells grown in monolayer culture, *Am. J. Physiol.* **246:**C355–C359.

Colthorpe, P., Farr, S. J., Taylor, G., Smith, I., and Wyatt, D., 1992, The pharmacokinetics of pulmonary-delivered insulin: A comparison of intratracheal and aerosol administration to the rabbit, *Pharm. Res.* **9:**764–768.

Corrales, R. J., Coleman, D. L., Jacoby, D. B., Leikauf, G. D., Hahn, H. L., Nadel, J. A., and Widdicombe, J. H., 1986, Ion transport across cat and ferret tracheal epithelia, *J. Appl. Physiol.* **61:**1065–1070.

Cott, G. R., Walker, S. R., and Mason, R. J., 1987, The effect of substratum and serum on the lipid synthesis and morphology of alveolar type II cells *in vitro*, *Exp. Lung Res.* **13:**427–447.

Cotton, C. U., Lawson, E. E., Boucher, R. C., and Gatzy, J. T., 1983, Bioelectric properties and ion transport of airways excised from adult and fetal sheep, *J. Appl. Physiol.* **55:**1542–1549.

Cozens, A. L., Yezzi, M. J., Chin, L., Simon, E. M., Friend, D. S., and Gruenert, D. C., 1991, Chloride ion transport in transformed normal and cystic fibrosis epithelial cells, *Adv. Exp. Med. Biol.* **290:**187–196.

Cozens, A. L., Yezzi, M. J., Yamaya, M., Steiger, D., Wagner, J. A., Garber, S. S., Chin, L., Simon, E. M., Cutting, G. R., Gardner, P., Friend, D. S., Basbaum, C. B., and Gruenert, D. C., 1992, A transformed human epithelial cell line that retains tight junctions post crisis, *In Vitro Cell. Dev. Biol.* **28A:**735–744.

Cozens, A. L., Yezzi, M. J., Kunzelmann, K., Ohrui, T., Chin, L., Eng, K., Finkbeiner, W. E., Widdicombe, J. H., and Gruenert, D. C., 1994, CFTR expression and chloride secretion in polarized immortal human bronchial epithelial cells, *Am. J. Respir. Cell Mol. Biol.* **10:**38–47.

Crandall, E. D., and Kim, K.-J., 1981, Transport of water and solutes across bullfrog alveolar epithelium, *J. Appl. Physiol.* **50:**1263–1271.

Crandall, E. D., and Kim, K. J., 1991, Alveolar epithelial barrier properties, in: *The Lung: Scientific Foundations*, Vol. 1 (R. G. Crystal, P. Barnes, and J. B. West, eds.), Raven Press, New York, pp. 273–287.

Crapo, J. D., Barry, B. E., Gehr, P., Bachofen, M., and Weibel, E. R., 1982, Cell numbers and characteristics of the normal human lung, *Am. Rev. Respir. Dis.* **125:**332–337.

Croxton, T. L., 1993, Electrophysiological properties of guinea pig tracheal epithelium determined by cable analysis, *Am. J. Physiol.* **265:**L38–L44.

Croxton, T. L., Takahashi, M., and Hirshman, C. A., 1994, Decreased ion transport by tracheal epithelium of the basenji-greyhound dog, *J. Appl. Physiol.* **76:**1489–1993.

Culp, D. J., Lee, D. K., Penney, D. P., and Marin, M. G., 1992, Cat tracheal gland cells in primary culture, *Am. J. Physiol.* **263:**L264–L275.

Danto, S. I., Zabski, S. M., and Crandall, E. D., 1992, Reactivity of alveolar epithelial cells in primary culture with type I cell monoclonal antibodies, *Am. J. Respir. Cell Mol. Biol.* **6:**296–306.

Debs, R. J., Fuchs, H. J., Philips, R., Montgomery, A. B., Brunette, E. N., Liggitt, D., Patton, J. S., and Shellito, J. E., 1988, Lung-specific delivery of cytokines induces sustained pulmonary and systemic immunomodulation in rats, *J. Immunol.* **140:**3482–3488.

Deffebach, M. E., Islami, H., Price, A., and Webber, S. E., 1990, Prostaglandins alter methacholine-induced secretion in ferret *in vitro* trachea, *Am. J. Physiol.* **258:**L75–L80.

Dobbs, L. G., 1990, Isolation and culture of alveolar type II cells, *Am. J. Physiol.* **258:**L134–L147.

Dobbs, L. G., Williams, M. C., and Brandt, A. E., 1985, Changes in biochemical characteristics and pattern of lectin binding of alveolar type II cells with time in culture, *Biochim. Biophys. Acta* **846:**155–166.

Dobbs, L. G., Gonzalez, R., and Williams, M. C., 1986, An improved method for isolating type II cells in high yield and purity, *Am. Rev. Respir. Dis.* **134:**1'41–145.

Dobbs, L. G., Williams, M. C., and Gonzalez, R., 1988, Monoclonal antibodies specific to apical surface of rat alveolar type I cells bind to surfaces of cultured, but not freshly isolated type II cells, *Biochim. Biophys. Acta* **970:**146–156.

Durand, J., Durand-Arczynska, W., and Schoenenweid, F., 1986, Oxygen consumption and active sodium and chloride transport in bovine tracheal epithelium, *J. Physiol.* **372:**51–62.

Egan, M. E., Wagner, M. H., Zeitlan, P. L., and Guggino, W. B., 1992, Modulation of ion transport in cultured rabbit tracheal epithelium by lipoxygenase metabolites, *Am. J. Respir. Cell Mol. Biol.* **7:** 500–506.

Evans, M. J., and Shami, S. G., 1989, Lung cell kinetics, in: *Lung Cell Biology* (D. Massaro, ed.), Marcel Dekker, New York, pp. 1–36.

Evans, M. J., Cabral, L. J., Stephens, R. L., and Freeman, G., 1975, Transformation of alveolar type II cells to type I cells following exposure to NO_2, *Exp. Mol. Pathol.* **22:**142–150.

Finkelstein, J. N., and Shapiro, D. L., 1982, Isolation of type II alveolar epithelial cells using low protease concentrations, *Lung* **160:**85–98.

Folkesson, H. G., Westroem, B. R., Dahlbaeck, M., Lundin, S., and Karlsson, B. W., 1992, Passage of aerosolized BSA and nonapeptide dDAVP via the respiratory tract in young and adult rats, *Exp. Lung Res.* **18:**595–614.

Gil, J., Silage, D. A., and McNiff, J. M., 1971, Distribution of vesicles in cells of air–blood barrier in the rabbit, *Am. J. Physiol.* **50:**334–340.

Goodman, B. E., Kim, K. J., and Crandall, E. D., 1987, Evidence for active sodium transport across alveolar epithelium of isolated rat lung, *Am. J. Physiol.* **62:**2460–2466.

Graham, A., Steel, D. M., Alton, E. W., and Geddes, D. M., 1992, Second-messenger regulation of sodium transport in mammalian airway epithelia, *J. Physiol.* **453:**475–491.

Graham, A., Steel, D. M., Wilson, R., Cole, P. J., Alton, E. W., and Geddes, D. M., 1993, Effects of purified *Pseudomonas* rhamnolipids on bioelectric properties of sheep tracheal epithelium, *Exp. Lung Res.* **19:**77–89.

Gruenert, D. C., Basbaum, C. B., and Widdicombe, J. H., 1990, Long-term culture of normal and cystic fibrosis epithelial cells grown under serum-free conditions, *In Vitro Cell. Dev. Biol.* **26:**411–418.

Haies, D. M., Gil, J., and Weibel, E. R., 1981, Morphometric study of rat lung cells. I. Numerical and dimensional characteristics of parenchymal cell population, *Am. Rev. Respir. Dis.* **123:**533–541.

Hoover, J. L., Rush, B. D., Wilkinson, K. F., Day, J. S., Burton, P. S., Vidmar, T. J., and Ruwart, M. J., 1992, Peptides are better absorbed from the lung than the gut in the rat, *Pharm. Res.* **9:**1103–1106.

Hubbard, R. C., Casolaro, M. A., Mitchell, M., Sellers, A., Arabia, F., Matthay, M. A., and Crystal, R. G., 1989, Fate of aerosolized recombinant DNA-produced $alpha_1$-antitrypsin: Use of the epithelial surface of the lower respiratory tract to administer proteins of therapeutic importance, *Proc. Natl. Acad. Sci. USA* **86:**680–684.

Jarnigan, F., Davis, J. D., Bromberg, P. A., Gatzy, J. T., and Boucher, R. C., 1983, Bioelectric properties and ion transport of excised rabbit trachea, *Am. J. Physiol.* **55**:1884–1892.

Jefferson, D. M., Valentich, J. D., Marini, F. C., Grubman, S. A., Iannuzzi, M. C., Dorkin, H. L., Li, M., Klinger, K. W., and Welsh, M. J., 1990, Expression of normal and cystic fibrosis phenotypes by continuous airway epithelial cell lines, *Am. J. Physiol.* **259**:L496–L505.

Johnson, L. G., Cheng, P. W., and Boucher, R. C., 1989, Albumin absorption by canine bronchial epithelium, *Am. J. Physiol.* **66**:2772–2777.

Kawada, H., Shannon, J. M., and Mason, R. J., 1990, Improved maintenance of adult rat alveolar type II cell differentiation *in vitro*: Effect of serum-free, hormonally-defined medium and a reconstituted basement membrane, *Am. J. Respir. Cell Mol. Biol.* **3**:33–43.

Kim, K.-J., 1990, Active Na$^+$ transport across *Xenopus* lung alveolar epithelium, *Respir. Physiol.* **81**: 29–40.

Kim, K.-J., and Crandall, E. D., 1983, Heteropore populations in alveolar epithelium, *J. Appl. Physiol.* **54**:140–146.

Kim, K.-J., and Crandall, E. D., 1988, Sodium-dependent lysine flux across bullfrog alveolar epithelium, *J. Appl. Physiol.* **65**:1655–1661.

Kim, K.-J., LeBon, T. R., Shinbane, J. S., and Crandall, E. D., 1985, Asymmetric [^{14}C]albumin transport across bullfrog alveolar epithelium, *J. Appl. Physiol.* **59**:1290–1297.

Kim, K.-J., Cheek, J. M., and Crandall, E. D., 1990, Contribution of Na$^+$ and Cl$^-$ fluxes to net ion transport by alveolar epithelium, *Respir. Physiol.* **85**:245–256.

Kim, K.-J., Suh, D. J., Lubman, R. L., Danto, S. I., Borok, Z., and Crandall, E. D., 1992, Studies on the mechanisms of active ion fluxes across alveolar epithelial cell monolayers, *J. Tissue Culture Methods* **14**:187–194.

Kitano, S., Wells, U. M., Webber, S. E., and Widdicombe, J. G., 1992, The effects of intraluminal and extraluminal drug application on secretion and smooth muscle tone in the ferret liquid-filled trachea *in vitro*, *Pulm. Pharmacol.* **5**:167–174.

Knowles, M. R., Buntin, W. H., Bromberg, P. A., Gatzy, J. T., and Boucher, R. C., 1982, Measurements of transepithelial electric potential differences in the trachea and bronchi of human subjects *in vivo*, *Am. Rev. Respir. Dis.* **126**:108–112.

Knowles, M. R., Clarke, L. L., and Boucher, R. C., 1991, Activation by extracellular nucleotides of chloride secretion in the airway epithelia of patients with cystic fibrosis, *N. Engl. J. Med.* **325**: 533–538.

Kondo, M., Finkbeiner, W. E., and Widdicombe, J. H., 1991, Simple technique for culture of highly differentiated cells from dog tracheal epithelium, *Am. J. Physiol.* **261**:L106–L117.

Kondo, M., Finkbeiner, W. D., and Widdicombe, J. H., 1993, Cultures of bovine tracheal epithelium with differentiated ultrastructure and ion transport, *In Vitro Cell. Dev. Biol.* **29A**:19–24.

Langridge-Smith, J. E., 1986, Interaction between sodium and chloride transport in bovine tracheal epithelium, *J. Physiol.* **376**:299–319.

Langridge-Smith, J. E., Rao, M. C., and Field, M., 1984, Chloride and sodium transport across bovine tracheal epithelium: Effects of secretagogues and indomethacin, *Pflügers Arch. Eur. J. Physiol.* **402**:42–47.

Lazo, J. S., Merrill, W. W., Pham, E. T., Lynch, T. J., McCallister, J. D., and Ingbar, D. H., 1984, Bleomycin hydrolase activity in pulmonary cells, *J. Pharmacol. Exp. Ther.* **231**:583–588.

Lee, V. H. L., 1991, *Peptide and Protein Drug Delivery*, Marcel Dekker, New York, pp. 1–56.

Liu, M., Xu, J., Tanswell, A. K., and Post, M., 1993, Stretch-induced growth-promoting activities stimulate fetal rat lung epithelial cell proliferation, *Exp. Lung Res.* **19**:505–517.

Mangum, J. B., Everitt, J. I., Bonner, J. C., Moore, L. R., and Brody, A. R., 1990, Co-culture of primary cells to model alveolar injury and translocation of proteins, *In Vitro Cell. Dev. Biol.* **26**:1135–1143.

Mason, R. J., Williams, M. C., Widdicombe, J. H., Sanders, M. J., Misfeldt, D. S., and Berry, L. C., 1982, Transepithelial transport by pulmonary alveolar type II cells in primary culture, *Proc. Natl. Acad. Sci. USA* **79**:6033–6037.

Mason, R. J., Walker, S. R., Shields, B. A., Henson, B. A., and Williams, M. C., 1985, Identification of rat alveolar type II epithelial cells with a tannic acid and polychrome stain, *Am. Rev. Respir. Dis.* **131:** 786–788.

Massey, T. E., Geddes, B. A., and Forkert, P. G., 1987, Isolation of nonciliated bronchiolar epithelial (Clara) cells and alveolar type II cells from mouse lungs, *Can. J. Physiol. Pharmacol.* **65:**2368–2372.

McBride, R. K., Stone, K. K., and Marin, M. G., 1993, Oxidant injury alters barrier function of ferret tracheal epithelium, *Am. J. Physiol.* **264:**L165–L174.

McLaughlin, G. E., Kim, K. J., Berg, M. M., Agoris, P., Lubman, R. L., and Crandall, E. D., 1993, Measurements of solute fluxes in isolated rat lungs, *Respir. Physiol.* **91:**321–334.

Mochizuki, H., Morikawa, A., Tokuyama, K., Kuroume, T., and Chao, A. C., 1994, The effect of non-steroidal anti-inflammatory drugs on the electrical properties of cultured dog tracheal epithelial cells, *Eur. J. Pharmacol.* **252:**183–188.

Morimoto, K., Yamahara, H., Lee, V. H. L., and Kim, K.-J., 1993, Dipeptide transport across rat alveolar epithelial cell monolayers, *Pharm. Res.* **10:**1668–1674.

Morimoto, K., Yamahara, H., Lee, V. H. L., and Kim, K. J., 1994, Thyrotropin-releasing hormone transport across rat alveolar epithelial cell monolayers, *Life Sci.* **54:**2083–2092.

Nathanson, I., Widdicombe, J. H., and Nadel, J. A., 1983, Effects of amphotericin B on ion and fluid movement across dog tracheal epithelium, *Am. J. Physiol.* **55:**1257–1261.

Niven, R. W., Rypacek, F., and Byron, P. R., 1990, Solute absorption from the airway of the isolated rat lung. II. Absorption of several peptidase-resistant, synthetic polypeptides: Poly-(2-hydroxyethyl)-aspart-amides, *Pharm. Res.* **7:**990–994.

Okumara, K., Iwakawa, S., Yoshida, T., Seki, T., and Komada, F., 1992, Intratracheal delivery of insulin: Absorption from solution and aerosol by rat lung, *Int. J. Pharm.* **88:**63–73.

Olsen, J. C., Johnson, L. G., Stutts, M. J., Sarkadi, B., Yankaskas, J. R., Swanstrom, R., and Boucher, R. C., 1992, Correction of the apical membrane chloride permeability defect in polarized cystic fibrosis airway epithelia following retroviral-mediated gene transfer, *Hum. Gene Ther.* **3:**253–266.

Olver, R. E., and Robinson, E. J., 1986, Sodium and chloride transport by the tracheal epithelium of fetal, new-born and adult sheep, *J. Physiol.* **375:**377–390.

Olver, R. E., Davis, B., Marin, M. G., and Nadel, J. A., 1975, Active transport of Na^+ and Cl^- across the canine tracheal epithelium *in vitro*, *Am. Rev. Respir. Dis.* **112:**811–815.

Patton, J. S., and Platz, R. M., 1992, Routes of delivery: Case study. Pulmonary delivery of peptides and proteins for systemic action, *Adv. Drug Deliv. Res.* **8:**179–196.

Patton, J. S., McCabe, J. G., Hansen, S. E., and Daugherty, A. L., 1990, Absorption of human growth hormone from the rat lung, *Biotech. Ther.* **1:**213–228.

Pfleger, R. C., 1977, Type II epithelial cells from the lungs of Syrian hamsters: Isolation and metabolism, *Exp. Mol. Pathol.* **27:**152–166.

Price, A. M., Webber, S. E., and Widdicombe, J. G., 1990, Transport of albumin by the rabbit trachea *in vitro*, *Am. J. Physiol.* **68:**726–730.

Price, A. M., Webber, S. E., and Widdicombe, J. G., 1993, Osmolality affects ion and water fluxes and secretion in the ferret trachea, *Am. J. Physiol.* **74:**2788–2794.

Rannels, D. E., and Rannels, S. R., 1989, Influence of the extracellular matrix on type II cell differentiation, *Chest* **96:**165–173.

Robinson, P. C., Voelker, D. R., and Mason, R. J., 1984, Isolation and culture of human alveolar type II epithelial cells: Characterization of their phospholipid secretion, *Am. Rev. Respir. Dis.* **130:**1156–1160.

Robison, T. W., and Kim, K. J., 1994, Air-interface cultures of guinea pig airway epithelial cells: Effects of active sodium and chloride transport inhibitors on bioelectric properties, *Exp. Lung Res.* **20:**101–117.

Robison, T. W., and Kim, K. J., 1995, Dual effect of nitrogen oxide on barrier properties of guinea pig tracheobronchial epithelial monolayers cultured in an air-interface, *J. Toxicol. Environ. Health* **44:** 57–71.

Robison, T. W., Dorio, R. G., and Kim, K. J., 1993, Tight airway epithelial cell monolayers cultured in an air-interface: Bioelectric properties, *BioTechniques* **15:**468–473.

Saha, P., Kim, K. J., Yamahara, H., Crandall, E. D., and Lee, V. H. L., 1994, Transport of beta-blockers across rat alveolar epithelial cell monolayers, *J. Controlled Release* **32**:191–200.

Sakr, F. M., 1992, A new approach for insulin delivery via the pulmonary route: Design and pharmacokinetics in non-diabetic rabbits, *Int. J. Pharm.* **86**:1–7.

Sannes, P. L., 1991, Structural and functional relationships between type II pneumocytes and components of extracellular matrices, *Exp. Lung Res.* **17**:639–659.

Schneeberger, E. E., and Lynch, R. D., 1994, Ultrastructure of the distal pulmonary epithelium, in: *Fluid and Solute Transport in the Airspaces of the Lungs* (Lung Biology in Health and Disease, Vol. 70, C. Lenfant, exec. ed.; R. M. Effros and H. K. Chang, ed.), Marcel Dekker, New York, pp. 1–25.

Scothorne, R. J., 1987, The respiratory system, in: *Cunningham's Textbook of Anatomy*, 12th ed. (G. J. Romanes, ed.), Oxford University Press, Oxford, pp. 491–529.

Shannon, J. M., Mason, R. J., and Jennings, S. D., 1987, Functional differentiation of alveolar type II epithelial cells *in vitro*: Effects of cell shape, cell–matrix interactions and cell–cell interactions, *Biochim. Biophys. Acta* **931**:143–156.

Sikpi, M. O., Nair, C. R., Johns, A. E., and Das, S. K., 1986, Metabolic and ultrastructural characterization of guinea pig alveolar type II cells isolated by centrifugal elutriation, *Biochim. Biophys. Acta* **877**: 20–30.

Smith, F. B., Kikkawa, Y., Diglio, C. A., and Dalen, R. C., 1980, The type II epithelial cells of the lung. VI. Incorporation of ^{3}H-choline and ^{3}H-palmitate into lipids of cultured type II cells, *Lab. Invest.* **42**: 296–301.

Smith, J. J., and Welsh, M. J., 1993, Fluid and electrolyte transport by cultured human airway epithelia, *J. Clin. Invest.* **91**:1590–1597.

Smith, J. J., Karp, P. H., and Welsh, M. J., 1994, Defective fluid transport by cystic fibrosis airway epithelia, *J. Clin. Invest.* **93**:1307–1311.

Smith, R. M., Traber, L. D., Traber, D. L., and Spragg, R. G., 1989, Pulmonary deposition and clearance of aerosolized alpha$_1$-proteinase inhibitor administered to dogs and sheep, *J. Clin. Invest.* **84**:1145–1154.

Steel, D. M., Graham, A., Geddes, D. M., and Alton, E. W., 1994, Characterization and comparison of ion transport across sheep and human airway epithelium, *Epithel. Cell Biol.* **3**:24–31.

St. George, J. A., Harkema, J. R., Hyde, D. M., and Plopper, C. G., 1988, Cell populations and structure–function relationships of cells in the airways, in: *Toxicology of the Lung* (D. E. Gardner, J. D. Crapo, and E. J. Massaro, eds.), Raven Press, New York, pp. 71–102.

Tanswell, K. A., Byrne, P. J., Han, R. N. N., Edelson, J. D., and Han, V. K., 1991, Limited division of low-density adult rat type II pneumocytes in serum-free culture, *Am. J. Physiol.* **260**:L395–L402.

Taylor, A. E., and Gaar, K. A., 1970, Estimation of equivalent pore radii of pulmonary capillary and alveolar membrane, *Am. J. Physiol.* **218**:1133–1140.

Theodore, J., Robin, E. D., Gaudio, R., and Acevedo, J., 1975, Transalveolar transport of large polar solutes (sucrose, inulin, and dextran), *Am. J. Physiol.* **229**:989–996.

Tournier, J. M., Merten, M., Meckler, Y., Hinnrasky, J., Fuchey, C., and Puchelle, E., 1990, Culture and characterization of human tracheal gland cells, *Am. Rev. Respir. Dis.* **141**:1280–1288.

Van Scott, M. R., and Paradiso, A. M., 1992, Intracellular Ca^{2+} and regulation of ion transport across rabbit Clara cells, *Am. J. Physiol.* **263**:L122–L127.

Van Scott, M. R., Yankaskas, J. R., and Boucher, R. C., 1986, Culture of airway epithelial cells: Research techniques, *Exp. Lung Res.* **11**:75–94.

Van Scott, M. R., Hester, S., and Boucher, R. C., 1987, Ion transport by rabbit nonciliated bronchiolar epithelial cells (Clara cells) in culture, *Proc. Natl. Acad. Sci. USA* **84**:5496–5500.

Van Scott, M. R., Lee, N. P., Yankaskas, J. R., and Boucher, R. C., 1988, Effect of hormones on growth and function of cultured canine tracheal epithelial cells, *Am. J. Physiol.* **255**:C237–C245.

Van Scott, M. R., McIntire, M. R., and Henke, D. C., 1990, Arachidonic acid metabolism and regulation of ion transport in rabbit Clara cells, *Am. J. Physiol.* **259**:L213–L221.

Vulliemin, P., Durand-Arczynska, W., and Durand, J., 1983, Electrical properties and electrolyte transport in bovine tracheal epithelium: Effects of ion substitutions, transport inhibitors and histamine, *Pflügers Arch. Eur. J. Physiol.* **396:**54–59.

Webber, S. E., and Widdicombe, J. G., 1989, The transport of albumin across the ferret *in vitro* whole trachea, *J. Physiol.* **408:**457–472.

Webber, S. E., Lim, J. C., and Widdicombe, J. G., 1991, The effects of calcitonin gene-related peptide on submucosal gland secretion and epithelial albumin transport in the ferret trachea *in vitro*, *Br. J. Pharmacol.* **102:**79–84.

Weibel, E. R., Gehr, P., Haies, D., Gil, J., and Bachofen, M., 1976, The cell population of the normal lung, in: *Lung Cells in Disease* (A. Bouhuys, ed.), Elsevier, Amsterdam, pp. 3–16.

Weller, N. K., and Karnovsky, M. J., 1986, Isolation of pulmonary alveolar type I cells from adult rats, *Am. J. Physiol.* **125:**448–456.

Welsh, M. J., 1985, Ion transport by primary cultures of canine tracheal epithelium: Methodology, morphology, and electrophysiology, *J. Membr. Biol.* **88:**149–163.

Welsh, M. J., 1986, Adrenergic regulation of ion transport by primary cultures of canine tracheal epithelium: Cellular electrophysiology, *J. Membr. Biol.* **91:**121–128.

Welsh, M. J., Smith, P. L., and Frizzell, R. A., 1982, Chloride secretion by canine tracheal epithelium: II. The cellular electrical potential profile, *J. Membr. Biol.* **70:**227–238.

West, D. C., Sattar, A., and Kumar, S., 1985, A simplified *in situ* solubilization procedure for the determination of DNA and cell number in tissue cultured mammalian cells, *Anal. Biochem.* **147:** 289–295.

Whitcutt, M. J., Adler, K. B., and Wu, R., 1988, A biphasic chamber system for maintaining polarity of differentiation of cultured respiratory tract epithelial cells, *In Vitro Cell Dev. Biol.* **24:**420–428.

Widdicombe, J. H., 1986, Ion transport by tracheal epithelial cells in culture, *Clin. Chest Med.* **7:**299–305.

Widdicombe, J. H., 1990, Use of cultured airway epithelial cells in studies of ion transport, *Am. J. Physiol.* **258:**L13–L18.

Widdicombe, J. H., Basbaum, C. B., and Highland, E., 1981, Ion contents and other properties of isolated cells from dog tracheal epithelium, *Am. J. Physiol.* **241:**C184–C192.

Widdicombe, J. H., Coleman, D. L., Finkbeiner, W. E., and Tuet, I. K., 1985, Electrical properties of monolayers cultured from cells of human tracheal mucosa, *J. Appl. Physiol.* **58:**1729–1735.

Widdicombe, J. H., Coleman, D. L., Finkbeiner, W. E., and Friend, D. S., 1987, Primary cultures of the dog's tracheal epithelium: Fine structure, fluid, and electrolyte transport, *Cell Tissue Res.* **247:**95–103.

Wu, R., and Smith, D., 1982, Continuous multiplication of rabbit tracheal epithelial cells in a defined, hormone-supplemented medium, *In Vitro* **18:**800–812.

Yamahara, H., Morimoto, K., Lee, V. H. L., and Kim, K. J., 1994a, Effects of protease inhibitors on vasopressin transport across rat alveolar epithelial cell monolayers, *Pharm. Res.* **11:**1619–1624.

Yamahara, H., Lehr, C. M., Lee, V. H. L., and Kim, K. J., 1994b, Fate of insulin during transit across the alveolar epithelial cell monolayers, *Eur. J. Pharm. Biopharm.* **40:**294–298.

Yamaya, M., Finkbeiner, W. E., and Widdicombe, J. H., 1991a, Ion transport by cultures of human tracheobronchial submucosal glands, *Am. J. Physiol.* **261:**L485–L490.

Yamaya, M., Finkbeiner, W. E., and Widdicombe, J. H., 1991b, Altered ion transport by tracheal glands in cystic fibrosis, *Am. J. Physiol.* **261:**L491–L494.

Yamaya, M., Finkbeiner, W. E., Chun, S. Y., and Widdicombe, J. H., 1992, Differentiated structure and function of cultures from human tracheal epithelium, *Am. J. Physiol.* **262:**L713–L724.

Yamaya, M., Ohrui, T., Finkbeiner, W. E., and Widdicombe, J. H., 1993, Calcium-dependent chloride secretion across cultures of human tracheal surface epithelium and glands, *Am. J. Physiol.* **265:**L170–L177.

Yankaskas, J. R., and Boucher, R. C., 1990, Transformation of airway epithelial cells with persistence of cystic fibrosis or normal ion transport phenotypes, *Methods Enzymol.* **192:**565–571.

Yankaskas, J. R., Gatzy, J. T., and Boucher, R. C., 1987, Effects of raised osmolarity on canine tracheal epithelial ion transport function, *Am. J. Physiol.* **62:**2241–2245.

Yankaskas, J. R., Haizlip, J. E., Conrad, M., Koval, D., Lazarowski, E., Paradiso, A. M., Rinehart, C. A., Jr., Sarkadi, B., Schlegel, R., and Boucher, R. C., 1993, Papilloma virus immortalized tracheal epithelial cells retain a well-differentiated phenotype, *Am. Rev. Respir. Dis.* **264:**C1219–C1230.

Zeitlin, P. L., Loughlin, G. M., and Guggino, W. B., 1989a, Ion transport in cultured fetal and adult rabbit tracheal epithelia, *Am. J. Physiol.* **254:**C691–C698.

Zeitlin, P. L., Wagner, M., Markakis, D., Loughlin, G. M., and Guggino, W. B., 1989b, Steroid hormones: Modulators of Na^+ absorption and Cl^- secretion in cultured tracheal epithelia, *Proc. Natl. Acad. Sci. USA* **86:**2502–2505.

Chapter 18

Drug Transport across *Xenopus* Alveolar Epithelium *in Vitro*

Doris Wall and Doreen Pierdomenico

1. INTRODUCTION

Biopharmaceutical polypeptides are usually relatively large, hydrophilic molecules with considerable susceptibility to hydrolase degradation and very low epithelial permeability. These features result in poor oral and transdermal absorption and limit most compounds presently on the market to injectable formulations. Recently, data illustrating relatively high bioavailability for polypeptides administered via the pulmonary route (Adjei and Gupta, 1994; Patton *et al.*, 1993; Wall, 1995) and the feasibility of generating small-particle aerosols of some of these molecules (Niven, 1993; Cipolla *et al.*, 1994) have increased interest in mechanisms of macromolecular transport across the lung epithelium. Although many polypeptides have much higher bioavailability in animals when administered by the pulmonary than by the oral route, this does not apply to all compounds, particularly those susceptible to proteolytic cleavage (Adjei and Gupta, 1994; Patton *et al.*, 1993; Wall, 1995). In addition, the time course of absorption across the lung is quite variable, with some small molecules (e.g., the cationic antibiotic pentamidine) having very little absorption compared to much larger compounds (Montgomery *et al.*, 1988). Systematic evaluation of the factors determining rate and extent of transport across pulmonary epithelium is needed to understand and predict when pulmonary delivery may be a successful approach to consider for drug molecules.

The pulmonary epithelial surface of mammals is relatively inaccessible due to

Doris Wall and Doreen Pierdomenico • Pharmaceutical Technologies, SmithKline Beecham Pharmaceuticals, King of Prussia, Pennsylvania 19406.

Models for Assessing Drug Absorption and Metabolism, Ronald T. Borchardt *et al.*, eds., Plenum Press, New York, 1996.

the anatomic complexity of the multiply branched airways of their lungs. This precludes mounting of this tissue in Ussing transport chambers, an approach that has allowed study of absorptive pathways across tissues such as gastrointestinal and nasal epithelia. Microscopic anatomy of the air–blood barrier is similar in frogs and mammals (Meban, 1973; Dierichs, 1975), but the simpler gross structure of amphibian lungs allows the organ to be spread as a flat sheet of tissue, enabling *in vitro* transport studies. This chapter describes procedures for establishing and characterizing an *in vitro* system to examine transport across lungs of the South African frog *Xenopus*, including examples of its use in analysis of amino acid and peptide transport mechanisms.

2. METHODS

2.1. Materials

Female South African clawed frogs were obtained from either Nasco (Fort Atkinson, WI) or Xenopus I (Ann Arbor, MI). Females are preferred to males because they are larger and their lung tissue is easier to mount. Although early studies of amphibian lung transport utilized even bigger bullfrogs, substitution of *Xenopus* allows use of laboratory-bred animals, which are easier to obtain at all times of year and avoids depleting natural amphibian populations.

Amiloride, ouabain, and unlabeled transport marker compounds were purchased from Sigma Chemical Co. (St, Louis, MO). Radiochemicals were obtained from New England Nuclear Research Products (Dupont Co., Wilmington, DE) or from the Department of Radiochemistry, SmithKline Beecham Pharmaceuticals (radiolabeled peptides). All other chemicals were reagent-grade materials obtained from standard suppliers.

Ussing chambers are modified for pulmonary transport studies by addition of soft neoprene rubber O-ring seals inside the tissue-mounting pins of chambers commonly used for studies of transport across tissues such as intestine (modified chambers obtained from Penn Century, Philadelphia, PA). The O-rings provide a better seal with this delicate tissue, reducing edge damage and allowing demonstration of higher transepithelial resistance. The chambers have an exposed surface area of 1.13 cm^2.

2.2. Tissue Preparation

Animals are anesthetized by either hypothermia (immersion in an ice-water bath) or by immersion in a cold anesthetic solution of 0.1% tricaine (3-aminobenzoic acid methyl ester, Sigma, St. Louis, MO). Lungs are exposed by a ventral incision and excised by severing the tracheoglottis. Each lung is filled with approximately 3 ml of Ringer solution (see below), and the organ is cut open to form a sheet. The luminal side is rinsed gently with Ringer solution before mounting in Ussing chambers, using gentle stretching to fit the lung over the pins which lie outside of the O-ring seal. Tissue is allowed to equilibrate for 30–45 min before radiolabeled compounds are added to begin transport studies.

Lung tissue is bathed on both sides with 10 ml of amphibian Ringer's solution, composed of 110 mM NaCl, 2.4 mM $KHCO_3$, 1 mM Ca-D-gluconate, 1 mM $MgSO_4$, and 10 mM *N*-2-hydroxyethylpiperazine-*N'*-2-ethanesulfonic acid (HEPES), pH 7.4 (Kim, 1990). Temperature of the solution is maintained at 20–22°C, and the reservoirs are gassed continuously with 100% O_2, which also serves to stir the reservoir fluid.

2.3. Electrical Parameters

Mounted tissues are continuously short-circuited with an automatic voltage clamp (JWT, Kansas City, KS). Transepithelial potential difference (PD) with reference to the mucosal bathing solution and short-circuit current (I_{sc}) are monitored throughout the course of experiments. Although resistance (R_t) levels determined from these data are usually maintained well during at least 4 hr of tissue incubation, initial values vary considerably, with normal mean values of 700–800 $\Omega \cdot cm^2$.

Short-circuit current also exhibits a range of initial values, from less than 5 to 30 $\mu A/cm^2$. Average values are usually 8–9 $\mu A/cm^2$ and are normally maintained for at least 5 hr. Short-circuit current across *Xenopus* lung is due primarily to Na^+ absorption (Fischer *et al.*, 1989; Kim, 1990). Measurement of I_{sc} provides a convenient, rapid way to monitor tissue viability at the end of an experiment by determining the effect of inhibitors of this process. Addition of amiloride to a final concentration of 10 μM on the alveolar side of the tissue causes a rapid drop in current, falling to 50% at 10 min after addition. Similarly, 100 μM ouabain on the pleural side of *Xenopus* lung tissue results in an even greater but more gradual drop in current, reducing I_{sc} to <5% of initial values by 2 hr after inhibitor addition.

2.4. Transport of Model Compounds

A major advantage of *in vitro* transport studies over *in vivo* absorption measurements is the ability to distinguish passive and active transport mechanisms through manipulation of experimental parameters such as composition of the medium, addition of inhibitors, and assessment of transport in both directions across tissues. Both measurement of electrical parameters (described above) and examination of the behavior of marker compounds with well-established transport mechanisms provide useful means of determining whether the mounted tissue is functioning normally.

Mannitol provides a small (182 Da), hydrophilic marker which crosses epithelial barriers by a passive, paracellular route. In *Xenopus* lung, mannitol is typically transported at a rate of 0.01–0.03 %/(hr·cm^2) in both the alveolar to pleural and the reverse direction, and the transport rate is unaffected by concentration within the range of 10 μM to 10 mM (Wall *et al.*, 1993). Higher rates of transport suggest loss of epithelial barrier patency. Addition of amiloride or ouabain has little effect on the transport rate of this compound, as expected for passively transported molecules.

Passive transcellular transport is characteristic of hydrophobic compounds capable of diffusing across the membrane bilayer of epithelial cells. An example is antipyrine, which is transported across *Xenopus* lung in both directions at rates of 1.5–4 %/(hr·cm^2), much faster than rates seen for hydrophilic compounds, even when the latter are utilizing a carrier-mediated mechanism. As expected for passively transported molecules, antipyrine flux is unaffected by concentration or addition of metabolic inhibitors of ion transport (Wall *et al.*, 1993).

Active absorption of amino acids across amphibian lung occurs in both bullfrog (Kim and Crandall, 1988) and *Xenopus* (Wall *et al.*, 1993). Flux is more rapid than in the case of mannitol, is greater in the alveolar to pleural direction [about 0.2 %/(hr·cm^2)], is partially inhibited by ouabain or by eliminating sodium from the bathing medium (Kim and Crandall, 1988, and data presented below), and saturates at increasing amino acid concentration (Kim and Crandall, 1988). In *Xenopus*, absorptive amino acid transport is more pronounced in tissues from some animals, with alveolar to pleural transport occurring at 4 to 20 times the rate of transport in the opposite direction. The reason for this experimental difference is not known.

2.5. Electron Microscopy

Comparison of the ultrastructural appearance of tissue mounted in Ussing chambers with unmounted control lung provides another means to assess the status of the experimental tissue and to directly visualize transport of large macromolecular tracers such as cationized ferritin. Normal morphology is maintained for at least 3 hr after mounting in Ussing chambers (Wall *et al.*, 1993).

Tissue mounted in Ussing chambers is fixed by immersion in 2% or 3% glutaraldehyde in 0.1 M sodium cacodylate, pH 7.4, after removal from the chambers. Unmounted whole lungs are fixed by filling with approximately 3 ml of cold glutaraldehyde solution, after which they are cut into pieces for rinsing and postfixation processing. After incubation for 1 hr on ice, lungs are cut into small pieces of approximately 2 mm^3, then rinsed with three changes of 0.1 M sodium cacodylate, pH 7.4. This is followed by postfixation with 1% osmium tetroxide in the same buffer for 1 hr at room temperature. The tissue is again rinsed with cacodylate buffer, dehydrated in ethanol, and embedded in PolyBed 812 (Polysciences, Fort Washington, PA). Grids are examined following staining with lead citrate and uranyl acetate.

3. EXPERIMENTAL PROTOCOLS

3.1. Transport Measurements

After mounted tissue has equilibrated for 30–45 min, radiolabeled tracer compounds are added to the appropriate chamber. In a typical experiment, 10 mM nonradioactive mannitol is added to both alveolar and pleural bathing solutions, with 5 μCi of [^{14}C]mannitol added to the medium on either the alveolar side of the lung, for alveolar to pleural transport studies (a–p), or to the pleural side, for pleural to alveolar (p–a) transport studies. Flux of a second tracer molecule can be studied in the same experiment by adding unlabeled compound at the same concentration on both sides and [^{3}H]-radiolabeled compound on the radioactive side. Addition of unlabeled material on both sides of the tissue prevents loss of small amounts of transported molecules by adsorption to the chamber walls. Transport is monitored for up to 5.5 hr by taking 100-μl samples from the donor (radioactive) side of the chamber at 0, 60, and 180 min, and at 300 min in longer experiments (these volumes are not replaced since they represent a small percent of the total chamber volume and their loss does not affect the results), and 1-ml samples from the transport (nonradioactive) side at 15 and 30 min and every 30 min there after for the duration of the experiment (these volumes are replaced with appropriate buffer solution to maintain a constant volume in the reservoir). The samples are mixed with 10 ml of ReadySafe scintillation fluid (Beckman Instruments, Inc., Fullerton, CA), and radioactivity is measured in a scintillation counter.

For concentration effect studies, the experiment is begun at the lowest concentration of compound (e.g., 10 μM mannitol), and samples are collected over 60 min to determine the transport rate at this concentration. Additional unlabeled compound is then added to both sides of the tissue (by adding a small amount of a concentrated solution) to raise the final concentration in the chambers to the next desired level (e.g., 100 μM mannitol), and samples are again collected to determine transport rate at this concentration. The process is repeated at 120 min to raise the concentration to the final level (e.g., 10 mM mannitol) and measure transport rates at this level.

3.2. Experimental Approaches to Distinguish Active from Passive Transport

Comparison of the rates of transport in both directions across the tissue often provides the first indication of active transport mechanisms, by demonstrating that a vectorial process exists. However, interpretation of such data can be complicated by metabolism of the parent compound to smaller metabolites. For example, studies of model peptide transport across rat alveolar epithelial cell monolayers are complicated by exopeptidases present on the alveolar epithelial cell surface, which hydrolyze dipeptides to amino acids that are transported across the tissue, probably via an amino acid carrier (Morimoto *et al.*, 1993). This phenomenon results in a much higher rate of absorptive flux of radioactivity across the tissue, presumably due to asymmetric distribution of aminopeptidase activity on the apical (alveolar) surface of the pulmonary epithelium and/or the vectorial nature of amino acid transport across alveolar epithelium. Since aminopeptidase activity is detectable on the alveolar side of mounted *Xenopus* lung also (unpublished data), the possibility that a similar phenomenon could occur in this system should be considered if the molecule being studied is susceptible to peptidase cleavage.

Energy dependence of active transport processes is most commonly demonstrated by addition of metabolic inhibitors of either ion transport or oxidative metabolism. Blockage of ion transport is a more satisfactory procedure in the *Xenopus* lung system, since it allows complete abolition of short-circuit current with relatively little change in permeability of the paracellular route (see below). Inhibition of oxidative metabolism in *Xenopus* lung with a combination of 2 mM sodium azide and 2 mM iodoacetamide also results in complete abolition of short-circuit current. However, these inhibitors also cause a marked increase in passive permeability of hydrophilic markers such as mannitol across the tissue, resulting in a rapid rise in passive background flux, which complicates interpretation of the experimental data.

Indirect evidence for active transport via a membrane-associated carrier or transporter can also be obtained by demonstrating that the rate of flux plateaus as the concentration of the compound in question rises or by competitive inhibition with a related, but not identical, compound. Provided the slower transport rate is not due to unrelated (e.g., cytotoxic effects) at the higher concentrations, the presence of a saturable carrier mechanism can be inferred and affinity of the carrier for the transported compound estimated. For example, total L-lysine flux decreases with increasing lysine concentration in bullfrog lung, with a K_t of 7.3 mM (Kim and Crandall, 1988). L-Leucine inhibited absorptive net flux of lysine, while α-methylaminoisobutyric acid did not (Kim and Crandall, 1988).

Another indication of specialized transport mechanisms for charged molecules is lack of effect of changes in transepithelial voltage on their permeability, as observed, for example, in the case of albumin transport across bullfrog lung *in vitro* (Kim *et al.*, 1985).

3.3. Determination of Tissue-Associated Radioactivity

In some cases, a compound will appear to disappear from the donor side of the chamber without an equivalent amount of material appearing in the opposite chamber, as the result of binding of the compound either to the tissue or to the walls of the apparatus itself. Assessment of tissue-associated activity can provide an indication of complications such as tissue binding or metabolism of the marker compound. Lung tissue is dissolved in 2–3 ml of 0.5 M KOH solution by heating overnight to 45°C in a shaking water bath. Samples (0.25–0.5 ml) are removed, mixed with an equal volume of 30% H_2O_2, neutralized with an equal volume of 0.5 M HCl, and mixed with 10 ml of ReadySafe scintillation fluid for determination of radioactivity.

3.4. Calculation of Data

Resistance values are calculated directly from experimental data by dividing PD in mV by $\mu A/cm^2$ and multiplying by 10^3 to give resistance in $\Omega \cdot cm^2$.

Transport data are plotted as percent transport/cm^2 versus time, and the rate of transport is determined from the slope of the best fit of data points obtained by linear regression, ignoring zero time points because of the 15-min lag period typically seen in these experiments.

4. APPLICATIONS TO STUDIES OF ABSORPTION MECHANISMS

Examination of leucine flux across *Xenopus* lung provides a good example of experimental evidence for an active transport mechanism. In the first study, 20 μM unlabeled leucine and 10 mM mannitol were added to both chambers, with 5 μCi of [^{3}H]leucine and [^{14}C]mannitol also added on the donor side (either alveolar or pleural, depending on the chamber). Time points were taken over 5.5 hr, and rates of transport of both the amino acid and mannitol were determined. As seen in Fig. 1, percent cumulative transport was highly asymmetric, with rates of 0.195 ± 0.02 %/(hr·cm^2) in the a–p direction and 0.042 ± 0.002 %/(hr·cm^2) in the p–a direction (n = 3 tissues for each direction). Mannitol transport rates in the same tissues were 0.016 0.004 %/(hr·cm^2) in the a–p direction and 0.012 0.001 %/(hr·cm^2) in the p–a direction.

To provide further evidence for an active transport mechanism, 100 μM ouabain was added to the pleural side of the tissue, and the effect on leucine transport monitored. As seen in Fig. 2, leucine transport rates were considerably reduced in the a–p direction within 60 min of ouabain addition, but leucine transport in the p–a direction and mannitol transport in both directions were unaffected by this inhibitor. Short-circuit current was gradually reduced to zero in the same tissues with no change in mannitol flux, indicating that ouabain was effective in inhibiting Na$^+$/K$^+$-ATPase activity with little effect on paracellular permeability. The aqueous solubility of leucine was too low to allow measurement of transport rates at much higher concentrations, precluding experiments to demonstrate saturation of the presumed carrier.

Partial reduction of a–p leucine transport in the presence of ouabain indicates that part of the total flux is dependent on active Na$^+$ transport. The rate of a–p transport in the presence of ouabain was reduced by 51% (calculated from the slopes

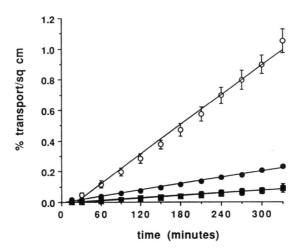

Figure 1.   Transport of leucine and mannitol across *Xenopus* lung. Cumulative transport of 20 μM leucine is much faster in the alveolar to pleural than in the reverse direction and remains linear over 5.5 hr. Mannitol (10 mM) flux across the same tissues is similar in both directions and always slower than that of leucine. (The symbols for a–p and p–a transport of mannitol are superimposed.) Transport in each direction was studied with tissues from three different animals. Correlation coefficients (R^2) determined by linear regression analysis ranged from 0.972 to 0.996.

before and after ouabain addition), bringing it to a similar level as the p–a flux. The uninhibited portion of the total flux may therefore represent the contribution of a passive component to the overall transport rate, most likely paracellular given the hydrophilicity and small size of these molecules. Inhibition of a portion of amino acid transport by ouabain indicates that maintenance of a Na^+ gradient at the basolateral membrane is essential for this transport process. Our data do not address whether this is a direct dependence due to Na^+–amino acid cotransport or an indirect dependence (i.e., a secondary active transport mechanism).

Passive transport of a growth hormone-releasing hexapeptide (ImAc-D-Trp-Ala-Trp-D-Phe-Lys-NH2; GHRP) occurs in the same tissue. As in the leucine transport experiments, 20 μM peptide and 10 mM mannitol were added to each side of the chamber, with 5 μCi of [³H]-GHRP and [¹⁴C]mannitol added to either the alveolar or the pleural side, as appropriate. Figure 3 shows that the percent cumulative transport of this peptide and of mannitol were similar in both directions: peptide flux was 0.022 ± 0.005 %/(hr·cm²) in the a–p direction and 0.031 ± 0.016 %/(hr·cm²) in the p–a direction, while mannitol transport rates in the same tissues were 0.012 ± 0.003 %/(hr·cm²) in the a–p direction and 0.022 ± 0.011 %/(hr·cm²) in the p–a direction. In contrast to amino acid transport, peptide transport was not affected by addition of 100 μM ouabain to the pleural side of the tissue (data not shown). These data strongly indicate that transport of this peptide occurs by a passive mechanism, most likely by the paracellular route since this compound is hydrophilic at physiological pH.

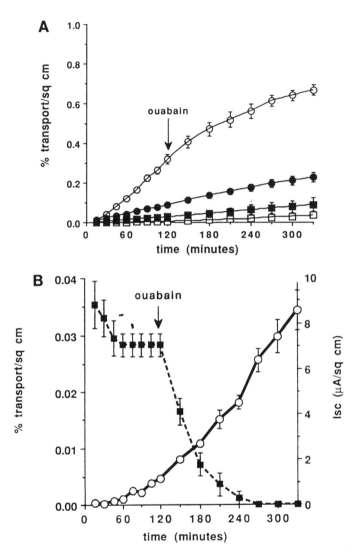

Figure 2. Effect of ouabain on leucine and mannitol transport across frog lung. Transport of leucine and mannitol was allowed to proceed under the same conditions as in Fig. 1 for 2 hr; then 100 μM ouabain was added to the pleural side chamber. Transport was monitored for another 3.5 hr. (A) Ouabain markedly slowed the rate of a–p leucine transport, but had little effect on p–a leucine transport or on mannitol transport in either direction. (B) The same data for a—p mannitol transport shown in (A) are plotted on an expanded scale, together with I_{sc} data from the same experiment. Tissue from three animals was used in these studies.

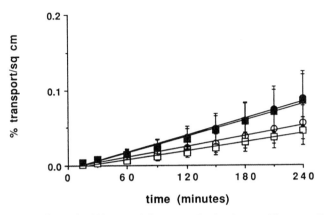

Figure 3. Transport of a hydrophilic growth hormone-releasing hexapeptide across *Xenopus* lung. Percent cumulative transport of the peptide at 20 μM concentration was 0.022 ± 0.005 %/(hr·cm)^2 in the a–p direction and 0.031 ± 0.016 %/(hr·cm)^2 in the p–a direction, similar to the rate of 10 mM mannitol transport in both directions across the same tissue. Flux was linear over a 4-hr period. Tissues were obtained from three animals. Correlation coefficients (R^2) determined by linear regression analysis ranged from 0.987 to 0.990.

5. ADVANTAGES AND DISADVANTAGES OVER OTHER METHODS

The utility of any *in vitro* transport system in biopharmaceutical development is ultimately very limited if data obtained from studies of it do not mimic behavior of the same compounds *in vivo* sufficiently to predict the likely outcome in human patients. Establishment of a correlation between *in vitro* transport rates and *in vivo* absorption from lung in experimental animals is the first step in demonstrating that a system has predictive utility. Although data are presently limited, comparison of the transport of a variety of compounds across *Xenopus* lung with rate of loss from rat lung after intratracheal instillation demonstrates a good correlation between these two parameters (Table I). Active transport of amino acids provides the best current evidence for a similar transport mechanism in amphibian and mammalian lung. However, further experiments to expand this database will be necessary to reach firm conclusions regarding the heuristic value of this system.

In vitro transport may be studied using analytical methods developed for detection of molecules *in vitro*, without need to develop methods for quantitation of the compound in plasma. Control of experimental parameters with *in vitro* systems allows determination of transport mechanisms, a very difficult question to address with *in vivo* studies. Nevertheless, correlations between absorption and transport do not always occur. For example, complexation with cyclodextrins slows transport of some hydrophobic compounds across *Xenopus* lung *in vitro* but has no effect on rate of absorption from rat lung *in vivo* (Wall *et al.*, 1994). This may be due to rapid removal

Table I
Comparison of Rate of Alveolar to Pleural Transport
across *Xenopus* Lung *in Vitro* with Rate of Loss
from Rat Lung after Intratracheal Instillation *in Vivo*

Compound	Loss from lung in rat $(1/t_{1/2})$	Transport in *Xenopus* $[\%/(\text{hr}\cdot\text{cm}^2)]$
Inulin	0.0045[a]	0.0010
Sucrose	0.011[a]	0.0061
p-Aminohippuric acid	0.022[a]	0.0113
Tetraethylammonium	0.018[a]	0.0130
Mannitol	0.017[a]	0.01–0.03
Urea	0.086[a]	0.035
Benzylpenicillin	0.03[a]	0.056
Leucine/cycloleucine[b]	0.36[a]	0.195
Testosterone	0.5	0.56
Antipyrine	4.0[a]	1.5–4.0
Rolipram	3–4[c]	2.9

[a]Values determined from published data (Brown and Schanker, 1983; Lin and Schanker, 1981; Schanker and Hemberger, 1983).
[b]Leucine was used in *Xenopus* experiments, cycloleucine in rat experiments.
[c]Value for $t_{1/2}$ estimated at 15–20 sec from data indicating that more than half of administered rolipram was lost from rat lung by 30 sec after administration (Wall *et al.*, 1994).

of uncomplexed molecules from lung *in vivo* by the circulation, a phenomenon that is not readily mimicked *in vitro* where equilibrium conditions exist (Wall *et al.*, 1994). In vitro transport across alveolar epithelium can also be studied with primary cultures of mammalian alveolar epithelial cells (Dobbs *et al.*, 1988; Kawada *et al.*, 1990; Danto *et al.*, 1992), or in isolated perfused lungs, usually from rat or dog (Byron *et al.*, 1992). Both approaches have the potential advantage of utilizing mammalian systems, which may more closely mimic human physiology. However, considerable similarity exists between *Xenopus* lung and mammalian lung, including similar alveolar cell morphology and overall dimensions of the air–blood barrier (Meban, 1973; Dierichs, 1975), active Na^+ and amino acid absorption (Kim and Crandall, 1988; Fischer *et al.*, 1989; Kim, 1990), surfactant composition (Hallman and Gluck, 1976; Vergara and Hughes, 1980), high transepithelial resistance, and presence of large- and small-radius pore populations of similar dimensions and relative frequency (Crandall and Kim, 1981).

Primary cell culture is a more labor-intensive system than use of amphibian lung tissue, requiring isolation of fresh cells each week owing to their relatively short-term viability. Perfused lungs possess some of the advantages of *in vitro* systems for controlling experimental parameters such as perfusion medium composition, but accurate sampling of the alveolar fluid and uniform deposition of administered compounds are as difficult to achieve as *in vivo*. Potential influence of the absence of other cell types when type I cultures are used (e.g., type II cells producing surfactant, alveolar macrophages) is difficult to assess in the absence of additional data, since all *in vitro* systems are in relatively early stages of development.

ACKNOWLEDGMENTS

We would like to thank Dr. Philip Smith and Mr. Frederick Ryan for assistance in applying the Ussing chamber technique to *Xenopus* lung.

REFERENCES

Adjei, A., and Gupta, P., 1994, Pulmonary delivery of therapeutic peptides and proteins, *J. Controlled Release* **29**:361–373.

Brown, R. A., and Schanker, L. S., 1983, Absorption of aerosolized drugs from the rat lung, *Drug Metab. Dispos.* **11**:355–360.

Byron, P. R., Rypacek, F., Sun, Z., and Katayama, H., 1992, Polypeptide absorption in the rat lung: Dose and charge dependence, *J. Biopharm. Sci.* **3**:227–232.

Cipolla, D. C., Gonda, I., and Shire, S. J., 1994, Characterization of aerosols of human recombinant deoxyribonuclease I (rhDNase) generated by jet nebulizers, *Pharm. Res.* **11**:491–498.

Crandall, E. D., and Kim, K.-J., 1981, Transport of water and solutes across bullfrog alveolar epithelium, *J. Appl. Physiol.: Respir. Environ. Exercise Physiol.* **50**:1263–1271.

Danto, S. I., Zabski, S. M., and Crandall, E. D., 1992, Reactivity of alveolar epithelial cells in primary culture with type I cell monoclonal antibodies, *Am. J. Respir. Cell Mol. Biol.* **6**:296–306.

Dierichs, R. ,1975, Electron microscopic studies of the lung of the frog, *Cell Tissue Res.* **160**:399–410.

Dobbs, L. G., Williams, M. C., and Gonzalez, R., 1988, Monoclonal antibodies specific to apical surface of rat alveolar type I cells bind to surfaces of cultured, but not freshly isolated type II cells, *Biochim. Biophys. Acta* **970**:146–156.

Fischer, H., Van Driessche, W., and Clauss, W., 1989, Evidence for apical sodium channels in frog lung epithelial cells, *Am. J. Physiol.* **256**:C764–C771.

Hallman, M., and Gluck, L., 1976, Phosphatidylglycerol in lung surfactant. III. Possible modifier of surfactant function, *J. Lipid Res.* **17**:257–262.

Kawada, H., Shannon, J. M., and Mason, R. J., 1990, Improved maintenance of adult rat alveolar type II cell differentiation *in vitro*: Effect of serum-free, hormonally-defined medium and a reconstituted basement membrane, *Am. J. Respir. Cell Mol. Biol.* **3**:33–43.

Kim, K.-J., 1990, Active Na^+ transport across *Xenopus* lung alveolar epithelium, *Respir. Physiol.* **81**:29–40.

Kim, K.-J., and Crandall, E. D., 1988, Sodium-dependent lysine flux across bullfrog alveolar epithelium, *J. Appl. Physiol.* **65**:1655–1661.

Kim, K.-J., LeBon, T. R., Shinbane, J. S., and Crandall, E. D., 1985, Asymmetric [^{14}C]albumin transport across bullfrog alveolar epithelium, *J. Appl. Physiol.* **59**:1290–1297.

Lin, Y.-J., and Schanker, L. S., 1981, Pulmonary absorption of amino acids in the rat: Evidence of carrier transport, *Am. J. Physiol.* **240**:C215–C221.

Meban, C., 1973, The pneumocytes in the lung of *Xenopus* laevis, *J. Anat.* **114**:235–244.

Montgomery, A. B., Debs, R. J., Luce, J. M., Corkery, K. J., Turner, J., Brunette, E. N., Lin, E. T., and Hopewell, P. C., 1988, Selective delivery of pentamidine to the lung by aerosol, *Am. Rev. Respir. Dis.* **137**:477–478.

Morimoto, K., Yamahara, H., Lee, V. H. L., and Kim, K.-J., 1993, Dipeptide transport across rat alveolar epithelial cell monolayers, *Pharm. Res.* **10**:1668–1674.

Niven, R. W., 1993, Delivery of biotherapeutics by inhalation aerosols, *Pharm. Technol.* **17:**72–82.

Patton, J. S., Trinchero, P., and Platz, R. M., 1993, Bioavailability of pulmonary delivered peptides and proteins: α-Interferon, calcitonins, and parathyroid hormones, *J. Controlled Release* **28:**79–85.

Schanker, L. S., and Hemberger, J. A., 1983, Relation between molecular weight and pulmonary absorption rate of lipid-insoluble compounds in neonatal and adult rats, *Biochem. Pharmacol.* **32:**2599–2601.

Vergara, G. A., and Hughes, G. M., 1980, Phospholipids in washings from the lungs of the frog (*Rana pipiens*), *J. Comp. Physiol.* **139:**117–120.

Wall, D. A., 1995, Pulmonary absorption of peptides and proteins, *Drug Target Deliv.* **2:**1–20.

Wall, D. A., Pierdomenico, D., and Wilson, G., 1993, An *in vitro* pulmonary epithelial system for evaluating peptide transport, *J. of Controlled Release* **24:**227–235.

Wall, D. A., Marcello, J., Pierdomenico, D., and Farid, A., 1994, Administration as hydroxypropyl β-cyclodextrin complexes does not slow rates of pulmonary drug absorption in rat, *S.T.P. Pharm. Sci.* **4:**63–68.

Chapter 19

In Situ and in Vivo Methods for Pulmonary Delivery

Mohammed Eljamal, Sudha Nagarajan, and John S. Patton

1. INTRODUCTION

The alveolar region of the mammalian lung seems to offer a promising route for the systemic delivery of certain protein and peptide biopharmaceuticals which otherwise must be injected (Bensch *et al.*, 1967; Byron, 1990; Dominquez *et al.*, 1967; Patton and Platz, 1992). The absorption of these molecules into the systemic circulation is thought to occur by diffusion in the conducting airways (Taylor and Gaar, 1970) and by diffusion and transcytosis in the alveolar region of the lungs (Patton and Platz, 1992). Diffusion of lipid-soluble drugs approximately parallels the lipid/water partition coefficients of the compounds as measured at pH 7.4, which suggests that diffusion is occurring through lipid structures. Drugs with very low lipid solubilities are absorbed at rates inversely related to the size of the molecule. This absorption is driven by a concentration gradient, suggesting the presence of "aqueous pores." The morphological correlate of aqueous pores is uncertain but may be tight junctions. Molecules greater than 2.3 nm in diameter, corresponding to molecular weights of 10 kDa, cannot diffuse through the tight junctions of the intestinal epithelial cells which are roughly similar to those in the airways (Madara, 1989; Taylor and Gaar, 1970). Transcytosis is a process where cells of the alveolar lining form endocytic sacs that carry fluid and solutes from the alveolar lumen into the interstitium. It is hypothesized

Mohammed Eljamal, Sudha Nagarajan, and John S. Patton • Inhale Therapeutic Systems, Palo Alto, California 94303.

Models for Assessing Drug Absorption and Metabolism, Ronald T. Borchardt *et al.*, eds., Plenum Press, New York, 1996.

that depending on the molecular size, molecules in the interstitium may transcytose through and/or diffuse between the capillary endothelial cells into the bloodstream. If the molecule is greater than 25–50 kDa in size, its transport across the capillary endothelium may be blocked by the basement membrane, and instead it will diffuse into the lymphatic system and eventually ends up in the circulation (Hubbard *et al.*, 1989; Taylor and Gaar, 1970).

To screen therapeutic candidates for pulmonary delivery, the pharmaceutical scientist is left with limited and experimentally challenging options: isolated perfused lung, intratracheal instillation, and aerosol deposition. These options are difficult to use, require extreme care to yield reasonable reproducibility, and very often demand sophisticated expertise and training. This chapter describes the preparations of the various models.

2. ISOLATED PERFUSED RAT LUNG MODEL (IPRL)

2.1. Introduction

Historically, isolated lung models have been used to obtain pharmacological (Niemeier and Bingham, 1972) and physiological (Fisher *et al.*, 1980) data. Because this model does not include first-pass elimination of the drug by the liver, it can be used to determine the absorption rate of pharmaceutical entities from the lungs provided they can be delivered in a reproducible fashion. Drug delivery to the isolated lungs is accomplished by either intratracheal instillation of a certain volume of liquid pharmaceutical or by aerosol deposition. The lack of dose reproducibility with intratracheal instillation of 100–200 µl of liquid pharmaceutical into the lungs is well established (Enna and Schanker, 1972; Fisher *et al.*, 1980; Niemeier and Bingham, 1972; Niven and Byron, 1987; Pritchard *et al.*, 1985). The major causes are (i) the uneven distribution of the liquid into the various lobes and the nonuniform distribution within each lobe, (ii) the varying degree of expectoration of liquid, and (iii) the unphysiological nature of injecting 200 µl of liquid into rats (equivalent to a half a liter in humans). To minimize these problems, Byron and Niven (1988) reproducibly dosed the lungs by using 25 µl of fluorocarbon propellant to expel the liquid dose while simultaneously inflating the lungs, thus preventing expectoration caused by the liquid plugging the tracheal and bronchial airways upon deflation. The isolated perfused rat lung (IPRL) model is thought to be viable for a maximum of 3 hr (Byron and Niven, 1988) before the epithelial barrier starts to break down. The absorption of most biopharmaceuticals (Patton and Platz, 1992) will take longer than 3 hrs limiting the use of the isolated perfused lung model to certain macromolecules that are quickly absorbed.

The method of drug delivery to the isolated perfused rat lung was previously described by a number of authors (Byron and Niven, 1988; Byron *et al.*, 1986; Enna and Schanker, 1972; Levey and Gast, 1966; Niemeier, 1984). The various preparations of this model were basically similar, but they differed in the way the test therapeutic was administered into the airways, which could be in the form of liquid instillation, nebulized liquid, or dry powder aerosol. In this section, a hypothetical preparation based on the reviewed literature (Byron and Niven, 1988; Byron *et al.*, 1986; Levey and Gast, 1966) of the IPRL model is described.

2.2. Materials and Methods

Male Sprague-Dawley rats (280–300 g) anesthetized with 60 mg of sodium pentobarbitone/kg injected intraperitoneally (Nembutal, 50 mg/ml, Abbott Laboratories, North Chicago, IL) are used in the IPRL model. In general, about a 3-cm incision in the skin at the neck is made and the trachea is exposed. A cross-sectional cut in mid-trachea between the fourth and fifth cartilage rings is made to allow the insertion of a stainless steel tracheal cannula (2–2.5 mm o.d., 1.8–2.0 mm i.d., and 3–5 cm long) about 5–10 mm. The cannula is fixed in place with surgical suture. The lungs are mechanically ventilated (25–35 breaths per minute, 2-ml tidal volume). The thorax is then opened at the diaphragm, the rib cage is severed at both sides, and the flaps are pushed backward. An injection of 0.1 mL of sodium heparin (1000 units/ml, Elkins-Sinn, Inc., Cherry Hill, NJ) is usually administered into the right ventricle to prevent blood clotting. A loose ligature is placed around the pulmonary artery and aorta, an incision is then made through the upper right ventricle. A blunt-tipped 16G gauge stainless steel needle connected to polyethylene tubing (Intramedic, Becton-Dickinson, NJ) is used to cannulate the pulmonary artery. It is fixed in place just before the arterial bifurcation by tightening the loose ligature. The atrium and the left ventricle are then cut so perfusate [Krebs–Henseleit buffer with 4% (w/v) bovine serum albumin (K4)] can be pumped freely. Ventilation is interrupted with the lungs partially inflated while they are severed, washed with 37°C K4, and suspended vertically in a jacketed glass thorax, which should be maintained at 37°C, 100% relative humidity, and slight negative pressure (1–2 cm H_2O). The slight negative pressure in the glass thorax is accomplished by drawing or adding air via a three-way valve and a 20-ml syringe. The perfusate reservoir should be maintained at 37 ± 0.2°C, pH 7.4 ± 0.1 and at a constant level, compensating for volume lost to evaporation by adding distilled water. Bubble-free perfusate is circulated through the pulmonary artery at 15 ml/min using a peristaltic pump (Masterflex, peristaltic pump, type 7553-20, Cole-Parmer Instrument Co., Chicago, IL). There are several techniques to deliver the test therapeutic into the lungs; the most common one is to instill 100–200 μl of the liquid formulation using a blunt-tipped 16G needle and syringe, by expelling the liquid as a coarse spray with the aid of a propellant (Byron and Niven, 1988) or by aerosol (Brown and Schanker, 1983; Byron *et al.*, 1986). Aliquots of perfusate are sampled at fixed time points after administration of the drug, and the concentrations of the therapeutic and/or its metabolites are determined using a suitable analytical assay.

2.3. Treatment of the Data

In the IPRL model the initial dose is known, and for drugs that do not metabolize or bind to cells in the lungs, the absorption rate can easily be determined assuming first-order kinetics using the following equation:

$$\frac{dC}{dt} = k \cdot A$$

where dC/dt is the change of amount absorbed (concentration in perfusate × volume, determined from the frequent sampling and subsequent analysis of perfusate) with respect to time, k is the first-order rate constant to be determined, and A is the amount of drug still in the lungs; if D is the total amount of drug delivered, then

$$A = D - C$$

Substituting for A and solving the above differential equation,

$$C = D \cdot (1 - e^{-k \cdot t})$$

The rate constant k is determined from the best fit of the experimental data to this model. The fit can either be determined mathematically by the least-squares method or one can plot the natural log of $\{(D - C)/D\}$ versus $\{t\}$ and best fit a straight line through the data. The slope of this line is k.

In cases in which the biopharmaceutical molecule can be metabolized in the lungs or, simply because of its size, cannot completely cross from the lumen into the blood side, the total amount delivered, D, cannot be used in the analysis. Instead, one should use only the amount that is available for absorption. An alternative would be to mathematically fit the experimental data to the above equation for first-order kinetics, that is, determine D and k simultaneously.

3. INTRATRACHEAL INSTILLATION MODEL

3.1. Introduction

Intratracheal instillation is the easiest of the three models described herein to prepare and use. In this model, drug is administered by the intratracheal instillation delivery technique described earlier for the *in vitro* model of the isolated perfused rat lung. Similarly, intratracheal instillation of biopharmaceutical solution suffers from the nonuniformity of dose distribution, expectoration, and the unphysiological nature of this mode of drug delivery. However, for the purpose of screening biopharmaceuticals, it has the advantage over the isolated lung model of being able to monitor absorption for as long as necessary—each time point can be determined independently from its own cohort of animals. Using a cohort is advantageous as it avoids the animal remaining under anesthesia for a long time. Also, in using a single animal, a jugular catheter has to be introduced by surgery for blood sampling, and the animal is left to recover overnight from the effect of anesthesia and surgery before the experiment is performed. This could become tedious and time-consuming. In addition, since the total blood volume in rats is relatively small, the use of a single animal limits sampling times. Furthermore, in prolonged studies, the effect of anesthesia has to be considered, and sometimes animals are moribund before the end of the experiment. Using independent cohorts to determine each time point eliminates the problems associated with catheterized animals such as anesthetic and volume effects. In addition, using separate animals for each time point provides very large blood samples for analysis and many lungs for lavage (clearance) studies. However, to obtain intravenous pharmacokinetics of rapidly cleared macromolecules, the catheterized animal is preferred for collection of the very early (i.e., 1–2 min) blood samples.

There are many ways of instilling drug into the rat lungs: (1) invasively, either by surgically cutting open the skin of the throat, pushing aside the muscle, and making an incision in the trachea, inserting a blunt-tipped needle, and instilling a solution or, without the tracheal incision, by injecting through the trachea, and (2) noninvasively, by inserting a blunt needle through the mouth into the trachea and instilling the drug. In our laboratory we have adopted the noninvasive approach for the intratracheal instillation of biopharmaceuticals to minimize the use of anesthesia. Pulmonary absorption of insulin instilled intratracheally into rat lungs is illustrated in this section.

3.2. Materials and Methods

Usually, drugs are either suspended or dissolved in an appropriate buffer. In this study we chose to instill a liquid formulation of insulin (human insulin, Eli Lilly, Indianapolis, IN) in the rat lung and determine the bioavailability of insulin in the circulation relative to that after subcutaneous administration.

3.2.1. INTRATRACHEAL ADMINISTRATION PROCEDURE

A total of 18 adult male Sprague-Dawley rats weighing between 280 and 300 g were fasted overnight but allowed free access to water. Each animal was lightly anesthetized for about 5 min in a small Plexiglas box containing absorbent paper soaked in methoxyflurane (Metofane, Pitman-Moore, Mundelein, IL). The lightly anesthetized rat was vertically held by hanging its upper jaw to a rubber band which was stretched using two buret stands. Approaching the suspended animal from the back, a blunt stainless steel 27G 10-cm-long needle for intratracheal instillation with a spray tip (PENN-CENTURY, Philadelphia, PA) was inserted through the mouth into the trachea just above the main carina, and 10 μg of insulin in 200 μl was sprayed into the lungs. The animal was allowed to recover from anesthesia on its own. When inserting the needle inside the trachea, one should feel with one's fingers for the roughness of the cartilage rings under the skin of the throat in contrast to the smoothness of the esophagus. Positioning the tip of the needle above the main carina was accomplished by first feeling for the resistance from the main bifurcation of the bronchi and by then sliding the syringe back about 5 mm before dosing. A cohort of 3 rats was assigned for each time point. At each time point, the designated animals were anesthetized with inhaled methoxyflurane followed by an intramuscular (i.m.) injection of anesthetic cocktail [a mixture of 1.5 ml of 100-mg/ml ketamine HCl (Ketaset, Aveco Co., Inc., Fort Dodge, IA) and 1.5 ml of 30-mg/ml xylazine (Rompun, Haver-Lockhart, Shenandoah, IA), mixed together in an empty aseptic vial (dose: 0.5–0.7 ml/kg)] before they underwent a single blood withdrawal from the descending aorta. The blood was withdrawn by opening the abdomen with a surgical blade, pushing the viscera aside to expose the aorta and vena cava. It is easy to distinguish between the aorta, which is dark red and pulsating, and the vena cava, which is dark blue. Blood samples were centrifuged (Centrifuge, RC5, Sorval, Wilmington, DE) for 10 min at 3000 rpm, and the resulting serum samples were saved at $-80°C$ until analyzed using a radioimmunoassay described later. Insulin serum concentrations for each time point (0, 15, 30, 60, 90, and 180 min post dosing) were averaged for each cohort. Baseline serum insulin levels were obtained from the zero-time-point animals that were not dosed.

3.2.2. SUBCUTANEOUS ADMINISTRATION PROCEDURE

A total of 18 adult male Sprague-Dawley rats weighing between 280 and 300 g fasted overnight but allowed free access to water were used in the subcutaneous administration study. Each animal was injected under the skin in the back of the neck with 200 μl of the same insulin formulation used in the intratracheal instillation. At the designated time point (0, 15, 30, 60, 90, and 180 min post dosing, 3 animals per time point), blood was withdrawn from the descending aorta, and the serum was separated as described earlier for the intratracheal instillation method. Similarly, insulin serum concentrations for each time point were averaged for each cohort. If the subcutaneous procedure is performed in conjunction with the intratracheal study, the same baseline data can be used, thus reducing the number of animals needed by 3.

3.3. Treatment of the Data

3.3.1. INSULIN

Insulin concentrations in the serum were determined a by radioimmunoassay (RIA) kit (COAT-A-COUNT RIA Kit, Diagnostic Products Corporation, Los Angeles, CA). In this assay, ^{125}I-labeled insulin competes with the serum insulin for sites on insulin-specific antibody immobilized to the wall of a polypropylene tube. Then the antibody-bound fraction is separated and counted in a gamma counter; the count is inversely related to the amount of insulin in the serum. The concentration of insulin is determined by comparing the count to a standard curve generated at the same time.

3.3.2. RESULTS

Averaged insulin concentrations of each cohort ± standard deviations were temporally plotted (serum profile). The serum profiles of intratracheal and subcutaneous administrations of insulin are shown in Fig. 1. A relative bioavailability of 8.3% was determined by dividing the area under the curve (AUC) of the intratracheal serum profile by the AUC of the dose-adjusted subcutaneous serum profile. Insulin serum levels for both subcutaneous and intratracheal administration appeared to return to baseline after 3 hr.

4. AEROSOL DEPOSITION MODEL

4.1. Introduction

Substances inhaled as aerosols are more uniformly distributed in the lungs and can show deeper penetration into the alveolar region than intratracheally administered solutions (Brain et al., 1976). In order to evaluate the bioavailability of aerosol delivery, it is important to be able to accurately estimate the deposited dose in the distal respiratory tract surface. Several direct and indirect methods to quantitate aerosol delivery have been described (Brain and Valberg, 1979; Stahlhofen et al., 1980; Smaldone et al., 1991; Smith et al., 1989; Dolovich, 1989; Ilowite et al., 1991; Eljamal et al., 1994). These direct estimates are usually made by using a surrogate tracer aerosol that can be detected in the lungs (radiolabeled colloid) or a readily absorbed one that can be detected in the systemic circulation (disodium fluorescein). Indirect estimates of the delivered dose are empirical and require the measurement of numerous parameters such as aerodynamic size distribution, aerosol concentration and flow rate, animal breathing rate, and tidal volume.

Many methods of exposure to aerosol formulations are available, such as the *positive pressure inhalation technique*, in which an anesthetized and intubated animal is exposed to aerosol from a generator integrated in the inspiratory arm of a ventilator; the *spontaneous breathing technique*, in which a lightly anesthetized and intubated animal breathes spontaneously from an aerosol generator through a one-way valve and exhales into a filter through another one-way valve; the *tracheotomy technique*, in which the animal undergoes a tracheotomy prior to study and is exposed to aerosol through the tracheotomy tube either through spontaneous breathing from a chamber or by positive pressure inhalation; and the *face mask technique*, in which the sedated animal breathes aerosol spontaneously from a face mask. For small rodents, the most

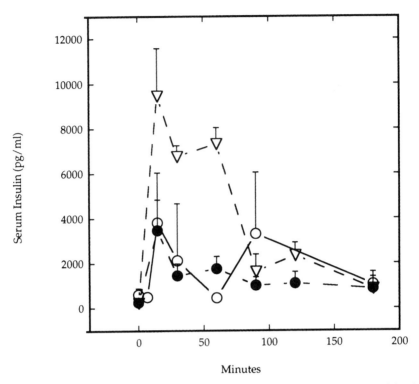

Figure 1.   Insulin serum profiles following subcutaneous (▽), intratracheal (●), and aerosol (○) administration.

popular method is to expose fully awake but contained animals to an aerosol. This section will describe spontaneous breathing nose-only aerosol exposure of rats.

4.2.   Materials and Methods

Adult male Sprague-Dawley rats weighing between 280 and 300 g were fasted overnight but allowed free access to water. A nose-only exposure chamber (In-Tox nose-only exposure chamber for 48 rats, In-Tox Products, Albuquerque, NM) was used to introduce aerosolized insulin to the animals. There are many ways to generate aerosols for the exposure chamber either as a mist from solution or suspension by using a jet or ultrasonic nebulizer or as a dry powder by blowing air through a loose mass of powder, the latter requiring elaborate arrangements to maintain constant output. Other methods in which the surface of a plug of compacted powder is abraded at a controlled rate by a mechanical scraper (Timbrell *et al.*, 1968; Wright, 1950) can also be used to generate concentrated dry-powder aerosol. In our exposure chamber we used a proprietary dry-powder aerosol generator.

The rats were placed inside holding tubes that were fitted to the exposure chamber, and air was provided to the nose of each animal at a flow rate of approximately 0.27 l/min. To ensure 0.27-l/min supply, a flow meter may be connected directly to the aerosol exposure outlet, the flow checked, and the inlet flow of air (do not use aerosol during this step) into the exposure system adjusted. Alternatively, the inlet flow of air into the exposure system may be adjusted to be equal to the number of exposure outlets times the flow rate at each outlet. A powder formulation of 20% insulin by weight was used, of which 255 mg was aerosolized over 14 min into the inlet air stream of the exposure chamber. Two exposure spots were reserved to determine the concentration and aerodynamic particle size distribution of the aerosol at the breathing zone. Aerosol concentration was determined by drawing 2 l/min through a glass fiber filter (type DV, 0.65-μm pore size, Millipore Corp., Bedford, MA), and the aerodynamic particle size distribution was determine using a Mercer-style seven-stage plus backup filter cascade impactor with a calibrated flow rate of 2 l/min. Both determinations were made gravimetrically using a balance (Mettler-Toledo, Inc., Hightstown, NJ). The aerosol concentration and aerodynamic size distribution were used to estimate the delivered dose. Animals were exposed to aerosol for 14 min, after which they were removed and blood was collected from a cohort of 3 rats at each designated time point (0, 7, 15, 30, 60, 90, 120, and 180 min). For each time point, the designated animals were anesthetized with inhaled methoxy-flurane followed by an injection (i.m.) of the anesthetic cocktail before they underwent a single blood withdrawal from the descending aorta. Blood samples were centrifuged for 10 min at 3000 rpm, and the resulting serum samples were saved at $-70°C$ until analyzed. To estimate the deposited dose of insulin, the lungs were lavaged as soon as possible after aerosol exposure. It took 7 minutes to prepare and lavage each animal; for molecules that are readily absorbed in the lung, a marker that is not cleared by absorption, such as radiotagged colloid, can be used to estimate the delivered dose. To lavage the lungs, a three-way stopcock was connected to a PE-50 tubing, to a 30-ml syringe filled with phosphate-buffered saline (PBS) for lavage, and to an empty 30-ml syringe for aspiration. The tubing was inserted through an incision in the trachea, a 5-ml aliquot of PBS for lavage was injected, and PBS was then aspirated for a total of 30 ml. Aliquots from the combined lavage solution were stored in polypropylene tubes at $-70°C$ until analyzed. Baseline serum insulin was determined from the zero-time point animals that were not dosed.

4.3.   Treatment of the Data

4.3.1.   AEROSOL

The concentration of insulin aerosol at the breathing zone was 1.3 mg/l of air. It was determined from the weight of powder deposited on the filter connected to one of the exposure ports, divided by the exposure time (14 min) and aerosol flow rate (2

l/min). Aerosol mass median aerodynamic diameter (MMAD) and percent less than
3.0 μm at the breathing zone were 1.4 μm and 70%, respectively (Fig. 2). The
following is a brief synopsis of how to construct the log-probability plot which is
commonly used in presenting the aerodynamic particle size distribution data. First,
find the mass of powder deposited at each stage and filter. Convert to percent fraction
of the total mass deposited on the stages and filter of the cascade impactor. Then,
calculate cumulative percents less than the cutoff diameters by adding the fractions
stepwise from the bottom up (see Table I). Using log-probability graph paper, plot the
cumulative percents on the probability scale and the cutoff diameters on the log scale
(Fig. 2). MMAD is the diameter corresponding to the 50th percentile on the probability scale. Cumulative percent less than 3.0 μm is also determined from the graph
(Fig. 2).

In Table I, the stages of the cascade impactor numbered 1 through 7 and the
backup filter are listed in column 1, the mass of deposited powder on each stage is
listed in column 2, percent of mass on each stage (mass of deposited powder on that
particular stage divided by the total mass in column 2) is listed in column 3, and

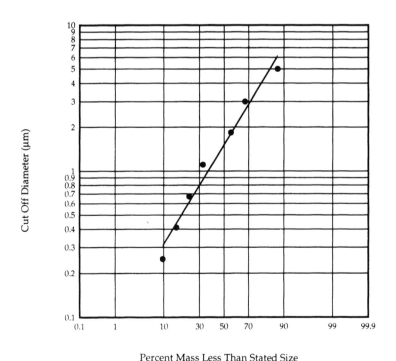

Percent Mass Less Than Stated Size

Figure 2.   Cascade impactor aerodynamic size distribution: cumulative mass percent less than stated size.

Table I
Cascade Impactor Aerosol Data

Stage	Deposited powder (mg)	Percent fraction	Cumulative percent	Cutoff diameter
1	351	12.60	87.40	5.00
2	560	20.10	67.30	3.00
3	320	11.49	55.81	1.84
4	649	23.30	32.51	1.11
5	270	9.69	22.82	0.67
6	202	7.25	15.57	0.41
7	167	5.99	9.58	0.25
Filter	267	9.58		

cumulative mass percent less than the corresponding cutoff diameter (provided by the manufacturer) is listed in column 4.

4.3.2. RESULTS

The absorption of insulin from the lung was studied after a single exposure to 255 mg of 20% insulin powder. The average deposited dose of insulin aerosol was estimated from lung lavage fluids (performed ~7 min after inhalation) to be 12.7 (± 6.9 μg of insulin (63.5 μg of powder), which corresponded to 0.02% of the total dose and 1.3% of the available dose (mass of aerosol at the breathing zone = 1.3 mg of powder/l $\times$ 0.27 l/min $\times$ 14 min = 4.91 mg powder). This illustrates the inefficiency of this aerosol exposure technique—aerosol is lost throughout the system: during generation (70% efficiency is considered good), in the exposure chamber; in the rat nose (a very efficient filter), and because of continuous aerosol flow to the nose which only is useful during inhalation. The aerosol deposited dose of 12.7 μg is minimal because some of the insulin is absorbed before the lavage can be completed and because the insulin cannot be completely washed out of the lung, and, therefore, the actual dose is definitely larger. This points out the need for a tracer technique to better estimate the aerosol deposited dose.

5. DISCUSSION

The described methods are commonly used to evaluate pulmonary bioavailability of biological macromolecules. Intratracheal instillation is easiest, quickest, and relatively inexpensive to utilize. It requires a small amount of drug for efficient administration. It enables precise and noninvasive dosing. It can determine whether a test macromolecule is absorbed from the lung. One drawback in the rodent intratracheal instillation model is the effect of interanimal variability on the absorption profile; different animals are often used to determine each time point. In contrast, aerosol delivery is expensive, very inefficient, and technically challenging, and it is very difficult to precisely quantify the delivered dose (Brown and Schanker, 1983); however, this technique has the advantages of being physiologic and providing a more even distribution of test molecules in the lung than the intratracheal administration method.

The rodent In-Tox aerosol exposure technique has several advantages over single-animal exposures. It allows the exposure of multiple animals simultaneously (up to 48), thus minimizing interanimal dose variability. It does not require anesthesia or sedation during aerosol exposure, which could alter or interfere with lung functions (e.g., depressing respiratory motor function), mucociliary clearance, lung secretions, and absorption. Also, it provides plenty of blood for assays and is very convenient for multiple exposures because animals get used to exposures. On the other hand, this technique suffers from low deposited dose; at best, around 2% of the dose charged in the nebulizer is deposited in the respiratory tracts of 48 animals. In large-animal aerosol exposure, around 32% deposition was achieved in dogs by positive pressure inhalation (Smith *et al.*, 1989). A small drawback in using the rodent In-Tox model is that different animals are used to determine blood levels at each time point increasing the effect of interanimal variability on the serum profile, whereas in large-animal aerosol exposure, a single animal is used, which provides a continuous temporal absorption profile and higher aerosol delivered dose.

Dry-powder insulin aerosol had a bioavailability of 29.8% relative to subcutaneous administration, which was higher than the 8.3% obtained following intratracheal instillation. Other macromolecules such as rhG-CSF and hGH had greater bioavailability following aerosol deposition than following liquid instillation (Niven *et al.*, 1994; Taylor *et al.*, 1994). The aerosol bioavailabilities of rhG-CSF and hGH were 66 ± 14% and 44.8 ± 11.2%, respectively, as compared to bioavailabilities of 27 ± 9% and 15.5 ± 2%, respectively, from intratracheal instillation of the same solution (Niven *et al.*, 1994; Taylor *et al.*, 1994). This disparity may be due to the difference in deposition patterns: central, which is mainly in the conducting airways, versus peripheral, which is in the alveoli. Following intratracheal administration of an insulin solution containing radioactive tracer to rabbit lungs, Colthorpe *et al.* (1991) showed a localized and a preferential central deposition pattern. Following aerosol administration of the same solution, they showed an evenly distributed peripheral deposition pattern of the tracer in the lungs. It follows to assume that more test macromolecules will be trapped in the mucus layer of the conducting airways during central rather than peripheral deposition pattern. Since the conducting airways are efficiently cleared by the mucociliary mechanism and are lined by an epithelium that is virtually impermeable to large macromolecules, one can safely assume that macromolecules trapped in the mucus layer of the conducting airways were cleared fast and were not available for absorption. Lower bioavailabilities should be expected following intratracheal instillation, where a localized and central deposition pattern is more evident, than following aerosol deposition, where an evenly distributed peripheral deposition pattern is observed.

ACKNOWLEDGMENTS

We thank Pat Trinchero for her technical support, and we are grateful to Linda Dulaney for reviewing the manuscript.

REFERENCES

Bensch, K. G., Dominquez, E. A. M., and Liebow, A. A., 1967, Absorption of intact protein molecules across the pulmonary air—tissue barrier, *Science* **157:**1204–1206.

Brain, J. D., and Valberg, P. A., 1979, Deposition of aerosol in the respiratory tract, *Am. Rev. Respir. Dis.* **120:**1325–1373.

Brain, J. D., Knudson, D. E., Sorokin, S. P., and Davis, M. A., 1976, Pulmonary distribution of particles given by intratracheal instillation or by aerosol inhalation, *Environ. Res.* **11:**13–33.

Brown, R. A., Jr., and Schanker, L. S., 1983, Absorption of aerosolized drugs from the rat lung, *Drug Metab. Dispos.* **11:**355–360.

Byron, P., 1990, Determinants of drug and polypeptide bioavailability from aerosols delivered to the lung, *Adv. Drug Deliv. Rev.* **5:**107–132.

Byron, P. R., and Niven, R. W., 1988, A novel dosing method for drug administration to the airway of the isolated rat lung, *J. Pharm. Sci.* **77:**693–695.

Byron, P. R., Roberts, N. S. R., and Clark A. R., 1986, An isolated perfused rat lung preparation for the study of aerosolized drug deposition and absorption, *J. Pharm. Sci.* **75:**168–171.

Colthorpe, P., Farr, S. J., Taylor, G., Smith, I. J., and Wyatt, D., 1991, The pharmacokinetics of pulmonary-delivered insulin: A comparison of intratracheal and aerosol administration to the rabbit, *Pharm. Research* **9:**764–768.

Dolovich, M., 1989, Physical principles underlying aerosol therapy. *J. Aerosol Med.* **2**(2):171–186.

Dominquez, E. A. M., Liebow, A. A., and Bensch, K. G., 1967, Studies on the pulmonary air—tissue barrier. I. Absorption of albumin by the alveolar wall, *Lab. Invest.* **16:**905–911.

Eljamal, M., Wong, L. B., and Yeates, D. B., 1994, Capsaicin-activated bronchial and alveolar-initiated pathways regulating tracheal ciliary beat frequency, *J. Appl. Physiol.* **77**(3):1239–1245.

Enna, S. J., and Schanker, L. S., 1972, Absorption of saccharides and urea from rat lung, *Am. J. Physiol.* **222:**409–414.

Fisher, A. B., Dodia, C., and Linask, J., 1980, Perfusate composition and edema formation in isolated rat lungs, *Exp. Lung Res.* **1:**13–21.

Hubbard, R. C., Casolaro, M. A., Mitchell, M., Sellers, S. E., Arabia, F., Matthay, M. A., and Crystal, R. G., 1989, Fate of aerosolized recombinant DNA-producing al-antitrypsin: Use of the epithelial surface of the lower respiratory tract to administer proteins of therapeutic importance, *Proc. Natl. Acad. Sci. USA* **86:**680–684.

Ilowite, J. S., Baskin, M. I., Sheetz, M. S., and Abd, A. G., 1991, Delivered dose and regional distribution of aerosolized pentamidine using different delivery systems, *Chest* **99:**1139–1144.

Levey, S., and Gast, R., 1966, Isolated perfused rat lung preparation, *J. Appl. Physiol.* **21:**313–316.

Madara, J. L., 1989, Loosening tight junctions: Lessons from the intestine, *J. Clin. Invest.* **83:**1089–1094.

Niemeier, R. W., 1984, The isolated perfused lung, *Environ. Health Perspect.* **56:**35–41.

Niemeier, R. W., and Bingham, E., 1972, An isolated perfused lung preparation for metabolic studies, *Life Sci.* **11:**807–820.

Niven, R. W., and Byron, P. R., 1987, Solute absorption from the airways of the isolated rat lung. I. The use of absorption data to quantify drug dissolution or release in the respiratory tract, *Pharm. Research* **5:**574–579.

Niven, R. W., Whitcomb, L., Wilson, J. V., Kinstler, O., and Shaner, L., 1994, Intratracheal instillation vs aerosol administration of rhG-CSF and PEGylated rhG-CSF, *Pharm. Res.* **11:**S289.

Patton, J. S., and Platz, R. M., 1992, Pulmonary delivery of peptide and proteins for systemic action, *Adv. Drug Deliv. Rev.* **8:**179–196.

Pritchard, J. N., Holmes, A., Evans, N., Evans, R. J., and Morgan, A., 1985, The distribution of dust in the rat lung following administration by inhalation and by single intratracheal instillation, *Environ. Res.* **36:**268–297.

Smaldone, G. C., Fuhrer, J., Steigbigel, R. T., and McPeck, M., 1991, Factors determining pulmonary deposition of aerosolized pentamidine in patients with human immunodeficiency virus infection, *Ann. Rev. Respir. Dis.* **143:**727–737.

Smith, R. M., Traber, L. D., Traber, D. L., and Spragg, R. G., 1989, Pulmonary deposition and clearance of aerosolized alpha-1-proteinase inhibitor administered to dogs and sheep, *J. Clin. Invest.* **84:**1145–1154.

Stahlhofen, W., Gebhart, J., and Heyder, J., 1980, Experimental determination of the regional deposition of aerosol particles in the human respiratory tract, *Am. Ind. Hyg. Assoc. J.* **41:**385–398.

Taylor, A. E., and Gaar, K. A., Jr., 1970, Estimation of equivalent pore radii of pulmonary and alveolar membranes, *Am. J. Physiol.* **218:**1133–1140.

Taylor, G., Colthorpe, P., and Farr, S. J., 1994, Human growth hormone pharmacokinetics in rabbits after selective regional pulmonary delivery, *Pharm. Res.* **11:**S289.

Timbrell, V., Hyett A. W., and Skidmore, J. W., 1968, A simple dispenser for generating dust clouds from standard reference samples of asbestos, *Ann. Occup. Hyg.* **11:**273– 281.

Wright, B. M., 1950, A new dust-feed mechanism, *J. Sci. Inst.* **27:**12–15.

Chapter 20

In Vitro Viable Skin Model

Robert L. Bronaugh

1. INTRODUCTION

Until recently, *in vitro* percutaneous absorption studies were conducted with nonviable skin. Early studies have shown that for many chemicals good *in vivo–in vitro* agreement can be obtained with nonviable skin (Bronaugh *et al.*, 1982a). This is most likely due to the fact that the nonliving upper layer of skin, the stratum corneum, is a major barrier to absorption. However, no information was obtained in these studies about first-pass metabolism in skin.

Absorption and metabolism of topically applied chemicals by skin can be readily measured by using *in vitro* techniques. A thin preparation of skin simulating the barrier layer is prepared and placed in a flow-through diffusion cell. A physiologic buffer maintains the viability of skin for at least 24 hr. The investigator can obtain information related to the absorption of the parent compound, as well as information on its biotransformation during the absorption process.

Although *in vitro* methods allow the study of the absorption and metabolism of potentially toxic chemicals by human skin, the permeability properties of human skin are unique and cannot be duplicated with animal skin (Bronaugh *et al.*, 1982b).

Robert L. Bronaugh • Office of Cosmetics and Colors, Food and Drug Administration, Laurel, Maryland 20708.

Models for Assessing Drug Absorption and Metabolism, Ronald T. Borchardt *et al.*, eds., Plenum Press, New York, 1996.

2. METHODS

2.1. Choice of Membrane

2.1.1. HUMAN OR ANIMAL SKIN

Human skin should be used to obtain the most accurate absorption data for regulatory concerns related to human health. The difficulty in obtaining viable human skin (after surgical procedures) may require that some studies be performed with animal skin. Experiments with animal skin can be conducted with greater confidence if some human skin studies are performed so as to "calibrate" the skin of the animal model with the test compound. Animal skin is more permeable to chemicals than is human skin (Bronaugh et al., 1982b), and therefore its use will give conservative values that overestimate human percutaneous absorption. The choice of an animal model depends in part on the ease of preparing the skin for the diffusion cells. The skin from a hairless guinea pig or rat is preferred because it can be cut into thin sections with a dermatome, so that most of the dermis is removed (Bronaugh and Stewart, 1986).

2.1.2. NUMBER OF SUBJECTS

Data from at least three animal or human subjects should be obtained and averaged to allow for biological variation among subjects. The variability in absorption is often small (less than twofold) for inbred strains of laboratory animals but can be fivefold in different specimens of human skin.

2.1.3. REGIONAL VARIABILITY

Variability in skin permeation occurs in different regions of human skin. The trunk (back and abdomen) and the extremities (arms and legs) have reasonably similar barrier properties (less than twofold differences). Enhanced absorption can be observed in regions of the face (fourfold) and especially the scrotum (20-fold). In dealing with absorption of a facial product, one should therefore expect faster absorption through facial skin than through abdominal skin. Small differences in regional absorption may be unimportant when one considers the large variability in skin permeation from subject to subject.

2.1.4. VALIDATION OF HUMAN SKIN BARRIER

Because human skin is obtained after trauma such as surgery, illness, or accident, it can be damaged before it is prepared for a study—without the knowledge of the investigator. Scrubbing skin with a detergent before surgery or an autopsy is a frequent cause of barrier alteration. For this reason, the barrier properties of the skin should be pretested with a standard compound such as tritiated water (Bronaugh *et al.*, 1986) before an experiment is conducted with the test compound.

[^{3}H]Water permeation has often been measured by applying an excess of the compound to the surface of the skin and measuring the steady-state rate of permeation, for example, by taking at least four to five measurements at hourly intervals following application of [^{3}H]water. A permeability constant can be determined by dividing this rate by the initial concentration of applied material.

We observed that a more rapid evaluation of water permeability could be made in what we called the 20-min test. By using diffusion cells with an exposed area of skin of 0.32 cm^2, 100 μl of [^{3}H]water (approximately 0.3 μCi) was applied to the surface of the skin so that it was completely covered. The tops of the cells were occluded with Parafilm. After 20 min, the unabsorbed material was blotted from the surface of the skin with a cotton-tipped applicator, and then the surface of the skin was rinsed once with distilled water. Effluent from the flow cell was collected for an additional 60 min, at which time radioactivity in the effluent had returned to baseline. [^{3}H]Water absorption was expressed as the percent of the applied dose absorbed. Values obtained with the 20-min test showed good correlation ($r = 0.98$; $P < 0.01$) with permeability constant values obtained from the same skin (Fig. 1).

2.2. Preparation of Membrane

Full-thickness skin should not be used. Since chemicals absorbed *in vivo* are taken up by blood vessels directly beneath the epidermis, an *in vitro* study should use a membrane with most of the dermis removed. This is particularly important for water-insoluble compounds that would diffuse slowly through the dermis.

The best way of preparing biological membranes for percutaneous absorption studies is to use the dermatome. Unlike other methods (such as those using heat or chemical separation), a dermatome can be used with hairless or haired skin without adversely affecting the viability of the membrane. We have prepared membranes almost exclusively with a Padgett Electro Dermatome (Padgett Instruments, Kansas City, MO) (Bronaugh and Stewart, 1984, 1986).

Full-thickness skin from a human subject or an animal is pinned (epidermis side up) to the surface of a block for cutting. Styrofoam is convenient because it can be readily shaped to the desired size with the aid of a knife, and pins can be easily punched into this material to anchor the skin. The width of the Styrofoam block must be less than the cutting edge of the dermatome blade so that the blade can rest on the surface of the skin. The piece of skin should overlap the edges of the block and be attached to the side of the block with the pins, which are out of the way of the dermatome blade.

The depth of the cut is controlled with a lever on the side of the dermatome head—calibrations are indicated in thousandths of an inch. The actual thickness of

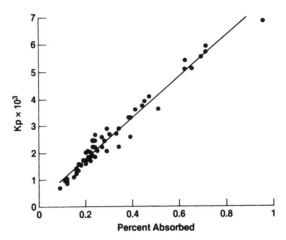

Figure 1. Correlation of results from two methods of measuring water permeation through skin: permeability constant (Kp) values and the percent dose absorbed (20-min test).

the membrane obtained is a result of the pressure applied and the angle at which the dermatome is held as it is pushed across the skin. We have found it helpful to check the thickness of each membrane prepared with the dermatome by using a micrometer (Mitutoyo micrometer, 0.01 to 9 mm, L. A. Benson Inc., Baltimore, MD). With a little practice, it is possible to make skin sections of reproducible thickness.

2.3. Diffusion Cell Design

Flow-through cells are necessary for maintaining viability of skin in diffusion cells since nutrient media must be continually replaced. Also, these cells are preferable for studies requiring round-the-clock testing since specimens can be collected automatically in a fraction collector. A schematic diagram of the flow-through cell used in our laboratory is shown in Fig. 2.

Important features in the design of a flow-through cell are discussed below under the following headings: receptor volume, construction material, maintenance of physiological temperature, ease of assembly of skin, and mixing of receptor contents.

2.3.1. RECEPTOR VOLUME

The most important single feature of flow cell design may be the volume of the diffusion cell receptor, which must be small (less than 0.5 ml) so that the receptor can be completely flushed out with a manageable volume of receptor fluid during test collection intervals. The flow rate generally should be about 5 to 10 times the volume

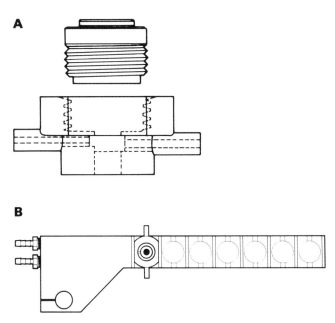

Figure 2. Flow-through cell and holding block. (A) Cross section of diffusion cell. (B) Aluminum holding block for cells.

of the receptor (i.e., a 0.5-ml receptor requires a flow rate of at least 2.5 ml/hr). Too often, investigators modify existing one-cell chambers, such as the Franz cell, that have receptor volumes as large as 5 ml and then pump receptor fluid through the cell at 1 or 2 ml per hour. Because the receptor contents are not rapidly removed from the cell following absorption through the skin, the time course of absorption will be skewed to the right, with absorption of a chemical appearing to occur at a later time than it actually happened. The importance of a small receptor was also stressed by Barry (1983) in his discussion of flow cells. In our laboratory, the receptor fluid is pumped beneath the skin through a chamber with a volume of only 0.13–0.26 ml (depending on the skin surface area of the diffusion cell). This small volume allows the receptor contents to be rapidly and completely flushed out at flow rates of 1.5 ml/hr or greater.

2.3.2. CONSTRUCTION MATERIAL

Cells should be made of a material that does not bind or retain test compounds during the course of a study. We initially prepared flow cells from Plexiglas because of its transparent properties, but we discovered that radiolabeled compounds diffused into this porous material and could not be washed off. The compounds also leached into the receptor fluid of subsequent experiments and confounded their results. Cells should preferably be constructed of glass or Teflon because of their inert properties.

The flow-through cells used in our laboratory are made from Teflon and are fitted with a glass window in the bottom through which we can view the contents of the receptor and verify the absence of air bubbles. Some very lipophilic molecules adhere to the surface of the cells but are easily removed by soaking the cells overnight in water.

2.3.3. MAINTENANCE OF PHYSIOLOGICAL TEMPERATURE

Skin surface temperature in a diffusion cell during an absorption/metabolism study should be maintained at a physiological temperature of about 32°C. This can be accomplished by placing the cells in a heated holder, jacketing the cells and running heated water through the compartment, or placing the cells in an environmental chamber heated to the correct temperature.

2.3.4. EASE OF ASSEMBLY OF SKIN

Skin must be easy to assemble in a suitable flow cell. Most commonly, diffusion cell halves have been clamped together in some way to assemble the cell before use. In the cell shown in Fig. 2 (Bronaugh and Stewart, 1985), the skin membrane is placed in the lower portion of the cell, and the cap is screwed into place. The inside portion of the cap swivels so that the skin is not twisted during the tightening process. This design was chosen because of the requirement for a small receptor volume.

2.3.5. MIXING OF RECEPTOR CONTENTS

Stirring bars are commonly used to mix the receptor contents of many types of diffusion cells. However, flow cells with small receptor volumes are unique. The receptor fluid flowing through the cell may be sufficient to provide adequate mixing. For water-soluble compounds, we have found that adequate mixing in our flow cell is achieved without stirring (Bronaugh and Stewart, 1985). For water-insoluble compounds, additional mixing promotes further partitioning of material from the skin into the receptor fluid.

2.4. Receptor Fluid

Skin viability should be maintained through the appropriate use of a balanced salt solution containing glucose (such as HEPES-buffered Hanks' balanced salt solution) or the use of a tissue culture medium (Collier et al., 1989). The use of viable skin in a diffusion cell study is warranted even if metabolism is not of interest. The credibility of in vitro data is enhanced by maintaining the skin in a viable state, which should be verified by techniques such as glucose metabolism monitoring or histological procedures.

In studies with water-insoluble test compounds, 4% bovine serum albumin (BSA) can be added to the receptor fluid to closely simulate blood by enhancing the partitioning of the compound from skin into the receptor fluid (see Section 2.9.2).

2.5. Temperature

Skin should be maintained at a physiological surface temperature of about 32°C. To achieve this skin temperature in the Bronaugh flow cells, water is heated to 35°C and pumped through the holding blocks. The required water temperature may vary if diffusion cells of different design are used. The percutaneous absorption of N,N-diethyl-m-toluamide was found to double when the air temperature above the skin was increased from 20 to 32°C (Hawkins and Reifenrath, 1984). Chang and Riviere (1991) found that the magnitude of the increase in absorption caused by raising the skin temperature depended on the concentration of parathion applied to the skin.

2.6. Vehicle

Generally, test compounds should be applied to skin in a vehicle that most closely simulates exposure conditions. Sometimes, absorption values are obtained from multiple vehicles to represent varied exposure conditions. The percutaneous absorption of N-nitrosodiethanolamine (NDELA), an impurity in some cosmetic products, was evaluated in three vehicles that were chosen to give a range of solubility properties (Bronaugh *et al.*, 1981). The polar nitrosamine was over 40 times more permeable from the lipoidal vehicle isopropyl myristate than from water. The vehicle effect can be explained, at least in part, by increased partitioning of NDELA into skin. The skin/vehicle partition coefficient was 127 greater when isopropyl myristate was used instead of water.

2.7. Dose

The dose of test compound applied to skin should simulate exposure conditions. Frequently, finite doses of chemicals are applied to skin, and therefore a linear extrapolation from one dose to another may not be accurate. If steady-state absorption is achieved with an infinite dose, then absorption is related linearly to concentration.

2.8. Duration of Study

The test compound should be left in contact with skin for a time that simulates exposure conditions. For many chemicals, a 24-hr exposure is appropriate. For chemicals that are washed off the skin soon after contact, a shorter exposure would be more relevant.

2.9. Measurement of Percutaneous Absorption

2.9.1. WATER-SOLUBLE TEST COMPOUND

Rates of percutaneous absorption are measured by analyzing receptor fluid. The skin surface is washed with soap and water (Bronaugh *et al.*, 1989) at the end of the experiment, and the amount of the test compound remaining in the skin is determined. Total absorption is the sum of the receptor fluid and skin levels of the test compound.

2.9.2. HYDROPHOBIC TEST COMPOUND

Lipid-soluble compounds with water solubility of less than about 10 mg/l do not freely partition from skin into an aqueous receptor fluid that maintains viability (Bronaugh and Stewart, 1984). BSA (4%) should be added to the receptor fluid to increase the solubility of hydrophobic compounds. Absorption of a compound by skin, measured at each collection time, is the sum of the levels of the compound in the receptor fluid and the absorbed compound that remains in the skin; unabsorbed compound is removed from the skin surface by washing gently with soap and water (Bronaugh *et al.*, 1989).

2.10. Expression of Data

Absorption data are most commonly expressed as the amount absorbed per unit of time. This can be done by calculating the percent of the applied dose absorbed per relevant specific time interval, e.g., 24 hr. Alternatively, actual amounts penetrating may be calculated (micrograms per hour per square centimeter). When an infinite dose is applied, dividing this dose by the concentration of applied compound results in a permeability constant.

3. APPLICATION OF MODEL TO SKIN ABSORPTION AND METABOLISM MEASUREMENTS

A recent study used the above techniques to characterize esterase and alcohol dehydrogenase activity in skin and examine the percutaneous absorption and metabolism of retinyl palmitate (Boehnlein *et al.*, 1994). Methyl salicylate and benzyl alcohol served as model compounds to study esterase and alcohol dehydrogenase activity, respectively.

No significant difference in the percutaneous absorption of methyl salicylate or benzyl alcohol through viable or nonviable hairless guinea pig skin (Table I) was found. Permeation of the compounds was similar through skin from the backs of animals of both sexes (Table I). Absorption of both compounds was rapid, with most of the absorbed compounds found in the initial 6-hr receptor fluid collection interval.

The metabolism of methyl salicylate differed with the state of viability of the skin and the sex of the animals whose skin was used in the experiments (Table II). Only esterase activity was observed in nonviable skin, resulting in the biotransformation of 38% of the absorbed parent compound to salicylic acid. In viable skin, esterase activity was significantly greater. Salicylic acid was further metabolized by glycine conjugation to salicyluric acid, with a total of 57% of the absorbed dose hydrolyzed. A marked difference in metabolism was observed between male and female hairless guinea pig skin (Table II). Similar amounts of radioactivity were absorbed through male and female skin, but the rate of total metabolism in male skin was more than twice that in female skin. At the end of the 24-hr study, the amount of salicylic acid formed by male skin (35.6% of absorbed dose) was significantly greater than that formed by female skin (12.3% of absorbed dose).

Oxidation of benzyl alcohol to benzoic acid was observed in viable and nonviable skin from animals of both sexes (Table III). However, approximately a threefold greater percentage of metabolism of the total absorbed compound occurred with male viable skin (marginally significant difference, $P > 0.07$). Only with viable skin was there further metabolism of benzoic acid to its glycine conjugate, hippuric acid.

Table I
Percutaneous Absorption of Methyl Salicylate
and Benzyl Alcohol in Hairless Guinea Pig Skin

Compound	Sex	Percentage of applied dose absorbed in 24 hr[a]	
		Viable skin[b]	Nonviable skin[b]
Methyl salicylate	Male	55.4 ± 5.9	46.6 ± 2.3
	Female	56.3 ± 15.9	50.1 ± 19.8
Benzyl alcohol	Male	61.0 ± 16.4	58.2 ± 16.0
	Female	63.0 ± 10.0	64.8 ± 3.2

[a]Mean ± SE of receptor fluid measurement using skin from 3 animals (3–4 repetitions per animal).
[b]The values obtained for viable and nonviable male and female guinea pig skin for each compound were not significantly different when compared by the two-tailed *t*-test ($P < 0.05$).

Table II

Metabolism of Methyl Salicylate in Hairless Guinea Pig Skin

| | Percentage of absorbed dose metabolized[a] | | | |
| | Viable skin | | | Nonviable skin |
Sex	Salicyluric acid	Salicylic acid	Total	Salicylic acid
Male	20.9 ± 5.4	35.6 ± 6.5[b]	56.5 ± 5.1[b,c]	38.3 ± 5.0[b,c]
Female	12.5 ± 3.5	12.3 ± 2.5[b]	24.8 ± 3.0[b,c]	13.4 ± 2.8[b,c]

[a]Mean ± SE of determinations in 3 animals (3–4 repetitions per animal).
[b]Significant male vs. female difference by the two-tailed t-test ($P < 0.01$).
[c]Significant viable vs. nonviable skin difference, same sex ($P < 0.05$).

The percutaneous absorption of the lipophilic compound retinyl palmitate was determined by summation of the absorbed material in the skin and in the receptor fluid at the end of the 24-hr study (Table IV). Even with 4% BSA added to the receptor fluid, less than 1% of the absorbed material partitioned into the receptor fluid. Substantial metabolism of retinyl palmitate to retinol was measured, but no additional metabolites were observed. The percent of the applied dose absorbed was lower when human skin was used in the diffusion cells. About 44% of the absorbed dose was metabolized to retinol in human skin. In human or guinea pig skin, the small amount of radioactivity in the receptor fluid ($<1\%$) was determined to be the metabolite retinol.

Our studies have demonstrated that retinol is formed in hairless guinea pig and human skin after topical application of retinyl palmitate and that if further metabolism to retinoic acid occurs, the amount present is too small to be observed. Any biological response of skin treated with retinyl palmitate formulations may be due to ester hydrolysis of the parent compound to retinol.

Table III

Metabolism of Benzyl Alcohol in Hairless Guinea Pig Skin

| | Percentage of absorbed dose metabolized[a] | | | |
| | Viable | | | Nonviable |
Sex	Hippuric acid	Benzoic acid	Total	Benzoic acid
Male	8.5 ± 1.9	44.2 ± 8.0[b]	52.7 ± 9.6[b]	30.2 ± 16.5
Female	4.1 ± 1.8	16.0 ± 8.4[b]	20.1 ± 9.6[b]	12.2 ± 6.0

[a]Mean ± SE of determinations in 3 animals (3–4 repetitions per animal).
[b]Marginally significant male vs. female difference by the two-tailed t-test ($p < 0.07$).

Table IV
Percutaneous Absorption and Metabolism of Retinyl Palmitate

	Skin[a]		Receptor fluid[a]	
Skin type	Radioactivity absorbed (%)[b]	Metabolized (%)[c]	Radioactivity absorbed (%)[b,d]	Metabolized (%)[c]
Guinea pig				
Male	29.8 ± 4.5	38.2 ± 13.0	0.5 ± 0.2	100
Female	33.4 ± 2.3	30.2 ± 16.3	0.6 ± 0.3	100
Human				
Female	17.9 ± 1.3	43.9 ± 5.0	0.2 ± 0.01	100

[a]Mean ± SE of determinations from 2 human donors (3–4 repetitions per donor) and 3 animals (3 repetitions per animal).
[b]Absorption is expressed as percent of applied dose.
[c]Metabolism is expressed as percent of the absorbed retinyl palmitate hydrolyzed to retinol.
[d]0–24-hr fractions were combined.

4. COMPARISON OF MODEL TO OTHER METHODS

Only *in vitro* diffusion cell techniques can reliably measure skin metabolism as well as skin absorption. Metabolism in skin usually cannot be determined during *in vivo* absorption studies since metabolism of the test compound by blood, liver, and other systemic tissues also occurs.

In vitro techniques are also important for the study of chemicals too toxic for *in vivo* human studies. Viable human skin assembled in a flow-through diffusion cell can provide valuable information about the skin absorption and metabolism of potential carcinogens and other highly toxic chemicals. As is generally true with *in vitro* methods, diffusion cell studies can be conducted more easily and less expensively than *in vivo* studies using animal or human subjects.

In vitro diffusion cell methods for measuring skin absorption cannot be used to assess the effects of certain biological responses on the skin absorption process. For example, the alteration in barrier properties resulting from an irritation or a sensitization reaction would be more suitably studied by using *in vivo* skin absorption methodologies.

REFERENCES

Barry, B. W., 1983, Methods for studying percutaneous absorption, in: *Dermatological Formulations: Percutaneous Absorption*, Marcel Dekker, New York, pp. 234–295.
Boehnlein, J., Sakr, A., Lichtin, J. L., and Bronaugh, R. L., 1994, Characterization of esterase and alcohol

dehydrogenase activity in skin. Metabolism of retinyl palmitate to retinol (vitamin A) during percutaneous absorption, *Pharm. Res.* **11:**1155–1159.

Bronaugh, R. L., and Stewart, R. F., 1984, Methods for *in vitro* percutaneous absorption studies III: Hydrophobic compounds, *J. Pharm. Sci.* **73:**1255–1258.

Bronaugh, R. L., and Stewart, R. F., 1985, Methods for *in vitro* percutaneous absorption studies IV: The flow-through diffusion cell, *J. Pharm. Sci.* **74:**64–67.

Bronaugh, R. L., and Stewart, R. F., 1986, Methods for *in vitro* percutaneous absorption studies VI: Preparation of the barrier layer, *J. Pharm. Sci.* **75:**487–491.

Bronaugh, R. L., Congdon, E. R., and Scheuplein, R. J., 1981, The effect of cosmetic vehicles on the penetration of *N*-nitrosodiethanolamine through excised human skin, *J. Invest. Dermatol.* **76:**94–96.

Bronaugh, R. L., Stewart, R. F., Congdon, E. R., and Giles, A. L., Jr., 1982a, Methods for *in vitro* percutaneous absorption studies I: Comparison with *in vivo* results, *Toxicol. Appl. Pharmacol.* **62:**474–480.

Bronaugh, R. L., Stewart, R. F., and Congdon, E. R., 1982b, Methods for *in vitro* percutaneous absorption studies II: Animal models for human skin, *Toxicol. Appl. Pharmacol.* **62:**481–488.

Bronaugh, R. L., Stewart, R. F., and Simon, M., 1986, Methods for *in vitro* percutaneous absorption VII: Use of excised human skin, *J. Pharm. Sci.* **75:**1094–1097.

Bronaugh, R. L., Stewart, R. F., and Storm, J. E., 1989, Extent of cutaneous metabolism during percutaneous absorption of xenobiotics, *Toxicol. Appl. Pharmacol.* **99:**534–543.

Chang, S. K., and Riviere, J. E., 1991, Percutaneous absorption of parathion in porcine skin: Effects of dose, temperature, humidity and perfusate composition on absorptive flux, *Fundam. Appl. Toxicol.* **17:** 494–504.

Collier, S. W., Sheikh, N. M., Sakr, A., Lichtin, J. L., Stewart, R. F., and Bronaugh, R. L., 1989, Maintenance of skin viability during *in vitro* percutaneous absorption/metabolism studies, *Toxicol. Appl. Pharmacol.* **99:**522–533.

Hawkins, G. S., and Reifenrath, W. G., 1984, Development of an *in vitro* model for determining the fate of chemicals applied to skin, *Fundam. Appl. Toxicol.* **4:**S133–S144.

Chapter 21

Isolated Perfused Porcine Skin Flap Systems

Jim E. Riviere

1. INTRODUCTION

The ultimate goal of an *in vitro* model system is to predict the behavior of the drug in the *in vivo* setting. Most *in vitro* skin models used to assess the percutaneous absorption or transdermal delivery of topically applied drugs are designed around the assumption that the stratum corneum and/or epidermis is the principal barrier to compound penetration through skin. Thus, all such models were usually avascular and, until recently, nonviable preparations. However, *in vivo*, this stratum corneum and living epidermal barrier resides on a well-vascularized and metabolically active dermal substrate offering ample biological targets for specific types of drugs. Drugs may be vasoactive and modulate the cutaneous microcirculation; they may serve as substrates of epidermal and dermal drug-metabolizing enzymes, or they may activate cytokine and/or other modulator receptors which result in changes in epidermal, dermal, or endothelial cell function. Therefore, the anatomical and physiological complexity of human skin is significantly greater than that modeled in existing *in vitro* systems, which thus do not afford the possibility of detecting these potential biologically relevant events.

One solution to this dilemma is to create an anatomically intact, viable, isolated perfused *in vitro* skin model that maintains many of the *in vivo* attributes in an *ex vivo* setting. Isolated organ perfusions have been a useful tool for pharmacological and toxicological studies of the kidney, liver, lung, intestine, and heart. These organs have

Jim E. Riviere • Cutaneous Pharmacology and Toxicology Center, North Carolina State University, Raleigh, North Carolina 27606.

Models for Assessing Drug Absorption and Metabolism, Ronald T. Borchardt *et al.*, eds., Plenum Press, New York, 1996.

lent themselves to perfusion techniques because of both an easily isolatable vascular supply and a "closed" anatomical structure (encapsulated or surrounded by serosa) amenable to perfusion. The skin does not possess either of these attributes. There have been sporadic reports of perfused skin studies in the literature (Feldberg and Paton, 1951; Kjaersgaard, 1954; Hiernickel, 1985), but no model has been fully developed and validated for transdermal drug delivery studies. Based on this lack of a suitable model, our laboratory developed an isolated perfused porcine skin flap (IPPSF) in 1984 specifically as a tool to study transdermal drug delivery and cutaneous toxicology (Riviere *et al.*, 1986; Monteiro-Riviere *et al.*, 1987). Since that time, some additional isolated perfused models have been described, including a perfused human skin flap (Kreidstein *et al.*, 1991), a perfused human tumor-bearing skin flap (Vaden *et al.*, 1993), perfused rabbit (Behrendt and Kampffmeyer, 1989; Celesti *et al.*, 1993) or pig (de Lange *et al.*, 1992) ears, and a perfused bovine udder (Kietzmann *et al.*, 1991). Although the perfused ear has recently been used by some investigators, we feel that a major limitation relates to the anatomical heterogeneity inherent to a preparation which, in addition to containing skin and fat, also includes perfused cartilage and muscle. This would add an additional level of complexity in defining pharmacokinetic models and interpreting release of biomarkers secondary to toxicosis or irritation. Additionally, because of its role in thermal regulation, the vasculature of the ear is different from that of other body sites, a fact reflected in the higher blood flow seen in ears of most species (Monteiro-Riviere *et al.*, 1990). It is thus our group's opinion that a more defined preparation is needed for an optimal model to be developed. The IPPSF will serve as a case example of perfused skin preparations. Methodology related to its use in studying transdermal drug delivery will be stressed, and the reader is referred to recent review articles for other uses of this model in toxicology (Monteiro-Riviere, 1992; Riviere and Monteiro-Riviere, 1991).

2. METHODS

The limitations inherent to perfusing skin may be overcome if a two-stage reconstructive surgical procedure is utilized to create a "closed" skin preparation with an easily isolatable vasculature. When such a tubed, pedicle flap is employed, skin may be perfused under ambient environmental conditions without concern about dermal dehydration. Such preparations may then be harvested by cannulating the artery, thus removing the confounding influence of systemic metabolic processes. The caudal superficial epigastric artery perfusing the abdominal skin of swine is ideally suited for this purpose.

2.1. Surgery

The IPPSF is a single-pedicle, axial-pattern tubed skin flap obtained from the ventral abdomen of female weanling Yorkshire swine (*Sus scrofa*). Two flaps per animal, each lateral to the ventral midline, can be created in a single surgical procedure. As depicted in Fig. 1, the procedure involves two steps; creation of the flap in stage I and harvest in stage II (Riviere *et al.*, 1986; Bowman *et al.*, 1991). Briefly, pigs weighing approximately 20–30 kg are premedicated with atropine sulfate and xylazine hydrochloride, anesthesia is induced with ketamine hydrochloride, and inhalational anesthesia is maintained with halothane. Each pig is prepared for routine

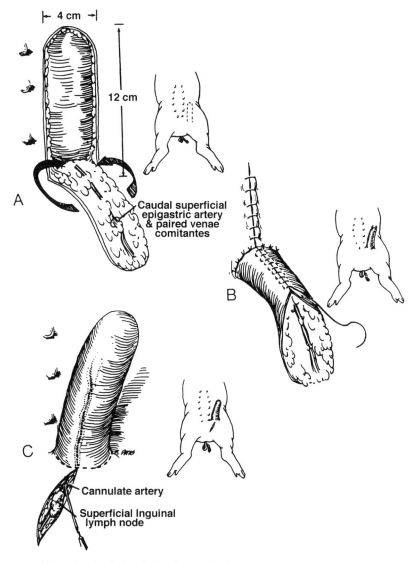

Figure 1. Surgical technique for creating isolated perfused porcine skin flaps.

aseptic surgery in the caudal abdominal and inguinal regions. A 4 cm × 12 cm area of skin, known from previous dissection and *in vivo* angiography studies, has been shown to be perfused primarily by the caudal superficial epigastric artery and its associated paired venae comitantes. Following incision and scalpel dissection of the subcutaneous tissue, the caudal incision is apposed and sutured, and the tubed skin flap edges are trimmed of fat and closed. Two days later, a second surgical procedure is used to cannulate the artery and harvest each of these skin flaps. The two-day period between flap creation and harvest was determined to be optimal from the standpoint of lack of viability, overall flap leakiness, normal histologic appearance, normal vascularization, and animal housing economics. The IPPSF is then transferred to the perfusion chamber illustrated in Fig. 2. The wound is flushed and allowed to heal, and pigs are generally returned to the housing facility.

2.2. Isolated Perfusion Technique

The isolated perfusion apparatus is a custom-designed temperature- and humidity-regulated chamber made specifically for this purpose. Perfusion pressure, flow, pH, and temperature are monitored. Flexibility is afforded in the experimental design by allowing both temperature and relative humidity (RH) to be maintained at specific set points (normally 37°C and 60–80% RH). The perfusion medium is a Krebs–Ringer bicarbonate buffer (pH 7.4, 350 mosmol/kg), containing albumin (45 g/l) (both to mimic *in vivo* plasma and to facilitate absorption of lipid-soluble penetrants) and supplied with glucose (80–120 mg/dl) as the primary energy source. Normal perfusate flow through the skin flap is maintained at 1 ml/min per flap (3–7 ml/min per 100 g) with a mean arterial pressure ranging from 30–70 mm Hg. These values are consistent with *in vivo* values reported in the literature. Both recirculating and nonrecirculating (single-pass) configurations are possible (Monteiro-Riviere, 1990).

2.3. Assessment of Viability

To date, our laboratory has perfused over 2200 IPPSFs. Viability has been assessed by monitoring perfusate flow, pressure, vascular resistance, pH, glucose utilization (arterial–venous glucose extraction), lactate production, and enzyme leakage. Viability for up to 24 hr has been confirmed through biochemical studies and extensive light- and electron-microscopic histological studies (Monteiro-Riviere *et al.*, 1987). In addition, specific biomarkers of inflammation, including prostaglandins and leukotrienes, have also been assessed in order to monitor chemical-induced irritation (Monteiro-Riviere, 1992; Srikrishna *et al.*, 1992; Zhang *et al.*, 1995a,b) and phototoxicity (Monteiro-Riviere *et al.*, 1994).

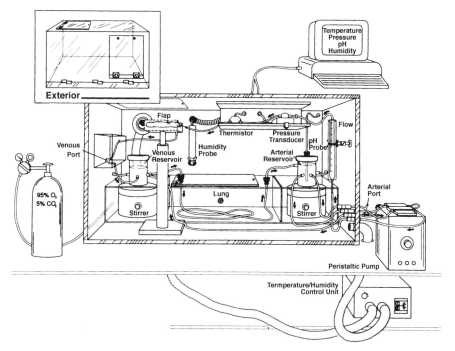

Figure 2. Perfusion chamber.

2.4. Design of Percutaneous Absorption and Transdermal Drug Delivery Studies

Percutaneous absorption studies are conducted by placing the study chemical on the surface of the IPPSF and assaying the venous effluent over time for absorbed compound. Compound may be applied neat or diluted in vehicle under ambient or occluded conditions. Various types of patches or transdermal delivery systems may also be employed. A relatively large dosing area of up to 10 cm^2 is available for compound application and is a major advantage of this system. IPPSFs are usually allowed to equilibrate for 1–2 hr prior to compound application. When experiments are designed to model uptake of compound from perfusate into skin (systemic distribution, outward transdermal migration, inverse penetration, etc.), drug is added to the arterial reservoir and infused into the IPPSF. Analysis of the venous efflux profile allows one to then study the kinetics of cutaneous uptake using pharmacokinetic models described below.

2.5. Data Analysis

The primary types of investigations conducted using the IPPSF are related to assessing the transdermal flux of a topically applied compound. Figures 3–5 depict an example of the kind of data typically collected. From the perspective of data analysis, one may represent the venous effluent fluxes as either individual flap data (Fig. 3), mean and variance of individual time points (Fig. 4), or as a variance envelope across all times (Fig. 5). It is best to plot the values on the dependent axis in flux units of either mass per unit time or % dose per unit time. Although perfusate flow is relatively constant and some prefer using concentration units alone, this method results in a loss of precision because it does not account for changes in flow. Depending on the experimental circumstances, one may also analyze paired treatment data for two IPPSFs from the same pig, where one flap is control (neat drug) and the other is the experimental treatment (e.g., enhancer). In such cases, a nested analysis may be appropriate.

There are two methods available to assess cumulative flux. The first is simply to sum all fluxes at each time interval (Σ mass/time), or, alternatively, one can determine the area under the flux versus time curve. Both of these methods give the cumulative amount of drug that has been absorbed into the perfusate. If the terminal perfusate flux is not down to baseline, suggesting that absorption is not complete, then a pharmacokinetic analysis of the data may allow extrapolation to later time points. It must be stressed that analysis of the venous perfusate allows *only* estimation of the amount of

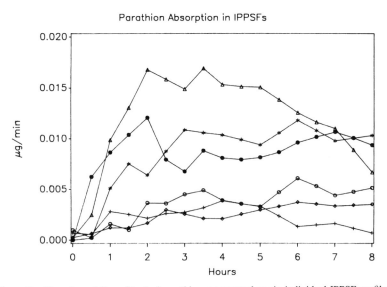

Figure 3. Transdermal flux of topical parathion represented as six individual IPPSF profiles.

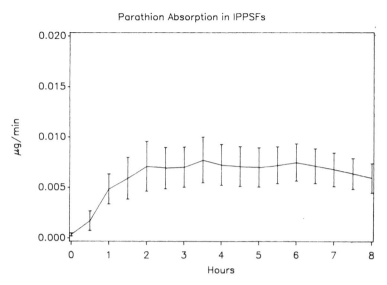

Figure 4. Transdermal flux of topical parathion plotted as mean ± standard error of six IPPSFs.

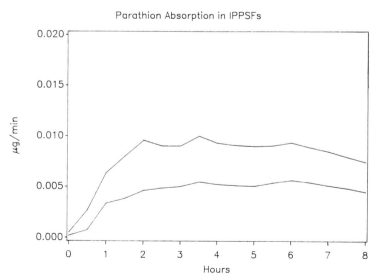

Figure 5. Transdermal flux of topical parathion presented as a variance envelope of two standard errors.

drug that has entered the vascular system. In many cases, significant amount of drug is retained in various levels of the skin.

There are a number of methods to assess this amount of *penetrated* but not *absorbed* drug, depending on the precision of the answer required relative to intracutaneous localization and available analytical techniques for determination of drug concentrations. Most of the studies designed to assess drug disposition within the skin use radiolabeled (preferably with a metabolically stable ^{14}C label) compound. The first step is to quantitate how much drug was left on the surface of the skin. This is usually quantitated by swabbing the surface with an appropriate detergent solution and then counting the activity in these rinses. This author strongly recommends against the use of a solvent (e.g., ethanol, acetone) to "wipe" the surface of the skin as instead one may in fact be promoting further absorption of surface chemical through a penetration-enhancing effect of the solvent (Williams *et al.*, 1994). If an application device is used, this must also be counted for mass balance. If the compound is volatile, either a trap may be used or this fraction of dose must just be discounted. Again, this depends upon the experimental design since use of trapping techniques (flowing air across the application site or occluding it) may significantly alter penetration by altering skin hydration and temperature (Chang and Riviere, 1991, 1993). There is also considerable debate about what one does with this nonabsorbed surface dose in the final calculations. Some workers believe that it should be subtracted from the applied dose since it was not absorbed. However, most, including the present author, feel that it is just the residual dose that was not absorbed and should *not* be considered as being "unavailable for absorption" at the beginning of the study because all events, including skin penetration, evaporation, and dose–device binding, are actually competing kinetic events driven by the applied dose.

Once the skin surface has been "cleaned," many options are available. The first is to just digest the entire IPPSF and count this as penetrated drug. Alternatively, the surface may be "stripped" with cellophane adhesive tape to estimate stratum corneum concentrations. The remaining epidermis and dermis may be separated to independently quantify drug penetration in these areas. The most precise way to accomplish this is to take a core biopsy of the stripped dosing site, snap freeze it with liquid nitrogen, and, using a cryostat, take serial sections. Each section is then digested and counted so that the resulting disk then represents drug concentrations in a specifically localized area of skin. This technique has been employed in our laboratory (Riviere *et al.*, 1992a).

Because the IPPSF is an isolated and closed system, more extensive sampling and collateral data collection is possible. That is, in parallel to assessing drug absorption, one may also monitor physiological or biochemical parameters, measure inflammatory mediator production secondary to drug irritation, or directly sample tissue for drug concentrations or morphological assessment of irritation. If the endpoint of a drug's activity is within the skin, then measured concentrations may be directly correlated *in the same tissue preparation* with indices of biological effect. This approach has recently been adopted with studies of chemical vesicants, where in addition to monitoring chemical penetration and distribution within skin, assessments of markers of vascular perfusion and histological endpoints of vesication and biochemical assays of inflammatory mediator production were simultaneously performed. This is a unique advantage of such an isolated perfused system.

2.6. Pharmacokinetic Modeling and *in Vitro* to *in Vivo* Extrapolation

There are a number of areas in which pharmacokinetics may be applied to IPPSF experiments. These may be principally broken down into two applications: (1) prediction of *in vivo* percutaneous absorption, and (2) defining quantitative endpoints for experiments designed to study the mechanisms of chemical and drug penetration and absorption. In some cases experiments may be designed to address both simultaneously.

The primary difference between the type of modeling approach used relates to whether the emphasis of the study is to predict a drug serum concentration–time profile using the IPPSF "efflux" profile as the "input" profile for a systemic pharmacokinetic model, or alternatively whether the focus is on identifying the processes within skin that are responsible for producing a specific efflux profile. A knowledge of the shape of this flux profile (mass/time over time) is sufficient to predict *in vivo* absorption. This can either be determined experimentally (see Fig. 6) or be simulated using the mean profile from an IPPSF-based dermatopharmacokinetic model.

The basic strategy is outlined in Fig. 6 and has been fully described in the literature. The IPPSF profile simply serves as a variable input into the central compartment of a classic systemic pharmacokinetic model or the circulatory system of a physiological-based pharmacokinetic model. This can best be visualized by considering the IPPSF as a "living infusion pump." This approach also works if the compound is metabolized within the skin, in which case parent drug and metabolite fluxes are now used as multiple inputs into the systemic model. A problem with this approach relates to the statistics of integrating the IPPSF efflux profile with the systemic pharmacokinetic data. The original approach involved using the mean ± SEM of the input flux profile and the mean ± SEM of the volume of distribution and the elimination rate constant (K_{el}) of a one-compartment pharmacokinetic model (Riviere *et al.*, 1992b). For some drugs such as iontophoretically delivered luteinizing hormone-releasing hormone (LHRH; Heit *et al.*, 1993), this approach overestimated the width of the observed *in vivo* serum concentration–time window despite accurately predicting the mean profile (Fig. 7). Our laboratory has found a superior approach which produces predicted serum concentration–time profile envelopes closer to those observed *in vivo*. We term this the "full space" method (Williams and Riviere, 1994). This method assumes that the cutaneous input function is independent of the drug's systemic disposition. To use this technique, one simulates all possible

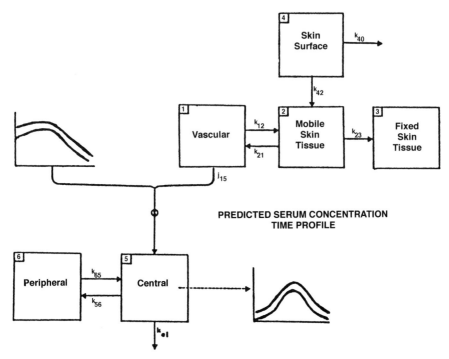

Figure 6. Pharmacokinetic strategy for coupling IPPSF profile (*top left*) or model-predicted fluxes (*top right*) with systemic pharmacokinetics to predict a serum concentration–time profile.

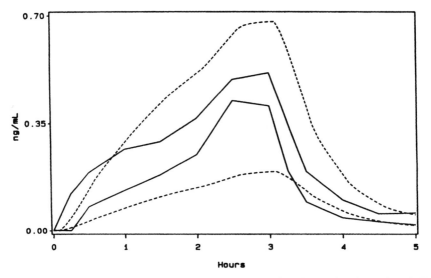

Figure 7. IPPSF predicted vs. observed *in vivo* plasma concentration–time profile of iontophoretically delivered LHRH in pigs.

combinations of IPPSF input profiles onto all individual systemic pharmacokinetic parameters. For example, assume that one had 6 IPPSF profiles and 8 individual systemic pharmacokinetic data sets. A full simulation would result in 48 different predicted serum concentration–time profiles. The mean ± SEM of these would then be calculated to produce an estimated *in vivo* concentration–time envelope. This model is especially useful when the systemic pharmacokinetic model is more complex as it was with the LHRH example above. A strength of these methods is that they are robust relative to the nature of the pharmacokinetic model used to describe the systemic data and are particularly useful in drug development studies where the goal is to predict *in vivo* behavior. In these cases, the IPPSF data is used to assess the cutaneous input function while intravenous pharmacokinetic studies in humans are used for the systemic functions. This eliminates the need for human volunteers in early preclinical dosage formulation trials.

More complex pharmacokinetics are encountered when the goal of a study is to assess the mechanisms of drug absorption and distribution within the skin. In these cases, the IPPSF venous efflux profile is analyzed in order to gain insight into the biophysical and physiological processes in skin that acted on the topically applied drug to produce a profile of the observed shape. In order to create pharmacokinetic models with relatively unique solutions, we initiated this work using studies where drug was infused into the arterial system of the IPPSF and disposition into the skin was modeled based on an analysis of the arterial and venous drug concentration gradient over time (Williams and Riviere, 1989a). This first pharmacokinetic model describing drug movement from the vasculature into the extracellular and intracellular compartments was shown to be mathematically identifiable. Actual volumes of physiological spaces were then estimated using inulin and albumin infusion studies (Williams and Riviere, 1989b). This utilization of multiple biological markers in the same preparation is another strength of this model.

The next step was to add an absorption component from the surface of the skin. A typical model is illustrated at the top right of Fig. 6 (Carver *et al.*, 1989; Williams *et al.*, 1990). In order to optimize modeling and restrict the solution space, additional samples other than perfusate, as described in Section 2.5 above (tape strips, core biopsies, etc.), may also be analyzed at the termination of an experiment. The complexity of the resulting model will be dependent upon the number and nature of the samples collected. Similarly, if parent drug and metabolites are analyzed, a metabolism component must be incorporated into the model. Such a complex model, incorporating both IPPSF and *in vivo* pharmacokinetics, is presented in the discussion of the pesticide application below (Section 3.1). Another area that has received attention is the role of the vasculature on the percutaneous absorption and transdermal delivery of drugs. Dermatopharmacokinetic modeling is especially useful for such studies because the vascular compartments may be quantitatively studied.

Finally, it is widely acknowledged that penetration of a topically applied compound through the stratum corneum is often the rate-limiting step in percutaneous absorption. The latest focus of IPPSF pharmacokinetic studies is to specifically incorporate principles of lipid biophysics into the absorption components of the model. Additionally, it is known that the penetration of a chemical is often very dependent upon the vehicle used to apply the drug. The vehicle may interact with the drug at multiple levels of the absorption process by various mechanisms ranging from surface evaporation, partitioning into the stratum corneum lipids, and altering the diffusional resistance of the drug through the lipid barrier to affecting the cutaneous biotransformation of metabolized drugs. Figure 8 depicts our initial attempt to incorporate these principles into a more biophysically and physiologically realistic model (Williams and Riviere, 1995). The drawback to this approach is that significantly more experiments are required to obtain reasonable estimates of its many parameters. For many chemicals , all components of the model may not be necessary. Many of the parameters are also estimated using independent *in vitro* studies conducted in porcine skin (Williams *et al.*, 1994). By using this approach, even small differences between porcine and human skin could be incorporated into the appropriate component of the model.

The major advantage of this approach is that the model is constructed based upon the mechanism of interaction between a penetrating chemical and the skin. The model is essentially used as a tool to quantitate this interaction. Most steps in the model are experimentally verifiable due to the unique sampling access inherent to the IPPSF. The model also lends itself directly to developing linked pharmacodynamic models since the pharmacokinetic models will establish drug concentration profiles in specific compartments and many drug effects can be simultaneously evaluated. Work on defining relevant vascular pharmacodynamic endpoints has begun (Rogers and Riviere, 1994). Finally, we are presently extending the binary penetrant/solvent modeling approach to more complex mixtures selected on the basis of having a mechanism of action that could alter a compound's absorption. This approach, which we term mechanistically defined chemical mixtures (MDCM), will be a direct extension of the binary model and will identify the type of components of a topical mixture that could significantly affect the absorption of an active chemical. There are direct applications of this approach to the topical formulation field.

3.   APPLICATIONS

As discussed in Section 1, the IPPSF system has been used in numerous applications in percutaneous absorption and cutaneous toxicology. The two most pertinent and illustrative examples relate to the absorption and biotransformation of pesticides and studies in iontophoretic drug delivery.

3.1.   Passive Percutaneous Absorption and Biotransformation of Pesticides

One of the major applications of the IPPSF has been in the field of pesticide toxicology, specifically in assessing systemic exposure after topical application.

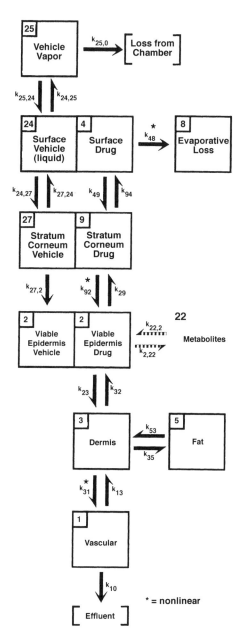

Figure 8. Dermatopharmacokinetic model coupling chemical and vehicle absorption parameters. Output of the model is into the IPPSF venous effluent.

Initial studies utilized a simple multicompartmental model to assess the absorption of ^{14}C-labeled malathion and parathion in a recirculating IPPSF configuration. Using pharmacokinetic models fitted to 8-hr IPPSF experiments, this system accurately predicted *in vivo* 6-day total absorption in pigs (Carver *et al.*, 1989). When the more physiologically relevant modeling approach, similar to that depicted in Fig. 6, was used, the IPPSF precisely predicted the *in vivo* data [parathion: 5.9% vs. 5.2%; malathion: 6.6% vs. 6.4% (IPPSF vs. *in vivo*); Williams *et al.*, 1990]. In fact, for a series of seven diverse compounds, the correlation coefficient between IPPSF and *in vivo* pig absorption was high ($R^2 = 0.95$). Similarly, the correlation between IPPSF predicted and reported *in vivo* human absorption for a series of eight compounds [benzoic acid, caffeine, carbaryl, diisopropyl fluorophosphidate (DFP), malathion, parathion, progesterone, and testosterone] was excellent ($R^2 = 0.94$), supporting the utility of not only the IPPSF, but also the pig, to predict percutaneous absorption in humans. Additional studies have also modeled the percutaneous absorption of paraquat (Srikrishna *et al.*, 1992) and carbaryl, lindane, malathion, and parathion (Chang *et al.*, 1994b) in nonrecirculating IPPSF systems. These studies have clearly demonstrated the applicability of the IPPSF to predict the percutaneous absorption of a wide variety of pesticides in humans.

The most exciting aspects of the pesticide work done to date reflect on the metabolism of the pesticides in the skin. Work has focused on the biotransformation of parathion to paraoxon and ρ-nitrophenol (Carver *et al.*, 1990; Chang *et al.*, 1994a) and carbaryl to naphthyl (Chang *et al.*, 1994b). Initial studies indicated that the method of application (occluded vs. nonoccluded) was important because the fraction of absorbed parathion metabolized was increased under occlusive dressings. After confirming these findings with classical *in vitro* flow-through diffusion cell studies (Riviere and Chang, 1992), we then created an integrated *in vitro–in vivo* pharmacokinetic model which described the absorption and cutaneous metabolism of parathion in pigs (Qiao and Riviere, 1995; Qiao *et al.*, 1994). As can be seen in Fig. 9, the approach is very similar to that discussed in Section 2.6, where the skin and systemic phases of the model are clearly separated. In this cases, the IPPSF and other *in vitro* data were used to determine the structure of the skin component of the overall model. Although parathion was dosed, *in vitro* studies determined that there is always a ρ-nitrophenol contaminant present which must be accounted for, or otherwise metabolism would be overestimated. This is made more complicated by the finding that ρ-nitrophenol is absorbed faster than parathion and actually enhances parathion absorption (Chang *et al.*, 1994a). Unless these *in vitro* data were explicitly included in the model, the determination of the amount of parathion that was metabolized in skin would be confounded by the topical ρ-nitrophenol influx. This model also illustrates that for a topically applied compound that is metabolized by skin, fluxes of parent drug and metabolites must be used as inputs into the systemic model.

In the complete model presented, both topical and intravenous parathion experiments were conducted, with serum, urine, and tissues being analyzed for parent drug and metabolites. The structure of the model was then validated in independent

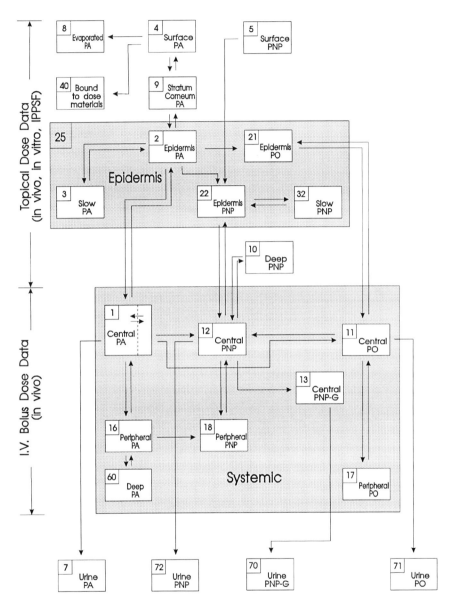

Figure 9. Comprehensive pharmacokinetic model of parathion absorption and disposition in pigs, illustrating complexity encountered when biotransformation occurs both systemically and in the skin (PA, parathion; PO, paraoxon; PNP, para-nitrophenol; PNP-G, PNP-glucuronide).

intravenous ρ-nitrophenol experiments. Note that we could not detect glucuronidation of ρ-nitrophenol in skin and thus could only attribute glucuronide formation to systemic biotransformation. Although the construction and experimental validation of such hybrid *in vitro–in vivo* models is costly and labor intensive, it is the only approach possible if one is interested in studying cutaneous biotransformation independent of systemic effects. In this study, the finding of increased cutaneous metabolism secondary to occlusion was confirmed at two separate body sites (back and IPPSF abdomen site). Additionally, site differences in both the extent of absorption and percent metabolized were detected. These findings would have significant impact on the design and interpretation of more limited single-site/single-mode-of-application *in vivo* and *in vitro* studies.

3.2. Iontophoresis

Another area that has received significant attention has been quantification of the transdermal iontophoretic delivery of drugs. The IPPSF iontophoretic experiments with arbutamine in humans (Riviere *et al.*, 1992b), LHRH in pigs (Heit *et al.*, 1993), and a number of other proprietary molecules in humans clearly demonstrate the ability of this model to accurately predict serum concentration–time profiles in humans. It was largely in these studies that the techniques discussed in Section 2.6 above for *in vitro–in vivo* extrapolations were developed.

It was this research that led to the characterization of the importance of the cutaneous vasculature in predicting *in vivo* drug delivery for vasoactive compounds. In an initial set of studies using lidocaine as a model drug, we demonstrated that co-iontophoresis of a vasoactive compound modulated the transdermal flux of lidocaine *in vivo* and in the IPPSF (Fig. 10) but not in avascular *in vitro* systems (Riviere *et al.*, 1991). This ultimately led to the realization that modulation of the cutaneous vasculature could have a significant impact on transdermal flux of drugs (Riviere and Williams, 1992). To quantitate these effects in skin, a specific pharmacokinetic model (Fig. 11) was then reported (Williams and Riviere, 1993). As with other models, the output (K_{10}) may serve as the input for predicting systemic profiles as depicted in Fig. 6.

It is appropriate at this conjecture to make a comment about our pharmacokinetic modeling philosophy. In order to make data between these vastly different experimental conditions (pesticides vs. active transdermal delivery) comparable, the pharmacokinetic models used have the same underlying structure so that advances made in one area (e.g., metabolism or lipid interactions with pesticides; vascular activity with iontophoresis) will aid interpretation of another. However, when actually modeling one specific effect, the model is generally collapsed to contain only the relevant components for the study at hand.

The crux of these studies with iontophoretic delivery of vasoactive drugs

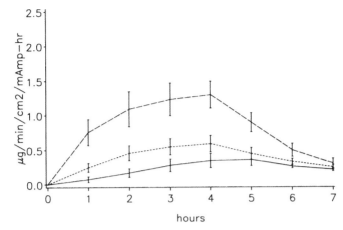

Figure 10. IPPSF venous efflux profiles of iontophoretically delivered lidocaine HCl administered alone (———) or with the vasodilator tolazoline (—————) or the vasoconstrictor norepinephrine (————).

suggests that the effect of vascular modulation on transdermal drug delivery relates to the volume of perfused dermal tissue which is available for absorbing drug that has penetrated the epidermal barrier. This so-called involved capillary surface area (ICSA) can be increased by capillary recruitment or decreased by shunting secondary to modulation of arterial-venous anastomoses function (Williams and Riviere, 1995). As demonstrated in vasoactive drug infusion studies (Rogers and Riviere, 1994), both of these effects are possible depending on the vasoactive drug's mechanism of action and degree of vasomotor tone present in the tissue. These effects may significantly

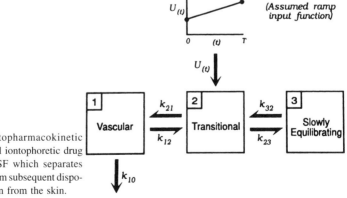

Figure 11. Dermatopharmacokinetic model of transdermal iontophoretic drug delivery in the IPPSF which separates electrode delivery from subsequent disposition and elimination from the skin.

alter the shape of the IPPSF venous efflux profile. For rapidly delivered iontophoretic drugs or labile biological molecules, such changes in cutaneous residence time may significantly affect the achieved serum concentration–time profile and even biological effect.

The IPPSF has now been adopted by a number of pharmaceutical companies as a preclinical screen for the development of human transdermal iontophoretic systems and by a contract research organization for cutaneous toxicology. It has also been used to investigate the irritation associated with passive chemical and active iontophoretic drug delivery (including electroporation). In this mode, markers of irritation may be assessed simultaneously with the determination of cutaneous and transdermal drug fluxes and, at the end of the experiment, with morphological markers of cutaneous damage. As increased numbers of drugs are studied under similar experimental conditions, molecular factors required for optimal iontophoretic delivery for a number of different classes of drugs (e.g., organics, peptides, oligonucleotides) are being identified. Similarly, the reaction of skin to this myriad of drug and delivery conditions is being defined.

4. ADVANTAGES AND DISADVANTAGES OF THE IPPSF

As one can appreciate from the above discussion, the IPPSF has been developed to specifically occupy a niche between classic *in vitro* excised skin culture and/or diffusion cell systems and *in vivo* studies. This juxtaposition results in it having similar advantages and disadvantages to both.

The major advantages relate to the fact that the IPPSF is an *in vitro* isolated system which has the experimental access and control inherent to other *in vitro* systems but maintains some of the broad range of biological functions normally only found in *in vivo* systems. Based upon the studies reviewed above, in most cases the model is predictive of the *in vivo* data but does not have the associated confounding factors. A wide range of experimental designs are possible with the IPPSF, and different endpoints (drug flux, biomarkers of irritation, histology) may be monitored in the same preparation. Most transdermal systems are compatible with the model. The model is also an accepted alternative humane animal model. Finally, the development of integrated pharmacokinetic models at all stages of development allows data obtained in the IPPSF to be easily extrapolated to humans.

The major disadvantages are a direct extension of the complexity of the IPPSF. These relate to the surgical expertise required to create the preparation, animal housing needs, and perfusion equipment and expertise. We have routinely designated college-trained technicians, *without* prior surgery experience, to perform all of the surgery. It must be noted that microsurgical expertise is *not* required. A supervised training period of one month is generally adequate. The actual cost of an experiment is similar to that of an *in vivo* pig or dog study. An IPPSF study is more expensive than an excised skin *in vitro* study, only slightly more expensive than some human skin-equivalent studies, and significantly less expensive than any *in vivo* human study. Certain surface skin manipulations that result in loss of epidermal integrity (punctures, aspiration) cannot be done during an experiment, since with the IPPSF, unlike intact animals, clotting does not occur and leakage ensues. However, this limitation is shared by all *in vitro* models.

In conclusion, the IPPSF is a sophisticated isolated tissue preparation that occupies a unique niche in the hierarchy of experimental models related to skin absorption. Its main advantage is its similarity to the *in vivo* situation while maintaining the access and control of an *in vitro* system.

ACKNOWLEDGMENTS

The author wishes to acknowledge the technical and intellectual input of Drs. Nancy Monteiro, Patrick Williams, and Karl Bowman, whose collaborations were essential to the development of this model.

REFERENCES

Behrendt, H., and Kampffmeyer, H. G., 1989, Absorption and ester cleavage of methyl salicylate by skin of single-pass perfused rabbit ears, *Xenobiotica* **19**:131–141.

Bowman, K. F., Montero-Riviere, N. A., and Riviere, J. E., 1991, Development of surgical techniques for preparation of *in vitro* isolated perfused porcine skin flaps for percutaneous absorption studies, *Am. J. Vet. Res.* **25**:75–82.

Carver, M. P., Williams, P. L., and Riviere, J. E., 1989, The isolated perfused porcine skin flap (IPPSF). III. Percutaneous absorption pharmacokinetics of organophosphates, steroids, benzoic acid and caffeine, *Toxicol. Appl. Pharmacol.* **97**:324–337.

Carver, M. P., Levi, P. E., and Riviere, J. E., 1990, Parathion metabolism during percutaneous absorption in perfused porcine skin. *Pestic. Biochem. Physiol.* **38**:245–254.

Celesti, L., Murratzu, C., Valoti, M., Sgaragli, G., and Corti, P., 1993, The single-pass perfused rabbit ear as a model for studying percutaneous absorption of clonazepam, *Methods Find. Exp. Clin. Pharmacol.* **15**:49–56.

Chang, S. K., and Riviere, J. E., 1991, Percutaneous absorption of parathion *in vitro* in porcine skin. Effects of dose, temperature, humidity and perfusate composition on absorptive flux, *Fundam. Appl. Toxicol.* **17**:494–504.

Chang, S. K., and Riviere, J. E., 1993, Effect of humidity and occlusion on the percutaneous absorption of parathion *in vitro*, *Pharm. Res.* **10**:152–155.

Chang, S. K., Dauterman, W. C., and Riviere, J. E., 1994a, Percutaneous absorption of parathion and its metabolites paraoxon and *p*-nitrophenol administered alone or in combination: *In vitro* flow through diffusion cell system, *Pestic. Biochem. Physiol.* **48**:56–62.

Chang, S. K., Williams, P. L., Dauterman, W. C., and Riviere, J. E., 1994b, Percutaneous absorption, dermatopharmacokinetics, and related biotransformation studies of carbaryl, lindane, malathion and parathion in isolated perfused porcine skin, *Toxicology* **91**:269–280.

de Lange, J., van Eck, P., Elliott, G. R., de Kort, W. L. A. M., and Wolthius, O. L., 1992, The isolated blood-perfused pig ear: An inexpensive and animal saving model for skin penetration studies, *J. Pharmacol. Toxicol. Methods* **27**:71–77.

Feldberg, W., and Paton, W. D. M., 1951, Release of histamine from skin and muscle in the cat by opium alkaloids and other histamine liberators, *J. Physiol.* **114:**490–509.

Heit, M., Williams, P., Jayes, F. L., Chang, S. K., and Riviere, J. E., 1993, Transdermal iontophoretic peptide delivery. *In vitro* and *in vivo* studies with luteinizing hormone releasing hormone (LHRH), *J. Pharm. Sci.* **82:**240–243.

Hiernickel, H., 1985, An improved method for *in vitro* perfusion of human skin, *Br. J. Dermatol.* **112:** 299–305.

Kietzmann, M., Arens, D., Loscher, W., and Lubach, D., 1991, Studies on the percutaneous absorption of dexamethasone using a new *in vitro* model, the isolated perfused bovine udder, in: *Prediction of Percutaneous Penetration* (R. C. Scott, R. H. Guy, J. Hadgraft, and H. E. Bodee, eds.), IBC Technical Services, Ltd., London, pp. 519–526.

Kjaersgaard, A. R., 1954, Perfusion of isolated dog skin, *J. Invest. Dermatol.* **22:**135–141.

Kreidstein, M. L., Pang, C. Y., Levine, R. H., and Knowlton, R. J., 1991, The isolated perfused human skin flap: Design, perfusion technique, metabolism and vascular reactivity, *Plast. Reconstr. Surg.* **87:** 741–749.

Monteiro-Riviere, N. A., 1990. Specialized technique: The isolated perfused porcine skin flap (IPPSF), in: *Methods for Skin Absorption* (B. W. Kemppainen and W. G. Reifenrath, eds.), CRC Press, Boca Raton, Florida, pp. 175–189.

Monteiro-Riviere, N. A., 1992, Use of isolated perfused skin model in dermatotoxicology, *In Vitro Toxicol.* **5:**219–233.

Monteiro-Riviere, N. A., Bowman, K. F., Scheidt, V. J., and Riviere, J. E., 1987, The isolated perfused porcine skin flap (IPPSF): II. Ultrastructural and histological characterization of epidermal viability, *In Vitro* Toxicol. **1:**241–252.

Monteiro-Riviere, N. A., Bristol, D. G., Manning, T. O., Rogers, R. A., and Riviere, J. E., 1990, Interspecies and interregional analysis of the comparative histological thickness and laser Doppler blood flow measurements at five cutaneous sites in nine species, *J. Invest. Dermatol.* **95:**582–586.

Monteiro-Riviere, N. A., Inman, A. O., and Riviere, J. E., 1994, Development and characterization of a novel skin model for phototoxicology, *Photodermatol, Photoimmunol. Photomed.* **11:**235–243.

Qiao, G. L., and Riviere, J. E., 1995, Significant effects of application site and occlusion on the pharmacokinetics of cutaneous penetration and biotransformation of parathion *in vivo* in swine, *J. Pharm. Sci.* **84:**425–432.

Qiao, G. L., Williams, P. L., and Riviere, J. E., 1994, Percutaneous absorption, biotransformation and systemic disposition of parathion *in vivo* in swine. I. Comprehensive pharmacokinetic model, *Drug Metab. Dispos.* **22:**459–471.

Riviere, J. E., and Chang, S., 1992, Transdermal penetration and metabolism of organophosphate insecticides, in: *Organophosphates: Chemistry, Fate and Effects* (J. E. Chambers and P. L. Levi, eds.), Academic Press, New York, pp. 241–253.

Riviere, J. E., and Monteiro-Riviere, N. A., 1991, The isolated perfused porcine skin flap as an *in vitro* model for percutaneous absorption and cutaneous toxicology, *Crit. Rev. Toxicol.* **21:**329–344.

Riviere, J. E., and Williams, P. L., 1992, Pharmacokinetic implications of changing blood flow in skin, *J. Pharm. Sci.* **81:**601–602.

Riviere, J. E., Bowman, K. F., Monteiro-Riviere, N. A., Carver, M. P., and Dix, L. P., 1986, The isolated perfused porcine skin flap (IPPSF). I. A novel *in vitro* model for percutaneous absorption and cutaneous toxicology studies, *Fundam. Appl. Toxicol.* **7:**444–453.

Riviere, J. E., Sage, B. S., and Williams, P. L., 1991, The effects of vasoactive drugs on transdermal lidocaine iontophoresis, *J. Pharm. Sci.* **80:**615–620.

Riviere, J. E., Monteiro-Riviere, N. A., and Inman, A. O., 1992a, Determination of lidocaine concentration in skin after transdermal iontophoresis: Effects of vasoactive drugs, *Pharm. Res.* **9:**211–214.

Riviere, J. E., Williams, P. L., Hillman, R., and Mishky, L., 1992b, Quantitative prediction of transdermal iontophoretic delivery of arbutamine in humans using the *in vitro* isolated perfused porcine skin flap (IPPSF), *J. Pharm. Sci.* **81:**504–507.

Rogers, R. A., and Riviere, J. E., 1994, Pharmacologic modulation of cutaneous vascular resistance in the isolated perfused porcine skin flap (IPPSF), *J. Pharm. Sci.* **83:**1682–1689.

Srikrishna, V., Riviere, J. E., and Monteiro-Riviere, N. A., 1992, Cutaneous toxicity and absorption of paraquat in porcine skin, *Toxicol. Appl. Pharmacol.* **115:**89–97.

Vaden, S. L., Page, R. L., Peters, B. P., Cline, J. M., and Riviere, J. E., 1993, Development and characterization of an isolated and perfused tumor and skin preparation for evaluation of drug disposition, *Cancer Res.* **53:**101–105.

Williams, P. L., and Riviere, J. E., 1989a, Definition of a physiologic pharmacokinetic model of cutaneous drug distribution using the isolated perfused porcine skin flap (IPPSF), *J. Pharm. Sci.* **78:**550–555.

Williams, P. L., and Riviere, J. E., 1989b, Estimation of physiological volumes in the isolated perfused porcine skin flap, *Res. Commun. Chem. Pathol. Pharmacol.* **66:**145–158.

Williams, P. L., and Riviere, J. E., 1993, A model describing transdermal iontophoretic delivery of lidocaine incorporating consideration of cutaneous microvascular state, *J. Pharm. Sci.* **82:**1080–1084.

Williams, P. L., and Riviere, J. E., 1994, A "full-space" method for predicting *in vivo* transdermal plasma drug profiles reflecting both cutaneous and systemic variability, *J. Pharm. Sci.* **83:**1062–1064.

Williams, P. L., and Riviere, J. E., 1995, A biophysically-based dermatopharmacokinetic compartment model for quantifying percutaneous penetration and absorption of topically applied agents. I. Theory, *J. Pharm. Sci.* **84:**599–608.

Williams, P. L., Carver, M. P., and Riviere, J. E., 1990, A physiologically relevant pharmacokinetic model of xenobiotic percutaneous absorption utilizing the isolated perfused porcine skin flap (IPPSF), *J. Pharm. Sci.* **79:**305–311.

Williams, P. L., Brooks, J. D., Inman, A. I., Monteiro-Riviere, N. A., and Riviere, J. E., 1994, Determination of physicochemical properties of phenol, paranitrophenol, acetone and ethanol relevant to quantitating their percutaneous absorption in porcine skin, *Res. Commun. Chem. Pathol. Pharmacol.* **83:**61–75.

Zhang, A., Riviere, J. E., and Monteiro-Riviere, N. A., 1995a, Evaluation of protective effects of sodium thiosulfate, cysteine, niacinamide and indomethacin on sulfur mustard-treated isolated perfused porcine skin, *Chem.-Biol. Interact.* **96:**249–262.

Zhang, A., Riviere, J. E., and Monteiro-Riviere, N. A., 1995b, Topical sulfur mustard induces changes in prostaglandins and interleukin 1α in isolated perfused porcine skin, *In Vitro Toxicol.* **8:**149–158.

Chapter 22

Vaginal Epithelial Models

Sy-Juen Wu and Joseph R. Robinson

1. INTRODUCTION

The vaginal route of drug administration has historically been used for treating local female-related conditions. Examples include the administration of steroid hormones for contraception, oxytocin for labor induction, or antibacterial, antifungal agents for treatment of infection. The vaginal route also has considerable potential for delivering systematically acting drugs in the female population. The vagina has a reasonably large surface area, good blood supply, and acceptable permeability to a wide range of drugs. Unfortunately, the vagina is also subject to cyclic changes both in women and in some animal models (Okada, 1991).

In this chapter, we will discuss the experimental methods in detail, the suitability of various animal models used in vaginal absorption or permeation studies, and the future application of controlled release in vaginal drug delivery.

2. TISSUE PERMEABILITY

In common with other membrane delivery routes, transport of vaginally administered drugs across the vaginal membrane can occur by three possible mechanisms as illustrated in Fig. 1 (Okada, 1991). A number of drugs cross vaginal tissue by an active transport mechanism. Thus, in the vagina, which is an estrogen-responsive tissue, estradiol will first bind to a cytoplasmic receptor to form an estrogen–receptor

Sy-Juen Wu and Joseph R. Robinson • School of Pharmacy, University of Wisconsin, Madison, Wisconsin 53706.

Models for Assessing Drug Absorption and Metabolism, Ronald T. Borchardt *et al.*, eds., Plenum Press, New York, 1996.

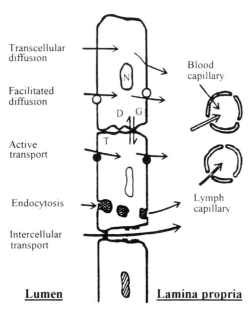

Figure 1. Vaginal epithelium transport pathways. T, Tight junction; D, desomsome; G, gap junction; N, nucleus (Okada, 1991).

complex, which will be translocated to the nucleus to perform its effects. Therefore, the vagina has greater ability to absorb estradiol than other nonestrogen-target tissues (Aref *et al.*, 1978).

Most vaginally absorbed drugs are transported by simple diffusion. It is thought that lipophilic substances are absorbed transcellularly, whereas hydrophilic substances are absorbed intercellularly, or across pores that exist in vaginal tissue. These large pores allow diffusion of high-molecular-weight immune material and water. For lipophilic substances, the partition coefficient of the penetrant is the primary factor affecting permeability. Several studies have shown that in rabbits and monkeys, vaginal permeability increases with increasing chain length, and, more specifically, permeability is directly related to partition coefficient. The more lipophilic the substance is, the higher the permeability.

Permeability is also influenced by physiologic factors, such as tissue thickness and porosity of the vaginal epithelium. Several studies have shown that vaginal absorption of estradiol and progesterone in postmenopausal women who have thinner, atrophic epithelia is significantly higher than in premenopausal women (Psychera *et al.*, 1989). Aside from the epithelium, the volume, viscosity, and pH of vaginal fluids may also affect dissolution, dilution, diffusion, and hence vaginal absorption. The greater the volume of the fluid, the more drug is dissolved and absorbed. On the other hand, the viscosity of the fluid may be a barrier for absorption (Richardson and Illum,

1992). Finally, the acidic pH (pH ≈ 5.7) (Kistner, 1978) of the vagina may affect absorption of ionizable drugs.

2.1. Materials

Buffers: 0.9% NaCl; phosphate buffer, pH 7.4; Krebs–Ringer buffer (KRB), pH 7.4.

UW Preservative Solution*: Lactobionic acid, 0.1 M; KH_2PO_4, 0.25 M; $MgSO_4$, 0.005 M; raffinose, pentahydrate, 0.3 M; adenosine, 0.005 M; glutathione, reduced form, 0.003 M; allopurinol, 0.001 M; hydroxyethyl starch, 10% solution.

2.2. *In Vitro* Model

As a prelude to our discussion of various *in vitro* techniques, we mention here that our personal experience suggests that excised tissue remains viable for about two hours post surgery and that any *in vitro* technique should be limited to approximately two hours and perhaps no longer than three hours. In addition, monitoring of tissue during permeability experiments, such as with electrophysiological measurements of tissue resistance, is advised.

Diffusion cells for *in vitro* experiments have been described by Hsu *et al.* (1983). The female mouse (or other experimental animal) is sacrificed, and the lower abdomen cut open. The fat tissue around the area is carefully removed to reveal the Y-shaped reproductive system. A pair of forceps is clamped ~0.5 cm above the cervix on the uterus before the pubic bone is cut open. The surrounding connective tissue is then carefully removed. The vagina is located between the cervix and the orifice. The tube-shaped vagina is cut off and immediately placed in ice-cold buffer. The vaginal epithelium of the mouse (or other rodent animal model) is cornified on the mucosal side. This cornified layer can be removed using a pair of tweezers to obtain a layer of noncornified membrane that is similar to a human vaginal membrane.

The vaginal tissue is then mounted onto a diffusion cell which is specially designed for the small available area of the mouse vaginal epithelium (~0.8–1.0 cm²). As shown in Fig. 2, it contains two ports, one for the stirrer and the other for sampling. The diameter of the cell opening is 0.6 cm, which provides an effective diffusional area of 0.28 cm² for a cell volume of 1.0 ml. The vaginal epithelium is sandwiched between two diffusion cells with the epithelial side facing the donor solution as depicted in Fig. 3. Equal volumes (0.9 ml) of normal saline at 37°C are added to the donor and the receiver chamber, and 100 μl of the solution of interest is then added to the donor side and an equal volume of normal saline is added to the receiver side. Aliquots are taken from the receiver side periodically, and the drug concentration is

*UW Preservative Solution was designed to preserve organs and tissues for transplant.

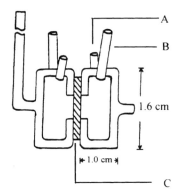

Figure 2. Diffusion cells for permeation experiments. A, sampling port; B, stirrer port; C, membrane (Hsu *et al.*, 1983).

determined. In this experiment, the steady-state flux across the membrane is equal to the product of the apparent permeability coefficient, P_{app}, and the concentration gradient:

$$\left(\frac{dC_t}{dt}\right)\left(\frac{V}{A}\right) = P_{app}(C_t^D - C_t^R) \qquad (1)$$

where C_t is the concentration of the reference at time t, C^D and C^R are the concentrations in the donor and the receiver chamber, respectively, A is the area, and V is the solution volume.

$$\frac{1}{P_{app}} = \frac{1}{P_{vaginal}} + \frac{1}{2P_{aq}} \qquad (2)$$

where $P_{vaginal}$ and P_{aq} are the permeabilities of the membrane and the aqueous layer, respectively.

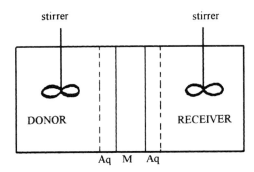

Figure 3. Schematic diagram of the diffusion cell setup (Hsu *et al.*, 1983).

The transport resistance arising from aqueous diffusion layers generally does not greatly influence the overall transport; in cases in which the aqueous layer is thick, its influence on both steady-state transport and lag time may be appreciable (Yu *et al.*, 1979). The permeability of the aqueous diffusion layer can be obtained from the following equation:

$$P_{aq} = \frac{D_a}{h_{aq}} \tag{3}$$

where D_a is the diffusivity of the layer, and h_{aq} is layer thickness. The thickness may be determined by conducting a dissolution rate experiment with a reference solute (such as benzoic acid) for which both the solubility and the diffusivity are known. The data are plotted as $\ln[C_s/(C_s - C_t)]$ versus time, from which D/h can be computed from the slope according to the dissolution rate equation:

$$\ln\left(\frac{C_s}{C_s - C_t}\right) = \left(\frac{D}{h}\right)\left[\frac{A}{V}(t - t_l)\right] \tag{4}$$

where C_s is the solubility of the reference compound, C_t is the concentration of the reference at time t, t_l is lag time, A is the area exposed to the solution, V is the bulk solution volume, and D is the aqueous diffusivity of the reference. Therefore, h_{aq} is obtained from the reference. The aqueous diffusivity of the drug can also be estimated from that of the reference:

$$D_a = \left(\frac{M_R}{M_a}\right)^{1/3} D_R \tag{5}$$

where D_a and D_R are the diffusivities of the drug and reference, respectively, and M_a and M_R are their molecular weights.

However, when only initial steady-state flux is used and $C_t^R\, S < C_t^D$ (i.e., $C_t^D - C_t^R \approx C_0$, where C_0 is the initial donor side drug concentration), Eq. (1) can be rewritten as (Yu *et al.*, 1979)

$$C_t = \left(\frac{A}{V}\right)C_0\left(\cfrac{1}{\cfrac{1}{P_{vaginal}} + \cfrac{1}{2P_{aq}}}\right)(t - t_l) \tag{6}$$

Other investigators have employed a similar approach using Ussing chambers (Bechgaard and Jørgensen, 1994; Bechgaard and Larsen, 1992). The Ussing chamber consists of two acrylic half-chambers connected to voltage-sensing electrodes (for measuring membrane resistance) and a temperature-adjustable water bath (Fig. 4). After the vaginal tissue was mounted and the cambers were filled with solution, aeration and circulation were provided by bubbling 95% O_2/5% CO_2 mixture into the solution on both sides. All processes were maintained at 37°C throughout the study (Rojanasakul *et al.*, 1992).

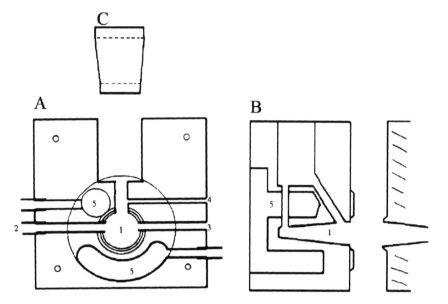

Figure 4. The Ussing chamber: (A) cross section, (B) side view, (C) funnel. 1, Chamber; 2, glucose–Ringer agar bridges which connect the voltage sensing electrodes to the bathing compartments; 3, current-sensing electrode (Ag/AgCl); 4, gas lift system (95% O_2/5% CO_2); 5, water jacket (37°C) (Jørgensen, 1992).

2.3. *In Situ* Model

Totsuyanagi *et al.* (1975) have described an *in situ* perfusion system to determine vaginal permeability for a series of aliphatic alcohols and carboxylic acids. Figures 5 and 6 illustrate the perfusion system used with rabbits.

Rabbits are popular laboratory animals because of their cost, size, and ease of handling. In rabbits, ovulation is dependent on coitus; this means that it is inducible, and not spontaneous. Normally, they do not show regular estrus cycles in the absence of males, and therefore, vaginal tissue of rabbits is nearly constant in histological, biochemical, and physiological properties. Rabbit vaginal epithelia is expected to show minimum variability in membrane permeability studies. However, the anatomy and histology of the rabbit vagina is quite different from that of the human female. The rabbit vagina is lined with columnar epithelium in the upper two-thirds of the vaginal tract, and the epithelium consists of both ciliated and nonciliated cells (Richardson and Illum, 1992). Only the lower third of the vagina is lined by a stratified and squamous epithelium that is similar to human vaginal epithelium. This may affect the suitability of using rabbits for studying permeability *in vivo*.

Mature female rabbits whose vaginal tract was about 8 cm long and 2 cm in

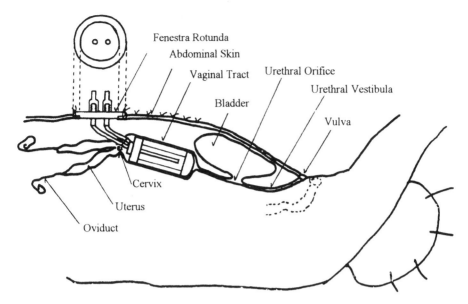

Figure 5.   Position of implanted rib-cage cell in rabbit vaginal tract (Totsuyanagi *et al.*, 1975).

diameter were obtained. The perfusion system consists of two parts. The first part is the "rib-cage" cell, which is surgically implanted in the vaginal tract of rabbits and is designed to fit vaginal dimensions in such a way as to provide a constant volume and surface area. The cell consists of two Teflon ends connected by eight stainless steel rods. The total volume of the cell is about 8.1 cm^3, and the surface area is about 22.5 cm^2. Perfusion solutions are introduced through one Teflon end which is connected to the second section of the perfusion system. The second section, external to the animal, consists of a rotating and reciprocating pump and a constant-temperature solution reservoir. During the experiment, these two parts are securely attached to provide a closed system for perfusion (Totsuyanagi *et al.*, 1975). Three days after surgery to implant the vaginal "rib-cage" cell, an absorption experiment can be performed. The rabbit is anesthetized with pentobarbital, the "rib-cage" cell opening is connected to the rotating pump, and a heating pad is placed under the rabbit to maintain body temperature. Before the start of the experiment, a 0.9% sodium chloride solution is passed through the vagina at a flow rate of 35 ml/min for 10 min to remove any exfoliated cells and secretions. Then, the sodium chloride solution is replaced with the buffer solution used in the experiment, warmed to 37°C, to wash the vagina for an additional 5 min. Lastly, the solution of interest is introduced into the reservoir, which is eventually introduced into the vaginal circuit at a flow rate of 35 ml/min at 37°C. Samples (0.05 ml) are withdrawn at various time intervals over a total experimental

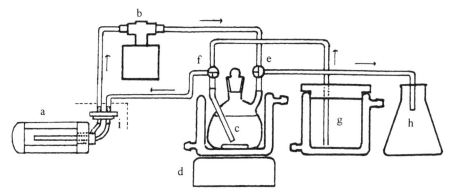

Figure 6. Diagram of perfusion system. a, Rib-cage cell; b, perfusion pump; c, solution reservoir; d, magnetic stirrer; e, f, three-way stopcocks; g, washing solution reservoir; h, drain beaker; i, fenestra rotunda (Totsuyanagi *et al.*, 1975).

duration of 80 min. After the experiment, the system is washed with normal saline for 15 min and then with buffer for 5 min.

The apparent permeability constant is calculated from the following equations, based on the assumption that the drug disappearance rate follows first-order kinetics:

$$\frac{dC_b}{dt} = -K_u C_b \tag{7}$$

$$K_u = \frac{A}{V} P_{app} \tag{8}$$

where C_b is the concentration of drug in the bulk solution, K_u is the first-order rate constant, A is the effective surface area of the vaginal membrane exposed to the solution, V is the total volume of the drug solution, and P_{app} is the apparent permeability coefficient.

A similar approach has also been applied to rhesus monkeys (Owada *et al.*, 1977). Each "rib-cage" cell was adjusted to fit each monkey's vaginal dimensions, and the cell could be inserted directly into the vagina through the vulval orifice without surgery (Fig. 7). In genetic and physiologic resemblance to humans, primates possess advantages over other animal species as an experimental animal model. Female primates are the only species that have menstrual cycles, other than human. The menstrual cycle of primates is about 28 days in duration like that of humans, and similar vaginal epithelial changes occur during the cycle in primates and humans (epithelial thickening, desquamation, etc.). Table I contains data on the apparent permeability of a series of alcohols through the vaginal tissue of rabbits and monkeys (Hwang, 1976, 1977), showing that the vaginal tissue of rabbits has higher permeability than that of monkeys. Chen *et al.* (1993) obtained similar results for peptide

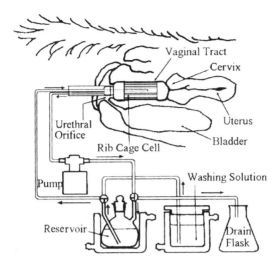

Figure 7. Vaginal perfusion system used in rhesus monkeys (Owada *et al.*, 1977).

drugs. They showed that the percent absorption of recombinant human relaxin (rhRlx) was 3.1 ± 1.4% in rabbits but only 0.2–1.4% in monkeys. It was also found that the permeability was highest right after menstruation and lowest at mid cycle around ovulation. It should be noted that a menopausal primate model is difficult to obtain, except by castration, given that extremely old animals are needed.

Another *in situ* approach, described by Okada *et al.* (1983a), utilized a mini-

Table I
Vaginal Permeability Coefficients
of a Series of Aliphatic Alcohols
in Rabbits and Monkeys

Alcohol	P_{app} ($\times 10^4$ cm/sec) at pH 6	
	Rabbit	Monkey
Methanol	1.32 ± 0.249	0.90 ± 0.224
1-Propanol	1.46 ± 0.287	—
1-Butanol	1.39 ± 0.250	1.39 ± 0.407
1-Hexanol	2.53 ± 0.666	—
1-Octanol	2.98 ± 0.462	2.85 ± 0.670

[a]Data from Hwong *et al.* (1976) and Owada *et al.* (1977).

pump. They inserted an osmotic minipump into the vagina of diestrous rats by setting the outlet of the pump toward the uterocervical canal under anesthesia. The flow rate was about 1 µl/hr and concentration of the drug [leuprolide, a luteinizing hormone-releasing hormone (LHRH) analog] was 150 µg/24 ml. Blood samples were collected at various intervals. The experimental duration was 150 hr and serum drug levels were maintained as high as with subcutaneous infusion. The absolute bioavailability was about 25.8%. This procedure does not require surgery.

2.4. *In Vivo* Model

More recently, researchers have tended to use *in vivo*, or nearly *in vivo*, methods. Drugs of interest are inserted into the vagina of rats, rabbits, monkeys, or women directly as a gel, cream, film, or suppository dosage form, and blood samples withdrawn. If the drugs are in solution, several approaches can be used. In one approach, shown in Fig. 8 (Yang and Schumacher, 1979), a plastic sponge (1.5 cm × 2.0 cm cylinder) was filled with the drug solution of interest and placed in the upper part of the vagina of a rhesus monkey against the ectocervix in a prone position. Subsequently, another sponge covered with Parafilm and a dry sponge were introduced into the vagina to prevent leakage from the first sponge. All the plugs were exchanged after 48–72 hr. Blood samples were taken from an appropriate vein, and drug concentrations determined.

Another approach is to instill the drug solution of interest and apply cyanoacrylate glue over the vaginal opening. This also reduces the possibility of producing blood drug levels as a result of oral ingestion through grooming. In a similar method, Okada *et al.* (1983b) inserted a cotton ball soaked with the drug solution of interest into the vagina and then closed the opening with an adhesive. Blood samples were then withdrawn.

Richardson and Illum (1989) described the insertion of a short length of polyethylene tubing (0.58 mm i.d., 0.96 mm o.d.) into the vagina of a rat. The tubing was attached to a 100-µl syringe and filled with the drug solution of interest, then gently inserted into the vagina, and secured in position with an adhesive. The drug solution was instilled into the vaginal tract, and the tubing was then clamped to prevent leakage. Blood samples were taken after administration, and drug concentrations determined.

Vaginal rings were also used by Radomsky *et al.* (1992). These investigators first anesthetized the animal, cut open the abdomen, and located the vaginal tract. Then a nonabsorbable nylon suture was firmly attached to the ring, which contained the antibodies (or drug of interest), as shown in Fig. 9 and pulled through the vaginal wall into the abdomen and secured in place. Blood samples were taken after the procedure. This method can be used for long study periods.

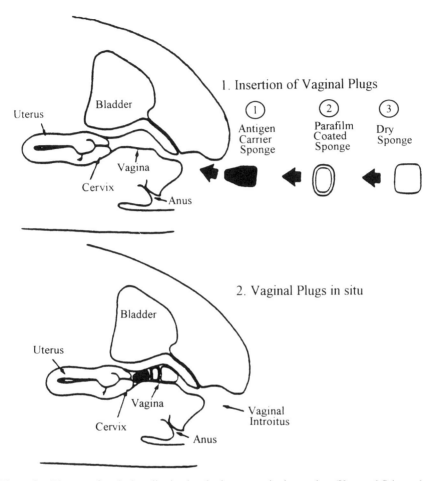

Figure 8. Diagram of vaginal application by plastic sponges in the monkey (Yang and Schumacher, 1979).

2.5. Ovariectomized Rat Model

In rodent species, such as the mouse, rat, and guinea pig, the vaginal epithelium is a stratified, squamous epithelium. The estrous cycles in rodents are usually quite short (4–5 days per cycle for rats and mice, 15–17 days for guinea pig) and clear, and the vaginal epithelium changes during each estrous cycle (similar to the human menstrual cycle). The epithelium thickens when the proestrous stage is entered, with an increase in estrogen concentration, and reaches a maximum at the time of estrus.

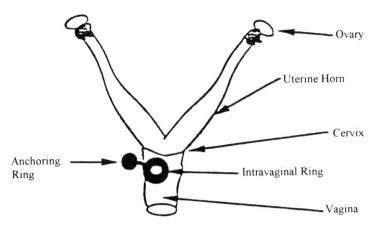

Figure 9.   Position of vaginal rings in the female mouse reproductive tract (Radamsky *et al.*, 1992).

After estrus, the epithelium again thins. In rodents, the stratified squamous epithelium thickens and is cornified in the superficial layer. The cyclic changes in the vaginal epithelium of rats is reported to have a substantial effect on vaginal absorption of hydrophilic substances. As the epithelial thickness increases, absorption declines at proestrous and estrous (Okada, 1983). Similar results were found in *in vitro* studies in mice (Hsu, 1983). However, since the vaginal epithelium of these rodents would be cornified at some stage of the cycle, rodents may not be representative for human vaginal absorption.

In order to be more representative of human vaginal epithelial tissue, more recent studies (Richardson and Illum, 1989) have used ovariectomized rats. Female rats were anesthetized using halothane. The bilateral ovaries were removed surgically. The wounds were closed with Michel clips, which were removed 7–10 days later. The animals were allowed to recover for at least 2 weeks before being used in experiments. After ovariectomy, the estrogen concentration is very low, and the vaginal epithelium becomes thin and atrophic with only two cell layers. This provides a consistent epithelial model for the study of vaginal absorption and a reasonable model for the menopausal human female. On the other hand, by giving low doses of estradiol to ovariectomized rats 24 hr before the experiments, the vagina epithelium recovers to a 41 μm thickness with basal cuboidal cells and several flattened cell layers, similar to the human vaginal epithelium, and can be used as another constant epithelium for vaginal drug absorption.

2.6. Metabolic Enzyme Activity Study

Bioavailability of drugs depends not only on permeability across the tissue, but also on degradation of the drugs before or during absorption. Vaginal enzymes

(Schmidt, 1978) can be generally divided into three groups: hydrolytic enzymes, such as phosphatases, aminopeptidases, endopeptidases; the oxydoreductase, such as succinic dehydrogenase; and some fibrinolytic enzymes. The low bioavilability of vaginally administered drugs (especially peptides and proteins) may also be due to the enzyme barrier in the vaginal lumen and mucosa. The enzymatic degradation of peptides and proteins after vaginal administration has been studied by using mucosal homogenates (Stratford and Lee, 1986).

Rabbits were sacrificed by overdosing pentobarbital solution through the ear vein and vaginal tissue was removed as described in the section on the *in vitro* model. The tissue was rinsed with 0.9% NaCl and stored at $-70°C$. It was thawed to room temperature before use for 10 min, and rinsed twice in 0.05 M Tris maleate buffer (pH 7.4) (Stratford and Lee, 1986) or isotonic KCl (Kashi and Lee, 1986). It was then homogenized in several milliliters of buffer at 4°C using a Teflon-glass homogenizer. The homogenate was centrifuged at 3020g and 4°C for 10 min to remove cellular and nuclear debris. The supernatant containing cytosol, plasma, and intracellular membrane fractions was collected and its total protein concentration determined by a dye-binding assay using rabbit serum albumin as a standard. One hundred microliters of supernatant was added to 2.8 ml of buffer at 37°C in preparation for the aminopeptidase activity assay. One hundred microliters of substrate solution was added to the mixture after 15 min. The substrates in this specific study, to test for aminopeptidase activity, were non-fluorescent 4-methoxy-2-naphthylamides of L-leucine, L-alanine, L-glutamic acid, and L-arginine. Fluorescence, from the formation of a fluorescent leaving group after the aminopeptidase cleaved the substrate, was monitored at an excitation wavelength of 342 nm and an emission wavelength of 426 nm. It was found that the amount of vaginal aminopeptidases was lower than in the ileum, but not much different from in the duodenum (Stratford, 1986). Furthermore, the hydrolysis of 3 pentapeptides, Met-enkephalin, Leu-enkephalin, and [D-Ala^2]Met-enkephalinamide, in homogenates of vaginal mucosa was the lowest among nasal, buccal, rectal, and vaginal mucosa; however, the half-life of the peptides in these homogenates did not vary substantially from that in the ileal homogenate.

The activity of several vaginal enzymes was found to change with stages of the menstrual cycle, the concentration of estrogen, or with the vaginal pH value (Schmidt, 1978). Obviously, the presence of all these enzymes decreases the bioavailability of metabolically sensitive drugs. Furthermore, fluctuation of enzyme activity with cyclic changes or hormonal changes adds to the difficulty of predicting bioavailability.

3. APPLICATIONS

Desirable features of a vaginal delivery system would be absence of tissue irritation, ease of application, absence of offensive odor or staining, and compatibility with other systems, e.g., contraceptives. The dosage forms used were creams, gels, solutions, tablets, powders, suppositories, vaginal rings, and aerosol foams, etc., with the aid of an applicator.

The most commonly used systems for a controlled-release are vaginal rings, cylinders, or discs. They are usually made from silicone polymer and can be designed in different forms, such as homogeneous rings, bended rings, shell rings, and core rings, depending on where or how drugs are released from the rings (Nash and Jackanicz, 1982). Similarly, vaginal pessaries which are made of porous polyurethane sponge can be used for slow-release of progestin (Chen, 1993). For a more rate-controlled release sponge, a layer of rate-controlled silicone device containing drug reservoir can be added to the sponge.

More recently, a gel slab has been marketed for prostaglandin E2. This PEG-hexane trioldiisocyanate hydrogel forms a 3-dimensional lattice which swells when exposed to water and in this way can be loaded with drug solution. After drying, the drug is trapped into the polymer lattice and after administration into the vagina, the gel reswells and releases drugs (McNeill, 1984 and Embrey, 1986).

4. ADVANTAGES AND DISADVANTAGES

In vitro models (diffusion cells) are popular because they are easy to use. They are useful for a rough approximation of drug permeability, the potential effectiveness of a enhancer, and as a means to study the mechanism of drug permeation. Since the tissue is isolated, it is possible to select the parts of the membrane that are similar to that in humans, e.g., the lower one third of the rabbit vaginal epithelium, or with some modification to eliminate differences e.g., removing cornified vaginal epithelium of rats. On the other hand, isolated tissue viability is the greatest concern for diffusion cell studies, so that studies of long duration are not possible. Furthermore, the enzyme activity may change after the tissue is isolated, which can affect the permeability dramatically, especially for peptides and proteins. In addition, the limited surface area of tissue exposed to the drug solution for a diffusion cell study can be a problem.

The *in situ* model (perfusion) seems more reasonable in terms of tissue viability and surface area. However, the "rib-cage" cell applies a mechanical force to the vaginal epithelium. This outer force may damage the epithelium or affect the per-meability in many ways (Diamond, 1995). In addition, a variety of physiological factors that may affect the vaginal epithelium, such as the menstrual cycle, the different types of epithelial cells, or cornification, cannot be controlled in a perfusion study. Thus, it may be hard to interpret the experimental results without considering all these factors.

The *in vivo* model seems to be the most relevant model. It is easy to obtain the pharmacokinetic results and predict how efficient the drug delivery system is through direct measurement of blood samples. However, as in the case of the *in situ* model, there are a lot of physiological factors involved in the study that cannot be controlled.

By understanding the advantages and disadvantages of each model, it is possible to choose a model to suit the purposes of the study.

REFERENCES

Aref, I., El-Sheikha, Z., and Hafez, E. S. E., 1978, Absorption of drugs and hormones in the vagina, in: *The Human Vagina* (E. S. E. Hafez and T. N. Evans, eds.), Elsevier/North-Holland Biomedical Press, Amsterdam, pp. 179–191.

Bechgaard, E., Gizurarson, S., Jørgensen, L., and Larsen, R., 1992, The viability of isolated rabbit nasal mucosa in the Ussing chamber, and the permeability of insulin across the membrane, *Int. J. Pharm.* **87:**125–132.

Bechgaard, E., Riis, K. J., and Jørgensen, L., 1994, The development of an Ussing chamber technique for isolated human vaginal mucosa, and the viability of the *in vitro* system, *Int. J. Pharm.* **106:**237–242.

Burgos, M. H., and Roig de Vargas-Linares, C. E., 1978, Ultrastructure of the vaginal mucosa, in: *The Human Vagina* (E. S. E. Hafez and T. N. Evans, eds.), Elsevier/North-Holland Biomedical Press, Amsterdam, pp. 63–93.

Chen, S. A., Reed, B., Nguyen, T., Gaylord, N., Fuller, G. B., and Mordenti, J., 1993, The pharmacokinetics and absorption of recombinant human relaxin in nonpregnant rabbits and rhesus monkeys after intravenous and intravaginal administration, *Pharm. Res.* **10**(2)**:**223–227.

Diamond, J. M., 1995, How to be physiological, *Nature* **376:**117–118.

Ho, N. F. H., Suhardja, L., Hwang, S., Owada, E., Flynn, G. L., Higuchi, W. I., and Park, J. Y., 1976, Systems approach to vaginal delivery of drugs III: Simulation studies interfacing steroid release from silicone matrix and vaginal absorption in rabbits, *J. Pharm. Sci.* **65**(11)**:**1578–1585.

Hsu, C. C., Park, J. Y., Ho, N. F. H., Higuchi, W. I., and Fox, J. L., 1983, Topical vaginal drug delivery I: Effect of the estrous cycle on vaginal membrane permeability and diffusivity of vidarabine in mice, *J. Pharm. Sci.* **72:**674–680.

Hwang, S., Owada, E., Yotsutanagi, T., Suhardja, L., Ho, N. F. H., Flynn, G. L., and Higuchi, W. I., 1976, Systems approach to vaginal delivery of drugs II: *In situ* vaginal absorption of unbranched aliphatic alcohols, *J. Pharm. Sci.* **65**(11)**:**1574–1578.

Kashi, S. D., and Lee, V. H. L., 1986, Enkephalin hydrolysis in homogenates of various absorptive mucosae of the albino rabbit: Similarities in rates and involvement of aminopeptidases, *Life Sci.* **38:**2019–2028.

Kistner, R. W., 1978, Physiology of the vagina, in: *The Human Vagina* (E. S. E. Hafez and T. N. Evans, eds.), Elsevier/North-Holland Biomedical Press, Amsterdam, pp. 109–120.

Knuth, K., Amiji, M., and Robinson, J. R., 1993, Hydrogel delivery systems for vaginal and oral applications: Formulation and biological considerations, *Adv. Drug Deliv. Rev.* **11:**137–167.

Li, V. H. K., and Robinson, J. R., 1987, Influence of drug properties and routes of drug administration on the design of sustained and controlled release systems, in: *Controlled Drug Delivery* (J. R. Robinson and V. H. L. Lee, eds.), 2nd ed., Marcel Dekker, New York, pp. 3–61.

Morimoto, K., Takeeda, T., Nakamoto, Y., and Morisaka, K., 1982, Effective vaginal absorption of insulin in diabetic rats and rabbits using polyacrylic acid aqueous gel bases, *Int. J. Pharm.* **12:**107–111.

Nash, H. A., and Jackanicz, T. M., 1982, Contraceptive vaginal rings, in: *Advances in Fertility Research* (D. R. Mishell, ed.), Raven Press, New York, pp. 129–144.

Okada, H., 1991, Vaginal route of peptide and protein drug delivery, in: *Peptide and Protein Drug Delivery* (V. H. L. Lee, ed.), Marcel Dekker, New York, pp. 633–666.

Okada, H., Yamazaki, I., Ogawa, Y., Hirai, S., Yashiki, T., and Mima, H., 1982, Vaginal absorption of a potent luteinizing hormone-releasing hormone analogue (Leuprolide) in rats I: Absorption by various routes and absorption enhancement, *J. Pharm. Sci.* **71:**1367–1371.

Okada, H., Yamazaki, I., Sakura, Y., Yashiki, T., Shimamoto, T., and Mima, H., 1983a, Desensitization of gonadotropin-releasing response following vaginal consecutive administration of leuprolide in rats, *J. Pharmacobio.-Dyn.* **6:**512–522.

Okada, H., Yamazaki, I., Yashiki, T., and Mima, H., 1983b, Vaginal absorption of a potent luteinizing hormone-releasing hormone analogue (Leuprolide) in rats II: Mechanism of absorption enhancement with organic acids, *J. Pharm. Sci.* **72:**75–78.

Okada, H., Yashiki, T., and Mima, H., 1983c, Vaginal absorption of a potent luteinizing hormone-releasing hormone analogue (Leuprolide) in rats III: Effect of estrous cycle on vaginal absorption of hydrophilic model compounds, *J. Pharm. Sci.* **72:**173–176.

Okada, H., Yamazaki, I., Yashiki, T., Shimamoto, T., and Mima, H., 1984, Vaginal absorption of a potent luteinizing hormone-releasing hormone analogue (Leuprolide) in rats IV: Evaluation of the vaginal absorption and gonadotropin responses by radioimmunoassay, *J. Pharm. Sci.* **73:**298–302.

Owada, E., Behl, C. R., Hwang, S., Suhardja, L., Flynn, G. L., Ho, N. F. H., and Higuchi, W. I., 1977, Vaginal drug absorption in rhesus monkeys I: Development of methodology, *J. Pharm. Sci.* **66:** 216–219.

Parasad, R. N. V., Roy, A. C., Kottegoda, S. R., Ratnam, S. S., and Karim, S. M. M., 1985, Plasma levels of 13,14-dihydro-15 keto PGE_2 after vaginal application of a new PGE_2 film, *Prostaglandins* **29**(2): 269–272.

Platzer, W., Poisel, S., and Hafez, E. S. E., 1978, Functional anatomy of the human vagina, in: *The Human Vagina* (E. S. E. Hafez and T. N. Evans, eds.), Elsevier/North-Holland Biomedical Press, Amsterdam, pp. 39–53.

Psychera, H., Hjerpe, A., and Carlstrom, K., 1989, Influence of the maturity of the vaginal epithelium upon the absorption of vaginally administered estradiol-17-β and progesterone in postmenopausal women, *Gynecol. Obstet. Invest.* **27:**204–207.

Radomsky, M. L., Whaley, K. J., Cone, R. A., and Saltzman, W. M., 1992, Controlled vaginal delivery of antibodies in the mouse, *Biol. Reprod.* **47:**133–140.

Richardson, J. L., and Illum, L., 1992, Routes of delivery: Case studies. The vaginal route of peptide and protein drug delivery, *Adv. Drug Deliv. Rev.* **8:**341–361.

Richardson, J. L., Minhas, P. S., Thomas, N. W., and Illum, L., 1989, Vaginal administration of gentamicin to rats. Pharmaceutical and morphological studies using absorption enhancers, *Int. J. Pharm.* **56:**29–35.

Richardson, J. L., Illum, L., and Thomas, N. W., 1992, Vaginal absorption of insulin in the rat: Effect of penetration enhancers on insulin uptake and mucosal histology, *Pharm. Res.* **9:**878–883.

Ritschel, W. A., and Hussain, A. S., 1989, "Body burden" of phosphonoformic acid after topical and vaginal administration to rabbits and beagle dogs, *Methods Find. Exp. Clin. Pharmacol.* **ll**(2):111–114.

Rojanasakul, Y., Wang, L., Bhat, M., Glover, D. D., Malanga, C. J., and Ma, J. K. H., 1992, The transport barrier of epithelia: A comparative study on membrane permeability and charge selectivity in the rabbit, *Pharm. Res.* **9:**1029–1034.

Schmidt, E. H., and Beller, F. K., 1978, Biochemistry of the vagina, in: *The Human Vagina* (E. S. E. Hafez and T. N. Evans, eds.), Elsevier/North-Holland Biomedical Press, Amsterdam, pp. 139–149.

Solleveld, H. A., McAnulty, P., Ford, J., Peters, P. W. J., and Tesh, J., 1986, Breeding, housing, and care of laboratory animals, in: *Laboratory Animals: Laboratory Animal Models for Domestic Animal Production* (E. J. Ruitenberg and P. W. J. Peters, eds.), Elsevier Science Publishing, Amsterdam, pp. 15–25.

Steger, R. W., and Hafez, E. S. E., 1978, Age-associated changes in the vagina, in: *The Human Vagina* (E. S. E. Hafez and T. N. Evans, eds.), Elsevier/North-Holland Biomedical Press, Amsterdam, pp. 95–106.

Stratford, R. E., and Lee, V. H. L., 1986, Aminopeptidase activity in homogenates of various absorptive mucosae in the albino rabbit: Implications in peptide delivery, *Int. J. Pharm.* **30:**73–82.

Thapar, M. A., Parr, E. L., and Parr, M. B., 1990, The effect of adjuvants on antibody titers in mouse vaginal fluid after intravaginal immunization, *J. Reprod. Immunol.* **17:**207–216.

Totsuyanagi, T., Molokhia, A., Hwang, S., Ho, N. F. H., Flynn, G. L., and Higuchi, W. I., 1975, Systems approach to vaginal delivery of drugs I: Development of *in situ* vaginal drug absorption procedure, *J. Pharm. Sci.* **64:**71–76.

Yang, S., and Schumacher, G. F., 1979, Immune response after vaginal application of antigens in the rhesus monkey, *Fertil. Steril.* **32:**588–598.

Yu, C. D., Fox, J. L., Ho, N. F. H., and Higuchi, W. I., 1979, Physical model evaluation of topical prodrug delivery—simultaneous transport and bioconversion of vidarabine-5′-valerate II: Parameter determination, *J. Pharm. Sci.* **68:**1347–1357.

Chapter 23

Ocular Epithelial Models

Vincent H. L. Lee

1. INTRODUCTION

Next to the brain, the eye is probably the most guarded organ against the entry of all but the essential nutrients. This is credited to the simple yet highly efficient protective machinery comprised of rapid removal of the applied dose through drainage (Chrai *et al.*, 1973, 1974) or tear turnover (Mishima *et al.*, 1966); diversion of drugs into the systemic circulation via blood vessels in the conjunctival and the nasal mucosae (Chang and Lee, 1987); a practically impermeable corneal barrier (Sieg and Robinson, 1976); and, to a lesser extent, metabolism of drugs, notably those containing ester (Lee, 1983; Lee *et al.*, 1983a,b), peptide (Stratford and Lee, 1985), and ketone linkages (Ashton *et al.*, 1991b), during and following transport. The net result is that typically less than 1% of the applied dose reaches the anterior segment of the eye (Lee and Robinson, 1986) and that virtually none is available to act on the posterior segment tissues except when under iontophoresis (Lam *et al.*, 1994). It is therefore not surprising that a major activity in ocular drug development has been focused on identifying means to improve ocular drug bioavailability (Lee *et al.*, 1994; Lehr *et al.*, 1994; Naveh *et al.*, 1994; Pleyer et al., 1993; Zimmer *et al.*, 1994). The realization that topically applied drugs can be absorbed systemically (Lee *et al.*, 1993; Liu and Chiou, 1994; Podder *et al.*, 1992) to elicit serious side effects in some instances has provided yet another compelling incentive toward meeting this goal. Through dose reduction in proportion to the gain in ocular absorption, the systemic drug load can be minimized (Potter *et al.*, 1988). The focus of this chapter will, however, be on ocular drug absorption in the context of animal and experimental models following topical

Vincent H. L. Lee • Department of Pharmaceutical Sciences, School of Pharmacy, University of Southern California, Los Angeles, California 90033.

Models for Assessing Drug Absorption and Metabolism, Ronald T. Borchardt *et al.*, eds., Plenum Press, New York, 1996.

dosing. Subconjunctival (Conrad and Robinson, 1980) and intravitreal administration (Rahimy et al., 1994) will not be considered.

2. CHOICE OF ANIMAL MODELS

Ideally, the animal model selected must be predictive of behavior of a drug as well as performance of its delivery system in humans. In reality, the choice of an animal model is often dictated by the experimental technique involved, the process being studied, ease of handling of the animal, and cost. Over the years, monkeys, rabbits, dogs, cats, guinea pigs, rats, mice, chickens, and several other animals have been used. Of these, the albino rabbit is the most widely used primarily because of ease of handling, low cost, comparable size of its eyes to human eyes, and extensive information about its ocular biochemistry, physiology, pharmacokinetics, and pharmacodynamics. While, overall, the rabbit is an adequate model for understanding the mechanisms of ocular drug disposition and for predicting the influence of drug properties on ocular drug disposition (Sugaya and Nagataki, 1978), it falls short in its predictability of vehicle effect on ocular drug bioavailability. Specifically, the careful work of Saettone and associates (Saettone et al., 1980, 1982a,b, 1984, 1985) has revealed that the rabbit is less sensitive than human in this regard. This can be attributed, at least in part, to the 50% lower tear turnover rate and the much lower blinking frequency in rabbits as compared with that in humans. Whether the nictitating membrane in the rabbit also contributes to its the rabbit's sensitivity to vehicle effects is as yet unclear (Anderson, 1980; DeSantis and Schoenwald, 1978; Mindel et al., 1984).

Although the albino rabbit is commonly used in ocular drug penetration studies, there is growing evidence that the pigmented rabbit may be a more suitable animal to use for ocular pharmacokinetic studies with drugs demonstrating high binding potential (Lee and Robinson, 1982). Aside from the obvious difference in the degree of iris pigmentation, with its pharmacokinetic implications (Araie et al., 1982; Atlasik et al., 1980; Larsson and Tjalve, 1979; Patil and Jacobowitz, 1974; Shimada et al., 1976), the pigmented rabbit appears to differ from the albino rabbit in its drug-metabolizing enzyme profile. The pigmented rabbit is more active in ocular esterase activity (Lee, 1983; Lee et al., 1980, 1983b; Redell et al., 1983) but is lower in ocular ketone reductase activity (Lee et al., 1988). Where the difference in enzymatic activity resides in the corneal epithelium—the gateway of ocular drug transport—it is expected to affect the intraocular disposition of the drugs involved.

A major deficiency of most ocular drug pharmacokinetic studies is that experiments are rarely performed in animals with the disease state against which the drug is being tested. It is conceivable that marked discrepancies in ocular drug pharmacokinetics exist between animals with and without a certain disease state, especially when the absorptive barrier [cornea (Cox et al., 1972; Kupferman et al., 1974; Schoenwald and Houseman, 1982)] and elimination mechanism [tear and aqueous humor turnover (Bito, 1974; Kane *et al.*, 1981)] are involved. Unfortunately, information in this area is very limited.

3. TYPES OF EXPERIMENTAL MODELS

The assessment of ocular pharmacokinetics of a drug candidate is usually carried out in two parts: *in vitro* and *in vivo*.

3.1. *In Vitro* Models

The *in vitro* part of an ocular pharmacokinetic study is primarily concerned with evaluation of a drug's ability to traverse the various layers of the cornea; mechanism of transport (i.e., passive diffusion, carrier-mediated transport, or endocytosis); and effect of formulation pH, tonicity, and the presence of adjuvants such as chelating agents and preservatives on corneal drug penetration. The focus has been on the cornea because it is the major pathway of drug entry into the eye from topical dosing for most drugs, with the exception of the very polar drugs (Ahmed and Patton, 1985, 1987). These experiments are usually conducted using freshly excised corneas in a modified Ussing chamber arrangement (Burstein and Anderson, 1985). The same construct has also been used to evaluate drug transport across the conjunctiva (Ashton *et al.*, 1991a; Hayakawa *et al.*, 1992).

In a typical experiment, the freshly excised corneal or conjunctival tissue is sandwiched between the two compartments of the Ussing chamber. Two and a half milliliters (corresponding to the volume of the chamber) of glutathione bicarbonate Ringer's (GBR) solution (Ubels and Edelhauser, 1982), preadjusted to pH 7.4, are added to the endothelial side. This is followed by the addition of the same volume of drug solution to the epithelial side. The contents of both reservoirs are mixed by bubbling a 95% O_2/5% CO_2 mixture at the rate of 3–4 bubbles per second. The temperature within each reservoir is maintained at $35 \pm 1°C$, the corneal temperature. Periodically, 50-μl aliquots are removed from the endothelial side for assay of drug and are immediately replaced by an equal volume of GBR solution. The amount of drug accumulated on the endothelial side is plotted against time. The apparent permeability coefficient of each drug (P_{app}) can be calculated from the slope of the linear portion of such a plot (i.e., the flux) with normalization to the diffusional surface area (A) and the initial drug concentration (C_o), as follows: $P_{app} = \text{slope}/(C_o \cdot A)$ (Schoenwald and Huang, 1983). In the author's experience, variability on the order of 15–20% can routinely be obtained from a sample size of 4–6 eyes.

The GBR solution is made of 111.56 mM NaCl, 4.82 mM KCl, 1.04 mM $CaCl_2$, 0.78 mM $MgCl_2$, 0.86 mM NaH_2PO_4, 29.3 mM $NaHCO_3$, 5.01 mM glucose, and 0.30 mM reduced glutathione (Ubels and Edelhauser, 1982). This solution is essential for the proper functioning of the corneal endothelial pump (Edelhauser *et al.*, 1965; Lux and Dikstein, 1985), hence minimizing corneal swelling. Even under this optimal condition, meaningful transport data can only be collected for up to 4–6 hr (Hull *et al.*, 1974; Schoenwald and Ward, 1981). At the same time, care must be taken not to inadvertently damage the superficial corneal epithelia in any way. While these superficial corneal defects may not affect the transport of lipophilic drugs significantly (Shih and Lee, 1990), such may not be the case with hydrophilic drugs that tend to opt for the paracellular pathway for transport (Keller *et al.*, 1980; Lee *et al.*, 1983c,d, 1986; Stratford *et al.*, 1983). On the other hand, deliberate stripping of the corneal epithelial layer prior to the start of the experiment would yield useful information on the maximum extent to which corneal drug penetration can be enhanced by formulation changes. The factor of increase is 44 for hydrophilic atenolol (Ashton *et al.*, 1991a) and 192 for hydrophilic phenylephrine (Ashton *et al.*, 1992). Not surprisingly, there is no improvement for lipophilic betaxolol (Ashton *et al.*, 1991a).

There are three concerns associated with the use of diffusion chambers to evaluate formulation effects on corneal and conjunctival penetration. First and foremost is the unrealistically long exposure of the corneal and conjunctival surfaces to the drug when compared with the minutes of contact time seen *in vivo* (Chrai *et al.*, 1973). Richman and Tang-Liu (1990) attempted to address this concern by miniaturizing the donor chamber volume to 6% of that in the receiver chamber and by incorporating a fluid pumping mechanism in the donor chamber to simulate physiological tear turnover. A second concern with the original design of the diffusion chambers is the extent to which the adherent mucus remains intact (Dilly, 1985; Nichols *et al.*, 1985), as it can function as a diffusional barrier to the penetration of charged molecules and macromolecules (proteins) (Hui *et al.*, 1984). A third concern with the use of diffusion chambers is that permeability is determined under pseudo-steady-state conditions, which are not established *in vivo*. Nevertheless, reasonably good *in vitro–in vivo* correlations are to be expected since the terms which comprise P_{app}—the buffer/cornea partition coefficient and the diffusion coefficient within the cornea—also determine absorption *in vivo*. Moreover, provided that the corneal epithelium is saturated with drug within minutes to establish the concentration gradient for drug diffusion across the cornea, the *in vitro* model theoretically should mimic the *in vivo* situation reasonably well (Ashton *et al.*, 1991a). Notwithstanding the above concerns, the *in vitro* results, when used in conjunction with the *in vivo* results, would allow the delineation of the relative role of the formulation-induced changes in corneal and conjunctival penetration and the changes in precorneal retention of the instilled dose in affecting overall drug bioavailability.

3.2. *In Vivo* Models

An essential element in the pharmacokinetic assessment of drug candidates is the topical instillation of a formulation to the eyes of live rabbits. The purpose of these experiments is threefold: first, to define the influence of precorneal drug removal factors in ocular drug absorption; second, to determine the relative contributions of the corneal and the noncorneal routes to ocular drug absorption; and third, to determine intraocular drug distribution. Due to the often overlooked factors known to affect tear and instilled solution dynamics, including age of the animal (Nzekwe and Maurice, 1994; Patton and Robinson, 1976; Redell *et al.*, 1983), degree of anesthesia of the animal (Patton and Robinson, 1975; Sieg and Robinson, 1974), manner in which the animal is handled (Sieg and Robinson, 1974), method of instillation (Chrai *et al.*, 1974), and the time when the experiment is carried out (Ohdo *et al.*, 1991), it is not uncommon that the results from otherwise identical ocular drug studies vary from one laboratory to another or from one worker to another in the same laboratory. As evidence, Sieg and Robinson (1974) demonstrated that the degree to which the rabbit was anesthetized and the positioning of the animal (i.e., upright or lateral) affected the extent of absorption of fluorometholone from a suspension into the eye. Moreover, Ohdo *et al.* (1991) demonstrated that a two- to threefold difference in the ocular bioavailability of topically applied timolol in the pigmented rabbit would occur as the result of differences in the time of drop instillation.

3.2.1. GENERAL EXPERIMENTAL CONDITIONS

Even though an optimal (i.e., chemically stable) formulation may be available, it is recommended that the initial experiments be conducted with preservative-free aqueous solutions at physiological pH and isotonicity to minimize drug loss through induced lacrimation. Whenever possible, unanesthetized animals should be used. In a typical experiment, either a 25- or 50-μl drop is instilled onto the cornea, collecting in the cul-de-sac. At predetermined times, the rabbit is euthanized, and the eyes are dissected for isolation of tissues for assay of drug. Approximately 11 time points should be used. These typically include the 5-, 10-, 15-, 30-, 60-, 90-, 120-, 150-, 180-, 240-, and 360-min time points, which are appropriately spaced to define the absorption, distribution, and elimination phases of the drug. In reality, the duration over which drug levels can be measured is limited principally by assay sensitivity, not a trivial problem in ocular drug studies given the small amount of drug that is able to reach the internal eye from topical dosing.

Whether one or both eyes of an experimental animal should be used depends on the contribution of systemically absorbed drug to ocular levels. This varies from negligible in the case of pilocarpine (Conrad and Robinson, 1980) to substantial in the case of prostaglandin (Bito and Baroody, 1982). The exact contribution must be determined in initial experiments in which only one eye is dosed and drug levels in the undosed eye are compared to those in the dosed eye. If systemic contribution at the last anticipated time point is 10% or less, both eyes can probably be used. Similarly, decisions on whether both eyes should be devoted to the same or different time points should be made on the basis of the magnitude of systemic drug contribution to the undosed eye.

3.2.2. TISSUES TO BE SAMPLED

While it is tempting to sample only the aqueous humor for assessing ocular drug bioavailability because of the simplicity of the procedure, it is imperative that anterior segment tissues such as the conjunctiva, corneal epithelium, corneal stroma-endothelium, sclera, iris, ciliary body, and lens be sampled as well. This is because the assumption often invoked in sampling only the aqueous humor, namely, that drug concentration in it is correlated with that at the receptor site, may not be valid in every case (Lee and Robinson, 1982; Lee et al., 1983c,d). While the choroid, retina, and vitreous humor may also be sampled, the concentrations there are expected to be low or undetectable.

3.2.3. NUMBER OF RABBITS REQUIRED

Typically, 10–12 rabbits per time point are required to properly characterize the pharmacokinetics of topically applied drugs. This large number of rabbits is necessary to obtain statistically valid information. Even then, coefficients of variation on the order of 25–50% are not unusual. Adding to this demand for rabbits is, as already mentioned, the need to use on the order of 10 time points to properly define the ocular pharmacokinetic behavior of the drug concerned. Thus, it is not unusual that about 120–150 animals are required to complete a single dose study to define the pharmacokinetics of a drug under typical physiological conditions. Clearly, although primates probably may be more predictive of drug behavior in humans than rabbits, rabbits are still preferred in the majority of ocular drug pharmacokinetic studies from the cost effectiveness point of view.

In an attempt to reduce the number of animals required and to reduce the variability of the data, a method has been devised to sample the aqueous humor serially in the same manner as serial blood sampling is performed in systemic drug pharmacokinetic studies (Tang-Liu et al., 1984). However, because the rabbit eye is easily traumatized by this procedure and the blood–aqueous humor barrier is breached (Weingeist, 1970), the pharmacokinetic behavior of a drug in the aqueous humor would be inevitably altered.

The only ocular fluid that lends itself to serial sampling without the eye being traumatized is tear. Unfortunately, tear drug concentration data are often imprecise due to the unavoidable tear stimulation effect of the sampling procedure (Mishima et al., 1966), the small volume of fluid that can be sampled for assay, and the inevitable sampling of the dosage form, notably ointments and gels, that is not in homogeneous solution with the tear fluid.

3.2.4. DATA ANALYSIS

3.2.4a. Compartmental Data Analysis

The time course of drug concentration in the various tissues can be subjected to compartmental analysis to yield various apparent rate constants of drug transfer between compartments (Francoeur et al., 1985; Himmelstein et al., 1978; Lee and Robinson, 1979; Makoid and Robinson, 1979; Miller et al., 1981; Sieg and Robinson, 1981). These rate constants can then be incorporated into models for simulations on existing software, as exemplified by iThink® (High Performance Systems, Lyme, NH) (Grass and Lee, 1993). Originally designed for business-oriented applications, this software has recently been used to simulate the ocular and systemic pharmaco-kinetics of topically applied timolol in the rabbit (Grass and Lee, 1993). The attrac-tiveness of this program is that knowledge of advanced mathematical principles is not required for constructing the pharmacokinetic models diagrammatically and making modifications afterward. In essence, the program calculates all of the movements between compartments at user-specified time intervals using user-specified input functions and initial values.

A possible complication in compartmental data analysis is that it may not be possible to calculate the true drug absorption rate constant across the cornea. This is because of the overwhelming contribution of the other powerful precorneal loss rate constants to the overall apparent absorption rate constant. This is an example of the "parallel loss process" (Makoid et al., 1976). In an attempt to overcome this limitation, Eller et al. (1985) developed a topical infusion method, whereby a constant drug concentration in 700 µl is maintained over the cornea of an anesthetized rabbit through the use of a plastic cylinder secured over the limbal conjunctiva until steady-state ocular concentrations are reached. Rabbits are euthanized at various time intervals, ocular tissues are excised, and the excised tissues are then assayed for drug content. This topical infusion method permits an estimate of the true absorption rate constant as well as apparent volume of distribution at steady state and ocular drug clearance. However, this method has not been widely used.

3.2.4b. Model-Independent Data Analysis

In recent years, a model-independent approach has gained popularity in describ-ing the concentration–time profile of a drug. In addition to C_{max} (maximum drug concentration), t_{max} (time when the maximum drug concentration is reached), and AUC (area under the concentration–time curve), a key parameter in this approach is the mean residence time (MRT). The MRT can be defined as the time for 63.2% of the drug to be eliminated from a given tissue or simply the average length of time a typical drug molecule resides in that tissue (Gibaldi and Perrier, 1982). It is a ratio of two areas, AUMC/AUC, where AUMC is the area under the curve of a plot of the *product* of concentration and time versus time from zero time to infinity, and AUC is the area under the curve of a plot of concentration versus time, also from zero time to infinity. Gibaldi and Perrier (1982) have outlined a procedure to determine these areas from experimental data. By comparing the MRT in a given ocular tissue for an experimental formulation against that for a reference formulation, one can readily discern the effect of formulation changes on ocular drug absorption and accumulation (Eller *et al.*, 1985).

3.2.5. PHARMACODYNAMIC MEASUREMENTS

As an alternative to ocular drug level measurements, one may monitor the time course of changes in a drug's pharmacological response using noninvasive techniques, as succinctly reviewed by Maurice and Mishima (1984). This approach is necessarily limited to drugs that yield measurable pharmacological responses such as changes in pupil diameter, intraocular pressure, and size of corneal wound. The advantages of this approach are that (a) it provides a realistic measure of drug concentration at its effector site, (b) it may require a much smaller number of experimental animals, and (c) it can be conducted in human subjects. Its major disadvantage is that it does not provide mechanistic insight into the mechanism of drug movement in nontarget tissues, such as the conjunctiva, corneal epithelium, and corneal stroma, which collectively affect the amount of drug ultimately reaching the target tissue where the response is initiated. Moreover, dose–response curves are usually far less sensitive than dose–concentration profiles so that minor to modest changes in drug bioavailability are not readily discerned. As an example, the slope of the dose–miosis response curve for pilocarpine is only one-tenth that of the dose–concentration profile (Chrai *et al.*, 1974).

4. CONCLUSIONS

The experimental methods for evaluating the corneal transport and ocular pharmacokinetics of topically applied ophthalmic drugs are relatively straightforward and have been in use for over two decades. Overall, they are useful in guiding the selection of drug candidates and the development of drug formulations for the optimization of topical ocular drug delivery. Future work needs to be focused on the development of cell culture systems for evaluation of drug transport under various formulation conditions, atraumatic methods for continuous sampling of the ocular fluid compartments *in vivo*, noninvasive methods for drug monitoring *in vivo*, and detection techniques with improved sensitivity.

ACKNOWLEDGEMENTS

This work was supported in part by grants EY3816, EY7389, and EY10421 from the National Institutes of Health, Bethesda, Maryland.

REFERENCES

Ahmed, I., and Patton, T. F., 1985, Importance of the noncorneal absorption route in topical ophthalmic drug delivery, *Invest. Ophthalmol. Visual Sci.* **26:**584–587.

Ahmed, I., and Patton, T. F., 1987, Disposition of timolol and inulin in the rabbit eye following corneal versus non-corneal absorption, *Int. J. Pharm.* **38:**9–21.

Anderson, J. A., 1980, Systemic absorption of topical ocularly applied epinephrine and dipivefrin, *Arch. Ophthalmol.* **98:**350–353.

Araie, M., Takase, M., Sakai, T., Ishii, Y., Yokoyama, Y., and Kitagawa, M., 1982, Beta-adrenergic blockers: Ocular penetration and binding to the uveal pigment, *Jpn. J. Ophthalmol.* **26:**248–263.

Ashton, P., Podder, S. K., and Lee, V. H. L., 1991a, Formulation influence on the conjunctival penetration of four beta blockers in the pigmented rabbit: Comparison with corneal penetration, *Pharm. Res.* **8:**1166–1174.

Ashton, P., Wang, W., and Lee, V. H. L., 1991b, Location of penetration and metabolic barriers to levobunolol in the pigmented rabbit, *J. Pharmacol. Exp. Ther.* **259:**719–724.

Ashton, P., Clark, D. S., and Lee, V. H. L., 1992, A mechanistic study on the enhancement of corneal penetration of phenylephrine by flurbiprofen in the rabbit, *Curr. Eye Res.* **11:**85–90.

Atlasik, B., Stepien, K., and Wilczok, T., 1980, Interaction of drugs with ocular melanin *in vitro*, *Exp. Eye Res.* **30:**325–331.

Bito, L., 1974, The effects of experimental uveitis on anterior uveal prostaglandin transport and aqueous humor composition, *Invest. Ophthalmol. Visual Sci.* **13:**959–966.

Bito, L. Z., and Baroody, R. A., 1982, The penetration of exogenous prostaglandin and arachidonic acid into, and their distribution within, the mammalian eye, *Curr. Eye Res.* **1:**659–668.

Burstein, N. L., and Anderson, J. A., 1985, Corneal penetration and ocular bioavailability of drugs, *J. Ocular Pharmacol.* **1:**309–326.

Chang, S. C., and Lee, V. H. L., 1987, Nasal and conjunctival contributions to the systemic absorption of topical timolol in the pigmented rabbit: Implications in the design of strategies to maximize the ratio of ocular to systemic absorption, *J. Ocular Pharmacol.* **3:**159–169.

Chrai, S. S, Patton, T. F., Mehta, A., and Robinson, J. R., 1973, Lacrimal and instilled fluid dynamics in rabbit eyes, *J. Pharm. Sci.* **63:**1218–1223.

Chrai, S. S., Makoid, M. C., Eriksen, S. P., and Robinson, J. R., 1974, Drop size and initial dosing frequency problems of topically applied ophthalmic drugs, *J. Pharm. Sci.* **63:**333–338.

Conrad, J. M., and Robinson, J. R., 1980, Mechanisms of anterior segment absorption of pilocarpine following subconjunctival injection in albino rabbits, *J. Pharm. Sci.* **69:**875–884.

Cox, W. V., Kupferman, A., and Leibowitz, H. W., 1972, Topically applied steroids in corneal disease. I. The role of inflammation in stromal absorption of dexamethasone, *Arch. Ophthalmol.* **88:**308–313.

DeSantis, L. M., and Schoenwald, R. D., 1978, Lack of influence of rabbit nictitating membrane on miosis effect of pilocarpine, *J. Pharm. Sci.* **67:**1189–1190.

Dilly, P. N., 1985, On the nature and the role of the subsurface vesicles in the outer epithelial cells of the conjunctiva, *Br. J. Ophthalmol.* **69:**447–481.

Edelhauser, J. F., Hoffert, J. R., and Fromm, P. O., 1965, *In vitro* ion and water movement in corneas of rainbow trout, *Invest. Ophthalmol.* **4:**290–296.

Eller, M. G., Schoenwald, R. D., Dixson, J. A., Segarra, T., and Barfknecht, C. F., 1985, Topical carbonic anhydrase inhibitors IV: Relationship between excised corneal permeability and pharmacokinetic factors, *J. Pharm. Sci.* **74:**525–529.

Francoeur, M. L., Sitek, S. J., Costello, B., and Patton, T. F., 1985, Kinetic disposition and distribution of timolol in the rabbit. A physiologically based ocular model, *Int. J. Pharm.* **25:**275–292.

Gibaldi, M., and Perrier, D., 1982, Noncompartmental analysis based on statistical moment theory, in: *Pharmacokinetics*, Marcel Dekker, New York, pp. 409–417.

Grass, G. M., and Lee, V. H. L., 1993, A model to predict aqueous humor and plasma pharmacokinetics of ocularly applied drugs, *Invest. Ophthalmol. Visual Sci.* **34:**2251–2259.

Hayakawa, E., Chien, D. S., Inagaki, K., Yamamoto, A., Wang, W., and Lee, V. H. L., 1992, Conjunctival penetration of insulin and peptide drugs in the albino rabbit, *Pharm. Res.* **9:**769–775.

Himmelstein, K. J., Guvenir, I., and Patton, T. F., 1978, Preliminary pharmacokinetic model of pilocarpine uptake and distribution in the eye, *J. Pharm. Sci.* **67:**603–606.

Hui, H. W., Zeleznick, L., and Robinson, J. R., 1984, Ocular disposition of topically applied histamine, cimetidine, and pyrilamine in the albino rabbit, *Curr. Eye Res.* **3:**321–330.

Hull, D. S., Hine, J. E., Edelhauser, H. F., and Hyndiuk, B. A., 1974, Permeability of the isolated rabbit cornea to corticosteroids, *Invest. Ophthalmol.* **13:**457–459.

Kane, A., Barza, M., and Baum, J., 1981, Intravitreal injection of gentamicin in rabbits: Effects of inflammation and pigmentation on half-life and ocular distribution, *Invest. Ophthalmol. Visual Sci.* **20:**593–597.

Keller, N., Moore, D., Carper, D., and Longwell, A., 1980, Increased corneal permeability induced by the dual effect of transient tear film acidification and exposure to benzalkonium chloride, *Exp. Eye Res.* **30:**203–210.

Kupferman, A., Pratt, M. V., Suckewer, K., and Leibowitz, H. M., 1974, Topically applied steroids in corneal disease. III. The role of drug derivative in stromal absorption of dexamethasone, *Arch. Ophthalmol.* **91:**373–376.

Lam, T. T., Fu, J., Chu, R., Stojack, K., Siew, E., and Tso, M. O. M., 1994, Intravitreal delivery of ganciclovir in rabbits by transscleral iontophoresis, *J. Ocul. Pharmacol.* **10:**571–575.

Larsson, B., and Tjalve, H., 1979, Studies on the mechanism of drug-binding to melanin, *Biochem. Pharmacol.* **28:**1181–1187.

Lee, V. H. L., 1983, Esterase activities in adult rabbit eyes, *J. Pharm. Sci.* **72:**239–244.

Lee, V. H. L., and Robinson, J. R., 1979, Mechanistic and quantitative evaluation of precorneal pilocarpine disposition in albino rabbits, *J. Pharm. Sci.* **68:**673–684.

Lee, V. H. L., and Robinson, J. R., 1982, Disposition of topically applied pilocarpine in the pigmented rabbit eye, *Int. J. Pharm.* **11:**155–165.

Lee, V. H. L., and Robinson, J. R., 1986, Topical ocular drug delivery: Recent developments and future challenges, *J. Ocul. Pharmacol.* **2:**67–108.

Lee, V. H. L., Hui, H. W., and Robinson, J. R., 1980, Corneal metabolism of pilocarpine in pigmented rabbits, *Invest. Ophthalmol. Visual Sci.* **9:**210–213.

Lee, V. H. L., Iimoto, D. S., and Takemoto, K. A., 1983a, Subcellular distribution of esterases in the bovine eye, *Curr. Eye Res.* **2:**869–876.

Lee, V. H. L., Stratford, R. E., Jr., and Morimoto, K. W., 1983b, Age related changes in esterase activity in rabbit eyes, *Int. J. Pharm.* **13:**183–195.

Lee, V. H. L., Swarbrick, J., Redell, M. A., and Yang, D. C., 1983c, Vehicle influence on ocular disposition of sodium cromoglycate in the albino rabbit, *Int. J. Pharm.* **16:**163–170.

Lee, V. H. L., Swarbrick, J., Stratford, R. E., and Morimoto, K. W., 1983d, Disposition of topically applied sodium cromoglycate in the albino rabbit eye, *J. Pharm. Pharmacol.* **35:**445–450.

Lee, V. H. L., Carson, L. W., and Takemoto, K. A., 1986, Macromolecular drug absorption in the albino rabbit eye, *Int. J. Pharm.* **29:**43–51.

Lee, V. H. L., Chien, D. S., and Sasaki, H., 1988, Ocular ketone reductase distribution and its role in the metabolism of ocularly applied levobunolol in the pigmented rabbit, *J. Pharmacol. Exp. Ther.* **246:**871–878.

Lee, V. H. L., Li, S. Y., Sasaki, H., Saettone, M. F., and Chetoni, P., 1994, Effect of polymeric ocular inserts on systemic timolol absorption in the pigmented rabbit is polymer dependent, *J. Ocul. Pharmacol.* **10:**421–429.

Lee, Y. H., Kompella, U. B., and Lee, V. H. L., 1993, Systemic absorption pathways of topically applied beta adrenergic antagonists in the pigmented rabbit, *Exp. Eye Res.* **57:**341–349.

Lehr, C. M., Lee, Y. H., and Lee, V. H. L., 1994, Improved ocular penetration of gentamicin by mucoadhesive polymer polycarbophil in the pigmented rabbit, *Invest. Ophthalmol. Visual Sci.* **35:**2809–2814.

Liu, S. X. L., and Chiou, G. C. Y., 1994, Feasibility of insulin eyedrops for human use, *J. Ocul. Pharmacol.* **10:**587–590.

Lux, O. N., and Dikstein, S., 1985, Survival of isolated rabbit cornea and free radical scavengers, *Curr. Eye Res.* **4:**153–154.

Makoid, M. C., and Robinson, J. R., 1979, Pharmacokinetics of topically applied pilocarpine in albino rabbit eye, *J. Pharm. Sci.* **68:**435–443.

Makoid, M. C., Sieg, J. W., and Robinson, J. R., 1976, Corneal drug absorption: An illustration of parallel first-order absorption and rapid loss of drug from absorption depot, *J. Pharm. Sci.* **65:**150–152.

Maurice, D. M., and Mishima, S., 1984, Ocular pharmacokinetics, in: *Pharmacology of the Eye* (M. Sears, ed.), Springer-Verlag, Berlin, pp. 19–116.

Miller, S. C., Himmelstein, K. J., and Patton, T. F., 1981, A physiologically based pharmacokinetic model for the intraocular distribution of pilocarpine in rabbits, *J. Pharmacokinet. Biopharm.* **9:**653–677.

Mindel, J. S., Smith, H., Jacobs, M., Kharlamb, A. B., and Friedman, A. H., 1984, Drug reservoirs in topical therapy, *Invest. Ophthalmol. Visual Sci.* **25:**346–350.

Mishima, S., Gasset, A., Klyce, S. D., and Baum, J. L., 1966, Determination of tear volume and tear flow, *Invest. Ophthalmol.* **5:**264–276.

Naveh, N., Muchtar, S., and Benita, S., 1994, Pilocarpine incorporated into a submicron emulsion vehicle causes an unexpectedly prolonged ocular hypotensive effect in rabbits, *J. Ocul. Pharmacol.* **10:**509–520.

Nichols, B. A., Chiappino, M. L., and Dawson, C. R., 1985, Demonstration of the mucus layer of the tear film by electron microscopy, *Invest. Ophthalmol. Visual Sci.* **26:**464–473.

Nzekwe, E. U., and Maurice, D. M., 1994, The effect of age on the penetration of fluorescein into the human eye, *J. Ocul. Pharmacol.* **10:**521–523.

Ohdo, S., Grass, G. M., and Lee, V. H. L., 1991, Improving the ocular: systemic ratio of topical timolol by varying the dosing time, *Invest. Ophthalmol. Visual Sci.* **32:**2790–2798.

Patil, P. N., and Jacobowitz, D., 1974, Unequal accumulation of adrenergic drugs by pigmented and nonpigmented iris, *Am. J. Ophthalmol.* **78:**470–477.

Patton, T. F., and Robinson, J. R., 1975, Influence of topical anesthesia on tear dynamics and ocular bioavailability in albino rabbits, *J. Pharm. Sci.* **64:**267–271.

Patton, T. F., and Robinson, J. R., 1976, Pediatric dosing considerations in ophthalmology, *J. Pediatr. Ophthalmol.* **13:**171.

Pleyer, U., Lutz, S., Jusko, W., Nguyen, K., Narawane, M., Ruckert, D., Mondino, B. J., and Lee, V. H. L., 1993, Ocular absorption of topically applied FK506 from liposomal and oil formulations in the rabbit eye, *Invest. Ophthalmol. Visual Sci.* **34:**2737–2742.

Podder, S. K., Moy, K. C., and Lee, V. H. L., 1992, Improving the safety of topically applied timolol in the pigmented rabbit through manipulation of formulation composition, *Exp. Eye Res.* **54:**747–757.

Potter, D. E., Shumate, D. J., Bundgaard, H., and Lee, V. H. L., 1988, Ocular and cardiac beta-antagonism by timolol, O-butyryl timolol, O-pivaloyl timolol and levobunolol, *Curr. Eye Res.* **7:**755–759.

Rahimy, M. H., Peyman, G. A., Fernandes, M. L., El-Sayed, S. H., Luo, Q., and Borhani, H., 1994, Effects of an intravitreal daunomycin implant on experimental proliferative vitreoretinopathy: Simultaneous pharmacokinetic and pharmacodynamic evaluations, *J. Ocul. Pharmacol.* **10:**561–570.

Redell, M. A., Yang, D. C., and Lee, V. H. L., 1983, The role of esterase activity in the ocular disposition of dipivalyl epinephrine in rabbits, *Int. J. Pharm.* **17:**299–312.

Richman, J. B., and Tang-Liu, D. D. S., 1990, A corneal perfusion device for estimating ocular bio-availability *in vitro, J. Pharm. Sci.* **79:**153–157.

Saettone, M. F., Giannaccini, B., Savigni, P., and Wirth, A., 1980, The effect of different ophthalmic vehicles on the activity of tropicamide in man, *J. Pharm. Pharmacol.* **32:**519–521.

Saettone, M. F., Giannaccini, B., Barattini, F., and Tellini, N., 1982a, The validity of rabbits for investigations on ophthalmic vehicles: A comparison of four different vehicles containing tropicamide in humans and rabbits, *Pharm. Acta. Helv.* **57:**47–55.

Saettone, M. F., Giannaccini, B., Teneggi, A., Savigni, P., and Tellini, N., 1982b, Vehicle effects on ophthalmic bioavailability: The influence of different polymers on the activity of pilocarpine in rabbit and man, *J. Pharm. Pharmacol.* **34:**464–466.

Saettone, M. F., Giannaccini, B., Ravecca, S., La Marca, F., and Tota, G., 1984, Polymer effects on ocular bioavailability—the influence of different liquid vehicles on the mydriatic response of tropicamide in humans and in rabbits, *Int. J. Pharm.* **20:**187–202.

Saettone, M. F., Giannaccini, B., Guiducci, A., La Marca, F., and Tota, G., 1985, Polymer effects on ocular bioavailability. II. The influence of benzalkonium chloride on the mydriatic response of tropicamide in different polymeric vehicles, *Int. J. Pharm.* **25:**73–83.

Schoenwald, R. D., and Houseman, J. A., 1982, Disposition of cyclophosphamide in the rabbit and human cornea, *Biopharm. Drug Dispos.* **3:**231–241.

Schoenwald, R. D., and Huang, H. S., 1983, Corneal penetration behavior of beta-blocking agents. I: Physicochemical factors, *J. Pharm. Sci.* **72:**1266–1272.

Schoenwald, R. D., and Ward, R. L., 1981, Relationship between steroid permeability across excised rabbit cornea and octanol water partition coefficients, *J. Pharm. Sci.* **67:**786–788.

Shih, R. L., and Lee, V. H. L., 1990, Rate limiting barrier to the penetration of ocular hypotensive beta-blockers across the corneal epithelium in the pigmented rabbit, *J. Ocul. Pharmacol.* **6:**329–336.

Shimada, K., Bawaja, R., Sokoloski, T., and Patil, P. N., 1976, Binding characteristics of drugs to synthetic levodopa melanin, *J. Pharm. Sci.* **65:**1057–1060.

Sieg, J. W., and Robinson, J. R., 1974, Corneal absorption of fluorometholone in rabbits. A comparative evaluation of corneal drug transport characteristics in anesthetized and unanesthetized rabbits, *Arch. Ophthalmol.* **92:**240–243.

Sieg, J. W., and Robinson, J. R., 1976, Mechanistic studies on transcorneal permeation of pilocarpine, *J. Pharm. Sci.* **65:**1816–1822.

Sieg, J. W., and Robinson, J. R., 1981, Mechanistic studies on transcorneal permeation of fluorometholone, *J. Pharm. Sci.* **70:**1026–1029.

Stratford, R. E., Jr., and Lee, V. H. L., 1985, Ocular aminopeptidase activity and distribution in the albino rabbit, *Curr. Eye Res.* **4:**995–999.

Stratford, R. E., Redell, M. A., Yang, D. C., and Lee, V. H. L., 1983, Ocular distribution of liposome-encapsulated epinephrine and inulin in the albino rabbit, *Curr. Eye Res.* **2:**377–386.

Sugaya, M., and Nagataki, S., 1978, Kinetics of topical pilocarpine in the human eye, *Jpn. J. Ophthalmol.* **22:**127–141.

Tang-Liu, D. D. S., Liu, S. S., and Weinkam, R. J., 1984, Ocular and systemic bioavailability of ophthalmic flurbiprofen, *J. Pharmacokinet. Biopharm.* **12:**611–626.

Ubels, J. L., and Edelhauser, H. F., 1982, Retinoid permeability and uptake in corneas of normal and vitamin A-deficient rabbits, *Arch. Ophthalmol.* **100:**1828–1831.

Weingeist, T. A., 1970, The structure of the developing and adult ciliary complex of the rabbit eye: A gross, light and electron microscopic study, *Doc. Ophthalmol.* **28:**205–375.

Zimmer, A., Mutschler, E., Lambrecht, G., Mayer, D., and Kreuter, J., 1994, Pharmacokinetic and pharmacodynamic aspects of an ophthalmic pilocarpine nanoparticle-delivery-system, *Pharm. Res.* **11:**1435–1442.

Index

437